Updates on Molecular Targeted Therapies for CNS Tumors

Updates on Molecular Targeted Therapies for CNS Tumors

Editor

Edward Pan

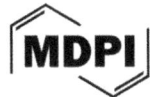

Basel • Beijing • Wuhan • Barcelona • Belgrade • Novi Sad • Cluj • Manchester

Editor
Edward Pan
UT Southwestern Medical
Center
Dallas, TX, USA

Editorial Office
MDPI
St. Alban-Anlage 66
4052 Basel, Switzerland

This is a reprint of articles from the Special Issue published online in the open access journal *Cancers* (ISSN 2072-6694) (available at: https://www.mdpi.com/journal/cancers/special_issues/Updates_Targeted_CNS).

For citation purposes, cite each article independently as indicated on the article page online and as indicated below:

Lastname, A.A.; Lastname, B.B. Article Title. *Journal Name* **Year**, *Volume Number*, Page Range.

ISBN 978-3-0365-8528-4 (Hbk)
ISBN 978-3-0365-8529-1 (PDF)
doi.org/10.3390/books978-3-0365-8529-1

© 2023 by the authors. Articles in this book are Open Access and distributed under the Creative Commons Attribution (CC BY) license. The book as a whole is distributed by MDPI under the terms and conditions of the Creative Commons Attribution-NonCommercial-NoDerivs (CC BY-NC-ND) license.

Contents

Edward Pan
Potential Molecular Targets in the Treatment of Patients with CNS Tumors
Reprinted from: *Cancers* 2023, 15, 3807, doi:10.3390/cancers15153807 1

Miranda M. Tallman, Abigail A. Zalenski, Ian Stabl, Morgan S. Schrock, Luke Kollin, Eliane de Jong, et al.
Improving Localized Radiotherapy for Glioblastoma via Small Molecule Inhibition of KIF11
Reprinted from: *Cancers* 2023, 15, 3173, doi:10.3390/cancers15123173 7

Vineeth Tatineni, Patrick J. O'Shea, Shreya Saxena, Atulya A. Khosla, Ahmad Ozair, Rupesh R. Kotecha, et al.
Combination of EGFR-Directed Tyrosine Kinase Inhibitors (EGFR-TKI) with Radiotherapy in Brain Metastases from Non-Small Cell Lung Cancer: A 2010–2019 Retrospective Cohort Study
Reprinted from: *Cancers* 2023, 15, 3015, doi:10.3390/cancers15113015 21

Vineeth Tatineni, Patrick J. O'Shea, Ahmad Ozair, Atulya A. Khosla, Shreya Saxena, Yasmeen Rauf, et al.
First- versus Third-Generation EGFR Tyrosine Kinase Inhibitors in EGFR-Mutated Non-Small Cell Lung Cancer Patients with Brain Metastases
Reprinted from: *Cancers* 2023, 15, 2382, doi:10.3390/cancers15082382 33

Ahmad Ozair, Vivek Bhat, Reid S. Alisch, Atulya A. Khosla, Rupesh R. Kotecha, Yazmin Odia, et al.
DNA Methylation and Histone Modification in Low-Grade Gliomas: Current Understanding and Potential Clinical Targets
Reprinted from: *Cancers* 2023, 15, 1342, doi:10.3390/cancers15041342 47

Isabele Fattori Moretti, Antonio Marcondes Lerario, Paula Rodrigues Sola, Janaína Macedo-da-Silva, Mauricio da Silva Baptista, Giuseppe Palmisano, et al.
GBM Cells Exhibit Susceptibility to Metformin Treatment According to TLR4 Pathway Activation and Metabolic and Antioxidant Status
Reprinted from: *Cancers* 2023, 15, 587, doi:10.3390/cancers15030587 69

Pushan Dasgupta, Veerakumar Balasubramanyian, John F. de Groot and Nazanin K. Majd
Preclinical Models of Low-Grade Gliomas
Reprinted from: *Cancers* 2023, 15, 596, doi:10.3390/cancers15030596 87

Atulya Aman Khosla, Shreya Saxena, Ahmad Ozair, Vyshak Alva Venur, David M. Peereboom and Manmeet S. Ahluwalia
Novel Therapeutic Approaches in Neoplastic Meningitis
Reprinted from: *Cancers* 2023, 15, 119, doi:10.3390/cancers15010119 101

Motoo Nagane, Koichi Ichimura, Ritsuko Onuki, Daichi Narushima, Mai Honda-Kitahara, Kaishi Satomi, et al.
Bevacizumab beyond Progression for Newly Diagnosed Glioblastoma (BIOMARK): Phase II Safety, Efficacy and Biomarker Study
Reprinted from: *Cancers* 2022, 14, 5522, doi:10.3390/cancers14225522 117

Valentina Bova, Alessia Filippone, Giovanna Casili, Marika Lanza, Michela Campolo, Anna Paola Capra, et al.
Adenosine Targeting as a New Strategy to Decrease Glioblastoma Aggressiveness
Reprinted from: *Cancers* 2022, 14, 4032, doi:10.3390/cancers14164032 135

Khoa Pham, Allison R. Hanaford, Brad A. Poore, Micah J. Maxwell, Heather Sweeney, Akhila Parthasarathy, et al.
Comprehensive Metabolic Profiling of MYC-Amplified Medulloblastoma Tumors Reveals Key Dependencies on Amino Acid, Tricarboxylic Acid and Hexosamine Pathways
Reprinted from: *Cancers* **2022**, *14*, 1311, doi:10.3390/cancers14051311 153

Akanksha Sharma, Lauren Singer and Priya Kumthekar
Updates on Molecular Targeted Therapies for Intraparenchymal CNS Metastases
Reprinted from: *Cancers* **2022**, *14*, 17, doi:10.3390/cancers14010017 179

Guangyang Yu, Ying Pang, Mythili Merchant, Chimene Kesserwan, Vineela Gangalapudi, Abdalla Abdelmaksoud, et al.
Tumor Mutation Burden, Expressed Neoantigens and the Immune Microenvironment in Diffuse Gliomas
Reprinted from: *Cancers* **2021**, *13*, 6092, doi:10.3390/cancers13236092 193

Thomas Larrew, Brian Fabian Saway, Stephen R. Lowe and Adriana Olar
Molecular Classification and Therapeutic Targets in Ependymoma
Reprinted from: *Cancers* **2021**, *13*, 6218, doi:10.3390/cancers13246218 209

Lauren D. Sanchez, Ashley Bui and Laura J. Klesse
Targeted Therapies for the Neurofibromatoses
Reprinted from: *Cancers* **2021**, *13*, 6032, doi:10.3390/cancers13236032 239

Elisha Hayden, Holly Holliday, Rebecca Lehmann, Aaminah Khan, Maria Tsoli, Benjamin S. Rayner and David S. Ziegler
Therapeutic Targets in Diffuse Midline Gliomas—An Emerging Landscape
Reprinted from: *Cancers* **2021**, *13*, 6251, doi:10.3390/cancers13246251 261

Lauren R. Schaff and Christian Grommes
Update on Novel Therapeutics for Primary CNS Lymphoma
Reprinted from: *Cancers* **2021**, *13*, 5372, doi:10.3390/cancers13215372 303

Kirit Singh, Kelly M. Hotchkiss, Kisha K. Patel, Daniel S. Wilkinson, Aditya A. Mohan, Sarah L. Cook and John H. Sampson
Enhancing T Cell Chemotaxis and Infiltration in Glioblastoma
Reprinted from: *Cancers* **2021**, *13*, 5367, doi:10.3390/cancers13215367 319

Maria-Magdalena Georgescu
Multi-Platform Classification of IDH-Wild-Type Glioblastoma Based on ERK/MAPK Pathway: Diagnostic, Prognostic and Therapeutic Implications
Reprinted from: *Cancers* **2021**, *13*, 4532, doi:10.3390/cancers13184532 343

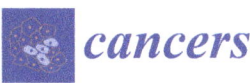

Editorial

Potential Molecular Targets in the Treatment of Patients with CNS Tumors

Edward Pan

Daiichi-Sankyo, Inc., 211 Mt. Airy Road, Basking Ridge, NJ 07920, USA; epan@dsi.com

Citation: Pan, E. Potential Molecular Targets in the Treatment of Patients with CNS Tumors. *Cancers* **2023**, *15*, 3807. https://doi.org/10.3390/cancers15153807

Received: 21 July 2023
Accepted: 25 July 2023
Published: 27 July 2023

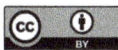

Copyright: © 2023 by the author. Licensee MDPI, Basel, Switzerland. This article is an open access article distributed under the terms and conditions of the Creative Commons Attribution (CC BY) license (https://creativecommons.org/licenses/by/4.0/).

The challenges in identifying effective therapies for CNS tumors continue to be daunting. Potentially effective targeted therapies must be able to penetrate the blood–brain barrier to reach the tumor, and in sufficient concentrations to result in meaningful treatment responses. Moreover, molecular targets must be key drivers in the growth and progression of CNS tumors. Numerous potentially efficacious therapies have failed in randomized clinical trials due to other factors, including subclonal genetic intratumoral heterogeneity (particularly within malignant gliomas), epigenetic heterogeneity, and failure to target important factors involved in the tumor microenvironment. Developing effective targeted therapies requires a thorough fundamental understanding of the genetic and epigenetic factors driving tumor progression, the interactions between CNS tumor cells and the tumor microenvironment, and the key mechanisms of tumor treatment resistance.

In this Special Issue entitled "Updates on Molecular Targeted Therapies for CNS Tumors", experts in the field of CNS tumors highlighted promising molecular targets in the development of treatments for patients with CNS tumors. The scope of this Special Issue includes multiple types of CNS tumors, translational and clinical studies, various treatment approaches (e.g., systemic therapies, radiotherapy, immunotherapies, etc.), as well as high-level reviews.

Brain metastases (BM) are the most common CNS tumors, with an estimated incidence of up to 40% in patients with metastatic cancer [1,2]. The most common solid tumor BM arises from lung cancer [3]. Tatineni et al. evaluated the efficacy of first versus third-generation EGFR TKIs in EGFR-mutated NSCLC BM in both first line and later line treatments [4]. Although no survival benefits between the first- and third-generation EGFR TKIs were found, larger prospective studies to confirm these findings are warranted. In another study, Tatineni et al. evaluated the combination of EGFR-Directed TKIs with radiotherapy in patients with NSCLC BM [5]. They found that these patients treated with EGFR TKIs plus stereotactic radiosurgery (SRS) had higher OS compared to those BM patients treated with EGFR TKIs plus whole brain radiation therapy (WBRT), suggesting that larger phase II/III clinical trials are warranted to investigate the synergy of EGFR TKIs with SRS in EGFR-mutated NSCLC BM. Sharma et al. reviewed other potential molecular targets (e.g., ALK, ROS-1, HER-2, etc.) in a tumor-agnostic fashion for BM harboring these specific mutations [6]. This article illustrates the need for continued evaluation of tumor tissue for their molecular profiles in addition to histologic diagnosis to improve our understanding of the molecular nature of BM.

Glioblastoma (GBM) is the most frequent primary malignant brain tumor in adults, with an incidence of 3–4 cases per 100,000 population, and often with poor prognoses (1 year survival rate of approximately 41%) [7]. Thus, there needs to be significant advances in our understanding of the molecular landscape of GBMs in order to make more meaningful clinical advances in GBM treatment. Georgescu described a multi-platform classification of an adult GBM cohort [8]. The study identified seven non-redundant IDH-wild type GBM molecular subgroups corresponding to the upstream RTK and RAS-RAF segment of the ERK/MAPK signal transduction pathway. Thus, this pathway may be utilized for potential targeted therapy approaches to GBMs. Singh et al. reviewed the role of T cell chemotaxis and infiltration in GBM [9]. This review discusses this process and the potential immunotherapeutic approaches to enhance T cell trafficking in GBM tumor cells, such as combinations of small-molecule inhibitors of the AKT1 and AKT2 isoforms with novel bispecific constructs with immune stimulatory cytokines. Bova et al. reviewed the role of adenosine and its interaction with its subtype receptions, as well as the potential efficacy of adenosine receptor antagonists (e.g., selective A2A receptor antagonists) to enhance immunotherapy effects in GBMs [10]. Moretti et al. analyzed the potential of targeting the metabolic status and tumor microenvironment in GBMs, specifically TLR4, in GBM cell lines. Metformin in combination with temozolomide (TMZ) demonstrated a response to a particular GBM cell line subtype with an activated TLR4 pathway, while another GBM cell line subtype (mitochondrial) with concomitant *CXCL8*/IL8 upregulation was more likely to respond to metformin combined with an antioxidant inhibitor (e.g., anti-SOD1) [11]. Thus, further exploration of the metabolic and antioxidant status of GBMs may yield another viable targeting strategy for GBMs. Another potential strategy is to decrease the resistance of GBMs to radiotherapy, which is currently the most effective treatment modality for GBM patients [12]. Tallman et al. evaluated the potential to increase sensitivity of GBM cells in mitosis to localized radiotherapy. A small molecular inhibitor of KIF11 (ispinesib) combined with radiotherapy demonstrated increased apoptosis in vivo compared to control plus radiotherapy [13]. Thus, the potential efficacy of ispinesib should be explored in GBM clinical trials. Nagane et al. completed a phase II trial that explored the effect of bevacizumab beyond progression in newly diagnosed GBM patients and evaluated predictors of response to bevacizumab. Although the primary endpoint was not met (2-year survival rate of 27%), RNA expression profiling identified Cluster 2 (enriched with genes involving microglia or macrophage activation) study patients as having longer OS and PFS independent of *MGMT* methylation status [14]. Thus, consideration may be given to complete a clinical trial evaluating bevacizumab in GBMs with the Cluster 2 subtype to determine if these specific GBM patients may derive increased benefit from antiangiogenic therapies.

Although low-grade gliomas (LGG) are less common (30% of all CNS tumors) and have better prognoses compared to GBMs, they eventually progress to high-grade gliomas and are ultimately fatal, with 5-year survival rates ranging from 30 to 80% [15]. Thus, there is an unmet need to develop novel therapeutics for patients with LGG. Dasgupta et al. reviewed the preclinical in vitro and in vivo models of LGG [16]. The review highlights the mechanistic challenges in generating accurate LGG models and summarizes potential strategies to overcome these challenges. Ozair et al. reviewed the role of epigenetics (specifically DNA methylation and histone modification) in LGG. This review summarizes the potential diagnostic and therapeutic targets for LGG (e.g., PARP, IDH, TERT, etc.) as well as the current clinical trial landscape for this patient population [17].

IDH-mutated gliomas have a distinct tumor biology compared to IDH-wildtype gliomas at both the genetic and epigenetic levels [18], with IDH-mutated gliomas having significantly more favorable outcomes compared to IDH-wildtype gliomas [19]. Yu et al. evaluated the association between tumor mutational burden (TMB), expressed neoantigens, and the tumor immune microenvironment in both IDH-mutant and IDH-wildtype gliomas to determine whether TMB may be a potential biomarker in diffuse gliomas [20]. The analysis of glioma samples determined that TMB was inversely correlated with immune score in IDH-wildtype gliomas with no correlation in IDH-mutant gliomas, suggesting further analyses of germline variants in a larger glioma cohort are warranted.

Ependymomas, although histologically classified as gliomas, behave differently from the typical gliomas. They originate from the lining of cerebral ventricles, occur more frequently in children than adults, are usually more chemotherapy-resistant, and have a different grading system than those of gliomas [21]. Larrew et al. discussed the molecular classifications of ependymomas and described potential therapeutic targets for patients with ependymomas based on their molecular classification (e.g., anti-YAP, FGFR3, anti-RELA, etc.) [22].

Primary CNS Lymphoma (PCNSL) is a rare variant of extra-nodal non-Hodgkin lymphoma affecting the CNS and/or vitreoretinal space without systemic involvement. It affects approximately 1600 people in the U.S. per year with a median age of diagnosis at 67 years [23]. Despite PCNSL typically being sensitive to chemotherapy and radiotherapy, relapse rates are high, especially for those who are not candidates for high-dose chemotherapy followed by autologous stem cell transplant, approximately 15% of patients have refractory disease, and median survival after first relapse is only 4.5 months [24]. Schaff and Grommes reviewed potential novel therapeutics for PCNSL, including targeting the BCR/TLR pathway, PI3K/mTOR pathway, and immunomodulatory drugs [25].

This Special Issue also includes studies involving pediatric CNS tumors. The most common malignant childhood brain tumor is medulloblastoma. Survival outcomes significantly depend on the molecular genetics and epigenetics of the medulloblastoma subtype [26]. Pham et al. discussed their metabolic studies of *MYC*-amplified medulloblastomas both in vitro and in vivo. They demonstrated that these specific medulloblastomas had upregulation of the TCA cycle and were dependent on several potentially targetable metabolic pathways, including tricarboxylic acid, amino acid, and hexosamine [27]. Another CNS tumor afflicting primarily children are the diffuse midline gliomas (DMG), which include diffuse intrinsic pontine gliomas (DIPG). They typically arise in the brainstem, thalamus, spinal cord, and cerebellum, which do not often allow for safe aggressive resections. They generally have dismal prognoses, with 5-year survival rates of less than 1% due to their high resistance to chemotherapy and radiotherapy, as well as their origins deep in the CNS structures [28]. Hayden et al. reviewed the underlying molecular landscape of DMG and discuss potential treatment targets, including HDAC, BET, and cell cycle inhibitors [29].

Finally, this Special Issue also includes reviews of rare neurologic diseases involving cancer, specifically neurofibromatoses and neoplastic meningitis. The neurofibromatoses, encompassing NF1, NF2, and schwannomatosis, are genetic tumor syndromes which cause affected patients to develop characteristic nerve-associated tumors both in the CNS and PNS (peripheral nervous system). Sanchez et al. review the clinical and molecular landscape of neurofibromatoses and discuss the recent treatment advances, particularly MEK inhibition with selumetinib and other potential therapeutic targets [30]. Neoplastic meningitis (NM) involves the spread of a primary tumor to the leptomeninges, dura, and subarachnoid space. The incidence of NM ranges from 5–8% (solid tumors) to 15% (hematologic malignancies), and typically has dismal prognoses with an overall survival of 2–4 months from diagnosis with treatment [31]. Khosla et al. reviewed the pathophysiology and current clinical trial landscape and highlighted potential targeted and immunotherapy strategies for the treatment of NM [32].

The goals of this Special Issue are to illustrate the various CNS tumor types and syndromes in both the adult and pediatric population and to highlight the shift in treatment strategies from traditional chemoradiotherapy approaches to target the key molecular drivers in these tumors. Increasing our understanding of the complex interactions within tumor cells as well as those of these cells with their tumor microenvironment will be crucial to the development of effective treatments for CNS tumors.

Conflicts of Interest: The author declares no conflict of interest.

References

1. Kromer, C.; Xu, J.; Ostrom, Q.T.; Gittleman, H.; Kruchko, C.; Sawaya, R.; Barnholtz-Sloan, J.S. Estimating the annual frequency of synchronous brain metastasis in the United States 2010–2013: A population-based study. *J. Neurooncol.* **2017**, *134*, 55–64. [CrossRef] [PubMed]
2. Schouten, L.J.; Rutten, J.; Huveneers, H.A.M.; Twijnstra, A. Incidence of brain metastases in a cohort of patients with carcinoma of the breast, colon, kidney, and lung and melanoma. *Cancer* **2002**, *94*, 2698–2705. [CrossRef]
3. Saad, A.G.; Yeap, B.Y.; Thunnissen, F.B.; Pinkus, G.S.; Pinkus, J.L.; Loda, M.; Sugarbaker, D.J.; Johnson, B.E.; Chirieac, L.R. Immunohistochemical markers associated with brain metastases in patients with non-small cell lung carcinoma. *Cancer* **2008**, *113*, 2129–2138. [CrossRef] [PubMed]

4. Tatineni, V.; O'Shea, P.J.; Ozair, A.; Khosla, A.A.; Saxena, S.; Rauf, Y.; Jia, X.; Murphy, E.S.; Chao, S.T.; Suh, J.H.; et al. First- versus Third-Generation EGFR Tyrosine Kinase Inhibitors in EGFR-Mutated Non-Small Cell Lung Cancer Patients with Brain Metastases. *Cancers* **2023**, *15*, 2382. [CrossRef]
5. Tatineni, V.; O'Shea, P.J.; Saxena, S.; Khosla, A.A.; Ozair, A.; Kotecha, R.R.; Jia, X.; Rauf, Y.; Murphy, E.S.; Chao, S.T.; et al. Combination of EGFR-Directed Tyrosine Kinase Inhibitors (EGFR-TKI) with Radiotherapy in Brain Metastases from Non-Small Cell Lung Cancer: A 2010–2019 Retrospective Cohort Study. *Cancers* **2023**, *15*, 3015. [CrossRef]
6. Sharma, A.; Singer, L.; Kumthekar, P. Updates on Molecular Targeted Therapies for Intraparenchymal CNS Metastases. *Cancers* **2021**, *14*, 17. [CrossRef] [PubMed]
7. Ostrom, Q.T.; Truitt, G.; Gittleman, H.; Brat, D.J.; Kruchko, C.; Wilson, R.; Barnholtz-Sloan, J.S. Relative survival after diagnosis with a primary brain or other central nervous system tumor in the National Program of Cancer Registries, 2004 to 2014. *Neuro-Oncol. Pr.* **2020**, *7*, 306–312. [CrossRef]
8. Georgescu, M.M. Multi-Platform Classification of IDH-Wild-Type Glioblastoma Based on ERK/MAPK Pathway: Diagnostic, Prognostic and Therapeutic Implications. *Cancers* **2021**, *13*, 4532. [CrossRef]
9. Singh, K.; Hotchkiss, K.M.; Patel, K.K.; Wilkinson, D.S.; Mohan, A.A.; Cook, S.L.; Sampson, J.H. Enhancing T Cell Chemotaxis and Infiltration in Glioblastoma. *Cancers* **2021**, *13*, 5367. [CrossRef]
10. Bova, V.; Filippone, A.; Casili, G.; Lanza, M.; Campolo, M.; Capra, A.P.; Repici, A.; Crupi, L.; Motta, G.; Colarossi, C.; et al. Adenosine Targeting as a New Strategy to Decrease Glioblastoma Aggressiveness. *Cancers* **2022**, *14*, 4032. [CrossRef]
11. Moretti, I.F.; Lerario, A.M.; Sola, P.R.; Macedo-da-Silva, J.; Baptista, M.D.S.; Palmisano, G.; Oba-Shinjo, S.M.; Marie, S.K.N. GBM Cells Exhibit Susceptibility to Metformin Treatment According to TLR4 Pathway Activation and Metabolic and Antioxidant Status. *Cancers* **2023**, *15*, 587. [CrossRef] [PubMed]
12. Stupp, R.; Mason, W.P.; van den Bent, M.J.; Weller, M.; Fisher, B.; Taphoorn, M.J.; Belanger, K.; Brandes, A.A.; Marosi, C.; Bogdahn, U.; et al. Radiotherapy plus concomitant and adjuvant temozolomide for glioblastoma. *N. Engl. J. Med.* **2005**, *352*, 987–996. [CrossRef]
13. Tallman, M.M.; Zalenski, A.A.; Stabl, I.; Schrock, M.S.; Kollin, L.; de Jong, E.; De, K.; Grubb, T.M.; Summers, M.K.; Venere, M. Improving Localized Radiotherapy for Glioblastoma via Small Molecule Inhibition of KIF11. *Cancers* **2023**, *15*, 3173. [CrossRef] [PubMed]
14. Nagane, M.; Ichimura, K.; Onuki, R.; Narushima, D.; Honda-Kitahara, M.; Satomi, K.; Tomiyama, A.; Arai, Y.; Shibata, T.; Narita, Y.; et al. Bevacizumab beyond Progression for Newly Diagnosed Glioblastoma (BIOMARK): Phase II Safety, Efficacy and Biomarker Study. *Cancers* **2022**, *14*, 5522. [CrossRef] [PubMed]
15. Ostrom, Q.T.; Cioffi, G.; Gittleman, H.; Patil, N.; Waite, K.; Kruchko, C.; Barnholtz-Sloan, J.S. CBTRUS Statistical Report: Primary Brain and Other Central Nervous System Tumors Diagnosed in the United States in 2012–2016. *Neuro. Oncol.* **2019**, *21* (Suppl. 5), v1–v100. [CrossRef]
16. Dasgupta, P.; Balasubramanyian, V.; de Groot, J.F.; Majd, N.K. Preclinical Models of Low-Grade Gliomas. *Cancers* **2023**, *15*, 596. [CrossRef]
17. Ozair, A.; Bhat, V.; Alisch, R.S.; Khosla, A.A.; Kotecha, R.R.; Odia, Y.; McDermott, M.W.; Ahluwalia, M.S. DNA Methylation and Histone Modification in Low-Grade Gliomas: Current Understanding and Potential Clinical Targets. *Cancers* **2023**, *15*, 1342. [CrossRef]
18. Turkalp, Z.; Karamchandani, J.; Das, S. IDH mutation in glioma: New insights and promises for the future. *JAMA Neurol.* **2014**, *71*, 1319–1325. [CrossRef]
19. Cancer Genome Atlas Research Network; Brat, D.J.; Verhaak, R.G.; Aldape, K.D.; Yung, W.K.; Salama, S.R.; Cooper, L.A.; Rheinbay, E.; Miller, C.R.; Vitucci, M.; et al. Comprehensive, Integrative Genomic Analysis of Diffuse Lower-Grade Gliomas. *N. Engl. J. Med.* **2015**, *372*, 2481–2498.
20. Yu, G.; Pang, Y.; Merchant, M.; Kesserwan, C.; Gangalapudi, V.; Abdelmaksoud, A.; Ranjan, A.; Kim, O.; Wei, J.S.; Chou, H.C.; et al. Tumor Mutation Burden, Expressed Neoantigens and the Immune Microenvironment in Diffuse Gliomas. *Cancers* **2021**, *13*, 6092. [CrossRef]
21. Wu, J.; Armstrong, T.S.; Gilbert, M.R. Biology and management of ependymomas. *Neuro-Oncology* **2016**, *18*, 902–913. [CrossRef] [PubMed]
22. Larrew, T.; Saway, B.F.; Lowe, S.R.; Olar, A. Molecular Classification and Therapeutic Targets in Ependymoma. *Cancers* **2021**, *13*, 6218. [CrossRef]
23. Ostrom, Q.T.; Patil, N.; Cioffi, G.; Waite, K.; Kruchko, C.; Barnholtz-Sloan, J.S. Corrigendum to: CBTRUS Statistical Report: Primary Brain and Other Central Nervous System Tumors Diagnosed in the United States in 2013–2017. *Neuro-Oncology* **2020**, *22*, iv1–iv96. [CrossRef]
24. Jahnke, K.; Thiel, E.; Martus, P.; Herrlinger, U.; Weller, M.; Fischer, L.; Korfel, A.; on behalf of the German Primary Central Nervous System Lymphoma Study Group (G-PCNSL-SG). Relapse of primary central nervous system lymphoma: Clinical features, outcome and prognostic factors. *J. Neuro-Oncol.* **2006**, *80*, 159–165. [CrossRef] [PubMed]
25. Schaff, L.R.; Grommes, C. Update on Novel Therapeutics for Primary CNS Lymphoma. *Cancers* **2021**, *13*, 5372. [CrossRef] [PubMed]

26. Weil, A.G.; Wang, A.C.; Westwick, H.J.; Ibrahim, G.M.; Ariani, R.T.; Crevier, L.; Perreault, S.; Davidson, T.; Tseng, C.-H.; Fallah, A. Survival in pediatric medulloblastoma: A population-based observational study to improve prognostication. *J. Neuro-Oncol.* **2016**, *132*, 99–107. [CrossRef] [PubMed]
27. Pham, K.; Hanaford, A.R.; Poore, B.A.; Maxwell, M.J.; Sweeney, H.; Parthasarathy, A.; Alt, J.; Rais, R.; Slusher, B.S.; Eberhart, C.G.; et al. Comprehensive Metabolic Profiling of MYC-Amplified Medulloblastoma Tumors Reveals Key Dependencies on Amino Acid, Tricarboxylic Acid and Hexosamine Pathways. *Cancers* **2022**, *14*, 1311. [CrossRef]
28. Louis, D.N.; Perry, A.; Wesseling, P.; Brat, D.J.; Cree, I.A.; Figarella-Branger, D.; Hawkins, C.; Ng, H.K.; Pfister, S.M.; Reifenberger, G.; et al. The 2021 WHO Classification of Tumors of the Central Nervous System: A summary. *Neuro-Oncology* **2021**, *23*, 1231–1251. [CrossRef] [PubMed]
29. Hayden, E.; Holliday, H.; Lehmann, R.; Khan, A.; Tsoli, M.; Rayner, B.S.; Ziegler, D.S. Therapeutic Targets in Diffuse Midline Gliomas-An Emerging Landscape. *Cancers* **2021**, *13*, 6251. [CrossRef]
30. Sanchez, L.D.; Bui, A.; Klesse, L.J. Targeted Therapies for the Neurofibromatoses. *Cancers* **2021**, *13*, 6032. [CrossRef]
31. Beauchesne, P. Intrathecal chemotherapy for treatment of leptomeningeal dissemination of metastatic tumours. *Lancet. Oncol.* **2010**, *11*, 871–879. [CrossRef] [PubMed]
32. Khosla, A.A.; Saxena, S.; Ozair, A.; Venur, V.A.; Peereboom, D.M.; Ahluwalia, M.S. Novel Therapeutic Approaches in Neoplastic Meningitis. *Cancers* **2022**, *15*, 119. [CrossRef]

Disclaimer/Publisher's Note: The statements, opinions and data contained in all publications are solely those of the individual author(s) and contributor(s) and not of MDPI and/or the editor(s). MDPI and/or the editor(s) disclaim responsibility for any injury to people or property resulting from any ideas, methods, instructions or products referred to in the content.

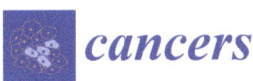

Article

Improving Localized Radiotherapy for Glioblastoma via Small Molecule Inhibition of KIF11

Miranda M. Tallman [1,2,†], Abigail A. Zalenski [1,3,†], Ian Stabl [1], Morgan S. Schrock [1], Luke Kollin [1], Eliane de Jong [1], Kuntal De [1], Treg M. Grubb [1], Matthew K. Summers [1] and Monica Venere [1,*]

[1] Department of Radiation Oncology, James Cancer Hospital and Comprehensive Cancer Center, College of Medicine, The Ohio State University, Columbus, OH 43210, USA; mmontgomery527@gmail.com (M.M.T.); azalenski18@gmail.com (A.A.Z.); moschrock@gmail.com (M.S.S.); luke.kollin@osumc.edu (L.K.); dejong.24@buckeyemail.osu.edu (E.d.J.); dek@miamioh.edu (K.D.); grubbt@ccf.org (T.M.G.); matthew.summers@osumc.edu (M.K.S.)
[2] Biomedical Sciences Graduate Program, The Ohio State University, Columbus, OH 43210, USA
[3] Neuroscience Graduate Program, The Ohio State University, Columbus, OH 43210, USA
* Correspondence: monica.venere@osumc.edu; Tel.: +1-614-685-7842
† These authors contributed equally to this work.

Simple Summary: Glioblastoma, IDH-wild type (GBM) is the most common malignant primary brain tumor. Advances in cancer therapy remain unsuccessful in the treatment of GBM patients and have not extended the median survival beyond 12–18 months with the current treatment of surgery, chemotherapy, and radiotherapy. A central issue to finding a curative treatment option is the radioresistant nature of GBM. The goal of our study was to validate the therapeutic efficacy of enriching GBM tumor cells in the phase of the cell cycle where they are most vulnerable to radiotherapy, mitosis, using a small molecule inhibitor to the mitotic kinesin, KIF11. We confirmed that KIF11 inhibition radiosensitized GBM cells and improved overall survival in preclinical mouse models of GBM. These findings offer a new therapeutic modality that can increase the efficacy of radiotherapy for GBM with the ultimate goal of improving patient outcomes.

Abstract: Glioblastoma, IDH-wild type (GBM) is the most common and lethal malignant primary brain tumor. Standard of care includes surgery, radiotherapy, and chemotherapy with the DNA alkylating agent temozolomide (TMZ). Despite these intensive efforts, current GBM therapy remains mainly palliative with only modest improvement achieved in overall survival. With regards to radiotherapy, GBM is ranked as one of the most radioresistant tumor types. In this study, we wanted to investigate if enriching cells in the most radiosensitive cell cycle phase, mitosis, could improve localized radiotherapy for GBM. To achieve cell cycle arrest in mitosis we used ispinesib, a small molecule inhibitor to the mitotic kinesin, KIF11. Cell culture studies validated that ispinesib radiosensitized patient-derived GBM cells. In vivo, we validated that ispinesib increased the fraction of tumor cells arrested in mitosis as well as increased apoptosis. Critical for the translation of this approach, we validated that combination therapy with ispinesib and irradiation led to the greatest increase in survival over either monotherapy alone. Our data highlight KIF11 inhibition in combination with radiotherapy as a new combinatorial approach that reduces the overall radioresistance of GBM and which can readily be moved into clinical trials.

Keywords: glioblastoma; radiotherapy; KIF11

Citation: Tallman, M.M.; Zalenski, A.A.; Stabl, I.; Schrock, M.S.; Kollin, L.; de Jong, E.; De, K.; Grubb, T.M.; Summers, M.K.; Venere, M. Improving Localized Radiotherapy for Glioblastoma via Small Molecule Inhibition of KIF11. *Cancers* **2023**, *15*, 3173. https://doi.org/10.3390/cancers15123173

Academic Editor: Edward Pan

Received: 15 May 2023
Revised: 31 May 2023
Accepted: 8 June 2023
Published: 13 June 2023

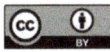

Copyright: © 2023 by the authors. Licensee MDPI, Basel, Switzerland. This article is an open access article distributed under the terms and conditions of the Creative Commons Attribution (CC BY) license (https:// creativecommons.org/licenses/by/ 4.0/).

1. Introduction

Less than 10% of glioblastoma (GBM, isocitrate dehydrogenase [IDH]-wild-type) patients survive longer than 5 years and the average length of survival after diagnosis is a dismal 12 to 18 months [1–4]. Standard of care for GBM includes radiotherapy, yet we and others have shown that GBM cells are refractory to this treatment, which contributes to tumor recurrence [5–9]. There is therefore a critical need to identify treatment modalities that can improve the efficacy of localized radiotherapy for GBM.

GBM is an inherently highly proliferative and mitotically active tumor and we and others have previously shown that perturbing mitosis is an effective means of limiting GBM tumor growth [10–15]. Specifically, we reported that the mitotic kinesin KIF11 (kinesin family member 11), required for bipolar spindle formation during mitosis, is elevated in GBM and portends poor prognosis [14]. We also demonstrated that the survival of mice bearing orthotopic GBM was prolonged using ispinesib, a small molecule inhibitor to KIF11 [14]. Notably, KIF11 inhibitors will arrest cells in mitosis, a phase of the cell cycle when cells are particularly vulnerable to radiotherapy [16–19]. Early studies indicated that this increased sensitivity to irradiation was linked to the compacted chromatin within mitosis being more vulnerable to DNA strand breaks, versus the dispersed chromatin of interphase cells [19]. More recent work has elucidated that, unlike the other phases of the cell cycle, DNA breaks that occur in mitosis do not trigger a cell cycle arrest unless the breaks are at telomeres or centromeres [20–22]. This leads to an overall increased sensitivity to DNA damage in mitosis [19,23,24]. The DNA lesions can be marked as damaged in mitosis and repaired in G1, but the increased chromosomal instability caused by mitotic progression in the presence of DNA breaks can also lead to an increase in cell death [20,23–30]. Hence, enriching GBM cells in mitosis prior to radiotherapy could serve to increase the level of tumor cell death. However, it is unknown if targeting KIF11 will radiosensitize GBM.

The goal of our study was to fill this gap by testing the hypothesis that KIF11 inhibition would serve to radiosensitize GBM by enriching the fraction of GBM cells within the radio-sensitive mitotic phase of the cell cycle. We were able to confirm KIF11 inhibition as a radiosensitizer using in vitro clonogenic assays. Our in vivo studies highlighted an increase in mitotic index following ispinesib treatment. Importantly, we confirmed that combinatorial treatment with ispinesib and radiotherapy significantly improved overall survival in our preclinical models. Taken together, our findings highlight enrichment in mitosis as a therapeutic paradigm that can enhance the efficacy of localized radiotherapy for GBM.

2. Materials and Methods

2.1. Cells and Cell Culture

All cells were obtained as de-identified specimens that were initially acquired as primary human brain tumor patient specimens in accordance with appropriate, approved Institutional Review Board (IRB) protocols. Of these cells, 3691 was a kind gift from Dr. Jeremy Rich (University of Pittsburgh), 1016 was a kind gift from Dr. Anita Hjelmeland, and NU757 was obtained from the Northwestern University Nervous System Tumor Bank.

Cells were cultured at 37 °C at 5% CO_2 in Neurobasal media (minus phenol red; Gibco, Grand Island, NY, USA) supplemented with B27 (minus Vitamin A; Gibco), human fibroblast growth factor-2 (10 ng/mL; Miltenyi Biotec, Bergisch Gladbach, Germany), human epidermal growth factor (10 ng/mL; Miltenyi Biotec), L-glutamine (2 mM; Gibco), sodium pyruvate (1 mM; Gibco), and penicillin/streptomycin (100 I.U./mL/100 μg/mL; Gibco). Cells plated adherently were on Geltrex LDEV-Free hESC-Qualified, Reduced Growth Factor Basement Membrane Matrix (Gibco), whereas in vivo studies were performed with cells grown in suspension as tumorspheres before dissociation and cell counting prior to implantation. TrypLE Express Enzyme was used to obtain single cell suspensions (no phenol red; Gibco). Mycoplasma testing was performed quarterly (Mycoplasma Detection Kit; Southern Biotech, Birmingham, AL, USA) and cell line verification was performed annually (microsatellite genotyping; Ohio State University Comprehensive Cancer Center Genomics Shared Resource).

2.2. Animals and In Vivo Studies

All animal studies described were approved by the Ohio State University Institutional Animal Care and Use Committee and conducted in accordance with the NIH Guide for the Care and Use of Laboratory Animals. Male and female athymic Nu/Nu mice were used for all studies and were obtained from the Ohio State University Comprehensive Cancer Center Target Validation Shared Resource. Cells at 1×10^4 were injected intracranially in a total volume of 2 µL Neurobasal media (no supplements) 2 mm into the right lateral part of bregma, and at a depth of 2.5 mm from the dura, in mice 6–8 weeks old. All mice were monitored daily for early removal criteria including neurological impairments and/or a drop in weight of more than 20% of their original weight. For single treatment studies, designed to compare mitotic index temporally and between delivery methods, tumor burden was established for 28 days and, then, mice were randomized into one of three treatment groups: vehicle, ispinesib (10 mg/kg, intraperitoneal), or ispinesib (10 mg/kg, intravenous via the tail vein), with mice from each group sacrificed 6 or 12 h after treatment. For full treatment and survival studies, mice were randomized into one of four treatment groups seven days after implantation: vehicle, ispinesib (10 mg/kg, intravenous), irradiation (2.5 Gy), or ispinesib and irradiation. Initiation of treatment was based on previous studies whereby tumor burden was known to have been established 7 days post-implantation for 3691 and 14 days post-implantation for 1016. Ispinesib or vehicle treatments were given once a week for four weeks (7, 14, 21, and 28 days after intracranial injection of 3691 and 14, 21, 28, and 35 for 1016). Irradiation was given to the tumor-bearing hemisphere 6 h after vehicle or ispinesib injections using the Small Animal Radiation Research Platform (SARRP; Xstrahl Medical and Life Sciences) for targeted dose delivery. All mice in the full treatment study were sacrificed 6 h after the irradiation was given to mice in those cohorts. For the survival study, mice were sacrificed upon meeting early removal criteria.

2.3. Small Molecule Inhibitor

Ispinesib was obtained from Selleck Chemicals (#S1452). For in vitro experiments, stock solutions of ispinesib were made in DMSO. Working concentrations were made immediately before use and diluted in cell media. DMSO served as the vehicle control. For in vivo work, working dilutions of ispinesib were made immediately before use in EtOH followed by Tween-80, and then sterile water at a ratio of 20:25:77.5, respectively. The EtOH, Tween-80, and sterile water mixture served as the vehicle control for in vivo studies.

2.4. Colony Formation Assays

Cells were plated at 250 cells per well onto Geltrex treated 6-well plates. The next day, cells were treated with ispinesib at 0.35 nM or with vehicle control (DMSO), and immediately left unirradiated (0 Gy) or irradiated with 1, 2, or 3 Gy. Irradiation was performed using a GammaCell 40 Irradiator (Best Theratronics). Sham irradiated control plates (0 Gy) were transported to the radiation facility, but not exposed. Media was changed 24 h later. Ten days post-treatment, cells were washed before being fixed and stained with a 0.5% crystal violet solution. Plates were imaged on the LI-COR Odyssey near infrared imaging system and analyzed via an ImageJ macro, which counts individual colonies, allowing for unbiased quantification.

2.5. Hematoxylin and Eosin Staining

Mice were perfused (1x PBS followed by 4% PFA) and tumor-bearing brains were harvested, fixed in 4% PFA overnight at 4 °C, sucrose sunk at 4 °C (30% sucrose solution), and then embedded in OCT compound. Sections of 10 µm were mounted onto slides (Superfrost Plus Microscope Slides; Fisherbrand, Pittsburgh, PA, USA) and stored at −20 °C till further processing. Sections were brought to room temperature for 30 min and then desiccated until dry (about 15 min). Sections were stained with hematoxylin (2 min) and eosin (20 s), followed by treatments with EtOH (20 s, three times) and xylenes (1 min, two times). Coverslips were mounted using Fluoromount-G Mounting Medium (Southern Biotech). Sections were imaged on an EVOS M7000 (AMF7000 Invitrogen, Software Version 2.0.2094.0) using the 10x objective.

2.6. Immunocytochemistry

Sections, as above, were warmed to room temperature for 2 h. Sections were then post-fixed with 4% PFA for 15 min, washed three times in 1x PBS, then blocked at room temperature for 1 h in 10% (w/v) BSA (for anti-cl-Caspase-3) or 10% goat serum (for anti-pH3Ser10) in PBS-Triton X-100 (0.2% v/v). After the block, sections were immunolabeled with anti-cleaved-Caspase-3 (cl-Caspase-3; 1:400; Cell Signaling 9664) or anti-phospho-Histone H3 Serine 10 (pH3S10; 1:1000; Cell Signaling 9706) overnight at 4 °C in a humidified chamber. The next day, slides were washed three times in PBS-Triton X-100 (0.2% v/v) followed by secondary detection with Alexa Fluor 594 (Invitrogen, Waltham, MA, USA) for 2 h at room temperature. Nuclei were counterstained with Hoechst. Coverslips were mounted using Fluoromount-G Mounting Medium (Southern Biotech, Birmingham, AL, USA). Images were acquired using EVOS M7000 (AMF7000 Invitrogen, Software Version 2.0.2094.0) and six images were taken per section (three random areas of the tumor rim and three random areas of the tumor core).

2.7. Image Analysis

Images were run through ImageJ (1.53f51) macros based on the marker. For pH3S10, we counted Hoechst-stained nuclei, and then calculated the percent of all cells that were positive for pH3S10. Cl-Caspase-3 was analyzed by taking the mean pixel intensity of the image.

2.8. Statistical Analysis

Statistical analyses were conducted using GraphPad Prism 9.4.1, unless otherwise stated. The statistical test used for each experiment is listed within the corresponding figure legend. For the colony formation assays, three biological repeats were performed for each specimen and each biological replicate included three technical replicates. For immunocytochemistry, tumors from three separate mice per condition were evaluated with six images taken per tumor for a total of eighteen separate images evaluated per condition.

3. Results

3.1. KIF11 Inhibition Radiosensitized Patient-Derived GBM Cells In Vitro

To begin to investigate if KIF11 inhibition was capable of radiosensitizing GBM cells, we utilized clonogenic assays to quantify reproductive cell survival after irradiation as this approach is associated with the clinical response of a tumor to radiotherapy [31–34]. GBM 3691 and GBM NU757 were treated with 0.35 nM ispinesib, a concentration that did not induce excessive cell death as a single treatment, and were then exposed to 0–3 Gy of irradiation. Clonogenic survival was reduced for both GBM specimens, with a resulting dose enhancement factor (DEF; DEF at surviving fraction 0.5 with a DEF greater than 1 indicating a synergistic effect) of 1.13 for GBM 3691 and 1.23 for GBM NU757 (Figure 1a,b). These data indicate that KIF11 inhibition via ispinesib prior to irradiation radiosensitized GBM cells.

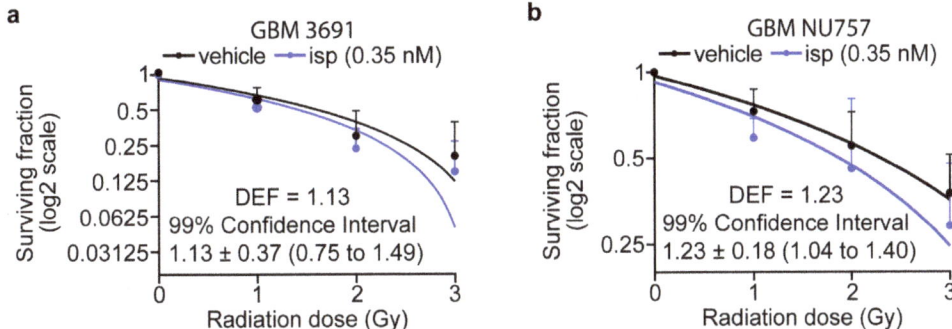

Figure 1. KIF11 inhibition combined with irradiation increased the radiosensitivity of GBM cells in vitro. (**a**) GBM 3691 and (**b**) GBM NU757 were treated with vehicle (DMSO) or 0.35 nM ispinesib (isp) and then irradiated (0–3 Gy). Colonies per well were normalized to 0 Gy and linear regression was used to model the effect of radiation on survival. Vehicle (black line) and ispinesib (blue line) data were graphed on log2 scale. n = 3 biological replicates per GBM specimen with n = 3 technical replicates per biological repeat. Dose enhancement factors (DEFs) were calculated by comparing doses at which the surviving fraction was 0.5 and the 99% confidence interval showed a DEF of above 1. Error bars represent standard deviation.

3.2. The Mitotic Index and Level of Apoptosis Were Increased in Tumors following a Single Treatment with Ispinesib

Having established KIF11 inhibition as an efficient approach to radiosensitize GBM cells in vitro, we then wanted to explore the in vivo efficacy of combination therapy. As a first step, we wanted to establish the drug delivery method and timing post-drug administration that would result in the greatest fraction of tumor cells arrested in mitosis and hence most vulnerable to irradiation. We previously found that repeated in vivo dosing of ispinesib at 10 mg/kg, given intraperitoneally (i.p.), was well tolerated, and so we chose this concentration for both i.p. and intravenous (i.v.) drug administration [14]. Mice bearing orthotopic tumors were given a single dose of vehicle or ispinesib 28 days post tumor cell implantation which, based on prior studies, is a time point with well-established tumor burden but prior to mice reaching early removal criteria [7]. Tumor-bearing brains were collected at 6 h and 12 h post-drug and evaluated for changes in the mitotic index via immunofluorescence to the mitotic marker pH3S10 (Figure 2a). Both i.v. and i.p. drug delivery, at both time points, resulted in increased mitotic indexes over the vehicle, with i.p. at 12 h having the least significance. Between i.v. and i.p. administration, the mitotic index was not statistically different between i.v. 6 h and 12 h and i.p. 6 h, but both i.v. timepoints had significantly higher mitotic indexes than the 12 h i.p. timepoint. For both i.v. and i.p. drug delivery, the earlier 6 h timepoint resulted in a significantly higher mitotic index over the later 12 h timepoint. As previous reports indicated that ispinesib concentrations were higher in the tumor core versus tumor rim, we wanted to further analyze our data to compare for differential mitotic arrest upon KIF11 inhibition between the tumor rim and the tumor core for the different delivery methods and time points (Figure 2b,c) [35]. Only the i.v. 12 h cohort had a significant difference in the mitotic index between the rim and the core. Overall, these data indicate that, despite potential differences in drug concentration across the bulk tumor, there are sufficient levels of ispinesib for target engagement and resulting mitotic arrest.

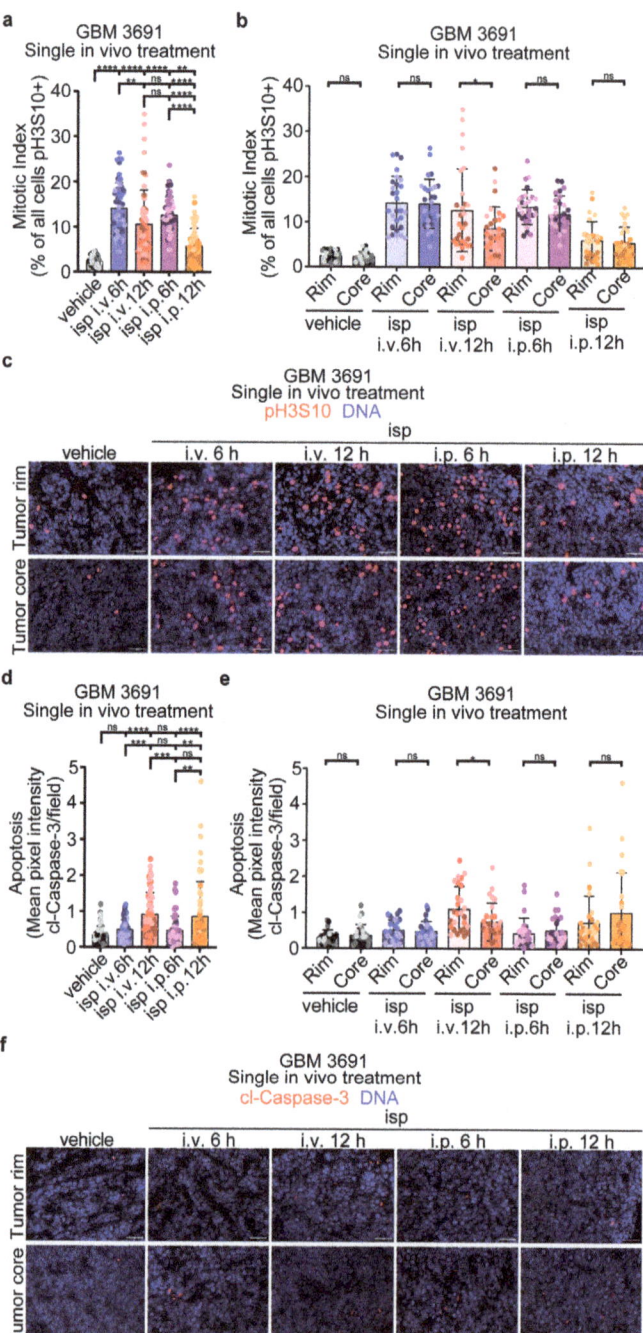

Figure 2. Single in vivo treatment with ispinesib increased the mitotic index and apoptosis of tumor cells. (**a**,**b**) Tumor-bearing mice were treated with vehicle or a single dose of ispinesib (isp), given intravenously (i.v.) or intraperitoneally (i.p.), and brains were harvested 6 or 12 h later. Tumor-bearing brains were sectioned and immunolabeled with anti-pH3S10 and DNA was counter-stained with Hoechst.

The percentage of pH3S10-positive tumor cells was calculated for each condition. (**c**) Representative images of mitotically arrested tumor cells in each condition. (**d**,**e**) Tumor sections were immunolabeled with anti-cl-Caspase-3 and DNA was counter-stained with Hoechst. The mean pixel intensity for cl-Caspase-3 per field was measured for each condition. (**f**) Representative images of apoptotic tumor cells in each condition. Tumors from three separate mice per condition were evaluated with six images taken per tumor (three at the tumor rim and three at the tumor core) for a total of eighteen separate images evaluated per condition. Each dot within the bar graphs represents the data from an individual image and the three different color shades each represents one of the three tumors evaluated. Data were analyzed in (**a**) and (**d**) by a one-way ANOVA with a Tukey's multiple comparison test and in (**b**) and (**e**) by Student's *t*-test. Error bars represent standard deviation. ns, no significance; *, $p < 0.05$; **, $p < 0.01$; ***, $p < 0.001$; ****, $p < 0.0001$.

To assess if even a single treatment of ispinesib can impact tumor cell viability, we evaluated for changes in apoptosis, via immunofluorescence, to the apoptotic marker cleaved-Caspase-3 (cl-Caspase-3) for both the whole tumor, and comparing the tumor rim to the tumor core (Figure 2d–f). Interestingly, although the mitotic index was higher for both i.v. and i.p. at the 6 h timepoint, apoptosis was highest at the 12 h timepoint for both delivery methods, potentially indicating that tumor cell death increases as more cells attempt to transit into mitosis in the presence of the drug (Figure 2d). For the tumor rim and tumor core, akin to the mitotic index, only the i.v. 12 h condition had a significant difference, albeit that the overall level of apoptosis, as measured by cl-Caspase-3, was very low in all treatment groups (Figure 2e,f). Given the maximal response in mitotic index at 6 h post i.v. administration, we chose this delivery method and timepoint post-drug to give radiotherapy for further in vivo studies. Taken together, these data indicate efficient KIF11 inhibition by ispinesib via different delivery methods and at different timepoints.

3.3. Repeated In Vivo Treatment with Ispinesib, with and without Radiotherapy, Led to Increased Mitotic Indexes and Tumor Cell Death

Having established the optimal delivery method and time post-administration for mitotic enrichment following ispinesib treatment, we next wanted to evaluate mitosis and apoptosis in tumors exposed to multiple drug treatments, as well as to combinatorial treatment with radiotherapy. We had four cohorts: vehicle, ispinesib (10 mg/kg), radiotherapy (2.5 Gy), or ispinesib and radiotherapy. For our treatment paradigm, we gave ispinesib or vehicle weekly for 4 weeks and radiotherapy 6 h following the administration of ispinesib or vehicle. The treatment started 7 days post tumor cell inoculation and tumors for all cohorts were harvested 6 h after the final administration of radiotherapy. Hematoxylin and eosin staining confirmed tumor burden for all treatment groups at time of harvest (Figure 3a). We next evaluted mitotic index by pH3S10 (Figure 3b,c) and apoptosis by cl-Caspase-3 (Figure 3d,e). Multiple treatments with ispinesib led to the greatest increase in mitotic index over vehicle (Figure 3b), whereas all treatment groups led to an increased level of apoptosis over the control (Figure 3d). Interestingly, the combination group had a lower mitotic index in comparison to ispinesib as a monotherapy, but had a significantly higher level of apoptosis over all treatment groups. The lower mitotic index in the combination group could indicate that more mitotic cells have died following irradiation, hence resulting in an overall decrease in mitotic index, but more refined temporal studies would be required to confirm this.

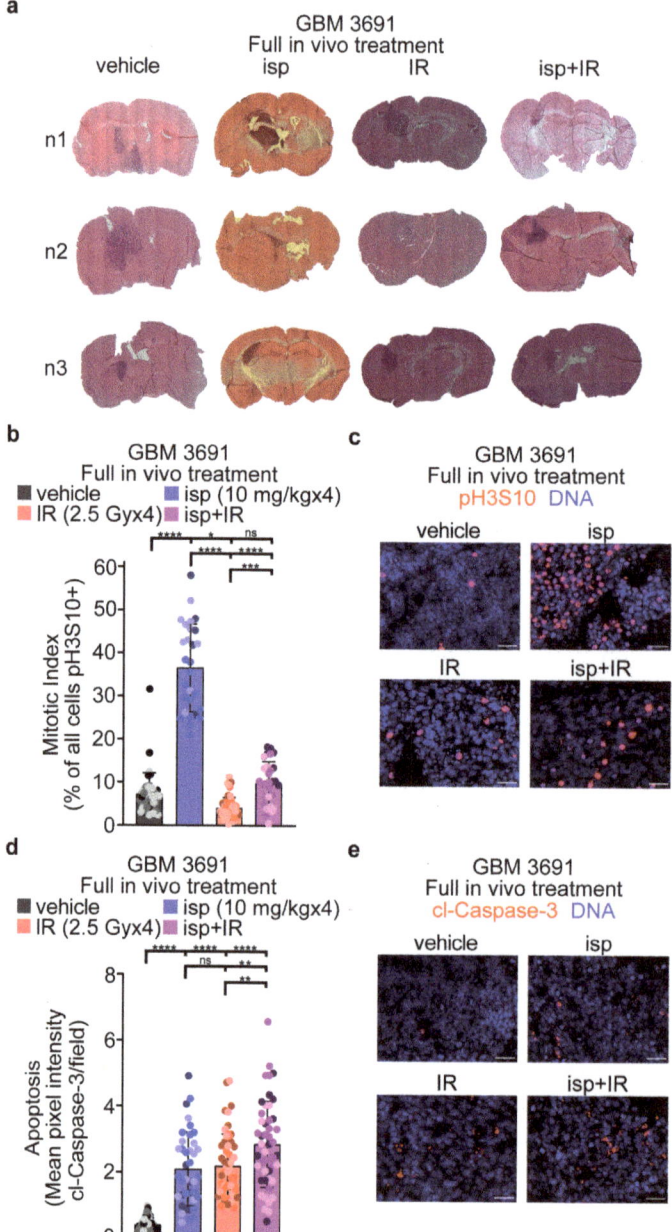

Figure 3. Multiple in vivo treatments with ispinesib increased the mitotic index and apoptosis of tumor cells. (**a**) Representative hematoxylin and eosin images of tumor-bearing brains following the full treatment timecourse for each cohort. (**b**) Tumor-bearing brains were sectioned and immunolabeled with anti-pH3S10 and DNA was counter-stained with Hoechst. The percentage of pH3S10-positive tumor cells was calculated for each condition. (**c**) Representative images of mitotically arrested tumor cells in each condition. (**d**) Tumor sections were immunolabeled with anti-cl-Caspase-3 and DNA was counter-stained with Hoechst. The mean pixel intensity for cl-Caspase-3 per field was measured for each condition. (**e**) Representative images of apoptotic tumor cells in each condition. Tumors from

three separate mice per condition were evaluated with six images taken per tumor for a total of eighteen separate images evaluated per condition. Each dot within the bar graphs represents the data from an individual image and the three different color shades each represents one of the three tumors evaluated. Data were analyzed in (**b**) and (**d**) by a one-way ANOVA with a Tukey's multiple comparison test. Error bars represent standard deviation. ns, no significance; *, $p < 0.05$; **, $p < 0.01$; ***, $p < 0.001$; ****, $p < 0.0001$.

3.4. Combination Treatment with Ispinesib and Radiotherapy Improved Survival in Preclinical Models of GBM

Given the positive in vitro data showing the radiosensitization of GBM cells via ispinesib, along with the in vivo data indicating an increase in cell death with the combination, we next wanted to evaluate if the combination treatment would provide a survival advantage. We had the same four cohorts and treatment schedule described above (i.e., vehicle, ispinesib (10 mg/kg), radiotherapy (2.5 Gy), or ispinesib and radiotherapy given every 7 days for 4 weeks with radiotherapy given 6 h post-ispinesib). The mice were then monitored for overall survival following cessation of treatments. We used both GBM 3691, which was used in previous in vivo mitotic index and apoptosis studies, as well as GBM 1016. For both patient-derived orthotopic models, the combinatorial therapy led to a significant increase in median survival in comparison to ispinesib or irradiation as a monotherapy as well as the vehicle cohort (Figure 4a,b). These data highlight that enriching GBM tumor cells in a radiosensitive cell cycle phase can lead to increased tumor cell death and improved survival.

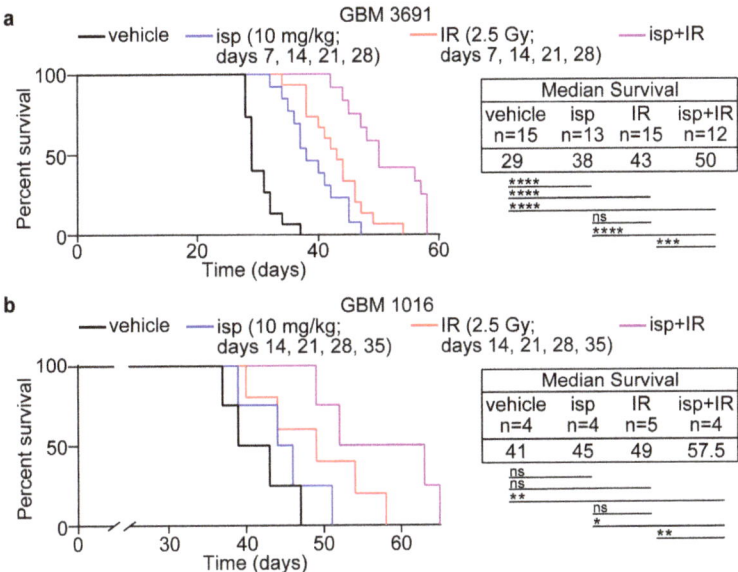

Figure 4. Combination treatment with ispinesib and radiothearpy increased survival in orthotopic preclinical mouse models of GBM. (**a**) GBM 3691 and (**b**) GBM 1016 orthotopic tumor bearing mice were treated with vehicle, ispinesib (isp; 10 mg/kg), irradiation (IR, 2.5 Gy) or ispinesib and IR (isp+IR) on the indicated days. Kaplan-Meier survival curves were generated for vehicle (black line), ispinesib (blue line), IR (red line), and isp+IR (purple line). The median survival and number of mice per group for each condition is indicated. Data were analyzed via independent log-rank (Mantel-Cox) tests between groups with a Bonferroni's post-hoc multiple comparison test. ns, no significance; *, $p < 0.05$; **, $p < 0.01$; ***, $p < 0.001$; ****, $p < 0.0001$.

4. Discussion

Given the inherent radioresistant nature of GBM, there have been numerous efforts to identify radiosensitizers that would serve to improve the overall efficacy of radiotherapy [36–39]. In our studies, we sought to evaluate if the enrichment of GBM cells in mitosis, using an inhibitor to the mitotic kinesin KIF11, could increase overall tumor cell death due to the increased sensitivity of mitotic cells to irradiation [16–19]. Indeed, our in vitro clonogenic assays confirmed the radiosensitization of GBM cells when pretreated with the KIF11 inhibitor ispinesib and then irradiated. We also confirmed mitotic enrichment in orthotopic preclinical mouse models of GBM, that was concomitant with an increase in cell death when tumors were also treated with radiotherapy. However, more in-depth temporal studies would serve to further strengthen the in vivo link between an increase in mitotic index and an increase in mitotic cell death following radiotherapy. Of key importance for translation, the combination therapy was able to extend survival in these mouse models.

The approach of using a KIF11 inhibitor to enrich tumor cells in mitosis prior to radiotherapy has strong rationale. However, to date, no KIF11 inhibitors have received FDA approval. This is despite the development of dozens of inhibitors with varying mechanisms of action for inhibition [40,41]. Ispinesib was the first KIF11 inhibitor to enter clinical trials and was reported to be well tolerated, but a lack of tumor response for ispinesib, and the other inhibitors that made it into clinical trials, has left the field with an overall disappointing outlook for clinical translation of KIF11 inhibitors. However, most of these studies were focused on KIF11 inhibition as a targeted, antiproliferative approach. Hence, many trials used the KIF11 inhibitor as a monotherapy. Combinatorial studies were also performed with a variety of chemotherapeutics, but none incorporated radiotherapy. Our approach of using KIF11, not only as an anti-proliferation strategy but also as a radiosensitizer, may therefore provide a new approach to achieving more positive clinical outcomes for KIF11 inhibition.

Should KIF11 inhibition plus radiotherapy move forward for GBM, which inhibitor to use and the design of the treatment schedule would be critical factors to consider. We used ispinesib in these studies based on our prior, promising work with this drug as a monotherapy for GBM [14]. Our current studies focused on human GBM models whereby we saw pronounced target engagement, as indicated by an increase in the mitotic index, following just a single dose of ispinesib. Most importantly, the combination with radiotherapy improved overall survival using multiple human GBM patient cell lines. Recent studies have reported a drug efflux of ispinesib by GBM cells and demonstrated that inhibition of the efflux pumps, in combination with ispinesib, improved efficacy in rodent and human models of GBM [35]. Although it is unknown if drug efflux is at play in our models, the combination of ispinesib and radiotherapy produced a significant impact on orthotopic tumors. For the dosing schedule, we chose a very conservative schedule for our studies, giving treatment only once a week. This treatment design nonetheless led to an overall increase in survival with the combination, demonstrating the utility of this strategy. Given that mice did succumb to tumor burden upon cessation of treatment, however, the efficacy of additional ispinesib plus radiotherapy cycles could be evaluated. Alternatively, the use of KIF11 inhibitors with a longer half-life, such as ARRY-520 with a half-life of more than 90 h, versus 16 h for ispinesib, could allow for a more frequent radiotherapy schedule to capitalize on the continued enrichment of cells in mitosis [42–44]. More frequent combinatorial radiotherapy could also be achieved with 4SC-205, which is an oral KIF11 inhibitor that can be administered daily [45]. Overall, our findings with ispinesib lay the foundation for future studies that could explore repeated and extended dosing of both KIF11 inhibition and radiotherapy to potentially achieve even great tumor cell death and further extension of survival if not, ideally, the full eradication of tumor burden.

5. Conclusions

Taken together, our work highlights a novel treatment approach for GBM that capitalizes on the radiosensitivity of cells in the mitotic phase of the cell cycle. Our work focuses on achieving this enrichment in mitosis via the inhibition of the mitotic kinesin, KIF11, but there are numerous small molecule inhibitors developed or in development for other mitotic regulators that could also be combined with radiotherapy and tested in the context of GBM. With no curative treatment options for this devastating tumor, this approach can be further explored to achieve better survival outcomes for GBM patients.

Author Contributions: Conceptualization, M.V.; methodology, M.V., M.M.T. and A.A.Z.; software, M.M.T. and I.S.; validation, M.M.T., A.A.Z. and I.S.; formal analysis, M.V., M.M.T., A.A.Z. and I.S.; investigation, M.M.T., A.A.Z., I.S., M.S.S., L.K., E.d.J., K.D. and T.M.G.; resources, M.V. and M.K.S.; data curation, M.V., M.M.T., A.A.Z. and I.S.; writing—original draft preparation, M.V., M.M.T. and A.A.Z.; writing—review and editing, M.V., M.M.T., A.A.Z., I.S., M.S.S., L.K., E.d.J., K.D., T.M.G. and M.K.S.; visualization, M.V. and M.M.T.; supervision, M.V. and M.K.S.; project administration, M.V.; funding acquisition, M.V. All authors have read and agreed to the published version of the manuscript.

Funding: This research was funded by an American Cancer Society Research Scholars Grant RSG-18-066-01-TBG, an Internal Research Program Grant from The Ohio State University Comprehensive Cancer Center, and funds from The Ohio State University Comprehensive Cancer Center/Department of Radiation Oncology (M.V.). Other funding includes the National Institute of General Medical Sciences of the National Institutes of Health under award number 2T32GM068412-11A1 (M.M.T.); an Ohio State University Graduate School Dean's Distinguished University Fellowship (A.A.Z.); the Pelotonia Fellowship Program (M.M.T. and A.A.Z.); an American Brain Tumor Association Basic Research Fellowship supported by an Anonymous Corporate Donor (M.S.S.); and the National Institute of General Medical Sciences of the National Institutes of Health under award numbers R01GM112895 and R01GM108743 (M.K.S.). The APC was funded by M.V and the Department of Radiation Biology. The Small Animal Radiation Research Platform was purchased via a National Institutes of Health shared instrument grant, 1S10OD020006-01. The research reported in this publication was supported by The Ohio State University Comprehensive Cancer Center and the National Institutes of Health under grant number P30 CA016058. Any opinions, findings, and conclusions expressed in this material are those of the authors and do not necessarily reflect those of the funding agencies or The Ohio State University.

Institutional Review Board Statement: All animal studies described were approved by the Ohio State University Institutional Animal Care and Use Committee and conducted in accordance with the NIH Guide for the Care and Use of Laboratory Animals.

Informed Consent Statement: Not applicable.

Data Availability Statement: No new data were created or analyzed in this study. Data sharing is not applicable to this article.

Acknowledgments: The authors thank Jeremy Rich (University of Pittsburg) for the kind gift of the GBM 3691 cells and Anita Hjelmeland (University of Alabama) for the kind gift of the GBM 1016 cells. We also thank members of The Ohio State University Comprehensive Cancer Center Target Validation Shared Resource, the Small Animal Imaging Core, and the Genomics Shared Resource.

Conflicts of Interest: The authors declare no conflict of interest. The funders had no role in the design of the study; in the collection, analyses, or interpretation of data; in the writing of the manuscript; or in the decision to publish the results.

References

1. Furnari, F.B.; Fenton, T.; Bachoo, R.M.; Mukasa, A.; Stommel, J.M.; Stegh, A.; Hahn, W.C.; Ligon, K.L.; Louis, D.N.; Brennan, C.; et al. Malignant astrocytic glioma: Genetics, biology, and paths to treatment. *Genes Dev.* **2007**, *21*, 2683–2710. [CrossRef] [PubMed]
2. Miller, K.D.; Ostrom, Q.T.; Kruchko, C.; Patil, N.; Tihan, T.; Cioffi, G.; Fuchs, H.E.; Waite, K.A.; Jemal, A.; Siegel, R.L.; et al. Brain and other central nervous system tumor statistics, 2021. *CA Cancer J. Clin.* **2021**, *71*, 381–406. [CrossRef] [PubMed]

3. Stupp, R.; Hegi, M.E.; Mason, W.P.; van den Bent, M.J.; Taphoorn, M.J.; Janzer, R.C.; Ludwin, S.K.; Allgeier, A.; Fisher, B.; Belanger, K.; et al. Effects of radiotherapy with concomitant and adjuvant temozolomide versus radiotherapy alone on survival in glioblastoma in a randomised phase III study: 5-year analysis of the EORTC-NCIC trial. *Lancet Oncol.* 2009, 10, 459–466. [CrossRef] [PubMed]
4. Stupp, R.; Mason, W.P.; van den Bent, M.J.; Weller, M.; Fisher, B.; Taphoorn, M.J.; Belanger, K.; Brandes, A.A.; Marosi, C.; Bogdahn, U.; et al. Radiotherapy plus concomitant and adjuvant temozolomide for glioblastoma. *N. Engl. J. Med.* 2005, 352, 987–996. [CrossRef]
5. Bao, S.; Wu, Q.; McLendon, R.E.; Hao, Y.; Shi, Q.; Hjelmeland, A.B.; Dewhirst, M.W.; Bigner, D.D.; Rich, J.N. Glioma stem cells promote radioresistance by preferential activation of the DNA damage response. *Nature* 2006, 444, 756–760. [CrossRef]
6. Hambardzumyan, D.; Squatrito, M.; Holland, E.C. Radiation resistance and stem-like cells in brain tumors. *Cancer Cell* 2006, 10, 454–456. [CrossRef]
7. Tallman, M.M.; Zalenski, A.A.; Deighen, A.M.; Schrock, M.S.; Mortach, S.; Grubb, T.M.; Kastury, P.S.; Huntoon, K.; Summers, M.K.; Venere, M. The small molecule drug CBL0137 increases the level of DNA damage and the efficacy of radiotherapy for glioblastoma. *Cancer Lett.* 2021, 499, 232–242. [CrossRef]
8. Tamura, K.; Aoyagi, M.; Wakimoto, H.; Ando, N.; Nariai, T.; Yamamoto, M.; Ohno, K. Accumulation of CD133-positive glioma cells after high-dose irradiation by Gamma Knife surgery plus external beam radiation. *J. Neurosurg.* 2010, 113, 310–318. [CrossRef]
9. Venere, M.; Hamerlik, P.; Wu, Q.; Rasmussen, R.D.; Song, L.A.; Vasanji, A.; Tenley, N.; Flavahan, W.A.; Hjelmeland, A.B.; Bartek, J.; et al. Therapeutic targeting of constitutive PARP activation compromises stem cell phenotype and survival of glioblastoma-initiating cells. *Cell Death Differ.* 2014, 21, 258–269. [CrossRef]
10. De, K.; Grubb, T.M.; Zalenski, A.A.; Pfaff, K.E.; Pal, D.; Majumder, S.; Summers, M.K.; Venere, M. Hyperphosphorylation of CDH1 in Glioblastoma Cancer Stem Cells Attenuates APC/C(CDH1) Activity and Pharmacologic Inhibition of APC/C(CDH1/CDC20) Compromises Viability. *Mol. Cancer Res.* 2019, 17, 1519–1530. [CrossRef]
11. Ding, Y.; Hubert, C.G.; Herman, J.; Corrin, P.; Toledo, C.M.; Skutt-Kakaria, K.; Vazquez, J.; Basom, R.; Zhang, B.; Risler, J.K.; et al. Cancer-Specific requirement for BUB1B/BUBR1 in human brain tumor isolates and genetically transformed cells. *Cancer Discov.* 2013, 3, 198–211. [CrossRef]
12. Godek, K.M.; Venere, M.; Wu, Q.; Mills, K.D.; Hickey, W.F.; Rich, J.N.; Compton, D.A. Chromosomal Instability Affects the Tumorigenicity of Glioblastoma Tumor-Initiating Cells. *Cancer Discov.* 2016, 6, 532–545. [CrossRef]
13. Mao, D.D.; Gujar, A.D.; Mahlokozera, T.; Chen, I.; Pan, Y.; Luo, J.; Brost, T.; Thompson, E.A.; Turski, A.; Leuthardt, E.C.; et al. A CDC20-APC/SOX2 Signaling Axis Regulates Human Glioblastoma Stem-like Cells. *Cell Rep.* 2015, 11, 1809–1821. [CrossRef]
14. Venere, M.; Horbinski, C.; Crish, J.F.; Jin, X.; Vasanji, A.; Major, J.; Burrows, A.C.; Chang, C.; Prokop, J.; Wu, Q.; et al. The mitotic kinesin KIF11 is a driver of invasion, proliferation, and self-renewal in glioblastoma. *Sci. Transl. Med.* 2015, 7, 304ra143. [CrossRef]
15. Xie, Q.; Wu, Q.; Mack, S.C.; Yang, K.; Kim, L.; Hubert, C.G.; Flavahan, W.A.; Chu, C.; Bao, S.; Rich, J.N. CDC20 maintains tumor initiating cells. *Oncotarget* 2015, 6, 13241–13254. [CrossRef]
16. Sinclair, W.K. Cyclic x-ray responses in mammalian cells in vitro. *Radiat. Res.* 1968, 33, 620–643. [CrossRef]
17. Sinclair, W.K.; Morton, R.A. X-ray sensitivity during the cell generation cycle of cultured Chinese hamster cells. *Radiat. Res.* 1966, 29, 450–474. [CrossRef]
18. Terasima, T.; Tolmach, L.J. Variations in several responses of HeLa cells to x-irradiation during the division cycle. *Biophys. J.* 1963, 3, 11–33. [CrossRef]
19. Stobbe, C.C.; Park, S.J.; Chapman, J.D. The radiation hypersensitivity of cells at mitosis. *Int. J. Radiat. Biol.* 2002, 78, 1149–1157. [CrossRef]
20. Bakhoum, S.F.; Kabeche, L.; Compton, D.A.; Powell, S.N.; Bastians, H. Mitotic DNA Damage Response: At the Crossroads of Structural and Numerical Cancer Chromosome Instabilities. *Trends Cancer* 2017, 3, 225–234. [CrossRef]
21. Hayashi, M.T.; Cesare, A.J.; Fitzpatrick, J.A.; Lazzerini-Denchi, E.; Karlseder, J. A telomere-dependent DNA damage checkpoint induced by prolonged mitotic arrest. *Nat. Struct. Mol. Biol.* 2012, 19, 387–394. [CrossRef] [PubMed]
22. Mikhailov, A.; Cole, R.W.; Rieder, C.L. DNA damage during mitosis in human cells delays the metaphase/anaphase transition via the spindle-assembly checkpoint. *Curr. Biol.* 2002, 12, 1797–1806. [CrossRef] [PubMed]
23. Audrey, A.; de Haan, L.; van Vugt, M.; de Boer, H.R. Processing DNA lesions during mitosis to prevent genomic instability. *Biochem. Soc. Trans.* 2022, 50, 1105–1118. [CrossRef] [PubMed]
24. Giunta, S.; Belotserkovskaya, R.; Jackson, S.P. DNA damage signaling in response to double-strand breaks during mitosis. *J. Cell Biol.* 2010, 190, 197–207. [CrossRef]
25. Harding, S.M.; Benci, J.L.; Irianto, J.; Discher, D.E.; Minn, A.J.; Greenberg, R.A. Mitotic progression following DNA damage enables pattern recognition within micronuclei. *Nature* 2017, 548, 466–470. [CrossRef]
26. Leimbacher, P.A.; Jones, S.E.; Shorrocks, A.K.; de Marco Zompit, M.; Day, M.; Blaauwendraad, J.; Bundschuh, D.; Bonham, S.; Fischer, R.; Fink, D.; et al. MDC1 Interacts with TOPBP1 to Maintain Chromosomal Stability during Mitosis. *Mol. Cell* 2019, 74, 571–583.e8. [CrossRef]
27. Pedersen, R.T.; Kruse, T.; Nilsson, J.; Oestergaard, V.H.; Lisby, M. TopBP1 is required at mitosis to reduce transmission of DNA damage to G1 daughter cells. *J. Cell Biol.* 2015, 210, 565–582. [CrossRef]

28. Suzuki, M.; Suzuki, K.; Kodama, S.; Watanabe, M. Phosphorylated histone H2AX foci persist on rejoined mitotic chromosomes in normal human diploid cells exposed to ionizing radiation. *Radiat. Res.* **2006**, *165*, 269–276. [CrossRef]
29. Van den Berg, J.; Manjón, A.G.; Kielbassa, K.; Feringa, F.M.; Freire, R.; Medema, R.H. A limited number of double-strand DNA breaks is sufficient to delay cell cycle progression. *Nucleic Acids Res.* **2018**, *46*, 10132–10144. [CrossRef]
30. Williams, R.S.; Moncalian, G.; Williams, J.S.; Yamada, Y.; Limbo, O.; Shin, D.S.; Groocock, L.M.; Cahill, D.; Hitomi, C.; Guenther, G.; et al. Mre11 dimers coordinate DNA end bridging and nuclease processing in double-strand-break repair. *Cell* **2008**, *135*, 97–109. [CrossRef]
31. Deacon, J.; Peckham, M.J.; Steel, G.G. The radioresponsiveness of human tumours and the initial slope of the cell survival curve. *Radiother. Oncol.* **1984**, *2*, 317–323. [CrossRef]
32. Fertil, B.; Dertinger, H.; Courdi, A.; Malaise, E.P. Mean inactivation dose: A useful concept for intercomparison of human cell survival curves. *Radiat. Res.* **1984**, *99*, 73–84. [CrossRef]
33. Fertil, B.; Malaise, E.P. Inherent cellular radiosensitivity as a basic concept for human tumor radiotherapy. *Int. J. Radiat. Oncol. Biol. Phys.* **1981**, *7*, 621–629. [CrossRef]
34. Fertil, B.; Malaise, E.P. Intrinsic radiosensitivity of human cell lines is correlated with radioresponsiveness of human tumors: Analysis of 101 published survival curves. *Int. J. Radiat. Oncol. Biol. Phys.* **1985**, *11*, 1699–1707. [CrossRef]
35. Gampa, G.; Kenchappa, R.S.; Mohammad, A.S.; Parrish, K.E.; Kim, M.; Crish, J.F.; Luu, A.; West, R.; Hinojosa, A.Q.; Sarkaria, J.N.; et al. Enhancing Brain Retention of a KIF11 Inhibitor Significantly Improves its Efficacy in a Mouse Model of Glioblastoma. *Sci. Rep.* **2020**, *10*, 6524. [CrossRef]
36. Aiyappa-Maudsley, R.; Chalmers, A.J.; Parsons, J.L. Factors affecting the radiation response in glioblastoma. *Neurooncol. Adv.* **2022**, *4*, vdac156. [CrossRef]
37. Ali, M.Y.; Oliva, C.R.; Noman, A.S.M.; Allen, B.G.; Goswami, P.C.; Zakharia, Y.; Monga, V.; Spitz, D.R.; Buatti, J.M.; Griguer, C.E. Radioresistance in Glioblastoma and the Development of Radiosensitizers. *Cancers* **2020**, *12*, 2511. [CrossRef]
38. Matsui, J.K.; Perlow, H.K.; Ritter, A.R.; Upadhyay, R.; Raval, R.R.; Thomas, E.M.; Beyer, S.J.; Pillainayagam, C.; Goranovich, J.; Ong, S.; et al. Small Molecules and Immunotherapy Agents for Enhancing Radiotherapy in Glioblastoma. *Biomedicines* **2022**, *10*, 1763. [CrossRef]
39. McAleavey, P.G.; Walls, G.M.; Chalmers, A.J. Radiotherapy-drug combinations in the treatment of glioblastoma: A brief review. *CNS Oncol.* **2022**, *11*, CNS86. [CrossRef]
40. Garcia-Saez, I.; Skoufias, D.A. Eg5 targeting agents: From new anti-mitotic based inhibitor discovery to cancer therapy and resistance. *Biochem. Pharmacol.* **2021**, *184*, 114364. [CrossRef]
41. Jiang, C.; You, Q. Kinesin spindle protein inhibitors in cancer: A patent review (2008–present). *Expert Opin. Ther. Pat* **2013**, *23*, 1547–1560. [CrossRef] [PubMed]
42. Khoury, H.J.; Garcia-Manero, G.; Borthakur, G.; Kadia, T.; Foudray, M.C.; Arellano, M.; Langston, A.; Bethelmie-Bryan, B.; Rush, S.; Litwiler, K.; et al. A phase 1 dose-escalation study of ARRY-520, a kinesin spindle protein inhibitor, in patients with advanced myeloid leukemias. *Cancer* **2012**, *118*, 3556–3564. [CrossRef] [PubMed]
43. Lee, H.C.; Shah, J.J.; Feng, L.; Manasanch, E.E.; Lu, R.; Morphey, A.; Crumpton, B.; Patel, K.K.; Wang, M.L.; Alexanian, R.; et al. A phase 1 study of filanesib, carfilzomib, and dexamethasone in patients with relapsed and/or refractory multiple myeloma. *Blood Cancer J.* **2019**, *9*, 80. [CrossRef] [PubMed]
44. Ocio, E.M.; Motllo, C.; Rodriguez-Otero, P.; Martinez-Lopez, J.; Cejalvo, M.J.; Martin-Sanchez, J.; Blade, J.; Garcia-Malo, M.D.; Dourdil, M.V.; Garcia-Mateo, A.; et al. Filanesib in combination with pomalidomide and dexamethasone in refractory MM patients: Safety and efficacy, and association with alpha 1-acid glycoprotein (AAG) levels. Phase Ib/II Pomdefil clinical trial conducted by the Spanish MM group. *Br. J. Haematol.* **2021**, *192*, 522–530. [CrossRef]
45. Masanas, M.; Masia, N.; Suarez-Cabrera, L.; Olivan, M.; Soriano, A.; Majem, B.; Devis-Jauregui, L.; Burgos-Panadero, R.; Jimenez, C.; Rodriguez-Sodupe, P.; et al. The oral KIF11 inhibitor 4SC-205 exhibits antitumor activity and potentiates standard and targeted therapies in primary and metastatic neuroblastoma models. *Clin. Transl. Med.* **2021**, *11*, e533. [CrossRef]

Disclaimer/Publisher's Note: The statements, opinions and data contained in all publications are solely those of the individual author(s) and contributor(s) and not of MDPI and/or the editor(s). MDPI and/or the editor(s) disclaim responsibility for any injury to people or property resulting from any ideas, methods, instructions or products referred to in the content.

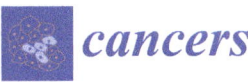

Article

Combination of EGFR-Directed Tyrosine Kinase Inhibitors (EGFR-TKI) with Radiotherapy in Brain Metastases from Non-Small Cell Lung Cancer: A 2010–2019 Retrospective Cohort Study

Vineeth Tatineni [1], Patrick J. O'Shea [1,2], Shreya Saxena [3], Atulya A. Khosla [3], Ahmad Ozair [3], Rupesh R. Kotecha [3], Xuefei Jia [1], Yasmeen Rauf [1,4,5], Erin S. Murphy [1,6], Samuel T. Chao [1,6], John H. Suh [1,6], David M. Peereboom [1,4] and Manmeet S. Ahluwalia [3,7,*]

1. Rosa Ella Burkhart Brain Tumor and Neuro-Oncology Center, Taussig Cancer Institute, Cleveland Clinic, Cleveland, OH 44106, USA
2. Case Western Reserve University School of Medicine, Cleveland, OH 44106, USA
3. Miami Cancer Institute, Baptist Health South Florida, Miami, FL 33176, USA; ahmad.ozair@baptisthealth.net (A.O.)
4. Department of Medical Oncology, Taussig Cancer Institute, Cleveland Clinic, Cleveland, OH 44106, USA
5. Division of Neuro-Oncology, University of North Carolina, Chapel Hill, NC 27599, USA
6. Department of Radiation Oncology, Taussig Cancer Institute, Cleveland Clinic, Cleveland, OH 44106, USA
7. Herbert Wertheim College of Medicine, Florida International University, Miami, FL 33199, USA
* Correspondence: manmeeta@baptisthealth.net; Tel.: +1-(216)-280-2412

Citation: Tatineni, V.; O'Shea, P.J.; Saxena, S.; Khosla, A.A.; Ozair, A.; Kotecha, R.R.; Jia, X.; Rauf, Y.; Murphy, E.S.; Chao, S.T.; et al. Combination of EGFR-Directed Tyrosine Kinase Inhibitors (EGFR-TKI) with Radiotherapy in Brain Metastases from Non-Small Cell Lung Cancer: A 2010–2019 Retrospective Cohort Study. *Cancers* **2023**, *15*, 3015. https://doi.org/10.3390/cancers15113015

Academic Editor: Edward Pan

Received: 20 January 2023
Revised: 17 May 2023
Accepted: 22 May 2023
Published: 1 June 2023

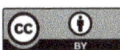

Copyright: © 2023 by the authors. Licensee MDPI, Basel, Switzerland. This article is an open access article distributed under the terms and conditions of the Creative Commons Attribution (CC BY) license (https://creativecommons.org/licenses/by/4.0/).

Simple Summary: Radiotherapy, in the form of either whole-brain radiotherapy (WBRT) or stereotactic radiosurgery (SRS), continues as the standard of care for patients of non-small cell lung cancer with brain metastases (NSCLCBM). Recently, targeted therapies have emerged as systemic options for brain metastases with certain genetic mutations. Tyrosine kinase inhibitors directed against EGFR protein (EGFR-TKI) have come forth as the preferred treatment of EGFR-mutated NSCLC and have also shown promise in NSCLCBM. However, there have been few studies comparing the synergistic effects of EGFR-TKIs and radiotherapy in NSCLCBM. This study is one of the few that investigates survival rates between standard radiotherapy modalities and a combination of radiotherapies and EGFR-TKIs. Our data may help guide clinicians in future treatment plans for EGFR-mutated NSCLCBM patients.

Abstract: Introduction: Traditionally, brain metastases have been treated with stereotactic radiosurgery (SRS), whole-brain radiation (WBRT), and/or surgical resection. Non-small cell lung cancers (NSCLC), over half of which carry EGFR mutations, are the leading cause of brain metastases. EGFR-directed tyrosine kinase inhibitors (TKI) have shown promise in NSCLC; but their utility in NSCLC brain metastases (NSCLCBM) remains unclear. This work sought to investigate whether combining EGFR-TKI with WBRT and/or SRS improves overall survival (OS) in NSCLCBM. Methods: A retrospective review of NSCLCBM patients diagnosed during 2010–2019 at a tertiary-care US center was performed and reported following the 'strengthening the reporting of observational studies in epidemiology' (STROBE) guidelines. Data regarding socio-demographic and histopathological characteristics, molecular attributes, treatment strategies, and clinical outcomes were collected. Concurrent therapy was defined as the combination of EGFR-TKI and radiotherapy given within 28 days of each other. Results: A total of 239 patients with EGFR mutations were included. Of these, 32 patients had been treated with WBRT only, 51 patients received SRS only, 36 patients received SRS and WBRT only, 18 were given EGFR-TKI and SRS, and 29 were given EGFR-TKI and WBRT. Median OS for the WBRT-only group was 3.23 months, for SRS + WBRT it was 3.17 months, for EGFR-TKI + WBRT 15.50 months, for SRS only 21.73 months, and for EGFR-TKI + SRS 23.63 months. Multivariable analysis demonstrated significantly higher OS in the SRS-only group (HR = 0.38, 95% CI 0.17–0.84, $p = 0.017$) compared to the WBRT reference group. There were no significant differences in overall survival for the SRS + WBRT combination cohort (HR = 1.30, 95% CI = 0.60, 2.82 $p = 0.50$), EGFR-TKIs and WBRT combination cohort (HR = 0.93, 95% CI = 0.41, 2.08, p = 0.85), or the EGFR-TKI + SRS cohort (HR = 0.46, 95% CI = 0.20, 1.09, p = 0.07). Conclusions: NSCLCBM patients treated with SRS had a significantly higher OS compared to patients treated with WBRT-only. While sample-size limitations and investigator-associated selection bias may limit the generalizability of these results, phase II/III clinicals trials are warranted to investigate synergistic efficacy of EGFR-TKI and SRS.

Keywords: epidermal growth factor receptor; brain metastasis; lung carcinoma; targeted therapy; molecular therapy; whole-brain radiation therapy; stereotactic radiosurgery

1. Introduction

Lung cancer is the second most common type of cancer worldwide, with non-small cell lung cancer (NSCLC) being the most common subtype and the most common cause of brain metastases [1,2]. In addition to lung cancer itself being a leading cause of cancer mortality, the development of brain metastases adds considerable symptoms, a poorer prognosis, and a much poorer quality of life [3,4]. Management of brain metastases with systemic therapies, particularly chemotherapies, has been challenging due to poor blood–brain-barrier penetration, leading to a low intracranial response rate [4]. Therefore, brain metastases have been historically treated with stereotactic radiosurgery (SRS), whole-brain radiation (WBRT), surgical resection, or a combination of these treatments [4].

In recent years, the management of NSCLCBM has shifted from traditional radiation and surgical therapy to targeted molecular therapies [5]. While several molecular agents have been studied, only a few have demonstrated meaningful utility as either therapeutic targets or prognostic markers [5]. Epidermal growth factor receptor (EGFR), a transmembrane growth factor receptor tyrosine kinase, is mutated in 40–60% of NSCLCs [6]. The risk of developing brain metastases is higher in patients with EGFR mutations, though, fortunately, EGFR signaling pathways have also become an effective targetable marker [7].

EGFR tyrosine kinase inhibitors (EGFR-TKIs) were first introduced in the early 2000s and have been proven to be more effective than standard chemotherapy [8,9]. First-generation EGFR-TKIs are limited by their ability to cross the blood–brain barrier (BBB) and are ineffective against certain tumor mutations [10,11]. This, of course, limits their ability to treat an EGFR-mutated lung tumor that has metastasized to the brain. Second-generation EGFR-TKIs have improved activity against exon 19 deletion mutations and therefore have better efficacy than first-generation agents [11–13]. Third-generation EGFR-TKIs have shown both better BBB penetration and efficacy against T790M mutations [13], making them, in theory, the most effective against metastatic lung tumors in the brain.

Though these new targeted therapies have shown great promise in NSCLC, there are few robust data when looking specifically at NSCLCBM [14,15]. Fan et al. conducted a systemic review of 16 clinical studies where the pooled analysis indicated EGFR-TKIs are effective for patients with NSCLCBM [16].

The development of resistance to EGFR-TKIs is inevitable, and a few trials have analyzed the efficacy of its combination with WBRT and SRS in patients with EGFR-mutated NSCLCBM [17,18]. In parallel to the increasing utility of EGFR-TKIs, stereotactic radiosurgery (SRS) has also emerged as a superior tool for radiotherapy in brain metastases, compared to whole-brain teletherapy approaches [19,20]. SRS is now commonly used as first-line local therapy for brain metastases [21]. The interaction of EGFR-TKI therapy and SRS together has been a topic of interest in recent years [22–24]. We look to add to this field of newer interest with our large, single-institution study.

As EGFR-TKI data in NSCLCBM becomes more comprehensive, synergistic therapies need to be looked at. There is no consensus on its management, and the efficacy of the combination regimen of EGFR-TKIs and radiotherapy remains unclear among patients with various mutation subtypes. Therefore, we aimed to evaluate the OS in NSCLCBM patients treated with WBRT only, SRS only, WBRT and SRS, and a combination of EGFR-TKIs and SRS and EGFR-TKIs and WBRT.

2. Methods

2.1. Study Design, Patient Population, and Selection

A multi-arm retrospective cohort study was conducted, after institutional review board (IRB) approval, and reported following the 'strengthening the reporting of observational studies in epidemiology' (STROBE) guidelines. We investigated all EGFR-mutated NSCLCBM patients diagnosed during 2010–2019 at Cleveland Clinic, Ohio, a tertiary-care institution in the US.

We included all patients >18 years of age with EGFR-mutated NSCLCBM who were treated with SRS, WBRT, or EGFR-TKIs, as first-line therapy after the diagnosis of brain metastases. We did not exclude patients who received intracranial surgery at any point in the disease course. We also did not exclude patients who received EGFR-TKIs or other systemic therapies before the diagnosis of brain metastases as long as there was a change in therapy after the diagnosis of brain metastases since our primary goal was to evaluate the OS rates after the diagnosis of brain metastases. Patients who were included in our study were followed in the outpatient setting approximately every 3 months. Overall survival (OS) was defined as the date of first therapy after the diagnosis of brain metastases until the date of the last progress note or date of death.

Patient characteristics, initial imaging, genomic analysis, and treatment details were collected from the institution's electronic medical records. Data were recorded in a secure online database and then exported for statistical analysis. Characteristic information collected includes the Karnofsky Performance Score (KPS), age, race, and sex. The treatment details collected include the date of therapy initiation and the line of therapy.

2.2. EGFR-TKI Data

Erlotinib, gefitinib, afatinib, and osimertinib were primarily investigated in this study, whereas dacomitinib was not evaluated as no patients received this drug in our cohort. There was no EGFR-TKI-only cohort because all patients who received EGFR-TKIs also received some form of radiation during their treatment course. It is possible that patients in the EGFR-TKIs cohorts received more than one line of EGFR-TKI throughout their treatment course after the diagnosis of brain metastases; however, OS was only calculated based on the initiation of EGFR-TKI therapy after the diagnosis of brain metastases.

2.3. SRS Data

Patients in the SRS-only cohort were treated with SRS as first-line therapy and did not receive WBRT or systemic therapies after diagnosing brain metastases. However, the patients may have received further treatments for SRS throughout their disease course. The number of lesions that were treated upfront was not subclassified. The combination cohort of EGFR-TKIs and SRS was used to investigate a synergistic treatment approach. Concurrence was defined as therapies given within 28 days of each other.

2.4. WBRT Data

Patients in the WBRT-only cohort were treated with WBRT as first-line therapy and did not receive SRS or any systemic therapies after diagnosing brain metastases. Patients in the WBRT-only cohort received one course of WBRT; no repeat treatment courses were given. The date of WBRT was defined as the first date of radiation treatment given to the patient over the full course of treatment. Concurrence for the combination EGFR-TKI + WBRT cohort was defined as treatments given within 28 days of each other. Nonconcurrent treatments were not investigated. The specific radiation dosage, length of WBRT course, or discontinuation of treatment due to symptoms were not subclassified. The WBRT-only cohort was the reference cohort due to its history as the traditional modality of treatment of brain metastases.

2.5. SRS + WBRT Data

Patients in the SRS + WBRT were treated concurrently with both modalities within 28 days of each other. Patients in this cohort were not treated with any form of systemic therapy after the diagnosis of brain metastases. This cohort may have received either SRS or WBRT further along in the disease treatment course. We again did not subclassify the number of lesions treated initially with SRS, the length of the WBRT course, or discontinuation of WBRT due to symptoms.

2.6. Data Analysis

Categorical clinicopathologic factors were summarized as frequency counts and percentages, and continuous factors as medians and ranges. OS was measured from the start date of the first treatment received to the date of the last follow-up or date of death and was summarized using the Kaplan–Meier method. The 1-year and 2-year survival rates and estimated median survival for each treatment cohort were reported. The Cox proportional hazard model with a two-sided Wald test was used to evaluate the impact of the treatment on OS. The survival model was adjusted by clinical variables selected using the random forest method. The primary model was adjusted by the variables mostly identified as prognostic factors in patients with NSCLCBM in previous studies [25]. These variables were age at diagnosis of brain metastases, gender, number of brain metastases, the existence of extracranial metastases, the existence of leptomeningeal metastases, KPS, symptomatic at time of brain metastases, and the duration from the date of diagnosis of brain metastases to the date of treatment.

Due to its historical use and previously being the standard of care, the WBRT-only cohort was used as the reference cohort to which we compared OS. Progression-free survival (PFS) was not calculated in our study due to the lack of specific magnetic resonance imaging (MRI) intracranial-lesion data and difficulty with consistent, unbiased alternative definitions of progression. Statistical significance was defined as a p-value (p) of <0.05. All statistical analyses were performed using R Statistical Software version 4.1.0 (R Foundation for Statistical Computing, Vienna, Austria).

3. Results

3.1. Patient Characteristics

Between 2010 and 2019, our retrospective study found a total of 239 patients who had NSCLCBM with EGFR mutations. Of these, a total of 32 patients received WBRT alone, another 51 patients received SRS alone, 36 patients were treated with SRS + WBRT combined, 29 patients received EGFR-TKI + WBRT, and 18 patients received combination EGFR-TKI + SRS.

The WBRT-only group had a median age of 68.4 years, with 62.5% being female. The SRS-only group had a median age of 62.7 years, with 70.6% female, while the SRS + WBRT cohort had a median age of 64.8 years, with 55.6% being female. The combination EGFR-TKI + SRS cohort had a median age of 70.5 years, with 50% being females, and the combination EGFR-TKI + WBRT cohort had a median age of 61.5 years with 58.6% being females. Further characteristics of the five subdivided cohorts are shown in Table 1.

There were statistically significant differences in the proportion of patients with single versus multiple brain metastases, the proportion of patients with versus without extracranial metastases, and the proportion of cases with and without leptomeningeal spread in each cohort.

Multivariable analysis permitted the selection of three key adjustment variables, all of which were significantly associated with poorer survival: KPS < 70 (p = 0.002), age (p = 0.042), and time from brain-metastases diagnosis to initiation of treatment (p = 0.005).

Table 1. Patient characteristics among each treatment cohort.

Characteristics	WBRT	SRS	WBRT + SRS	EGFR-TKIs + WBRT	EGFR-TKIs + SRS
Population (N)	32	51	36	29	18
Average age in years (N, range)	68.36 (38.91, 84.95)	62.66 (38.42, 89.50)	64.76 (40.79, 89.88)	61.49 (43.66, 83.25)	70.27 (28.44, 90.34)
Female (%)	20 (62.5)	36 (70.6)	20 (55.6)	17 (58.6)	9 (50.0)
Multiple brain metastases (N, %)	20 (83.3)	27 (55.1)	20 (69.0)	23 (88.5)	15 (83.3)
Single brain metastases (N, %)	4 (16.7)	22 (44.9)	9 (31.0)	3 (11.5)	3 (16.7)
Extracranial metastases (N, %)	25 (80.6)	28 (54.9)	21 (60.0)	23 (82.1)	13 (72.2)
Leptomeningeal spread (N, %)	5 (16.7)	4 (8.3)	10 (29.4)	4 (14.3)	0 (0.0)
Symptomatic at time of brain metastases (N, %)	22 (81.5)	23 (53.5)	24 (70.6)	12 (60.0)	10 (58.8)
Type of EGFR-TKI					
Erlotinib/gefitinib				19 (65.5)	8 (44.4)
Osimertinib/afatinib				10 (34.5)	10 (55.6)

WBRT: whole-brain radiation therapy, SRS: stereotactic radiosurgery, EGFR: epithelial growth factor receptor, TKI: tyrosine kinase inhibitors.

3.2. Single Therapies

The estimated median OS for the WBRT-only cohort was 3.23 months, with a 1-year OS rate of 35% (95% confidence interval (CI) = 17%, 54%) and a 2-year OS rate of 25% (95% CI = 10%, 44%). The estimated median OS for the SRS-only cohort was 21.73 months, with a 1-year OS rate of 68% (95% CI = 51%, 80%) and a 2-year OS rate of 39% (95% CI = 22%, 55%). Under multivariable analysis, when using the WBRT cohort as the reference cohort, the hazard ratio of the SRS-only group was 0.33 (95% CI = 0.17, 0.62), showing a statistically significant difference between the WBRT-only and the SRS-only cohorts ($p < 0.001$) (Table 2, Figure 1).

Table 2. Survival statistics for each treatment cohort.

Cohort	Median OS (Months)	1-Year OS (95% CI)	2-Year OS Rate (95% CI)
WBRT only	3.23	35% (17%, 54%)	25% (10%, 44%)
SRS only	21.73	68% (51%, 80%)	39% (22%, 55%)
WBRT + SRS	3.17	26% (12%, 42%)	6% (1%, 19%)
EGFR-TKI + WBRT	15.50	64% (42%, 79%)	28% (12%, 46%)
EGFR-TKI + SRS	23.63	71% (43%, 87%)	37% (12%, 62%)

WBRT: whole-brain radiation therapy, SRS: stereotactic radiosurgery, EGFR: epithelial growth factor receptor, TKI: tyrosine kinase inhibitors, OS: overall survival.

3.3. Combination Therapies

The estimated median OS for the WBRT + SRS combination cohort was 3.17 months, with a 1-year OS rate of 26% (95% CI = 12%, 42%) and a 2-year OS rate of 6% (95% CI = 1%, 19%).

The median OS for the EGFR-TKI + WBRT cohort was 15.50 months, and for the EGFR-TKI + SRS cohort was 23.63 months. The proportion of patients with 1-year OS for the two cohorts was 64% (95% CI = 42%, 79%) and 71% (95% CI = 43%, 87%), respectively. The 2-year OS rate was 28% (95% CI = 12%, 46%) and 37% (95% CI = 12%, 62%), respectively.

Through a multivariable analysis using the WBRT-only cohort as a reference, we found no significant difference in overall survival for the SRS + WBRT combination cohort (HR = 1.30, 95% CI = 0.60, 2.82, $p = 0.50$), the EGFR-TKIs and WBRT combination cohort (HR = 0.93, 95% CI = 0.41, 2.08, $p = 0.85$), and the EGFR-TKI + SRS cohort (HR = 0.46,

95% CI = 0.20, 1.09, p = 0.07). However, overall survival was much higher in the multivariate analysis for the SRS-only cohort (HR = 0.38, 95% CI = 0.17, 0.84, p = 0.017) (Table 3).

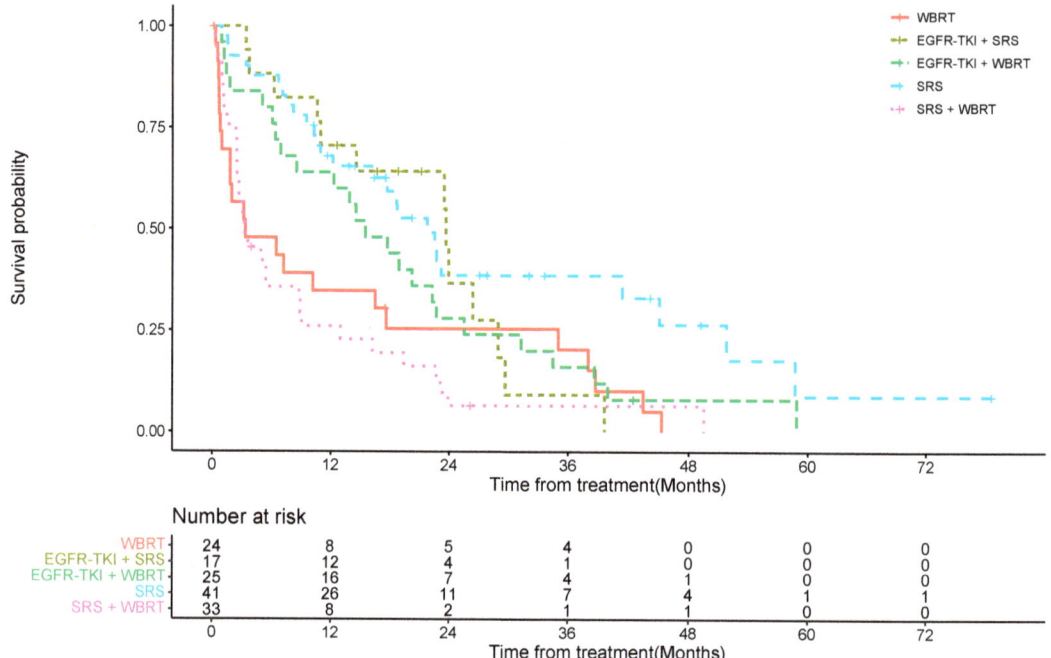

Figure 1. Kaplan–Meier curves demonstrating the overall survival in various cohorts. WBRT: whole-brain radiation therapy, SRS: stereotactic radiosurgery, EGFR: epithelial growth factor receptor, TKI: tyrosine kinase inhibitors.

Table 3. Multivariable analysis of survival using Cox's proportional hazards model with adjustment for KPS, age, time from brain-metastases diagnosis to initiation of treatment, symptomatic brain metastases, and number of brain metastases.

Cohort	Hazard Ratio (95% CI)	p-Value
Treatment		
WBRT only	Reference	
SRS only	0.38 (0.17, 0.84)	0.017
WBRT + SRS	1.30 (0.60, 2.82)	0.50
EGFR-TKI + WBRT	0.93 (0.41, 2.08)	0.85
EGFR-TKI + SRS	0.46 (0.20, 1.09)	0.077
Age	1.02 (1.00, 1.04)	0.03
Time from brain metastases to treatment	1.00 (1.00, 1.00)	0.012
KPS		
Greater than 70	Reference	
Lesser than 70	2.49 (1.10, 5.66)	0.029
Symptomatic at time of brain metastases		
Asymptomatic	Reference	
Symptomatic	1.42 (0.89, 2.27)	0.14
Number of brain metastases		
Multiple	Reference	
Single	0.92 (0.53, 1.62)	0.78

WBRT: whole-brain radiation therapy, SRS: stereotactic radiosurgery, EGFR: epithelial growth factor receptor, TKI: tyrosine kinase inhibitors.

4. Discussion
4.1. Relevance to Literature and Clinical Practice

In this large database of EGFR-mutated NSCLCBM patients treated at a tertiary-care center, SRS alone was found to have significantly better overall survival compared to WBRT alone, and to the SRS + WBRT, SRS + TKI cohorts, and TKI + WBRT cohorts. These findings expand on the previous studies that looked at the use of TKIs and radiotherapy in EGFR-mutated NSCLCBM [22–24]. Jia et al. compared the efficacy of combination of TKI with SRS or WBRT in NSCLCBM patients and reported an increased survival in the TKI + SRS cohort (25.1 months vs. 22.0 months, $p = 0.042$) [26].

Magnuson et al. specifically found that SRS combined with EGFR-TKI for upfront treatment resulted in the longest OS. However, our study compared combination therapies to WBRT only instead of combination therapies to a cohort of EGFR-only patients. Cheng et al. demonstrated increased survival in patients with NSCLCBM treated with SRS + 1st-gen TKI compared to TKI alone, and to addition of sequential 3rd-gen TKI: osimertinib further prolonged survival (43.5 vs. 24.3 months, $p < 0.001$) [27]. Similar to our results, WBRT in combination with TKI did not improve OS compared to WBRT alone (12.9 vs. 10.0 months, $p = 0.5$) in a multicenter phase III trial [28]. Zhai et al. also showed that the combination of WBRT and TKI did not increase the overall survival, but for the subset of patients with the EGFR L858R mutation, where the combination led to better survival ($p = 0.046$) [29]. A similar study by He et al. showed no improvement in OS in the cohort receiving the combination of WBRT and TKI compared to TKI alone, but the combination did improve intracranial PFS among patients with more than three brain metastases from NSCLC [30]. Finally, Chiou et al. reported improved intracranial tumor control rates in patients with NSCLCBM receiving a combination of TKI + SRS compared to TKI alone (79.8% vs. 31.2%, $p < 0.0001$) [31].

The BRAIN study was a phase III randomized clinical trial which compared the efficacy of icotinib, a first-gen EGFR-TKI with WBRT to treat NSCLCBM. After a median follow-up of 16.5 months, the intracranial PFS (iPFS) with icotinib was found to be 10.0 months vs. 4.8 months with WBRT, equating to a 44% reduction in event of intracranial progression ($p = 0.014$) [32]. In a retrospective study by Fan et al., icotinib was combined with RT in patients with NSCLCBM, and an improvement in iPFS was observed compared to the cohort receiving icotinib alone (22.4 vs. 13.9 months respectively, $p = 0.043$) [33]. Similar results were observed in studies utilizing erlotinib and gefitinib as first-generation EGFR-TKIs, which, when combined with RT, demonstrated superior outcomes than EGFR-TKIs alone [34,35].

Our study differs from previously mentioned studies as it also investigated an isolated SRS cohort, as opposed to radiotherapy more generally. Though our data showed the longest estimated OS for the combination of SRS and EGFR-TKIs, the SRS-only cohort also showed a statistical significance in OS rate. When available, SRS has become the prevailing first-line radiation for brain metastases; however, our data do not definitively conclude that the combination of EGFR-TKI and SRS therapy is superior to the SRS-only cohort [19–21].

With controlled variables, the current findings suggest that the improvement in OS is due to the improvement of CNS disease rather than selection bias or difference between patient cohorts. These findings advocate that a combination treatment of SRS + EGFR-TKIs may perhaps be the future standard of care for EGFR-mutated NSCLCBM. Though our data do not prove the superiority of combination treatment over SRS only, these results are likely the result of an underpowered cohort, and clinicians should consider using a combination approach with targeted therapy.

EGFR-TKIs provide a systemic approach, which has been proven to help control NSCLC and extracranial metastases [14,36]. Studies have also shown that EGFR-mutated NSCLC is highly sensitive to radiation, which can explain the benefit of using upfront SRS in these patients [37,38]. SRS has demonstrated high local control rates in EGFR-mutated brain metastases, with increasing utilization in this cohort [37,39]. SRS has also been shown with frequency to be an improved option over WBRT, with noninferior survival and decreased toxicity [24,40,41]. Kim et al. also similarly found no improvement in PFS between concurrent SRS + TKI and SRS alone; however, they noticed no additional adverse events related to concurrent therapy [42].

4.2. Limitations

Several limitations limit the generalizability of the current work. First, this was a retrospective study with limited adjustment for confounders, particularly the unknown ones. Second, given the observational setting, investigator-associated selection bias may have led to different group characteristics which likely impacted the results. Although certain variables were controlled for, patients were chosen for their specific treatment for several reasons, and these could have a confounding impact on survival. Third, this study was performed at a large academic tertiary-care center, and all places of care may not have access to the same treatments.

Finally, our study only evaluated OS; we were not able to evaluate PFS due to the lack of recorded MRI images in our database and difficulty with accurately evaluating progression without intracranial imaging. Without evaluating PFS, we were also unable to have an EGFR-TKI-alone cohort since all patients who received EGFR-TKI upfront also received radiotherapy at some point in their disease course, which may cause a confounding effect on estimated OS.

4.3. Potential Directions

For future studies, we believe an EGFR-TKI-alone cohort should be used along with the exploration of PFS based on the modified 'Response Assessment for Neuro-Oncology' (RANO) criteria for brain metastases [43,44]. This would provide more accurate and helpful data on whether there truly is a synergistic component to combining EGFR-TKIs and SRS treatments. Our work did not distinguish which treatment was given first and defined concurrence as within 28 days of each other. Future studies may consider utilizing randomized controlled trial design, or large prospective cohort studies should be used to investigate concurrent SRS and TKIs vs. SRS followed by TKIs vs. SRS alone.

Notably, a multi-institution retrospective study showed SRS followed by TKI was superior to TKI followed by SRS [24]. Another retrospective brain metastasis study showed minimal difference in OS between concurrent TKI and SRS treatment compared to SRS followed by TKI, but with a relatively small sample [45]. Until such investigations are performed to elucidate whether concurrent TKI/SRS is superior to SRS followed by TKI, upfront SRS may be considered the standard of care, with TKI use at clinical discretion.

5. Conclusions

This study demonstrates a significantly higher survival for NSCLCBM patients treated with SRS alone compared to patients treated with WBRT only. While sample-size limitations and investigator-selection bias may limit the validity of these results, phase II/III randomized controlled trials are warranted to demonstrate this synergistic effect through high-quality evidence.

Author Contributions: Conceptualization, J.H.S., D.M.P. and M.S.A.; Data curation, V.T., P.J.O., X.J. and M.S.A.; Formal analysis, A.A.K., A.O. and X.J.; Investigation, V.T. and P.J.O.; Resources, M.S.A.; Software, X.J.; Supervision, E.S.M., S.T.C., J.H.S., D.M.P. and M.S.A.; Writing—original draft, V.T., P.J.O., A.A.K., A.O., X.J. and M.S.A.; Writing—review and editing, V.T., P.J.O., S.S., A.A.K., A.O., R.R.K., Y.R., D.M.P. and M.S.A. All authors have read and agreed to the published version of the manuscript.

Funding: No funding for this manuscript.

Institutional Review Board Statement: This study was conducted in accordance with the Declaration of Helsinki. Ethical approval was obtained from the Cleveland Clinic (Ohio) Institutional Review Board (No. 09-911).

Informed Consent Statement: An IRB-approved waiver of consent and a waiver of HIPAA authorization were in effect, given this was a retrospective review of institutional outcomes with deidentified reporting.

Data Availability Statement: The study lead authors, and the senior author have access to the primary dataset. Data may be made available to interested investigators upon reasonable request to the senior author (manmeeta@baptisthealth.net) after approval by all required regulatory authorities.

Acknowledgments: The authors thank Cleveland Clinic staff for their help with the dataset and this manuscript.

Conflicts of Interest: Manmeet Singh Ahluwalia: Grants: AstraZeneca, BMS, Bayer, Incyte, Pharmacyclics, Novocure, MimiVax, Merck. **Consultation:** Bayer, Novocure, Kiyatec, Insightec, GSK, Xoft, Nuvation, Cellularity, SDP Oncology, Apollomics, Prelude, Janssen, Tocagen, Voyager Therapeutics, Viewray, Caris Lifesciences, Pyramid Biosciences, Varian Medical Systems, Cairn Therapeutics, Anheart Therapeutics, Theraguix. **Scientific Advisory Board:** Cairn Therapeutics, Pyramid Biosciences, Modifi Biosciences. **Stock shareholder:** Mimivax, Cytodyn, MedInnovate Advisors LLC. **David M. Peereboom: Consulting or Advisory Role:** Orbus Therapeutics, Sumitomo Dainippon Pharma Oncology Inc, Stemline Therapeutics, Novocure. **Research Funding:** Pfizer (Inst), Novartis (Inst), Neonc Technologies (Inst), Orbus Therapeutics (Inst), Bristol Myers Squibb (Inst), Genentech/Roche (Inst), Pharmacyclics (Inst), Bayer (Inst), Karyopharm Therapeutics (Inst), Apollomics (Inst), Vigeo Therapeutics (Inst), Global Coalition for Adaptive Research (Inst), MimiVax (Inst), Ono Pharmaceutical (Inst), Mylan (Inst). **R. R. Kotecha: Personal fees** from Accuray Inc., Elekta AB, ViewRay Inc., Novocure Inc., Elsevier Inc., Brainlab, Kazia Therapeutics, Castle Biosciences. **Institutional research funding** from Medtronic Inc., Blue Earth Diagnostics Ltd., Novocure Inc., GT Medical Technologies, AstraZeneca, Exelixis, ViewRay Inc., Brainlab, Cantex Pharmaceuticals, and Kazia Therapeutics. **Samuel Chao:** Honorarium: Varian Medical Systems, Stock: Merck. **John Suh:** Consultant: Abbvie. All other authors declare no conflict of interest.

References

1. Gelatti, A.C.Z.; Drilon, A.; Santini, F.C. Optimizing the sequencing of tyrosine kinase inhibitors (TKIs) in epidermal growth factor receptor (EGFR) mutation-positive non-small cell lung cancer (NSCLC). *Lung Cancer* **2019**, *137*, 113–122. [CrossRef] [PubMed]
2. Bray, F.; Ferlay, J.; Soerjomataram, I.; Siegel, R.L.; Torre, L.A.; Jemal, A. Global cancer statistics 2018: GLOBOCAN estimates of incidence and mortality worldwide for 36 cancers in 185 countries. *CA Cancer J. Clin.* **2018**, *68*, 394–424. [CrossRef] [PubMed]
3. Lee, K.E.; Nam, E.M.; Lee, H.J.; Nam, S.H.; Kim, D.Y.; Im, S.A.; Seong, C.M.; Lee, S.N.; Lee, K.J. Clinical Features and Prognosis of Lung Cancer with Brain Metastasis. *Cancer Res. Treat.* **2001**, *33*, 250–255. [CrossRef] [PubMed]
4. Ernani, V.; Stinchcombe, T.E. Management of Brain Metastases in Non-Small-Cell Lung Cancer. *J. Oncol. Pract.* **2019**, *15*, 563–570. [CrossRef] [PubMed]
5. Saad, A.G.; Yeap, B.Y.; Thunnissen, F.B.; Pinkus, G.S.; Pinkus, J.L.; Loda, M.; Sugarbaker, D.J.; Johnson, B.E.; Chirieac, L.R. Immunohistochemical markers associated with brain metastases in patients with nonsmall cell lung carcinoma. *Cancer* **2008**, *113*, 2129–2138. [CrossRef] [PubMed]
6. Rangachari, D.; Yamaguchi, N.; VanderLaan, P.A.; Folch, E.; Mahadevan, A.; Floyd, S.R.; Uhlmann, E.J.; Wong, E.T.; Dahlberg, S.E.; Huberman, M.S.; et al. Brain metastases in patients with EGFR-mutated or ALK-rearranged non-small-cell lung cancers. *Lung Cancer* **2015**, *88*, 108–111. [CrossRef]
7. Aiko, N.; Shimokawa, T.; Miyazaki, K.; Misumi, Y.; Agemi, Y.; Ishii, M.; Nakamura, Y.; Yamanaka, T.; Okamoto, H. Comparison of the efficacies of first-generation epidermal growth factor receptor tyrosine kinase inhibitors for brain metastasis in patients with advanced non-small-cell lung cancer harboring EGFR mutations. *BMC Cancer* **2018**, *18*, 1012. [CrossRef]
8. Rosell, R.; Carcereny, E.; Gervais, R.; Vergnenegre, A.; Massuti, B.; Felip, E.; Palmero, R.; Garcia-Gomez, R.; Pallares, C.; Sanchez, J.M.; et al. Erlotinib versus standard chemotherapy as first-line treatment for European patients with advanced EGFR mutation-positive non-small-cell lung cancer (EURTAC): A multicentre, open-label, randomised phase 3 trial. *Lancet Oncol.* **2012**, *13*, 239–246. [CrossRef]
9. Mitsudomi, T.; Morita, S.; Yatabe, Y.; Negoro, S.; Okamoto, I.; Tsurutani, J.; Seto, T.; Satouchi, M.; Tada, H.; Hirashima, T.; et al. Gefitinib versus cisplatin plus docetaxel in patients with non-small-cell lung cancer harbouring mutations of the epidermal growth factor receptor (WJTOG3405): An open label, randomised phase 3 trial. *Lancet Oncol.* **2010**, *11*, 121–128. [CrossRef]
10. Zhao, J.; Chen, M.; Zhong, W.; Zhang, L.; Li, L.; Xiao, Y.; Nie, L.; Hu, P.; Wang, M. Cerebrospinal fluid concentrations of gefitinib in patients with lung adenocarcinoma. *Clin. Lung Cancer* **2013**, *14*, 188–193. [CrossRef]
11. Remon, J.; Steuer, C.E.; Ramalingam, S.S.; Felip, E. Osimertinib and other third-generation EGFR TKI in EGFR-mutant NSCLC patients. *Ann. Oncol.* **2018**, *29*, i20–i27. [CrossRef] [PubMed]
12. Kim, Y.; Lee, S.H.; Ahn, J.S.; Ahn, M.J.; Park, K.; Sun, J.M. Efficacy and Safety of Afatinib for EGFR-mutant Non-small Cell Lung Cancer, Compared with Gefitinib or Erlotinib. *Cancer Res. Treat.* **2019**, *51*, 502–509. [CrossRef]

13. Ballard, P.; Yates, J.W.; Yang, Z.; Kim, D.W.; Yang, J.C.; Cantarini, M.; Pickup, K.; Jordan, A.; Hickey, M.; Grist, M.; et al. Preclinical Comparison of Osimertinib with Other EGFR-TKIs in EGFR-Mutant NSCLC Brain Metastases Models, and Early Evidence of Clinical Brain Metastases Activity. *Clin. Cancer Res.* **2016**, *22*, 5130–5140. [CrossRef]
14. Soria, J.C.; Ohe, Y.; Vansteenkiste, J.; Reungwetwattana, T.; Chewaskulyong, B.; Lee, K.H.; Dechaphunkul, A.; Imamura, F.; Nogami, N.; Kurata, T.; et al. Osimertinib in Untreated EGFR-Mutated Advanced Non-Small-Cell Lung Cancer. *N. Engl. J. Med.* **2018**, *378*, 113–125. [CrossRef]
15. Mok, T.S.; Wu, Y.L.; Ahn, M.J.; Garassino, M.C.; Kim, H.R.; Ramalingam, S.S.; Shepherd, F.A.; He, Y.; Akamatsu, H.; Theelen, W.S.; et al. Osimertinib or Platinum-Pemetrexed in EGFR T790M-Positive Lung Cancer. *N. Engl. J. Med.* **2017**, *376*, 629–640. [CrossRef]
16. Fan, Y.; Xu, X.; Xie, C. EGFR-TKI therapy for patients with brain metastases from non-small-cell lung cancer: A pooled analysis of published data. *Onco Targets Ther.* **2014**, *7*, 2075–2084. [CrossRef] [PubMed]
17. Welsh, J.W.; Komaki, R.; Amini, A.; Munsell, M.F.; Unger, W.; Allen, P.K.; Chang, J.Y.; Wefel, J.S.; McGovern, S.L.; Garland, L.L.; et al. Phase II trial of erlotinib plus concurrent whole-brain radiation therapy for patients with brain metastases from non-small-cell lung cancer. *J. Clin. Oncol.* **2013**, *31*, 895–902. [CrossRef]
18. Gerber, N.K.; Yamada, Y.; Rimner, A.; Shi, W.; Riely, G.J.; Beal, K.; Yu, H.A.; Chan, T.A.; Zhang, Z.; Wu, A.J. Erlotinib versus radiation therapy for brain metastases in patients with EGFR-mutant lung adenocarcinoma. *Int. J. Radiat. Oncol. Biol. Phys.* **2014**, *89*, 322–329. [CrossRef] [PubMed]
19. Niranjan, A.; Monaco, E.; Flickinger, J.; Lunsford, L.D. Guidelines for Multiple Brain Metastases Radiosurgery. *Prog. Neurol. Surg.* **2019**, *34*, 100–109. [CrossRef]
20. Achrol, A.S.; Rennert, R.C.; Anders, C.; Soffietti, R.; Ahluwalia, M.S.; Nayak, L.; Peters, S.; Arvold, N.D.; Harsh, G.R.; Steeg, P.S.; et al. Brain metastases. *Nat. Rev. Dis. Prim.* **2019**, *5*, 5. [CrossRef]
21. Specht, H.M.; Combs, S.E. Stereotactic radiosurgery of brain metastases. *J. Neurosurg. Sci.* **2016**, *60*, 357–366. [PubMed]
22. Dong, K.; Liang, W.; Zhao, S.; Guo, M.; He, Q.; Li, C.; Song, H.; He, J.; Xia, X. EGFR-TKI plus brain radiotherapy versus EGFR-TKI alone in the management of EGFR-mutated NSCLC patients with brain metastases. *Transl. Lung Cancer Res.* **2019**, *8*, 268–279. [CrossRef] [PubMed]
23. Chen, Y.; Wei, J.; Cai, J.; Liu, A. Combination therapy of brain radiotherapy and EGFR-TKIs is more effective than TKIs alone for EGFR-mutant lung adenocarcinoma patients with asymptomatic brain metastasis. *BMC Cancer* **2019**, *19*, 793. [CrossRef] [PubMed]
24. Magnuson, W.J.; Lester-Coll, N.H.; Wu, A.J.; Yang, T.J.; Lockney, N.A.; Gerber, N.K.; Beal, K.; Amini, A.; Patil, T.; Kavanagh, B.D.; et al. Management of Brain Metastases in Tyrosine Kinase Inhibitor-Naïve Epidermal Growth Factor Receptor-Mutant Non-Small-Cell Lung Cancer: A Retrospective Multi-Institutional Analysis. *J. Clin. Oncol.* **2017**, *35*, 1070–1077. [CrossRef] [PubMed]
25. Sperduto, P.W.; Yang, T.J.; Beal, K.; Pan, H.; Brown, P.D.; Bangdiwala, A.; Shanley, R.; Yeh, N.; Gaspar, L.E.; Braunstein, S.; et al. Estimating Survival in Patients With Lung Cancer and Brain Metastases: An Update of the Graded Prognostic Assessment for Lung Cancer Using Molecular Markers (Lung-molGPA). *JAMA Oncol.* **2017**, *3*, 827–831. [CrossRef] [PubMed]
26. Jia, F.; Cheng, X.; Zeng, H.; Miao, J.; Hou, M. Clinical research on stereotactic radiosurgery combined with epithermal growth factor tyrosine kinase inhibitors in the treatment of brain metastasis of non-small cell lung cancer. *J. Buon* **2019**, *24*, 578–584.
27. Cheng, W.C.; Shen, Y.C.; Chien, C.R.; Liao, W.C.; Chen, C.H.; Hsia, T.C.; Tu, C.Y.; Chen, H.J. The optimal therapy strategy for epidermal growth factor receptor-mutated non-small cell lung cancer patients with brain metastasis: A real-world study from Taiwan. *Thorac. Cancer* **2022**, *13*, 1505–1512. [CrossRef]
28. Yang, Z.; Zhang, Y.; Li, R.; Yisikandaer, A.; Ren, B.; Sun, J.; Li, J.; Chen, L.; Zhao, R.; Zhang, J.; et al. Whole-brain radiotherapy with and without concurrent erlotinib in NSCLC with brain metastases: A multicenter, open-label, randomized, controlled phase III trial. *Neuro-Oncology* **2021**, *23*, 967–978. [CrossRef]
29. Zhai, X.; Li, W.; Li, J.; Jia, W.; Jing, W.; Tian, Y.; Xu, S.; Li, Y.; Zhu, H.; Yu, J. Therapeutic effect of osimertinib plus cranial radiotherapy compared to osimertinib alone in NSCLC patients with EGFR-activating mutations and brain metastases: A retrospective study. *Radiat. Oncol.* **2021**, *16*, 233. [CrossRef]
30. He, Z.Y.; Li, M.F.; Lin, J.H.; Lin, D.; Lin, R.J. Comparing the efficacy of concurrent EGFR-TKI and whole-brain radiotherapy vs EGFR-TKI alone as a first-line therapy for advanced EGFR-mutated non-small-cell lung cancer with brain metastases: A retrospective cohort study. *Cancer Manag. Res.* **2019**, *11*, 2129–2138. [CrossRef]
31. Chiou, G.Y.; Chiang, C.L.; Yang, H.C.; Shen, C.I.; Wu, H.M.; Chen, Y.W.; Chen, C.J.; Luo, Y.H.; Hu, Y.S.; Lin, C.J.; et al. Combined stereotactic radiosurgery and tyrosine kinase inhibitor therapy versus tyrosine kinase inhibitor therapy alone for the treatment of non-small cell lung cancer patients with brain metastases. *J. Neurosurg.* **2022**, *137*, 563–570. [CrossRef]
32. Yang, J.J.; Zhou, C.; Huang, Y.; Feng, J.; Lu, S.; Song, Y.; Huang, C.; Wu, G.; Zhang, L.; Cheng, Y.; et al. Icotinib versus whole-brain irradiation in patients with EGFR-mutant non-small-cell lung cancer and multiple brain metastases (BRAIN): A multicentre, phase 3, open-label, parallel, randomised controlled trial. *Lancet Respir. Med.* **2017**, *5*, 707–716. [CrossRef]
33. Fan, Y.; Xu, Y.; Gong, L.; Fang, L.; Lu, H.; Qin, J.; Han, N.; Xie, F.; Qiu, G.; Huang, Z. Effects of icotinib with and without radiation therapy on patients with EGFR mutant non-small cell lung cancer and brain metastases. *Sci. Rep.* **2017**, *7*, 45193. [CrossRef] [PubMed]

34. An, N.; Wang, H.; Li, J.; Zhai, X.; Jing, W.; Jia, W.; Kong, L.; Zhu, H.; Yu, J. Therapeutic Effect Of First-Line EGFR-TKIs Combined With Concurrent Cranial Radiotherapy On NSCLC Patients With EGFR Activating Mutation And Brain Metastasis: A Retrospective Study. *Onco Targets Ther.* **2019**, *12*, 8311–8318. [CrossRef] [PubMed]
35. Zhu, Q.; Sun, Y.; Cui, Y.; Ye, K.; Yang, C.; Yang, D.; Ma, J.; Liu, X.; Yu, J.; Ge, H. Clinical outcome of tyrosine kinase inhibitors alone or combined with radiotherapy for brain metastases from epidermal growth factor receptor (EGFR) mutant non small cell lung cancer (NSCLC). *Oncotarget* **2017**, *8*, 13304–13311. [CrossRef] [PubMed]
36. Planchard, D.; Boyer, M.J.; Lee, J.S.; Dechaphunkul, A.; Cheema, P.K.; Takahashi, T.; Gray, J.E.; Tiseo, M.; Ramalingam, S.S.; Todd, A.; et al. Postprogression Outcomes for Osimertinib versus Standard-of-Care EGFR-TKI in Patients with Previously Untreated EGFR-mutated Advanced Non-Small Cell Lung Cancer. *Clin. Cancer Res.* **2019**, *25*, 2058–2063. [CrossRef]
37. Johung, K.L.; Yao, X.; Li, F.; Yu, J.B.; Gettinger, S.N.; Goldberg, S.; Decker, R.H.; Hess, J.A.; Chiang, V.L.; Contessa, J.N. A clinical model for identifying radiosensitive tumor genotypes in non-small cell lung cancer. *Clin. Cancer Res.* **2013**, *19*, 5523–5532. [CrossRef] [PubMed]
38. Spano, J.P.; Fagard, R.; Soria, J.C.; Rixe, O.; Khayat, D.; Milano, G. Epidermal growth factor receptor signaling in colorectal cancer: Preclinical data and therapeutic perspectives. *Ann. Oncol.* **2005**, *16*, 189–194. [CrossRef] [PubMed]
39. Wang, T.J.; Saad, S.; Qureshi, Y.H.; Jani, A.; Nanda, T.; Yaeh, A.M.; Rozenblat, T.; Sisti, M.B.; Bruce, J.N.; McKhann, G.M.; et al. Does lung cancer mutation status and targeted therapy predict for outcomes and local control in the setting of brain metastases treated with radiation? *Neuro-Oncology* **2015**, *17*, 1022–1028. [CrossRef]
40. Yamamoto, M.; Serizawa, T.; Shuto, T.; Akabane, A.; Higuchi, Y.; Kawagishi, J.; Yamanaka, K.; Sato, Y.; Jokura, H.; Yomo, S.; et al. Stereotactic radiosurgery for patients with multiple brain metastases (JLGK0901): A multi-institutional prospective observational study. *Lancet Oncol.* **2014**, *15*, 387–395. [CrossRef]
41. Habets, E.J.; Dirven, L.; Wiggenraad, R.G.; Verbeek-de Kanter, A.; Lycklama À Nijeholt, G.J.; Zwinkels, H.; Klein, M.; Taphoorn, M.J. Neurocognitive functioning and health-related quality of life in patients treated with stereotactic radiotherapy for brain metastases: A prospective study. *Neuro-Oncology* **2016**, *18*, 435–444. [CrossRef] [PubMed]
42. Kim, H.J.; Kim, W.S.; Kwon, D.H.; Cho, Y.H.; Choi, C.M. Effects of an Epithelial Growth Factor Receptor-Tyrosine Kinase Inhibitor Add-on in Stereotactic Radiosurgery for Brain Metastases Originating from Non-Small-Cell Lung Cancer. *J. Korean Neurosurg. Soc.* **2015**, *58*, 205–210. [CrossRef] [PubMed]
43. Okada, H.; Weller, M.; Huang, R.; Finocchiaro, G.; Gilbert, M.R.; Wick, W.; Ellingson, B.M.; Hashimoto, N.; Pollack, I.F.; Brandes, A.A.; et al. Immunotherapy response assessment in neuro-oncology: A report of the RANO working group. *Lancet Oncol.* **2015**, *16*, e534–e542. [CrossRef] [PubMed]
44. Lin, N.U.; Lee, E.Q.; Aoyama, H.; Barani, I.J.; Barboriak, D.P.; Baumert, B.G.; Bendszus, M.; Brown, P.D.; Camidge, D.R.; Chang, S.M.; et al. Response assessment criteria for brain metastases: Proposal from the RANO group. *Lancet Oncol.* **2015**, *16*, e270–e278. [CrossRef]
45. Wang, W.; Song, Z.; Zhang, Y. Efficacy of brain radiotherapy plus EGFR-TKI for EGFR-mutated non-small cell lung cancer patients who develop brain metastasis. *Arch. Med. Sci.* **2018**, *14*, 1298–1307. [CrossRef]

Disclaimer/Publisher's Note: The statements, opinions and data contained in all publications are solely those of the individual author(s) and contributor(s) and not of MDPI and/or the editor(s). MDPI and/or the editor(s) disclaim responsibility for any injury to people or property resulting from any ideas, methods, instructions or products referred to in the content.

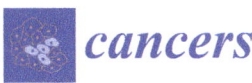

Article

First- versus Third-Generation EGFR Tyrosine Kinase Inhibitors in EGFR-Mutated Non-Small Cell Lung Cancer Patients with Brain Metastases

Vineeth Tatineni [1,†], Patrick J. O'Shea [1,2,†], Ahmad Ozair [3], Atulya A. Khosla [3], Shreya Saxena [3], Yasmeen Rauf [1,4,5], Xuefei Jia [1], Erin S. Murphy [1,6], Samuel T. Chao [1,6], John H. Suh [1,6], David M. Peereboom [1,5] and Manmeet S. Ahluwalia [1,3,7,*]

[1] Rosa Ella Burkhardt Brain Tumor & Neuro-Oncology Center, Cleveland Clinic, Cleveland, OH 44195, USA
[2] School of Medicine, Case Western Reserve University, Cleveland, OH 44106, USA
[3] Miami Cancer Institute, Baptist Health South Florida, Miami, FL 33176, USA
[4] Division of Neuro-Oncology, University of North Carolina, Chapel Hill, NC 27514, USA
[5] Department of Medical Oncology, Taussig Cancer Institute, Cleveland Clinic, Cleveland, OH 44106, USA
[6] Department of Radiation Oncology, Taussig Cancer Institute, Cleveland Clinic, Cleveland, OH 44106, USA
[7] Herbert Wertheim College of Medicine, Florida International University, Miami, FL 33199, USA
* Correspondence: manmeeta@baptisthealth.net; Tel.: +1-786-596-2000
† These authors contributed equally to this work.

Simple Summary: Targeted therapies have emerged as newer systemic options for certain cancers. EGFR-directed Tyrosine Kinase Inhibitors (EGFR-TKIs), which have several generations, have been found effective in a type of lung cancer called non-small cell lung cancer (NSCLC) when compared to conventional, platinum-based chemotherapy. More recently, EGFR-TKIs have shown promise in those NSCLC patients where the tumor has developed brain metastases. However, first-generation EGFR-TKIs and novel EGFR-TKIs have also been shown to differ regarding blood-brain-barrier penetration and mutation resistance. In this study, we analyzed the differences between the two generations of EGFR-TKIs in NSCLC patients with brain metastases. Our work did not find differences in overall survival and progression-free survival between the two generations of EGFR-TKIs. However, being a retrospective and single institutional analysis, this study had some limitations, which may have led to an underpowered comparison.

Abstract: Introduction: Up to 50% of non-small cell lung cancer (NSCLC) harbor EGFR alterations, the most common etiology behind brain metastases (BMs). First-generation EGFR-directed tyrosine kinase inhibitors (EGFR-TKI) are limited by blood-brain barrier penetration and T790M tumor mutations, wherein third-generation EGFR-TKIs, like Osimertinib, have shown greater activity. However, their efficacy has not been well-studied in later therapy lines in NSCLC patients with BMs (NSCLC-BM). We sought to compare outcomes of NSCLC-BM treated with either first- or third-generation EGFR-TKIs in first-line and 2nd-to-5th-line settings. **Methods:** A retrospective review of NSCLC-BM patients diagnosed during 2010–2019 at Cleveland Clinic, Ohio, US, a quaternary-care center, was performed and reported following 'strengthening the reporting of observational studies in epidemiology' (STROBE) guidelines. Data regarding socio-demographic, histopathological, molecular characteristics, and clinical outcomes were collected. Primary outcomes were median overall survival (mOS) and progression-free survival (mPFS). Multivariable Cox proportional hazards modeling and propensity score matching were utilized to adjust for confounders. **Results:** 239 NSCLC-BM patients with EGFR alterations were identified, of which 107 received EGFR-TKIs after diagnosis of BMs. 77.6% (83/107) received it as first-line treatment, and 30.8% (33/107) received it in later (2nd–5th) lines of therapy, with nine patients receiving it in both settings. 64 of 107 patients received first-generation (erlotinib/gefitinib) TKIs, with 53 receiving them in the first line setting and 13 receiving it in the 2nd–5th lines of therapy. 50 patients received Osimertinib as third-generation EGFR-TKI, 30 in first-line, and 20 in the 2nd–5th lines of therapy. Univariable analysis in first-line therapy demonstrated mOS of first- and third-generation EGFR-TKIs as 18.2 and 19.4 months, respectively, ($p = 0.57$), while

Citation: Tatineni, V.; O'Shea, P.J.; Ozair, A.; Khosla, A.A.; Saxena, S.; Rauf, Y.; Jia, X.; Murphy, E.S.; Chao, S.T.; Suh, J.H.; et al. First- versus Third-Generation EGFR Tyrosine Kinase Inhibitors in EGFR-Mutated Non-Small Cell Lung Cancer Patients with Brain Metastases. *Cancers* 2023, 15, 2382. https://doi.org/10.3390/cancers15082382

Academic Editor: Edward Pan

Received: 19 January 2023
Revised: 14 April 2023
Accepted: 18 April 2023
Published: 20 April 2023

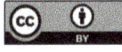

Copyright: © 2023 by the authors. Licensee MDPI, Basel, Switzerland. This article is an open access article distributed under the terms and conditions of the Creative Commons Attribution (CC BY) license (https:// creativecommons.org/licenses/by/ 4.0/).

unadjusted mPFS of first- and third-generation EGFR-TKIs was 9.3 and 13.8 months, respectively ($p = 0.14$). In 2nd–5th line therapy, for first- and third-generation EGFR-TKIs, mOS was 17.3 and 11.9 months, ($p = 0.19$), while mPFS was 10.4 and 6.08 months, respectively ($p = 0.41$). After adjusting for age, performance status, presence of extracranial metastases, whole-brain radiotherapy, and presence of leptomeningeal metastases, hazard ratio (HR) for OS was 1.25 (95% CI 0.63–2.49, $p = 0.52$) for first-line therapy. Adjusted HR for mOS in 2nd-to-5th line therapy was 1.60 (95% CI 0.55–4.69, $p = 0.39$). **Conclusions:** No difference in survival was detected between first- and third-generation EGFR-TKIs in either first or 2nd-to-5th lines of therapy. Larger prospective studies are warranted reporting intracranial lesion size, EGFR alteration and expression levels in primary tumor and brain metastases, and response rates.

Keywords: brain tumor; brain metastasis; lung cancer; lung malignancy; progression-free survival; epidermal growth factor receptor

1. Introduction

Lung cancer is the second most common type of cancer worldwide and the leading cause of cancer-related mortality in both male and female adults [1]. Non-small cell lung cancer (NSCLC) accounts for 80% of all lung cancers and is the most common cause of brain metastases [2]. With nearly 10–30% of patients with NSCLC developing brain metastasis, contributing to poorer prognosis and more symptoms, research in the field of brain metastasis has dramatically increased over the last decade [3].

In more recent years, the management of NSCLC has shifted from platinum-based chemotherapy to targeted molecular therapies. While multiple immunohistochemical markers have been studied, only a handful have been shown to be reliable targets and prognostic markers [3]. Epidermal growth factor receptor (EGFR) is a transmembrane receptor tyrosine kinase that is mutated in 40% to 60% of NSCLC with brain metastasis (NSCLC-BM) [4]. The signaling pathway, prompted by several growth factors, leads to autophosphorylation, causes tumor proliferation, and boosts cell survival [5]. The risk of developing brain metastases is higher in EGFR-altered patients, though providentially, the EGFR signaling pathway is being increasingly targeted [6]. There exist multiple known EGFR-related mutations, including deletion of exon 18, deletion of exon 19, exon 21-point mutation, and exon 20 insertion mutation [5]. Different mutations cause different structural alterations in the EGFR protein, which leads to differential sensitivities from targeted therapies [7].

While there exist multiple treatment options for treating NSCLC-BM, including whole-brain radiotherapy (WBRT), stereotactic radiosurgery (SRS), and, more rarely, surgical resection, the standard of care has shifted to the use of EGFR-directed tyrosine kinase inhibitors (EGFR-TKIs) [8–10]. EGFR-TKIs are reversible TKI inhibitors that target the adenosine triphosphate (ATP) cleft within the receptor [11]. First-generation EGFR-TKIs, such as erlotinib and gefitinib, were introduced in the early 2000s and have proven more effective than standard chemotherapy [12,13]. However, the efficacy of first-generation EGFR-TKIs for treating NSCLC-BM is limited by blood-brain barrier (BBB) penetration and exon 20 (T790M) tumor mutations [14,15]. Previous reports have shown the cerebrospinal fluid (CSF) concentration levels of first-generation EGFR-TKIs were low when given standard doses [5]. Though higher concentration levels could be achieved with higher doses, their peak was short-lived [5,15]. More frequent dosing, from weekly to daily, was also tested but was associated with more toxicity [16]. Even in patients with good responses to first-generation EGFR-TKIs, efficacy may be lost due to acquired resistance from T790M mutations [17]. Third-generation EGFR-TKIs, such as Osimertinib, introduced in the mid-2010s, have shown better BBB penetration and efficacy against T790M mutations [18].

Multiple studies, including the FLAURA and OCEAN trials, have demonstrated the efficacy of Osimertinib in NSCLC-BM. Data from the initial FLAUR publication and its follow-up demonstrated improved progression-free survival (PFS) and overall survival (OS) with Osimertinib compared to first-generation EGFR-TKIs. These findings have led to Osimertinib being increasingly used as first-line treatment in patients with EGFR-mutant NSCLC and NSCLC-BM [19,20]. These studies still leave a gap in comparing the efficacy of EGFR-TKI when given as first-line versus later-line therapies. Given the limited data and publications, we sought to compare the OS and PFS in NSCLC-BM patients treated with first versus third-generation EGFR-TKIs, in both first and later-line therapies.

2. Methods

2.1. Patient Selection and Data Collection

A retrospective cohort study involving EGFR-altered NSCLC-BM patients treated at Cleveland Clinic (Cleveland, OH, USA), a quaternary-care institution, was conducted and reported following 'strengthening the reporting of observational studies in epidemiology' (STROBE) guidelines. The work was approved by the Cleveland Clinic, Ohio Institutional Review Board (reference number 09-911) before commencement. Inclusion criteria for our study included all patients $\geq$18 years of age with EGFR-altered NSCLC-BM treated with erlotinib, gefitinib, or Osimertinib at any point after the diagnosis of brain metastases from 2010 to 2019 at our institution.

Patient demographics, initial diagnostic and genomic testing information, and treatment details were collected from the institution's electronic medical record. Among the information collected was Karnofsky Performance Score (KPS), age, race, and sex. Collected treatment details include the date of initiation, date of progress, line of therapy, and generation of EGFR inhibitor used. Data was recorded in REDCap, a secure database. Patients included in our study were followed in the outpatient setting every three months. The start of a new line of therapy, the use of SRS during EGFR inhibitor treatment, or death were also used to define disease progression. In patients with questionable pseudo-progression, the case was assessed at the hospital's interdisciplinary tumor board.

2.2. EGFR-TKI Data

Only patients treated with erlotinib, gefitinib, and Osimertinib were primarily investigated in this study. Treatment with first- versus third-generation EGFR-TKIs was primarily due to temporal effects. Third-generation TKIs are increasingly utilized as relevant literature, and recommendations gradually accumulated regarding their utility. We did not exclude patients who received erlotinib and gefitinib prior to the diagnosis of brain metastases if they received Osimertinib after the diagnosis of brain metastases, as we only evaluated response rates after the diagnosis of brain metastases. First-line therapy was defined as EGFR-TKI treatment given as the first systemic therapy after the diagnosis of brain metastases. Later (2nd to 5th) lines of therapy were defined as the initial EGFR-TKI given after the diagnosis of brain metastases but not as the first systemic therapy. Any patients experiencing breaks during the treatment due to symptoms were not excluded as long as there was no progression. We included patients who received EGFR-TKI, then had progression, and later also received EGFR-TKI. We also included patients who were taking EGFR-TKI, then had intracranial progression for which local control was attempted while EGFR-TKI was continued.

2.3. Statistical Methods

Categorical clinical and pathologic variables were summarized as frequency counts and percentages. Continuous variables were summarized as medians and ranges. Kruskal-Wallis Tests and Fisher's exact test was used to compare the quantitative and factor variables among treatment groups. OS was measured from the start date of the first treatment received to the date of the last follow-up or date of death and was summarized using the Kaplan-Meier method. PFS was measured from the start date of the treatment to the start date of a new line of therapy, the start date of the following SRS, or the date of the last follow-up or date of death. 1-year and 2-year survival rates and estimated median survivals for each treatment cohort were reported. Log-rank tests were used for univariable comparisons between treatments. The Cox proportional hazard model with a two-sided Wald test was used to evaluate the impact of the treatment on OS and PFS. The survival model was adjusted by clinical variables selected by the random forest method. The primary model was adjusted by the variables which were mostly identified as prognostic factors in patients with NSCLC-BM in previous studies [20]. These variables were age at diagnosis of brain metastases, gender, number of brain metastases, the existence of extracranial metastases, the existence of leptomeningeal metastases, KPS, and the duration from the date of diagnosis of brain metastases to the date of treatment. The first-generation EGFR-TKI cohort was used as the reference group for comparing OS and PFS due to being the older medication group with a long use history. Propensity score matching was also performed. Statistical significance was defined as a *p*-value of <0.05. All statistical analysis was performed using R Statistical Software version 4.1.0 (R Foundation for Statistical Computing, Vienna, Austria).

3. Results

3.1. Patient Characteristics

Between 2010 and 2019, we found 239 eligible patients who had NSCLC-BM with an EGFR alteration in the primary tumor. Overall, the median PFS (mPFS) was 6.3 months. The 1-year OS rate for EGFR-positive patients was 68% (95% confidence interval (CI) = 59%, 75%). The 2-year OS rate was 31% (95% CI = 23%, 40%). The 1-year PFS rate for the same overall encompassing group was 34% (95% CI = 27%, 42%), with a 2-year PFS rate of 14% (95% CI = 9%, 21%). The patient population was split into cohorts based on treatment with first-generation EGFR-TKIs and treatment with third-generation EGFR-TKIs (Figure 1, Table 1). 107 EGFR-mutant patients received EGFR-TKIs after diagnosis of BMs. 77.6% (83/107) received it as first-line treatment, and 30.8% (33/107) received it in later (2nd–5th) lines of therapy, with nine patients receiving it in both settings.

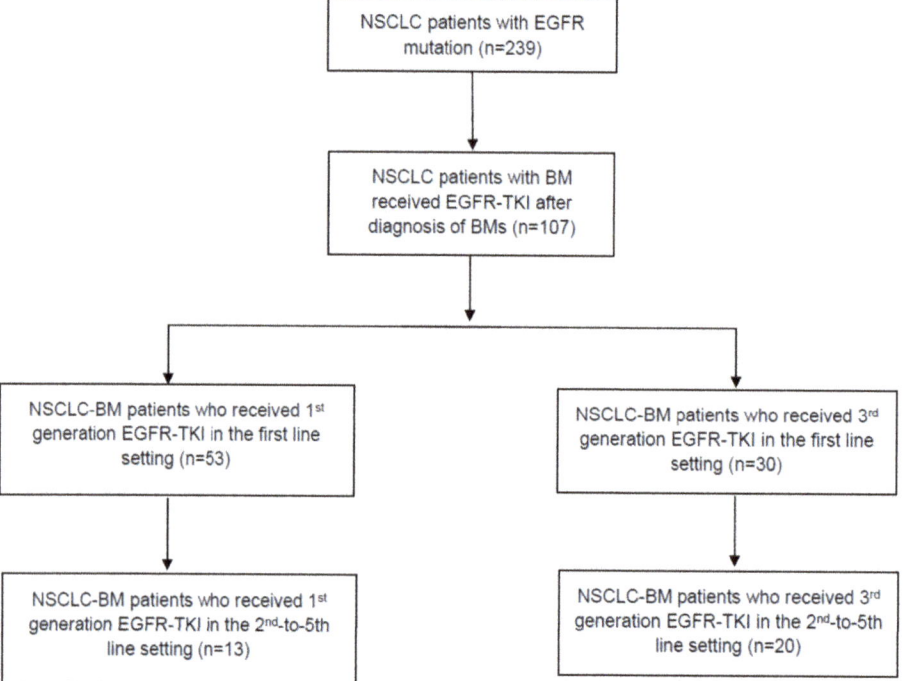

Figure 1. Flow diagram of the current study.

Table 1. Number of patients with EGFR-mutant NSCLC patients with brain metastases who received EGFR-TKI after BM diagnosis.

Group	n	Follow-Up Time
Total EGFR-mutant NSCLC patients treated with EGFR-TKI after BM diagnosis	107	17.1 months
Treated with first-generation EGFR-TKI (erlotinib/gefitinib), n	64	18.03 months
Treated with first-generation EGFR-TKI (Osimertinib), n	50	17.95 months

A total of 64 of 107 patients received first-generation (erlotinib/gefitinib) TKIs, with 53 receiving them in the first line setting and 13 receiving it in the 2nd–5th line of therapy (Table 2). 50 patients received Osimertinib as third-generation EGFR-TKI, 30 as first-line, and 20 as the 2nd–5th line of therapy. (Table 3). Later-line therapy was defined as systemic therapy given as the 2nd–5th line of therapy. The characteristics of the cohort are separately documented in Tables 2 and 3.

Table 2. Characteristics of patients with NSCLC brain metastases who received EGFR-directed Tyrosine Kinase Inhibitors (EGFR-TKIs) in the first-line setting.

Variable	Erlotinib/Gefitinib	Osimertinib
Cohort population (n)	53	30
Age in years, median (range)	63.1 (29.9, 90.7)	72.77 (31.92, 84.83)
Female, n (%)	32 (60.4)	23 (76.7)
KPS ≥70, n (%)	48 (96.0)	29 (96.7)
Multiple brain metastases, n (%)	42 (84.0)	21 (72.4)
Single brain metastases, n (%)	8 (16.0)	8 (27.6)
Extracranial metastases, n (%)	42 (80.8)	13 (44.8)
Leptomeningeal spread, n (%)	5 (9.4)	1 (3.3)
Received WBRT, n (%)	33 (62.3)	7 (23.3)
Received Surgery, n (%)	6 (11.3)	1 (3.3)
Received SRS, n (%)	29 (54.7)	20 (66.7)
Median Number of SRS (Range)	0 (0–10)	0 (0–8)

KPS, Karnofsky Performance Status; WBRT, Whole Brain Radiotherapy; SRS, Stereotactic Radiosurgery.

Table 3. Characteristics of patients with NSCLC brain metastases who received line EGFR-directed Tyrosine Kinase Inhibitors (EGFR-TKIs) in later (2nd to 5th) lines of therapy.

Variable	Erlotinib/Gefitinib	Osimertinib
Cohort population (n)	13	20
Age in years, median (range)	59.7 (46.8, 72.8)	62.7 (28.4, 83.5)
Female, n (%)	8 (61.5)	11 (55.0)
KPS ≥ 70, n (%)	11 (84.6)	19 (100.0)
Multiple brain metastases, n (%)	8 (72.7)	15 (78.9)
Single brain metastases, n (%)	3 (27.3)	4 (21.1)
Extracranial metastases, n (%)	9 (69.2)	18 (90.0)
Leptomeningeal spread, n (%)	1 (7.7)	1 (5.0)
Received surgery, n (%)	3 (23.1)	1 (5.0)
Received WBRT, n (%)	6 (46.2)	11 (55.0)
Received SRS, n (%)	9 (69.2)	14 (70.0)
Median Number of SRS (Range)	1 (0–3)	1 (0–5)

KPS, Karnofsky Performance Status; WBRT, Whole Brain Radiotherapy; SRS, Stereotactic Radiosurgery.

3.2. Overall Survival

When erlotinib or gefitinib was given as first-line therapy, the unadjusted median OS (mOS) was 18.2 months, while patients given Osimertinib in the first-line setting had an mOS of 19.4 months (Table 4). Kaplan-Meier curves for overall survival are provided in Figure 2. For the erlotinib/gefitinib cohort, the 1-year OS rate was 63% (95% CI 48%, 75%), and the 2-year OS rate was 32% (95% CI = 19%, 46%). The 1-year OS rate for the Osimertinib cohort was 82% (95% CI = 63%, 92%), and the 2-year OS rate for NSCLC-BM patients treated with Osimertinib as first-line therapy was 36% (95% CI = 13%, 61%).

Table 4. Overall survival (OS) of patients with NSCLC brain metastases treated with first-generation and third-generation EGFR-directed Tyrosine Kinase Inhibitors (EGFR-TKIs) in the first line and 2nd-to-5th line treatment settings. NA: Not Available.

Therapy	EGFR-TKI	Median OS (Months)	1-Year OS (95% CI)	2-Year OS (95% CI)
1st line	erlotinib/gefitinib	18.2	63% (48%, 75%)	32% (19%, 46%)
	Osimertinib	19.4	82% (63%, 92%)	36% (13%, 61%)
2nd–5th line	erlotinib/gefitinib	17.3	NA	NA
	Osimertinib	11.9	NA	NA

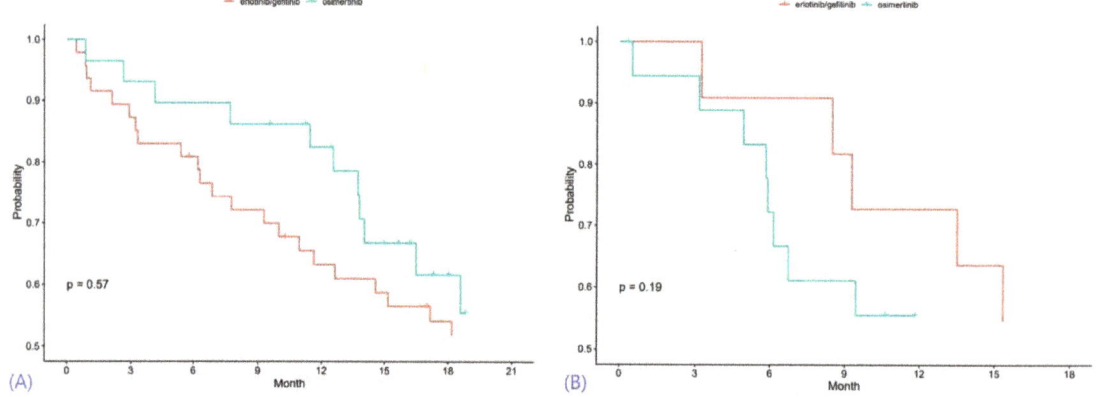

Figure 2. Kaplan-Meier curves for overall survival, with results of first-line therapy in (**A**) and outcomes of later-line therapy in (**B**).

Univariable Cox Proportional Hazards modeling of OS, using both categorical and continuous variables, is demonstrated in Table 5. After adjusting for age, KPS score, extracranial metastases, receipt of WBRT, and leptomeningeal metastases in multivariable analysis, there was no statistically significant OS difference found between the two first-line therapy cohorts (HR 1.25, 95% CI 0.63, 2.49, p = 0.52). For the 2nd-to-5th line of therapy, unadjusted comparison demonstrated no significant difference in mOS (p = 0.19). Multivariable analysis once again showed no statistical significance in mOS between the two cohorts (HR 1.60. 95% CI 0.55–4.69, p = 0.39) (Tables 6 and 7).

Table 5. Univariable Cox Proportional Hazards modeling of overall survival.

Variable	Level	1st Line		2nd-to-5th Line	
		HR (95% CI)	p-Value	HR (95% CI)	p-Value
Number of Brain Metastases	Multiple	Reference		Reference	
	Single	0.67 (0.42, 1.07)	0.09	0.24 (0.05, 1.05)	0.057
Extracranial Metastases Present at Time of Diagnosis	No	Reference		Reference	
	Yes	2.29 (1.44, 3.64)	<0.001	4.23 (0.92, 19.48)	0.064
Leptomeningeal metastases	No	Reference		Reference	
	Yes	1.83 (0.95, 3.52)	0.071	43.10 (3.81, 487.17)	0.002
Whole Brain Radiation Received	No	Reference		Reference	
	Yes	1.83 (1.24, 2.69)	0.002	2.13 (0.89, 5.10)	0.091
Surgery Received	No	Reference		Reference	
	Yes	0.96 (0.55, 1.69)	0.88	0.78 (0.26, 2.40)	0.67
Karnofsky Performance Status	≥70	Reference		Reference	
	70	1.92 (0.92, 4.03)	0.083	0.97 (0.13, 7.39)	0.98
SRS frequency	≥1	Reference		Reference	
	0	1.37 (0.92, 2.04)	0.12	1.24 (0.47, 3.29)	0.66
Sex	Female	Reference		Reference	
	Male	0.98 (0.67, 1.45)	0.93	0.58 (0.23, 1.47)	0.25
Generation of EGFR-TKI received	1st	Reference		Reference	
	3rd	0.84 (0.45, 1.55)	0.57	1.83 (0.74, 4.56)	0.19
Number of Brain metastases	-	1.06 (0.99, 1.12)	0.08	1.07 (0.88, 1.31)	0.51
SRS Total Number	-	0.78 (0.67, 0.92)	0.003	1.05 (0.73, 1.50)	0.79
Age	-	1.00 (0.98, 1.02)	0.99	0.98 (0.95, 1.02)	0.31

Table 6. Multivariable Cox-Proportional Hazards Modelling of overall survival (OS) for EGFR-altered NSCLC patients with brain metastases in first-line EGFR-TKI.

Variable	Level	HR (95% CI)	p-Value
Karnofsky performance status	≥70	Reference	
	<70	2.03 (0.57, 7.20)	0.28
Extracranial metastases at diagnosis	Absent	Reference	
	Present	3.10 (1.42, 6.76)	0.004
Whole-brain radiotherapy	No	Reference	
	Yes	1.58 (0.83, 3.01)	0.17
Age	-	1.01 (0.99, 1.03)	0.46
Leptomeningeal metastases	Absent	Reference	
	Present	0.71 (0.26, 1.92)	0.50
Generation of EGFR TKI	1st	Reference	
	3rd	1.25 (0.63, 2.49)	0.52

Table 7. Multivariable Cox-Proportional Hazards Modeling of overall survival (OS) for EGFR-altered NSCLC patients with brain metastases in 2nd-to-5th-line EGFR-TKI.

Variable	Level	HR (95% CI)	p-Value
Leptomeningeal metastases	Absent	Reference	
	Present	26.30 (1.91, 362.80)	0.015
Extracranial metastases at diagnosis	Absent	Reference	
	Present	4.06 (0.62, 26.71)	0.14
Generation of EGFR TKI	erlotinib/gefitinib	Reference	
	Osimertinib	1.60 (0.55, 4.69)	0.39
Sex	Female	Reference	
	Male	0.32 (0.10, 0.97)	0.045
Whole-brain radiotherapy	No	Reference	
	Yes	1.81 (0.62, 5.26)	0.28
Age	-	0.97 (0.93, 1.02)	0.23

3.3. Progression-Free Survival

For first-line therapy in NSCLC-BM patients, the unadjusted median PFS (mPFS) of first-generation and third-generation EGFR-TKIs was 9.27 months and 13.77 months, respectively, with no significant difference (Table 8). The 1-year PFS rate for first-generation EGFR-TKIs was 41% (95% CI 28%, 55%), while the 2-year PFS rate was 16% (95% CI 7%, 27%). NSCLC-BM patients treated with third-generation EGFR-TKIs as first-line therapy showed a 1-year PFS rate of 66% (95% CI = 46%, 80%) and a 2-year PFS rate of 34% (95% CI = 15%, 55%) (Figure 3).

Table 8. Unadjusted Progression-free survival (PFS) of patients with NSCLC brain metastases treated with first-generation and third-generation EGFR Tyrosine Kinase Inhibitors (EGFR-TKIs). NA: Not Available.

Therapy	EGFR-TKI	Median PFS (Months)	1-Year PFS (95% CI)	2-Year PFS (95% CI)
1st line	erlotinib/gefitinib	9.27	41% (28%, 55%)	16% (7%, 27%)
	Osimertinib	13.77	66% (46%, 80%)	34% (15%, 55%)
2nd–5th line	erlotinib/gefitinib	10.43	NA	NA
	Osimertinib	6.08	NA	NA

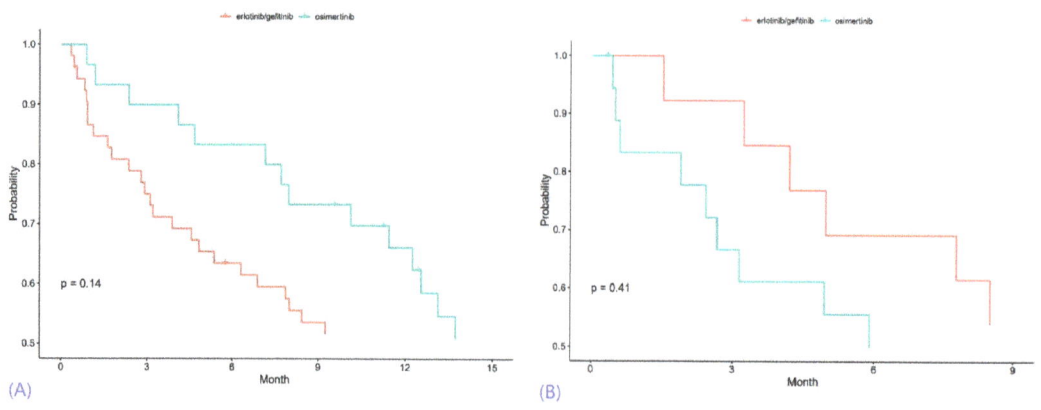

Figure 3. Kaplan-Meier curves for progression-free survival, with results of first-line therapy in (**A**) and outcomes of later-line therapy in (**B**).

Univariable Cox Proportional Hazards modeling of OS, using both categorical and continuous variables, is demonstrated in Table 9. There was also no statistically significant difference in PFS between the two cohorts when given as 1st line systemic therapy, with the adjustment of age, sex, extracranial mets, and WBRT treatment (HR 1.0, 95% CI 0.54–1.83, p = 0.99). When given as the 2nd to 5th line of systemic therapy in NSCLC-BM patients, the mPFS demonstrated no statistically significant difference (HR 1.12, 95% CI 0.43–2.93; p = 0.82) (Tables 10 and 11).

Table 9. Univariable Cox Proportional Hazards modeling of progression-free survival.

Variable	Level	1st Line		2nd-to-5th Line	
		HR (95% CI)	p-Value	HR (95% CI)	p-Value
Number of Brain Metastases	Multiple	Reference		Reference	
	Single	1.05 (0.70, 1.55)	0.82	0.20 (0.06, 0.70)	0.012
Extracranial Metastases Present at the time of diagnosis	No	Reference		Reference	
	Yes	1.68 (1.13, 2.49)	0.01	3.19 (0.94, 10.84)	0.064
Leptomeningeal metastases	No	Reference		Reference	
	Yes	0.82 (0.43, 1.53)	0.53	6.19 (1.27, 30.05)	0.024
Whole Brain Radiation Received	No	Reference		Reference	
	Yes	1.38 (0.97, 1.94)	0.07	2.94 (1.31, 6.64)	0.009
Received Surgery	No	Reference		Reference	
	Yes	1.20 (0.70, 2.06)	0.51	0.82 (0.28, 2.42)	0.72
Karnofsky Performance Status	≥70	Reference		Reference	
	70	1.42 (0.74, 2.72)	0.29	0.79 (0.18, 3.39)	0.75
SRS frequency	≥1	Reference		Reference	
	0	0.86 (0.60, 1.24)	0.41	0.73 (0.30, 1.73)	0.47
Sex	Female	Reference		Reference	
	Male	1.55 (1.10, 2.18)	0.013	1.12 (0.51, 2.45)	0.79
Generation of EGFR-TKI received	1st	Reference		Reference	
	3rd	0.66 (0.38, 1.15)	0.14	1.39 (0.63, 3.04)	0.41
Number of Brain metastases	-	1.05 (0.98, 1.12)	0.14	1.03 (0.89, 1.18)	0.72
SRS Total Number	-	0.95 (0.85, 1.07)	0.37	1.19 (0.88, 1.62)	0.25
Age	-	0.99 (0.98, 1.01)	0.29	0.98 (0.95, 1.01)	0.14

Table 10. Multivariable Cox-Proportional Hazards Modelling of progression-free survival (PFS) for EGFR-altered NSCLC patients with brain metastases in first-line EGFR-TKI.

Variable	Level	HR (95% CI)	p-Value
Sex	Female	Reference	0.016
	Male	1.9 (1.13, 3.23)	
Extracranial metastases at diagnosis	Absent	Reference	0.092
	Present	1.7 (0.91, 3.34)	
Whole-brain radiotherapy received	No	Reference	0.013
	Yes	2.1 (1.17, 3.93)	
Age	-	1.7 (0.91, 3.34)	0.95
Generation of EGFR TKI received	1st	Reference	>0.99
	3rd	1.0 (0.54, 1.83)	

Table 11. Multivariable Cox-Proportional Hazards Modelling of progression-free survival for EGFR-altered NSCLC patients with brain metastases in 2nd-to-5th-line EGFR-TKI.

Variable	Level	HR (95% CI)	p-Value
Leptomeningeal metastases	Absent	Reference	0.03
	Present	22.14 (1.35, 364.28)	
Extracranial metastases at diagnosis	Absent	Reference	0.35
	Present	1.96 (0.48, 7.98)	
Generation of EGFR TKI Received	1st	Reference	0.82
	3rd	1.12 (0.43, 2.93)	
Brain Metastases	Multiple	Reference	0.046
	Single	0.25 (0.07, 0.98)	
Age	-	1.12 (0.43, 2.93)	0.40

3.4. Outcomes after Propensity Score Matching

Propensity score matching was also performed to reduce baseline confounding, whose results are given in Table 12.

Table 12. Propensity score matching between first- and third-generation EGFR-TKI cohorts.

	EGFR-TKI	No. of Obs.	No. of Events	Median Duration (Month)	1-Year Rate (95% CI)	2-Year Rate (95% CI)	HR (95% CI)	p
OS	erlotinib/gefitinib	28	23	18.2	64% (44%, 79%)	28% (13%, 46%)	Reference	0.55
	Osimertinib	28	14	23.9	82% (62%, 92%)	38% (13%, 63%)	0.81 (0.40–1.63)	
PFS	erlotinib/gefitinib	28	26	9.37	43% (24%, 60%)	18% (6%, 35%)	Reference	0.26
	Osimertinib	28	17	13.77	64% (43%, 79%)	32% (12%, 55%)	0.69 (0.36–1.31)	

4. Discussion

In recent years, novel EGFR inhibitors, specifically Osimertinib, have taken precedence as the first-line treatment for EGFR-altered NSCLC over first-generation EGFR-TKIs [19,20]. In this work, we attempted to evaluate the efficacy of these drugs in NSCLC-BM patients at a single institution. Recent animal studies have shown better BBB penetration with Osimertinib than gefitinib, rociletinib, or afatinib, suggesting Osimertinib may have better survival outcomes in NSCLC-BM patients [18]. However, our study failed to show any statistically significant difference in PFS or OS between novel EGFR-TKI and erlotinib/gefitinib when treating EGFR-altered NSCLC-BM patients, either as first-line treatment or as a later line of treatment.

The FLAURA trial showed a clear survival benefit in NSCLC patients treated with third-generation EGFR-TKIs compared to first-generation EGFR-TKIs [20]. The FLAURA trial included patients with locally advanced or metastatic NSCLC, required to have proof of *EGFR* exon 19 deletions or p.Leu858Arg *EGFR* mutation. This Phase III trial randomized 556 patients in a 1:1 ratio to either Osimertinib or the standard of care (physician's choice of erlotinib or gefitinib). Osimertinib was found to improve median PFS from 10.2 months with the erlotinib/gefitinib to 18.9 months with Osimertinib (HR 0.46; 95% CI 0.37 to 0.57; $p < 0.001$). More specifically, when a subgroup of 116 patients with CNS metastases was evaluated, median PFS in NSCLC-BM patients treated with Osimertinib treatment (53 patients, PFS 15.2 months) was also found to be significantly higher than those provided the standard of care (63 patients, PFS 9.6 months) (HR 0.47; 95% CI 0.30–0.74;

$p < 0.001$). However, the FLAURA trial sub-analysis included patients who were treated previously with intracranial radiation [21,22]. The OCEAN study was a prospective study that evaluated Osimertinib in radiation-naive NSCLC-BM, again showing good efficacy with an overall response rate (ORR) of 40.5% and a median brain metastasis-related PFS of 25.2 months [23]. However, all the participants in the OCEAN trial were previously treated with older EGFR-TKIs [23]. The phase I BLOOM study further demonstrated Osimertinib's favorable CSF efficacy by analyzing radiological and symptomatic responses in NSCLC with leptomeningeal disease [24,25].

Only a few studies have evaluated the intracranial efficacy of EGFR-TKIs, generally reporting the benefit of 3rd generation EGFR-TKI use. Huang et al. compared the efficacy of Osimertinib and afatinib in treating EGFR-altered NSCLC and NSCLC-BM in the Taiwanese population. Interestingly, they reported a significant increase in PFS using Osimertinib (22.1 months vs. 12.9 months, $p = 0.045$) in patients with brain metastasis. However, there was no difference in median PFS in patients without brain metastasis (HR 1.02, 95% CI 0.56–1.85). When analyzed without subgroups, no statistically significant difference in median progression-free survival was found [26]. In another Asian cohort with NSCLC, Gen et al. studied 388 patients treated with EGFR-TKIs as 1st line therapy at five institutions. In a subgroup analysis of 118 patients with metastatic NSCLC disease in the brain, this study reported a longer PFS with Osimertinib compared to 1st gen TKIs erlotinib/gefitinib and 2nd gen TKI afatinib (16.3 vs. 7.9 vs. 8.3 months respectively). An improvement in OS was also noted to be trending towards significance with the use of Osimertinib compared to erlotinib/gefitinib (not reached vs. 20.9 months, $p = 0.0725$) [27].

Zhao et al. evaluated a Chinese cohort of 367 patients with NSCLC-BM subjected to either first-generation EGFR TKIs or Osimertinib as the first line of treatment. This study demonstrated a superior OS and intracranial ORR with the use of Osimertinib, despite the patients receiving it having a greater number and size of BMs than 1st gen TKIs (37.7 vs. 22.2 months, 68% vs. 50%, respectively) [28]. Meanwhile, Zhou et al. findings from a different approach. They chose a cohort of 813 diagnosed with EGFR-altered NSCLC without baseline CNS metastases who were treated with a 1st gen TKI or Osimertinib. 38 patients in the cohort developed CNS metastasis during treatment. They observed a decrease in risk of subsequent development of CNS metastases in patients treated with Osimertinib vs. 1st gen TKIs gefitinib or erlotinib. However, this result was not statistically significant ($p = 0.059$) [29]. In another study, Reungwetwattana et al. analyzed 200 brain metastases patients as a subset of the FLAURA trial. They found that the median CNS progression-free survival in patients with measurable or non-measurable CNS lesions was not reached with Osimertinib (95% CI, 16.5–NA) and 13.9 months (95% CI, 8.3–NA) with standard EGFR-TKIs (HR 0.48; 95% CI, 0.26–0.86; $p = 0.014$). These results were named nominally statistically significant, and further analysis showed that objective response rates were also improved in the patients receiving Osimertinib [30]. There are not many studies on this issue, and the existing studies have smaller sample sizes than would be ideal to fully elucidate the effect of 3rd generation EGFR TKIs in NSCLC-BM patients, as is our work. An underpowered comparison may partially explain the variability in outcomes, including progression-free survival.

The discrepancy between this work and prior literature may also be due to various reasons. First, our study had a small sample size of the first-line Osimertinib cohort; this led to a much higher median age, a known prognostic variable for brain metastases. However, interestingly the first-line Osimertinib treatment group also had fewer patients with extracranial metastasis and leptomeningeal spread. Secondly, there may have been confounding systemic therapies for EGFR-TKIs analyzed as 2nd to 5th line. Since our study was a retrospective cohort, considerable selection bias was likely present. Multivariable analysis, like the one performed in this work, can only adjust for the known confounders, typically just some of them. Finally, the complexity of defining PFS may have led to a lack of statistical difference between the two cohorts. PFS was defined as SRS after treatment, the start date of the next line of treatment, the date of death, or the date of the last follow-up.

No MRI brain metastases measurements were collected in our study, which would have provided the most accurate way to assess tumor progression. Nevertheless, our study provides another important data point in assessing targeted therapies in brain metastases from lung cancer.

Though some studies have shown promise for Osimertinib's BBB penetration, mutation resistance, and overall efficacy in NSCLC-BM, further studies need to be conducted to show intracranial efficacy by examining MRI measurements [18–20]. Large prospective studies are warranted that examine, along with the variables mentioned above, the determination of the genetic alteration(s) (e.g., EGFR) and level of expression in both primary tumors and brain metastasis. EGFR-altered NSCLC-BM treatments continue to evolve, as there are currently ongoing studies with Osimertinib and combination therapy, including SRS or immune checkpoint inhibitors [10,31]. With advances in precision medicine, strategic management approaches in the use of EGFR, especially for lung cancer-related metastasis in neuro-oncology, will continue to change.

5. Conclusions

This study found no survival benefit between the novel EGFR-TKIs and first-generation EGFR-TKIs when given either as first-line therapy or an alternative line of therapy in patients with EGFR-altered NSCLC with brain metastases. Larger studies, with rigorous, prospective data collection, are warranted, with reporting for intracranial lesion size, determination of the type of EGFR alteration, and level of EGFR expression in both primary tumors and brain metastases, along with intracranial and extracranial response rates.

Author Contributions: Conceptualization, E.S.M., S.T.C., J.H.S., D.M.P. and M.S.A.; Data curation, V.T., X.J. and A.O.; Formal analysis, P.J.O., A.A.K., A.O. and X.J.; Investigation, V.T., P.J.O., A.O. and X.J.; Methodology, P.J.O., X.J. and M.S.A.; Software, P.J.O. and X.J.; Supervision, E.S.M., S.T.C., J.H.S., D.M.P. and M.S.A.; Writing—original draft, V.T., P.J.O. and A.A.K.; Writing—review & editing, V.T., P.J.O., S.S., A.A.K., A.O., Y.R., E.S.M., S.T.C., J.H.S., D.M.P. and M.S.A. All authors have read and agreed to the published version of the manuscript.

Funding: This research received no external funding.

Institutional Review Board Statement: This work was conducted with approval from the Cleveland Clinic Institutional Review Board (reference code 09-911).

Informed Consent Statement: An IRB-approved waiver of consent and a waiver of HIPAA authorization were in effect, given this was a retrospective review of institutional outcomes with deidentified reporting.

Data Availability Statement: The study lead authors, and senior authors have access to the primary dataset. Data may be made available to interested investigators upon reasonable request to the corresponding author (manmeeta@baptisthealth.net) after approval by all required regulatory authorities.

Acknowledgments: The authors thank Cleveland Clinic staff for their help with the dataset and this manuscript.

Conflicts of Interest: Manmeet Singh Ahluwalia: Grants: AstraZeneca, BMS, Bayer, Incyte, Pharmacyclics, Novocure, MimiVax, Merck; Consultation: Bayer, Novocure, Kiyatec, Insightec, GSK, Xoft, Nuvation, Cellularity, SDP Oncology, Apollomics, Prelude, Janssen, Tocagen, Voyager Therapeutics, Viewray, Caris Lifesciences, Pyramid Biosciences, Varian Medical Systems, Cairn Therapeutics, Anheart Therapeutics, Theraguix; Scientific Advisory Board: Cairn Therapeutics, Pyramid Biosciences, Modifi Biosciences; Stock shareholder: Mimivax, Cytodyn, MedInnovate Advisors LLC. David M. Peereboom: Consulting or Advisory Role: Orbus Therapeutics, Sumitomo Dainippon Pharma Oncology Inc, Stemline Therapeutics, Novocure; Research Funding: Pfizer (Inst), Novartis (Inst), Neonc Technologies (Inst), Orbus Therapeutics (Inst), Bristol Myers Squibb (Inst), Genentech/Roche (Inst), Pharmacyclics (Inst), Bayer (Inst), Karyopharm Therapeutics (Inst), Apollomics (Inst), Vigeo Therapeutics (Inst), Global Coalition for Adaptive Research (Inst), MimiVax (Inst), Ono Pharmaceutical (Inst), Mylan (Inst). Samuel Chao: Honorarium: Varian Medical Systems, Stock: Merck. John Suh: Consultant: Abbvie. All other authors have no disclosures relevant to this manuscript.

References

1. Bray, F.; Ferlay, J.; Soerjomataram, I.; Siegel, R.L.; Torre, L.A.; Jemal, A. Global cancer statistics 2018: GLOBOCAN estimates of incidence and mortality worldwide for 36 cancers in 185 countries. *CA Cancer J. Clin.* **2018**, *68*, 394–424. [CrossRef]
2. Gelatti, A.C.Z.; Drilon, A.; Santini, F.C. Optimizing the sequencing of tyrosine kinase inhibitors (TKIs) in epidermal growth factor receptor (EGFR) mutation-positive non-small cell lung cancer (NSCLC). *Lung Cancer* **2019**, *137*, 113–122. [CrossRef]
3. Saad, A.G.; Yeap, B.Y.; Thunnissen, F.B.; Pinkus, G.S.; Pinkus, J.L.; Loda, M.; Sugarbaker, D.J.; Johnson, B.E.; Chirieac, L.R. Immunohistochemical markers associated with brain metastases in patients with non-small cell lung carcinoma. *Cancer* **2008**, *113*, 2129–2138. [CrossRef]
4. Rangachari, D.; Yamaguchi, N.; VanderLaan, P.A.; Folch, E.; Mahadevan, A.; Floyd, S.R.; Uhlmann, E.J.; Wong, E.T.; Dahlberg, S.E.; Huberman, M.S.; et al. Brain metastases in patients with EGFR-altered or ALK-rearranged non-small-cell lung cancers. *Lung Cancer* **2015**, *88*, 108–111. [CrossRef] [PubMed]
5. Rybarczyk-Kasiuchnicz, A.; Ramlau, R.; Stencel, K. Treatment of Brain Metastases of Non-Small Cell Lung Carcinoma. *Int. J. Mol. Sci.* **2021**, *22*, 593. [CrossRef]
6. Aiko, N.; Shimokawa, T.; Miyazaki, K.; Misumi, Y.; Agemi, Y.; Ishii, M.; Nakamura, Y.; Yamanaka, T.; Okamoto, H. Comparison of the efficacies of first-generation epidermal growth factor receptor tyrosine kinase inhibitors for brain metastasis in patients with advanced non-small-cell lung cancer harboring EGFR mutations. *BMC Cancer* **2018**, *18*, 1012. [CrossRef] [PubMed]
7. Passaro, A.; Mok, T.; Peters, S.; Popat, S.; Ahn, M.J.; de Marinis, F. Recent Advances on the Role of EGFR Tyrosine Kinase Inhibitors in the Management of NSCLC With Uncommon, Non Exon 20 Insertions, EGFR Mutations. *J. Thorac. Oncol.* **2021**, *16*, 764–773. [CrossRef] [PubMed]
8. Yen, C.T.; Wu, W.J.; Chen, Y.T.; Chang, W.C.; Yang, S.H.; Shen, S.Y.; Su, J.; Chen, H.Y. Surgical resection of brain metastases prolongs overall survival in non-small-cell lung cancer. *Am. J. Cancer Res.* **2021**, *11*, 6160–6172. [PubMed]
9. Patil, C.G.; Pricola, K.; Sarmiento, J.M.; Garg, S.K.; Bryant, A.; Black, K.L. Whole brain radiation therapy (WBRT) alone versus WBRT and radiosurgery for the treatment of brain metastases. *Cochrane Database Syst. Rev.* **2017**, *9*, CD006121.
10. Zhao, B.; Wang, Y.; Wang, Y.; Chen, W.; Zhou, L.; Liu, P.H.; Kong, Z.; Dai, C.; Wang, Y.; Ma, W. Efficacy and safety of therapies for EGFR-mutant non-small cell lung cancer with brain metastasis: An evidence-based Bayesian network pooled study of multivariable survival analyses. *Aging* **2020**, *12*, 14244–14270. [CrossRef]
11. Thomas, R.; Srivastava, S.; Katreddy, R.R.; Sobieski, J.; Zhang, W. Kinase-inactivated EGFR is required for the survival of wild-type EGFR-expressing cancer cells treated with tyrosine kinase inhibitors. *Int. J. Mol. Sci.* **2019**, *20*, 2515. [CrossRef]
12. Rosell, R.; Carcereny, E.; Gervais, R.; Vergnenegre, A.; Massuti, B.; Felip, E.; Palmero, R.; Garcia-Gomez, R.; Pallares, C.; Sanchez, J.M.; et al. Erlotinib versus standard chemotherapy as first-line treatment for European patients with advanced EGFR mutation-positive non-small-cell lung cancer (EURTAC): A multicentre, open-label, randomised phase 3 trial. *Lancet Oncol.* **2012**, *13*, 239–246. [CrossRef] [PubMed]
13. Mitsudomi, T.; Morita, S.; Yatabe, Y.; Negoro, S.; Okamoto, I.; Tsurutani, J.; Seto, T.; Satouchi, M.; Tada, H.; Hirashima, T.; et al. Gefitinib versus cisplatin plus docetaxel in patients with non-small-cell lung cancer harbouring mutations of the epidermal growth factor receptor (WJTOG3405): An open label, randomised phase 3 trial. *Lancet Oncol.* **2010**, *11*, 121–128. [CrossRef]
14. Yun, P.J.; Wang, G.C.; Chen, Y.Y.; Wu, T.H.; Huang, H.K.; Lee, S.C.; Chang, H.; Huang, T. Brain metastases in resected non-small cell lung cancer: The impact of different tyrosine kinase inhibitors. *PLoS ONE* **2019**, *14*, e0215923. [CrossRef] [PubMed]
15. Zeng, Y.D.; Liao, H.; Qin, T.; Zhang, L.; Wei, W.D.; Liang, J.Z.; Xu, F.; Dinglin, X.; Ma, S.; Chen, L. Blood-brain barrier permeability of gefitinib in patients with brain metastases from non-small-cell lung cancer before and during whole brain radiation therapy. *Oncotarget* **2015**, *6*, 8366–8376. [CrossRef] [PubMed]
16. Clarke, J.L.; Pao, W.; Wu, N.; Miller, V.A.; Lassman, A.B. High dose weekly erlotinib achieves therapeutic concentrations in CSF and is effective in leptomeningeal metastases from epidermal growth factor receptor mutant lung cancer. *J. Neurooncol.* **2010**, *99*, 283–286. [CrossRef]
17. Leonetti, A.; Sharma, S.; Minari, R.; Perego, P.; Giovannetti, E.; Marcello, T. Resistance mechanisms to osimertinib in EGFR-altered non-small cell lung cancer. *Br. J. Cancer* **2019**, *121*, 725–737. [CrossRef]
18. Ballard, P.; Yates, J.W.; Yang, Z.; Kim, D.W.; Yang, J.C.; Cantarini, M.; Pickup, K.; Jordan, A.; Hickey, M.; Grist, M.; et al. Preclinical Comparison of Osimertinib with Other EGFR-TKIs in EGFR-Mutant NSCLC Brain Metastases Models, and Early Evidence of Clinical Brain Metastases Activity. *Clin. Cancer Res.* **2016**, *22*, 5130–5140. [CrossRef]
19. Ramalingam, S.S.; Vansteenkiste, J.; Planchard, D.; Cho, B.C.; Gray, J.E.; Ohe, Y.; Zhou, C.; Reungwetwattana, T.; Cheng, Y.; Chewaskulyong, B.; et al. Overall Survival with Osimertinib in Untreated. *N. Engl. J. Med.* **2020**, *382*, 41–50. [CrossRef]
20. Soria, J.C.; Ohe, Y.; Vansteenkiste, J.; Reungwetwattana, T.; Chewaskulyong, B.; Lee, K.H.; Dechaphunkul, A.; Imamura, F.; Nogami, N.; Kurata, T.; et al. Osimertinib in Untreated EGFR-altered Advanced Non-Small-Cell Lung Cancer. *N. Engl. J. Med.* **2018**, *378*, 113–125. [CrossRef]
21. Goss, G.; Tsai, C.M.; Shepherd, F.A.; Ahn, M.J.; Bazhenova, L.; Crinò, L.; de Marinis, F.; Felip, E.; Morabito, A.; Hodge, R.; et al. CNS response to osimertinib in patients with T790M-positive advanced NSCLC: Pooled data from two phase II trials. *Ann. Oncol.* **2018**, *29*, 687–693. [CrossRef]
22. Wu, Y.L.; Ahn, M.J.; Garassino, M.C.; Han, J.Y.; Katakami, N.; Kim, H.R.; Hodge, R.; Kaur, P.; Brown, A.P.; Ghiorghiu, D.; et al. CNS Efficacy of Osimertinib in Patients With T790M-Positive Advanced Non-Small-Cell Lung Cancer: Data From a Randomized Phase III Trial (AURA3). *J. Clin. Oncol.* **2018**, *36*, 2702–2709. [CrossRef] [PubMed]

23. Yamaguchi, H.; Wakuda, K.; Fukuda, M.; Kenmotsu, H.; Mukae, H.; Ito, K.; Chibana, K.; Inoue, K.; Miura, S.; Tanaka, K.; et al. A Phase II Study of Osimertinib for Radiotherapy-Naive Central Nervous System Metastasis From NSCLC: Results for the T790M Cohort of the OCEAN Study (LOGIK1603/WJOG9116L). *J. Thorac. Oncol.* **2021**, *16*, 2121–2132. [CrossRef]
24. Yang, J.C.H.; Kim, S.W.; Kim, D.W.; Lee, J.S.; Cho, B.C.; Ahn, J.S.; Lee, D.H.; Kim, T.M.; Goldman, J.W.; Natale, R.B.; et al. Osimertinib in Patients With Epidermal Growth Factor Receptor Mutation-Positive Non-Small-Cell Lung Cancer and Leptomeningeal Metastases: The BLOOM Study. *J. Clin. Oncol.* **2020**, *38*, 538–547. [CrossRef]
25. Singhi, E.K.; Horn, L.; Sequist, L.V.; Heymach, J.; Langer, C.J. Advanced Non-small Cell Lung Cancer: Sequencing Agents in the EGFR-altered/ALK-Rearranged Populations. *Am. Soc. Clin. Oncol. Educ. Book* **2019**, *39*, e187–e197. [CrossRef] [PubMed]
26. Huang, Y.H.; Hsu, K.H.; Tseng, J.S.; Yang, T.Y.; Chen, K.C.; Su, K.Y.; Yu, S.L.; Chen, J.W.; Chang, J.C. The Difference in Clinical Outcomes Between Osimertinib and Afatinib for First-Line Treatment in Patients with Advanced and Recurrent EGFR-Mutant Non-Small Cell Lung Cancer in Taiwan. *Target. Oncol.* **2022**, *17*, 295–306. [CrossRef]
27. Gen, S.; Tanaka, I.; Morise, M.; Koyama, J.; Kodama, Y.; Matsui, A.; Hase, T.; Hibino, Y.; Yokoyama, T.; Kimura, T.; et al. Clinical efficacy of osimertinib in EGFR-mutant non-small cell lung cancer with distant metastasis. *BMC Cancer* **2022**, *22*, 654. [CrossRef] [PubMed]
28. Zhao, Y.; Li, S.; Yang, X.; Chu, L.; Wang, S.; Tong, T.; Chu, X.; Yu, F.; Zeng, Y.; Guo, T.; et al. Overall survival benefit of osimertinib and clinical value of upfront cranial local therapy in untreated EGFR-mutant non-small cell lung cancer with brain metastasis. *Int. J. Cancer* **2022**, *150*, 1318–1328. [CrossRef]
29. Zhou, Y.; Wang, B.; Qu, J.; Yu, F.; Zhao, Y.; Li, S.; Zeng, Y.; Yang, X.; Chu, L.; Chu, X.; et al. Survival outcomes and symptomatic central nervous system (CNS) metastasis in EGFR-mutant advanced non-small cell lung cancer without baseline CNS metastasis: Osimertinib vs. first-generation EGFR tyrosine kinase inhibitors. *Lung Cancer* **2020**, *150*, 178–185. [CrossRef]
30. Reungwetwattana, T.; Nakagawa, K.; Cho, B.C.; Cobo, M.; Cho, E.K.; Bertolini, A.; Bohnet, S.; Zhou, C.; Lee, K.; Nogami, N.; et al. CNS Response to Osimertinib Versus Standard Epidermal Growth Factor Receptor Tyrosine Kinase Inhibitors in Patients With Untreated EGFR-altered Advanced Non-Small-Cell Lung Cancer. *J. Clin. Oncol.* **2018**, *36*, 3290. [CrossRef]
31. Liang, H.; Liu, X.; Wang, M. Immunotherapy combined with epidermal growth factor receptor tyrosine kinase inhibitors in non-small-cell lung cancer treatment. *Oncol. Targets Ther.* **2018**, *11*, 6189–6196. [CrossRef] [PubMed]

Disclaimer/Publisher's Note: The statements, opinions and data contained in all publications are solely those of the individual author(s) and contributor(s) and not of MDPI and/or the editor(s). MDPI and/or the editor(s) disclaim responsibility for any injury to people or property resulting from any ideas, methods, instructions or products referred to in the content.

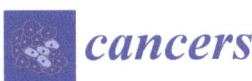

Review

DNA Methylation and Histone Modification in Low-Grade Gliomas: Current Understanding and Potential Clinical Targets

Ahmad Ozair [1,2,†], Vivek Bhat [3,†], Reid S. Alisch [4], Atulya A. Khosla [1], Rupesh R. Kotecha [1,5], Yazmin Odia [1,5], Michael W. McDermott [5,6,*] and Manmeet S. Ahluwalia [1,6,*]

- [1] Miami Cancer Institute, Baptist Health South Florida, Miami, FL 33176, USA
- [2] Faculty of Medicine, King George's Medical University, Lucknow 226003, India
- [3] St. John's Medical College, Bangalore 560034, India
- [4] Department of Neurosurgery, University of Wisconsin-Madison, Madison, WI 53792, USA
- [5] Herbert Wertheim College of Medicine, Florida International University, Miami, FL 33199, USA
- [6] Miami Neuroscience Institute, Baptist Health South Florida, Miami, FL 33176, USA
- * Correspondence: mwmcd@baptisthealth.net (M.W.M.); manmeeta@baptisthealth.net (M.S.A.)
- † These authors contributed equally to this work.

Simple Summary: Brain tumors comprise a large, varied group, with gliomas being the most common malignant tumors arising in the brain. This state-of-the-art review discusses the role of epigenetics in low-grade gliomas, i.e., those gliomas which are typically less invasive and have better survival rates than their high-grade counterparts. This paper is a summary of the current paradigms in DNA methylation and histone modification in low-grade gliomas, with their integration into the recently published WHO Classification for CNS Tumors, Fifth Edition. This paper, targeted towards a clinical audience, also describes the role of DNA methylation and histone modification in pathogenesis, clinical behavior, and outcomes of low-grade gliomas, with an emphasis on the potential therapeutic targets in associated cellular biomolecules, structures, and processes.

Abstract: Gliomas, the most common type of malignant primary brain tumor, were conventionally classified through WHO Grades I–IV (now 1–4), with low-grade gliomas being entities belonging to Grades 1 or 2. While the focus of the WHO Classification for Central Nervous System (CNS) tumors had historically been on histopathological attributes, the recently released fifth edition of the classification (WHO CNS5) characterizes brain tumors, including gliomas, using an integration of histological and molecular features, including their epigenetic changes such as histone methylation, DNA methylation, and histone acetylation, which are increasingly being used for the classification of low-grade gliomas. This review describes the current understanding of the role of DNA methylation, demethylation, and histone modification in pathogenesis, clinical behavior, and outcomes of brain tumors, in particular of low-grade gliomas. The review also highlights potential diagnostic and/or therapeutic targets in associated cellular biomolecules, structures, and processes. Targeting of MGMT promoter methylation, TET-hTDG-BER pathway, association of G-CIMP with key gene mutations, PARP inhibition, IDH and 2-HG-associated processes, TERT mutation and ARL9-associated pathways, DNA Methyltransferase (DNMT) inhibition, Histone Deacetylase (HDAC) inhibition, BET inhibition, CpG site DNA methylation signatures, along with others, present exciting avenues for translational research. This review also summarizes the current clinical trial landscape associated with the therapeutic utility of epigenetics in low-grade gliomas. Much of the evidence currently remains restricted to preclinical studies, warranting further investigation to demonstrate true clinical utility.

Keywords: methylation; methylomics; G-CIMP; MGMT; DNMT; ATRX; H3K27M; CpG island; tumor suppressor; methyltransferases; histone acetylation

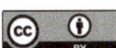

1. Introduction

Gliomas are a heterogenous group of central nervous system (CNS) tumors that are grouped based on their common origin from glial or precursor cells [1,2]. Gliomas include entities such as glioblastoma, astrocytoma, oligodendroglioma, ependymoma, and mixed gliomas amongst others. Taken together, they comprise over 60% of all primary brain tumors and nearly 25% of all malignant brain neoplasms [1,3–5].

Gliomas have been conventionally classified through Grades I-IV (now using 1–4) using the World Health Organization (WHO) schema, with low-grade gliomas typically referring to tumors belonging to Grade 1 or 2, even though some authors have infrequently referred to Grade 3 tumors as LGGs [1,3,5–7].

To discuss DNA methylation in LGGs, it is essential to (A) first recognize which entities are classified as LGGs currently, as their neuropathological classification has evolved in the last two decades, and (B) have a broad understanding of methylation processes. In general, Grade I gliomas, such as pilocytic astrocytoma, are typically localized, have low invasion potential, and remain amenable to surgical resection [1,8]. Grade 2 gliomas, also called diffuse LGGs (DLGGs), are more locally invasive and require adjuvant strategies for their curative therapy [1,2,4–6,8,9]. While the focus of the classification of gliomas has historically been on clinicopathological attributes, the recently released fifth edition of the CNS tumor classification (WHO CNS5) now characterizes brain tumors, including gliomas, using an integration of histological and molecular features, including DNA methylation [5].

2. Current Status of LGGs in the WHO Classification

Historically, gliomas were classified primarily based on their histologic attributes [1,3]. This practice continued until the 2007 WHO classification, which recognized seven different types of gliomas, based on differentiation along astrocytic and/or oligodendroglial lineages [10]. Further prognostic entities were later defined based on the histologic grading, with cellular features of mitoses and necroses associated with both higher grades and worse prognosis [10]. However, this classification system suffered from significant intra-observer and inter-observer variability, along with a lack of clarity regarding reproducible methods.

With advances in molecular analysis, glioma classification has undergone a paradigm shift, with significant molecular heterogeneity reported among each histologic type of glioma [1,6,11,12]. One such seminal advance was the discovery of mutations in the isocitrate dehydrogenase (IDH) 1 and 2 genes, with IDH1/2 mutations identified in over 70% of LGGs [13]. Furthermore, IDH1/2-mutant (IDHmt) tumors were found to have a demonstrably better prognosis than IDH1/2-wild type (IDHwt). In 2015, a study utilizing The Cancer Genome Atlas (TCGA) analyzed 293 LGGs and identified an additional molecular marker—the loss of chromosomes 1p and 19q—allowing subclassification into three prognostically distinct groups. Arranged from best to worst prognosis, LGGS can be fundamentally ordered into (A) IDH-mutant (IDHmt) LGGs with 1p/19q chromosomal codeletion, e.g., oligodendrogliomas, which are associated with gene mutations of Telomerase Reverse Transcriptase (TERT); (B) IDHmt LGGs without 1p/19q chromosomal codeletion, e.g., astrocytomas that are typically associated with mutations in Tumor Protein 53 (TP53) and ATP-Dependent Helicase ATRX (ATRX); and (C) IDH wild-type (IDHwt) LGGs [14]. Subsequent studies elucidated genetic signatures unique to each of these three groups [15,16].

Recognizing these advances, the WHO 2016 classification of gliomas emerged, which utilized a combination of histologic and molecular signatures for classification [17]. Here, six separate entities of glioma were identified, each with a unique molecular signature. While this was a welcome step, one persistent limitation was the continued reliance on 'brisk' mitotic activity to distinguish Grade 3 from Grade 2 gliomas, requiring subjective counting of specimens, something that was compounded by the fact that mitotic activity had little significance in IDHmt LGGs [18].

The most recent, fifth edition of the WHO Classification of Tumors of the Central Nervous System (WHO CNS5) took this one step further by incorporating the recommendations from the Consortium to Inform Molecular and Practical Approaches to CNS Tumor Taxonomy (cIMPACT-NOW) [14,19–22], along with the landmark DNA methylation-based classification of CNS tumors published in Nature [12]. The WHO CNS5 uses an integrated histo-molecular assessment, prioritizing genetic and molecular alterations, which were emphasized for several tumor types [5]. A summary of the view of the WHO CNS5 has been provided in Figure 1.

WHO CNS5 utilizes a hybrid approach with regard to tumor grouping [23]. While some tumor groups still find a lack of utilization for any molecular testing requirements such as meningiomas, several new types and subtypes are primarily characterized by molecular features such as medulloblastoma and ependymomas [5]. Gliomas currently fall under the group of "Gliomas, Glioneuronal and Neuronal Tumors". The grading of gliomas, now done using WHO Grade 1–4 instead of Grade I–IV, is to be based on a combination of histologic and molecular features [5]. Gliomas have also been separated into pediatric-type and adult-type, thus reorganizing and grouping entities with common genetic alterations (Table 1). Gliomas were also rearranged accounting for their prevalent genetic mutations, especially IDH 1/2 mutation (better prognosis), 1p/19q codeletion (better prognosis), and CDKN2A/B homozygous deletion (worse prognosis). Grading is now to be done within individual tumor types, instead of across tumor types. Perhaps the most landmark change for clinicians was the change in classification of glioblastomas (GBMs). As per WHO CNS5, GBM includes only IDH-wild type entities, while previously GBMs included both IDHmt (10%) and IDHwt (90%) [24].

As per WHO CNS5, diffuse astrocytic tumors can now be classified as Grade 2 (i.e., LGG), Grade 3, or Grade 4, the latter two being high-grade gliomas (HGGs). Diffuse astrocytic tumors with IDHwt, i.e., baseline more aggressive than IDHmt, that lack GBM-specific histology but have at least one of three particular genetic alterations would also be classified as GBMs [5]. These specific alterations are: (1) TERT promoter mutations (TERT-pmt), (2) EGFR gene amplifications, and/or (3) loss of chromosome 10 (+7/−10) [5,23]. On the other hand, IDHmt astrocytomas with CDKN2A/B homozygous deletions and related alterations can now be classified as WHO Grade 4, even if histologically lacking necroses or microvascular proliferation [5]. Thus, IDH mutation testing has become a key requirement for appropriate classification into LGG or HGG [23]. The characterization of methylomic attributes was added to diagnostic criteria, albeit as "desirable characteristics", acknowledging the general inaccessibility of these tools [25].

While recognizing newer or updated entities in the new classification, it is also essential to note that low-grade gliomas (LGG), in particular astrocytomas, can transform into higher-grade tumors or display more aggressive behavior after some time [2]. Nearly 70% of diffuse LGGs transform into a higher-grade type [26,27]. This is likely the result of the gradual accumulation of genetic and epigenetic alterations, which together allow cellular replication to take place in an unrestrained fashion. Epigenetic alterations in cancer cells have been demonstrated to increase genomic fragility, increase angiogenic capabilities, decrease the attribute of cellular adhesion, permit entry into the cell cycle, help avoid apoptosis and lead to defects in DNA repair, as further examined below [28].

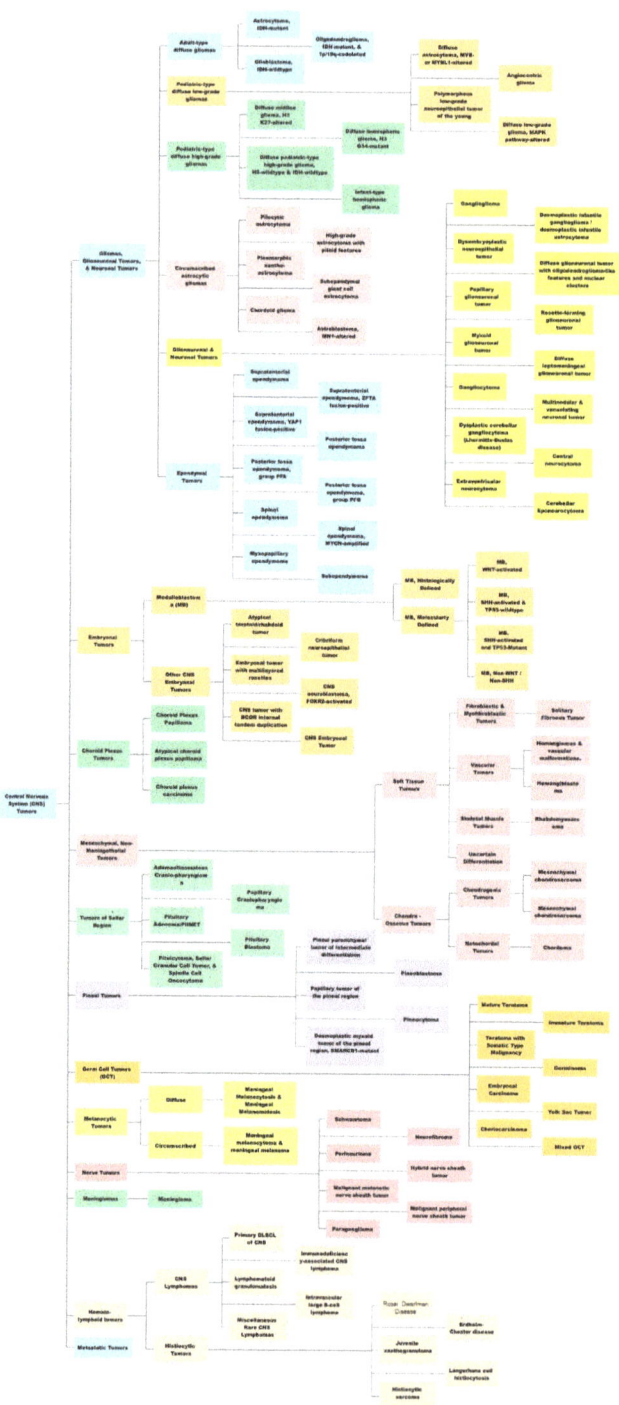

Figure 1. A summary view of the World Health Organization (WHO) 2021 classification of central nervous system (CNS) tumors. This original figure has been created using data available from the WHO CNS5 publication.

Table 1. Status of gliomas in the fifth edition of the WHO Classification of Tumors of the Central Nervous System (WHO CNS5). Adapted under Creative Commons Attribution-Noncommercial-Share Alike 4.0 License from [23]. Available from: https://www.ijpmonline.org/text.asp?2022/65/5/5/345057. Accessed on 15 December 2022.

Gliomas, Glioneuronal and Neuronal Tumors	WHO Grade	Remarks
Ependymal Tumors		
Adult-type diffuse gliomas		
Astrocytoma, IDH-mutant	2, 3, 4	"Diffuse" and "anaplastic" are terms no longer used; no tumor exists now that is called "astrocytoma, IDH-wild type".
Oligodendroglioma, IDH-mutant and 1p/19q-codeleted	2, 3	Similar grading approaches to WHO CNS4 (2016); tumor type "oligoastrocytoma" deleted.
Glioblastoma, IDH-wildtype	4	Terms such as "multiforme" and "Glioblastoma, IDH mutant" were removed from WHO CNS5. Three subtypes, namely giant cell type, gliosarcoma, and epithelioid type, are still discussed in the WHO CNS5 text but removed from the classification.
Pediatric-type diffuse low-grade gliomas (pDLGG)		
Diffuse astrocytoma, MYB- or MYBL1 altered	1	Newly recognized tumor type.
Angiocentric Glioma	1	First added in WHO 2007 classification under "neuroepithelial tumors", later moved in WHO 2016 classification to "other gliomas" and in WHO 2021 moved to "pDLGG"
Polymorphous low-grade neuroepithelial tumor of the young	1	Newly recognized tumor type.
Diffuse low-grade glioma, MAPK altered	Unassigned	Newly recognized tumor type.
Pediatric-type diffuse high-grade gliomas (HGG)		
Diffuse midline glioma (DMG), H3 K27-altered	4	Revised nomenclature: H3K27-altered instead of H3K27-mutant to recognize additional mechanisms.
Diffuse hemispheric glioma, H3 G34-mutant	4	Newly recognized tumor type.
Diffuse pediatric-type HGG, H3-wildtype and IDH-wildtype	4	Newly recognized tumor type.
Infant-type hemispheric glioma	Unassigned	Newly recognized tumor type.
Circumscribed astrocytic gliomas		
Pilocytic astrocytoma	1	-
High-grade astrocytoma with piloid features	Unassigned	Newly recognized tumor type.
Pleomorphic xanthoastrocytoma	2, 3	The term "anaplastic" is eliminated.
Subependymal giant cell astrocytoma	1	-
Chordoid glioma	2	Revised nomenclature – location modifier of "third ventricle" dropped.
Astroblastoma, MN1 altered	Unassigned	Revised nomenclature – genetic modifier added for specificity (MN1 altered).

Table 1. *Cont.*

Gliomas, Glioneuronal and Neuronal Tumors	WHO Grade	Remarks
Glioneuronal and neuronal tumors		
Ganglioglioma	1	-
Desmoplastic infantile ganglioglioma/astrocytoma	1	-
Dysembryoplastic neuroepithelial tumor	1	-
Diffuse glioneuronal tumor with oligodendroglioma-like features and nuclear clusters	Unassigned	Newly recognized tumor type.
Papillary glioneuronal tumor	1	-
Rosette-forming glioneuronal tumor	1	-
Myxoid glioneuronal tumor	1	Upgraded from a provisional status in 2016 to a distinct tumor type.
Diffuse leptomeningeal glioneuronal tumor (DLGNT)	2, 3	Three subtypes added: DLGNT-1q-gain, DLGNT-MC-1, and DLGNT-MC-2.
Gangliocytoma	1	-
Multinodular and vacuolating neuronal tumor	1	New tumor type in WHO 2021, after being upgraded from a mere pattern of ganglion cell tumors in WHO 2016.
Dysplastic cerebellar gangliocytoma (Lhermitte-Duclos disease)	1	-
Central neurocytoma	2	-
Cerebellar liponeurocytoma	2	-
Extraventricular neurocytoma	2	-

3. Overview of DNA Methylation and Demethylation

The importance of epigenetic processes in the clinical neurosciences may be amply demonstrated in the role of DNA methylation patterns in the physiological regulation of differentiation, in particular, through cellular, spatial and temporal specificities [29,30]. Notably, epigenetic deregulation has also been included amongst the updated hallmarks of cancer [31,32]. In the cancer cell, it acts in both a standalone fashion and synergistically with other genetic changes, in driving neoplastic evolution [29–32]. However, despite substantial advances in the understanding and the utility of investigating methylomics of various malignancies, considerably less headway has been made in the clinical utilization of epigenetics in brain tumors, especially in less aggressive tumors such as low-grade gliomas [30]. DNA methylation has been the most widely studied and most clinically explored epigenetic change in gliomas [28]. Given the complexity of the cellular processes involved, a brief review for clinicians of processes involved in DNA methylation follows.

The cellular DNA, including that of the cancer cell, is constructed out of four elements (DNA bases), namely, adenine (A), thymine (T), guanine (G), and cytosine (C). While adenine and guanine are purines, thymine and cytosine are pyrimidines. Base pairing occurs between AT and GC, but a methylated cytosine, with its corresponding CG base pairing, may undergo deamination to form a thymine.

DNA methylation is a process by which methyl (CH_3-) groups are added to the DNA bases, to allow for an additional layer of regulation of gene expression. This modification can change the activity of a DNA segment without changing the underlying sequence. DNA methylation typically occurs on cytosine bases, leading to the formation of 5-methylcytosine, often called the 'fifth DNA base'. It is estimated that 3–6% of cytosine bases in human cells carry methyl groups [28], where it is especially predominant in repetitive genomic sequences. The constant methylation status of these sequences has been reported to potentially play a role in the routine upkeep of healthy cells by averting chromosomal instability, translocations, and genetic disruptions. The latter, which may occur through the reactivation of certain transposon-derived sequences that have self-propagation and random site insertion properties, is prevented by hypermethylation [28,33]. Additionally, DNA methylation is one of the most reliable means to transmit epigenetic information across cellular replication [34–36]. Thus, maintaining the integrity of DNA methylation patterns is essential for proper cellular function, and disruptions to this process can have significant effects on health and disease.

Because cytosine is typically paired with guanine, a DNA sequence where several methylated cytosine and guanine pairs come together are known as 'CpG or CG Islands', where the highest amount of methylation is present in the genome [37]. CpG islands can be found throughout the genome, and their exact location and frequency can vary depending on the organism and the specific region of the genome [37]. CpG islands frequently occur near the 5' end of genes (~70%) that contain DNA sequences corresponding to the promoter, untranslated region (5'-UTR), and exon 1 (Figure 2). Unmethylated CpG sites permit the related sequences to be expressed when the required transcriptional activators are available [28,38,39].

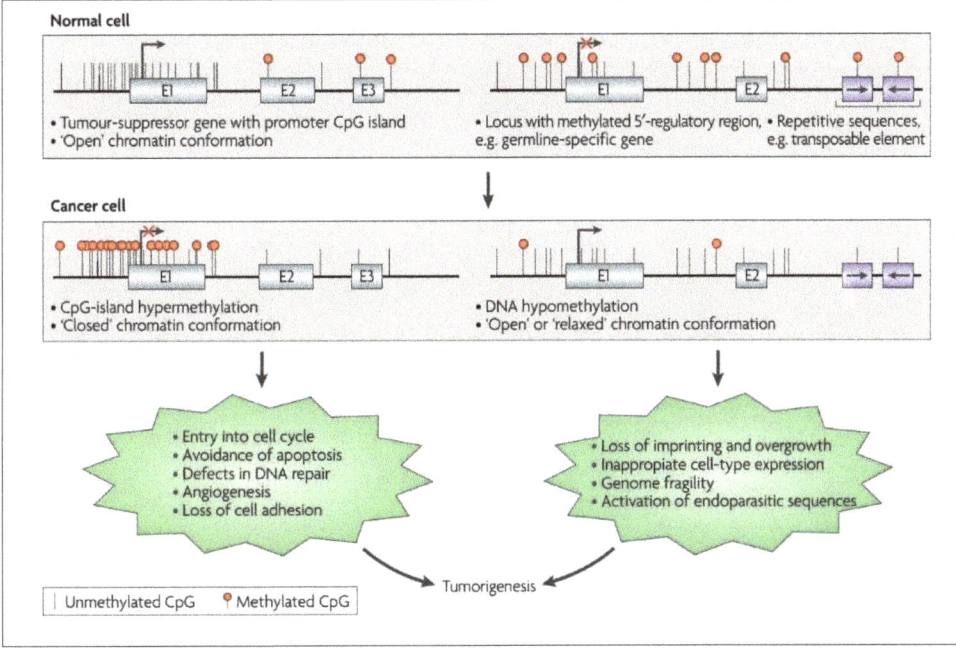

Figure 2. Altered DNA methylation and its downstream impact in the cancer cell. Reproduced with permission from [28].

The process of DNA methylation is carried out by DNA methyltransferases (DNMT), which transfer a methyl group from S-adenosyl methionine (SAM), a carrier molecule, to the DNA molecule, resulting in the addition of a methyl group to the cytosine base. While several of these enzymes exist, all of them utilize SAM as the carrier molecule. The proteins encoded by the *DNMT3* gene and its variants (*DNMT3A*, *DNMT3B*, regulatory *DNMT3L*) preferentially methylate unmethylated DNA strands and thus carry out a major part of de novo methylation [35]. Meanwhile, the proteins encoded by the *DNMT1* gene methylate DNA whose single strand has already been methylated (hemimethylated DNA) in a preferential fashion [35]. This permits it to maintain the methylation patterns across cellular replication [36,40].

To ensure the reliability of DNA methylation, cells have several mechanisms in place to monitor and repair methylation patterns. For example, enzymes of the Ten-Eleven Translocases (TET) family (*TET1, TET2, TET3*), can remove methyl groups from DNA, and help reverse the de novo methylation process, while other enzymes can recognize and repair damaged or improperly methylated DNA. TET enzymes, which are α-ketoglutarate-dependent dioxygenases, convert 5-methylCytosine (5mC) to 5-hydroxymethylCytosine (5hmC), 5-formylCytosine (5fC), and 5-carboxylCytosine (5caC) in a stepwise fashion [41,42], as part of the normal cytosine methylation cycle (Figure 3). The 5-carboxylcytosine is later removed by the human thymine-DNA glycosylase (hTDG) enzyme, in a process exemplifying "active DNA demethylation" [43,44]. This is immediately followed by the insertion of an unmethylated cytosine residue at the excision site, carried out by the DNA Base Excision Repair (BER) system [45]. The TET-hTDG-BER system is known to ensure that cells can actively and rapidly demethylate specific loci in response to environmental changes, such as cellular stressors. This active demethylation is in contrast to the passive demethylation process which occurs in locations where DNMT1 is not present to methylate DNA during replication [46]. Additionally, 5-hmC, by itself, has been hypothesized to play a role in the regulation of gene expression, given that it is noted to be present in both tissue-specific gene bodies and DNA enhancers, the latter being short regulatory sequences where transcription factors bind. Thus, dysregulation of this tightly controlled active methylation and active demethylation in healthy cells leads to errors that eventually permit the hallmark neoplastic features to manifest [32]. Efforts are underway to generate genome-wide 5-hmC profiles (tissue maps) of cells in various tumors [47].

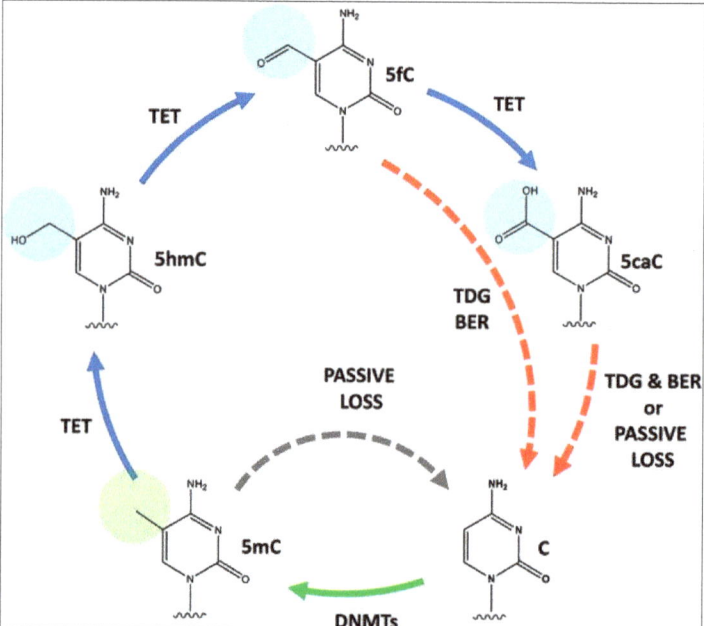

Figure 3. Cytosine methylation and demethylation cycle. C, cytosine; 5mc, 5-methylCytosine; 5hmC, 5-hydroxymethylCytosine; 5fc,5-formylCytosine; 5caC, 5-carboxylCytosine, TDG, thymine-DNA glycosylase; BER, Base Excision Repair, TET, Ten-Eleven Translocases, DNMT, DNA Methyltransferases. Reproduced with permission from [48].

4. DNA Methylation in Low-Grade Gliomas

The utility of studying DNA methylation was first identified in glioblastoma, due to its aggressiveness and poor prognosis. While such studies have begun to include low-grade gliomas (LGGs) as well, literature specific to LGGs remains scarce (Persico et al., 2022), even though there is wide recognition that DNA methylation is likely to play a key role in the next frontier of oncology diagnostics and therapeutics [49,50].

Fundamentally, methylation of a locus typically results in the repression of its expression level, which can then affect the expression level of other genes that are downstream targets. Methylated DNA sequences are less accessible to the cellular machinery that reads the genetic code. For example, if the locus has elements that repress expression (e.g., 5′ regulatory region) of the associated gene(s) (e.g., a DNA damage repair gene), then the methylated locus would become silenced, leading to an increase in gene expression of the associated gene (in this case higher production of DNA damage repair proteins).

In general, while cancer cells undergo a global loss of DNA methylation (Figure 2), CpG islands of tumor-suppressor genes (TSGs) undergo preferential hypermethylation [28]. The epigenetic silencing of TSGs permits the cancer cell to evade pro-apoptotic changes, proceed with unrestrained cellular replication, display angiogenesis and reduce cellular adhesion, amongst other mechanisms, thus contributing to the classically described hallmarks of cancer cells [28,35,51] (Figure 2). These unique DNA methylation changes are also accompanied by histone modifications, another epigenetic alteration that permits further silencing of TSGs and increased expression of oncogenes [52–54], as discussed later in the text. Hypermethylation of tumor suppressor genes is increasingly being explored as a prognostic marker in low-grade gliomas, for instance, testing for MGMT methylation status to predict response to chemotherapy [55]. O6-methylguanine-DNA methyltransferase (*MGMT*) is a protein involved in DNA repair. When the *MGMT* gene locus become methylated (i.e., hypermethylated), the amount of DNA repair across the genome reduces, leading to increased sensitivity to cytotoxic medications, making the tumor more responsive to chemotherapy [33]. Therefore, in gliomas, *MGMT* hypermethylation is associated with a better response to temozolomide, a DNA alkylating agent.

MGMT promoter hypermethylation is being increasingly explored as a clinical target in LGGs. It has been recently reported to be a predictor of hypermutation in LGGs at the time of recurrence. Mathur et al. demonstrated in 2020 that methylation-based silencing of *MGMT* expression enhances mutagenic processes caused by temozolomide in LGGs, thus leading to the development of hypermutation in these tumors. Further, analysis of DNA methylome of genes involved in DNA damage repair in the EORTC 22033 trial cohort has demonstrated that patients having a high MGMT-STP27 score, which measures methylation status, prognosticates those patients of IDHmt LGGs who are most likely to benefit from temozolomide chemotherapy [56]. Meanwhile, work from UCSF has demonstrated that temozolomide positively selects for tumor cells with *MGMT* hypermethylation in patients with LGGs lacking DNA mismatch repair (MMR) [57]. Given these and similar findings from the literature, *MGMT* promoter methylation is likely to serve as a useful biomarker for predicting response to therapy and risk of hypermutation at recurrence [56–58].

In addition to the involvement of DNA methylation in cellular processes in LGGs, errors in DNA methylation also predispose to mutations. Compared to cytosine (C), methylated cytosine residues (mC) are more prone to deamination, i.e., loss of the amine (-NH2) group, forming thymine residues, which are less likely to be repaired accurately [45]. This mutational event then changes the DNA sequence, which is the primary driver of the sequence of corresponding messenger RNA, leading to abnormalities in structure, quantity, or function in subsequent protein synthesis. Thus, 'CpG Islands' are more prone to mutations than human DNA sequences in general. One pertinent example is the glioma CpG island methylator phenotype (G-CIMP), a pattern of genetic changes that includes MGMT methylation, which is often associated with the presence of *IDH1* or *IDH2* gene mutations. G-CIMP, while quite underexplored in LGGs, likely represents a major avenue for future research given that Grade 2 astrocytoma (IDHmt) and oligodendroglioma (IDHmt, 1p/19q codeletion) are both characteristically associated with G-CIMP. This attribute gains importance given that, amongst WHO Grade 2/3 astrocytomas, oligodendrogliomas, and glioblastomas developing from these lower grade entities, IDH1 mutation occurs at codon number 132 in over two-thirds of these, with IDH2 mutations occurring in 6% of them [13]. Given that MGMT resides on chromosome 10, it has been reported that compared to GBM, where at least one copy of chromosome 10 is lost, IDHmt lower-grade gliomas do not lose either copy. Thus, sufficient silencing of the MGMT gene may not occur in these IDHmt gliomas, leading to MGMT expression, followed by remnant capacity for DNA repair. This is the likely cause behind the resistance of IDHmt gliomas to temozolomide chemotherapy, compared to GBM [45]. Additionally, the deletion of 1p36 has been demonstrated to occur in nearly 73% of oligodendrogliomas and 18% of astrocytomas, while the deletion of 19q13.3 chromosome has been found to occur in 73% of oligodendrogliomas and 38% of astrocytomas. 1p/19q-codeletion has been demonstrated to occur in nearly 64% of oligodendrogliomas and 11% of astrocytomas [59,60].

Additionally, methylation is known to alter the overall 3-dimensional organization of chromatin protein used for DNA compaction. Chromatin consists of loops or topology-associated domains (TADs), which are normally conserved and maintained across cells [45]. The architecture of TADs has been demonstrated to be disturbed in IDHmt gliomas, causing excessive oncogene and anti-apoptotic factor expression [61,62]. One example is the Cohesin and CCCTC-binding factor (CTCF), whose alteration affects the organization of TADs [45].

DNA methylation has also recently been implicated in the functioning of the Telomerase Reverse Transcriptase (TERT) gene, whose function is visually described in Figure 4. TERT-promoter mutations (TERT-pmt) are known to be amongst the most common and the earliest mutations in the most invasive gliomas [63–67]. TERT mutations have been reported to be closely associated with *IDH1/2* mutations and 1p/19q-codeletion in oligodendroglioma, but less well correlated in astrocytomas [68,69]. It has been hypothesized that TERT promoter mutations enhance the neoplastic potential of tumors with low rates of self-renewal, such as low-grade gliomas [70]. Where methylation additionally plays a role is in the regulation of the TERT gene, whose promoter region has elements called "GC boxes". These GC-base pair rich DNA sequences preferentially bind to the transcriptional activator SP1, leading to increased gene expression. These GC boxes are closely regulated through DNA methylation [71]. Furthermore, hypermethylation of the TERT promoter region has been demonstrated to be one factor behind the dysregulation of TERT function in cancer cells [72–74]. Uniquely, TERT hypermethylated oncological region (THOR), a 433-bp sequence, has been reported to be a region where methylation leads to increased transcriptional TERT activity. It is situated just upstream of the TERT promoter region and contains 52 CpG sites. THOR hypermethylation has been demonstrated to play a role in the pathogenesis and/or outcomes of several pediatric brain tumors, including gliomas [75–77].

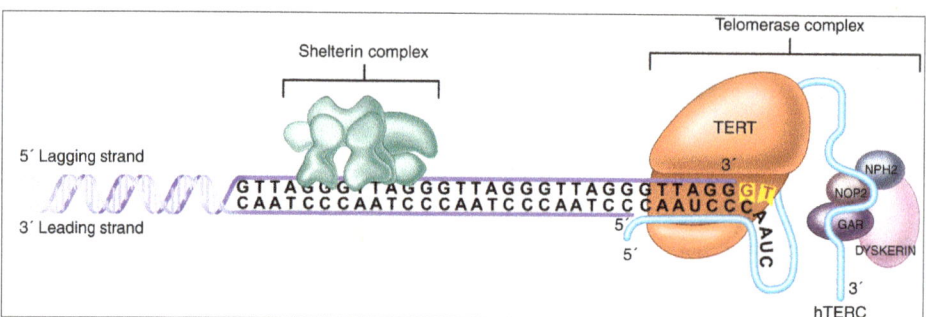

Figure 4. Mechanism of action of TERT enzyme, whose regulation is impacted by methylation of promoter and upstream THOR sequence. In the figure, TERT accesses the telomere complex at the terminal end of the DNA strand, through the Shelterin complex. It then catalyzes the addition of telomere repeat segments with the help of the hTERC enzyme, in a structure called Telomerase Complex. The latter's function of telomere elongation works against the routine telomere shortening that occurs during DNA replication. Figure reproduced under Creative Commons Attribution-Noncommercial 4.0 License from [74].

DNA methylation, within the context of low-grade gliomas, also plays a role in the regulation of the ADP-ribosylation factor-like (ARL) family of genes. The ADP-ribosylation factor (ARF) family of proteins, a part of the RAS superfamily, had been previously demonstrated to play a part in the pathogenesis of both glioblastoma and lower-grade gliomas [78–80]. Utilizing the TCGA database, Tan et al. recently identified low expression of ARL9 mRNA, along with ARL9 hypermethylation, which had hitherto been unexplored in LGGs, as positive prognostic factors in LGG [81]. The ARL9 protein expression was reported as correlating with CD8 T-cells in the LGG tissue, indicating the role of ARL9 methylation in tumor immune infiltration [81].

Broad prognostic signatures based on epigenetics have been very recently developed for low-grade gliomas. A two-CpG site DNA methylation signature (GALNT9 and TMTC4, both of whose expressions are highly dependent on methylation) has been recently identified that correlated highly with prognosis, regardless of the age, WHO grade, family history of cancer, and IDH mutation status [82]. Similarly, three methylation-driven genes (ARL9, CMYA5, STEAP3) have been recently identified as independent prognostic factors for survival in LGGs [83].

Overall, DNA methylation is an important mechanism for regulating gene expression in cancer cells, including LGGs, through several pathways (Figure 5). Alterations in DNA methylation lead to changes in gene expression that can result in neoplastic processes. The precise pattern of DNA methylation likely varies between cells of different grades and types of LGGs, being influenced by several factors, most of which are under investigation.

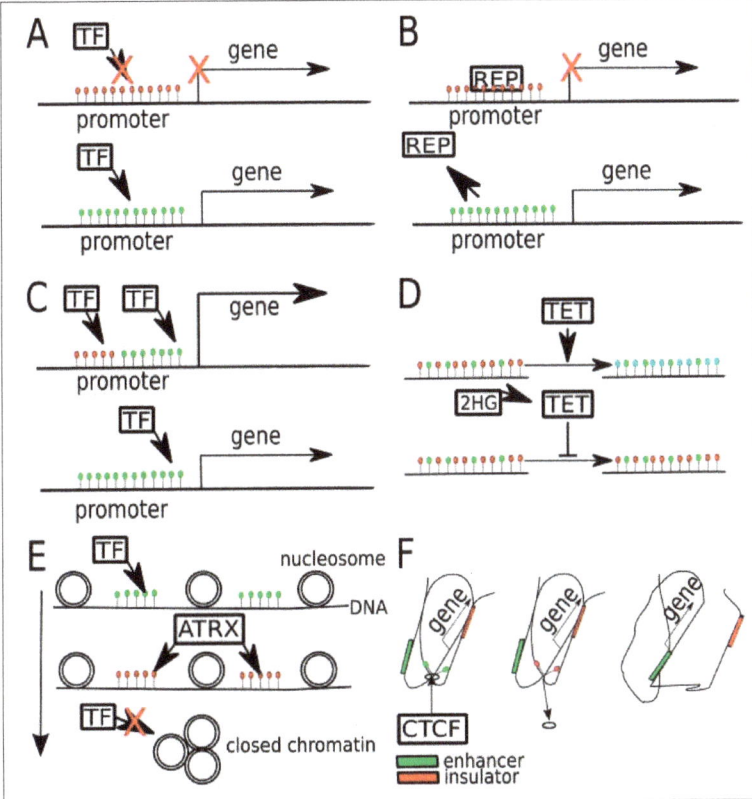

Figure 5. Potential targets in the various pathways where DNA methylation plays a role in regulating gene expression in gliomas. (Green dots are unmethylated Cytosine, red dots are 5-methylCytosine;

blue dots are 5-hydroxymethylcytosine). (**A**) Promoter hypermethylation may prevent the binding of transcriptional factors (TF), i.e., activator, leading to gene silencing. (**B**) In some other cases, a hypermethylated promoter may bind to the transcriptional repressor (REP) preferentially. When active demethylation occurs, REP is unable to bind and gene expression occurs. (**C**) In another gene, there may occur binding by two transcriptional factors (TFs), one to a methylated sequence and another to an unmethylated sequence. (**D**) In normal cells, TET enzymes convert 5mc to 5hmc and later into 5cac for maintenance purposes. When 2-Hydroxyglutarate (2-HG), a byproduct of mutant IDH enzymes, inhibits TET, a state of global hypermethylation occurs. (**E**) Relationship between DNA methylation and chromatin compaction. The latter is regulated by chromatin chaperones that are in turn affected by DNA methylation, histone methylation, and histone acetylation. ATRX binding to methylated gene sequences leads to an increased proportion of heterochromatin, thus reducing the binding of transcriptional factors (TFs) to DNA. (**F**) When CTCTF binding sites on the genome are methylated, then CTCF is unable to bind, leading to alteration in chromatin compaction. This causes an exchange of an insulator by an enhancer near the said sequence. Figure reproduced, with color correction, under Creative Commons Attribution-Noncommercial 4.0 license from [45].

5. Overview of Histone Modification

Histones are proteins that DNA is wrapped around to compact DNA in the nucleus. Together, an octamer of histones, with DNA wrapped around it, form a nucleosome, which is the functional unit of chromatin [84].

Histones are traditionally highly conserved across species. Post-translational modification of the histone typically occurs at one end, called the N-terminal tail, and is a significant epigenetic mechanism. This modification could be phosphorylation, ADP ribosylation, methylation, or acetylation, among others [85]. Methylation and acetylation, for example, are processes by which methyl and acetyl groups, respectively, are added to their amino acid residues in an enzyme-dependent fashion. These modifications can also change the expression of a DNA segment, without changing the underlying sequence.

Histone methylation is carried out by enzymes called histone methyltransferases, which transfer a methyl group from S-adenosylmethionine (SAM) to the histone protein. The particular residue that is methylated, and the number of methyl groups added, can vary and can have different effects on gene expression. For example, the addition of a single methyl group to a lysine residue on a histone protein (mono-methylation) can have a relatively mild effect on gene expression, while the addition of three methyl groups to the same residue (tri-methylation) can have a much stronger effect. Typically, methylation causes transcription dysregulation [85]. Figure 6 summarizes the differences in histone modification maps in healthy cells versus neoplastic ones.

Histone acetylation refers to the addition of an acetyl functional group, through a reaction between the hydrogen atom of a hydroxyl (-OH) group and an acetyl (CH3CO) group. This usually occurs on the lysine and arginine residues of histone proteins. Acetylation is carried out by histone acetyltransferases (HATs), while the reverse is carried out by histone deacetylases (HDACs). Acetylation of lysine weakens histone-DNA or inter-nucleosome interactions [86,87], altering chromatin conformation, and facilitating transcription. Conversely, deacetylation diminishes transcription. In normal cells, HATs and HDACs act in a dynamic equilibrium. Dysregulated acetylation, as in cancer cells, usually affects DNA transcription and repair [85].

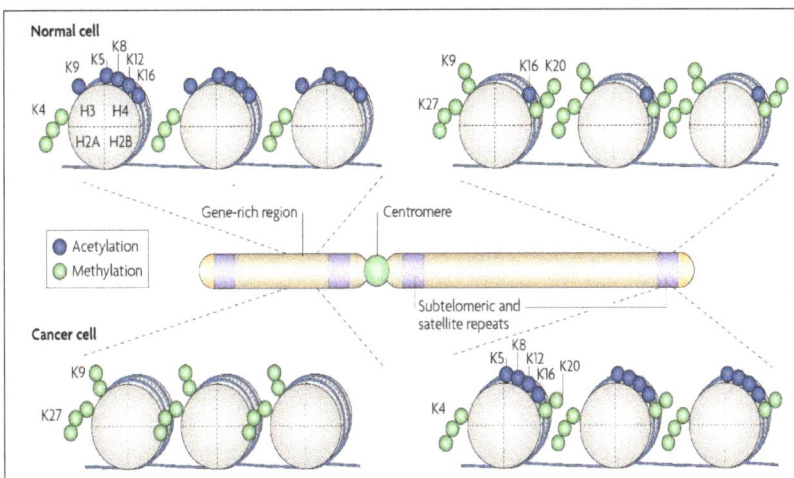

Figure 6. Histone modification maps for a typical chromosome in normal and cancer cells. In normal cells, DNA sequences that include the promoters of tumor-suppressor genes have more histone modification marks associated with active transcription, such as acetylation of H3 and H4 lysine residues (e.g., K5, K8, K9, K12, and K16) along with trimethylation of K4 residue of H3 protein. The normal cell also has DNA repeats and other heterochromatic regions having repressive histone marks, such as trimethylation of K27 residue and dimethylation of the K9 residue of H3, and trimethylation of K20 of H4. In cancer cells, there is a loss of the "active" histone marks on promoters of tumor-suppressor genes, leading to a tighter chromatin configuration. Additionally, the neoplastic cell has a loss of repressive marks at subtelomeric DNA and other repeat regions, causing a more "relaxed" chromatin conformation in these regions. Figure reproduced with permission from [28].

6. Histone Modification in LGGs

Histone modifications have been studied far more in high-grade gliomas, and the advances made there have not yet translated into the field of LGGs, but significant potential for translational research exists here. In particular, in diffuse midline gliomas, the H3K27M alteration has been shown to confer poor prognosis. Here, the H3 subunit, referring to either H3.1 or its variant H3.3, is subject to post-translational modifications, including methylation and acetylation. Typically, in the H3K27M alteration, methionine substitutes lysine at residue 27, resulting in halted post-transcriptional silencing by trimethylation. This modification resembles a gain-of-function mutation that enables the inhibition of polycomb repressive complex 2 (PRC2), as well as an increase in histone hypomethylation [88,89]. Additionally, it has become clear that the H3 variant also matters. H3.1K27M commonly co-occurs with activin-receptor type 1 (ACVR1) and phosphoinositide 3-kinase (PI3K), while the H3.3K27M commonly occurs with deletions of tumor suppressor 53 (TP53) and amplification of platelet-derived growth factor, with the latter shown to be significantly more aggressive and less differentiated [89,90]. Given the shared attributes of precursor cells of origin for LGGs and HGGs, these specific findings need investigation in LGGs as well.

Central to the advances made in histone modifications in LGGs has been the seminal discovery of IDH mutations as a genetic signature of most LGGs [91]. In IDHmt glioma cells, the disrupted metabolism of 2-hydroxyglutarate is key to their oncogenesis. As opposed to the conversion of isocitrate to alpha-ketoglutarate (α-KG) in IDHwt cells, IDHmt cells convert α-KG to 2-HG at supraphysiologic levels. This results in 2-HG levels several-fold higher than in IDHwt cells [92], with decreased levels of α-KG. 2-HG accumulation is likely a key step in gliomagenesis, which sets the stage for multiple later mutations [91]. 2-HG has been shown to alter DNA repair mechanisms, particularly the homologous recombination (HR) pathway, as well as multiple key cellular metabolic and oxidative pathways [93,94].

With respect to histones, 2-HG accumulation promotes methylation, through the inhibition of Jumonji-C-domain histone demethylases (JHDMs) [91,95–97]. These cumulative effects result in the G-CIMP phenotype of LGGs [91]. Further, as in pediatric diffuse gliomas, IDH1 mutations that cause H3K27 or H3K36 methylation have been implicated in progression from LGGs to GBM, i.e., secondary GBM [98].

7. Current State of Therapeutics

Table 2 summarizes ongoing (as of 13 January 2023) clinical trials in IDH-mutant LGGs, which broadly indicate that therapies targeting DNA and histone modification are gaining increasing cognizance.

Table 2. Ongoing clinical trials in IDH-mutant LGGs. Adapted under Creative Commons Attribution 4.0 International (CC BY 4.) License from [91].

NCT Number	Phase	Population	Study Medication	Current Status *
NCT04164901	3	Residual or recurrent IDH1/2-mt grade 2 gliomas	Vorasidenib (AG-881) versus placebo	Active, not recruiting
NCT03684811	1/2	Advanced IDH1-mt gliomas, GBM, other solid tumors (hepatocellular carcinoma; bile duct carcinoma; cholangiocarcinoma; other hepatobiliary carcinomas; chondrosarcoma)	FT-2102 with azacitidine (for gliomas)	Completed
NCT03991832	2	Advanced IDHmt gliomas, other solid tumors (cholangiocarcinoma and others)	Durvalumab and Olaparib	Recruiting
NCT03557359	2	Recurrent/progressive IDH-mut gliomas	Nivolumab	Active, not recruiting
NCT03718767	2	IDHmt gliomas	Nivolumab	Recruiting
NCT03212274	2	IDH1/2-mt gliomas (WHO grade 2, 3, GBM, recurrent), other solid tumors (cholangiocarcinoma, others)	Olaparib	Recruiting
NCT03561870	2	Recurrent IDHmt gliomas, high-grade gliomas	Olaparib	Completed
NCT03749187	1	IDH1/2-mt gliomas	PARP inhibitor (BGB-290) and TMZ	Recruiting
NCT03914742	1/2	Recurrent IDH1/2-mt gliomas	PARP inhibitor (BGB-290) and TMZ	Active, not recruiting
NCT03666559	2	Recurrent IDH1/2-mt gliomas	Azacitidine	Recruiting
NCT03922555	1	Recurrent/progressive non-enhancing IDHmt gliomas	ASTX727 (cedazuridine + cytidine antimetabolite decitabine)	Recruiting

NCT—National Clinical Trials, IDH—isocitrate dehydrogenase; IHDmt—IDH mutant, GBM—glioblastoma * As of 13 January 2023.

Based on the current understanding of the role of epigenetics in LGGs, several potential targets have emerged, albeit with preclinical data. Ongoing and completed trials remain in the early phases, and a long wait for definitive results is anticipated.

7.1. Therapeutics Targeting IDH1/2 Mutations

Given the central role of the IDH mutation in LGGs as a driver mutation and its role in downstream epigenetic modification, it is worth discussing attempts at targeting IDH1/2 mutations in LGGs. Data from completed clinical trials targeting IDH, all of which have been phase I trials, are summarized in Table 3.

Table 3. Completed clinical trials with IDH-targeted therapies in glioma cells. Adapted under Creative Commons Attribution 4.0 International (CC BY 4.0) License from [91].

Study	Drug	Population	Key Findings	Adverse Events (>10% Patients)
Mellinghoff et al., 2020 [99]	Ivosidenib (AG-120)	Advanced IDH1-mt solid tumors 35 non-enhancing recurrent gliomas, 31 enhancing recurrent gliomas	500mg once daily selected for expansion cohort DCR 88% vs. 45%; median PFS 13.6 vs. 1.4 months in non-enhancing vs. enhancing cohort	No DLT Headache, fatigue, nausea, vomiting, seizure, diarrhea, aphasia, hyperglycemia, neutropenia, depression, hypophosphatemia, paresthesia
Mellinghoff et al., 2021 [100]	Vorasidenib (AG-188)	Advanced IDH1/2mt solid tumors 22 non-enhancing recurrent gliomas, 30 enhancing recurrent gliomas	Recommended dose < 100 mg in gliomas Non-enhancing glioma: ORR 18% (1 PR; 3 minor responses; 17 SD) Enhancing glioma: ORR 0% (17 SD) Median PFS: 36.8 vs. 3.6 months in non-enhancing vs. enhancing groups	DLT (grade 2 ALT/AST increase) in 5 pts at 100 mg dose levels Headache, AST/ALT increase, fatigue, nausea, seizure, hyperglycemia, vomiting, constipation, dizziness, neutropenia, cough, diarrhea, aphasia, hypoglycemia
Mellinghoff et al., 2019 [101]	Perioperative Ivosidenib (n = 13) or Vorasidenib (n = 14)	Recurrent non-enhancing IDH1-mt LGGs undergoing craniotomy	2-HG concentration 92% (ivosidenib), 92.5% (vorasidenib) lower in resected tumor tissue of treated patients	Diarrhea, constipation, hypocalcemia, nausea, anemia, hyperglycemia, pruritus, headache, fatigue
Wick et al., 2021 [102]	BAY-1436032	Advanced IDH1-mt solid tumors 26 LGG astrocytoma, 13 LGG oligodendroglioma, 16 GBM	1500 mg twice daily selected for expansion cohorts LGG: ORR 11% (1 CR; 3 PR; 15 SD) GBM: ORR 0%, SD 29%. PFS-rate at three months: 0.31 vs. 0.22 in LGG vs. GBM	No DLT Fatigue, dysguesia
Natsume et al., 2019 [103]	DS-100b	Recurrent/progressive IDH1-mt glioma	125–1400 mg twice daily Non-enhancing glioma (n = 9): 2 minor responses; 7 SD Enhancing glioma (n = 29): 1 CR; 3 PR; 10 SD	DLT (grade 3 WBC decrease) at 1000mg twice daily Skin hyperpigmentation, diarrhea, pruritus, nausea, rash, headache
Platten et al., 2021 [104]	IDH1-vac	Newly diagnosed IDHmt grade 3/4 astrocytomas	93.3% IDH1-vac induced immune response 3 years PFS: 63%, 3 years OS: 84%	No RLTs Mild site reactions

2-HG—2-Hydroxyglutarate; ALT—alanine transaminase; AST—aspartate transaminase; CR—complete response; DCR—disease control rate; DLT—dose-limiting toxicity; GBM—glioblastoma; IDH—isocitrate dehydrogenase; LGG—low-grade glioma; ORR—objective response rate; OS—overall survival; PFS—progression-free survival; PR—partial response; RLT—regime-limiting toxicity; SD—stable disease; WBC—white blood cells.

IDH mutations, as well as the downstream accumulation of 2-HG [91], have been the focus of some of the earliest attempts for translating epigenetics from bench-to-bedside in LGGs, although preclinical results have been mixed. While Rohle et al. found reduced

2-HG levels and slowed growth in glioma xenografts by AG-5198 in 2013 [105], in later years, subsequent groups failed to show encouraging outcomes, be it regarding tumor size, DNA, or histone methylation [91]. In mouse IDHmt models, AG-120, a successor of AGI-5198, was found to be highly effective, leading to demonstrably lower levels of 2-HG, and reduced cell proliferation [106]. Later investigated drugs of the same class include BT142 and GB10, with only BT142 showing tumor growth inhibition in xenografts [107].

With discoveries that 2-HG greatly contributes to glioma immune escape and immunosuppressive mechanisms, immunotherapy targeting IDH mutations has been another promising avenue [91,108]. IDHmt vaccines targeting specific epitopes demonstrated efficacy in a glioma model [109]. More recently, Kadiyala et al. demonstrated significantly improved outcomes in IDH1-mt gliomas in mice, with the administration of a targeted inhibitor, either alone, or with radiation and TMZ [91,110].

Similarly, the effect of 2-HG on the HR pathway of DNA repair has been investigated [91,94]. IDHmt LGG cells have defective DNA repair, especially in the HR pathway, which is the most preferred mechanism of repair in most cells [93]. This, along with its backup mechanism, the alternative end-joining pathway of DNA repair, is highly dependent on poly(ADP-ribose) polymerase (PARP) [94]. Thus, PARP inhibitors are under investigation, particularly in combination with radiotherapy (RT) or temozolomide (TMZ). Wang et al. and Higuchi et al., in their preclinical models, demonstrated that PARP inhibition's efficacy may be enhanced by combination with TMZ or RT [111,112]. Recent clinical trials include a phase II trial investigating PARP inhibitors (Olaparib) alone for IDHmt advanced gliomas (NCT03212274), and a phase II trial investigating Olaparib in recurrent IDHmt gliomas (NCT03561870). Combinations of PARP inhibitors are also being investigated—NCT03749187 is a trial of BGB-290, a novel PARP inhibitor in combination with TMZ for IDHmt gliomas of all grades, while NCT03914742 is investigating the same combination for recurrent IDHmt gliomas, and NCT03991832 is investigating Olaparib in combination with a checkpoint inhibitor, Durvalumab [91] (Table 2).

Further, some hypothesized therapeutic pathways involve exploiting metabolic and apoptotic vulnerabilities in IDHmt cells [91,94]. However, the caveat remains that some of these results are from IDHmt GBM isolates, or isolates of other tumors, not from LGG-specific cell cultures. Tateishi et al. demonstrated that IDHmt glioma cells had lowered NAD+ levels, a crucial cofactor for cellular metabolism. Further, their team found that these cells were sensitive to inhibitors of nicotinamide phosphoribosyl transferase (NAMPT), an enzyme necessary for NAD+ synthesis [113]. NCT02702492 is an ongoing Phase I trial that is investigating KPT-9274, one such agent, in IDHmt solid tumors. In IDHmt tumor models, the presence of raised 2-HG levels was shown to trigger apoptosis by suppressing BCL-2, causing altered mitochondrial metabolism and apoptosis [65,91,94]. Another group of authors found that ABT263, a BCL-2 and BCL-xL inhibitor, was lethal to IDHmt glioma cells [94,114]. One avenue includes altering the production of 2-HG, by halting its production from α-KG. α-KG is produced from glutamate, and reducing glutaminase activity has been shown to reduce the growth and increase the sensitivity of IDHmt glioma cells to radiation [91]. Finally, IDHmt glioma cells have been shown to specifically exhibit greater levels of Notch ligand delta-like 3 (DLL3) RNA and were sensitive to anti-DLL3 antibodies [115]. The caveat to these advances, besides the fact that they are at the preclinical level, remains that most results are from studies on GBM-derived cells, or even IDHmt cells from other cancers. Regardless, they may provide some cause for cautious optimism.

7.2. Therapeutics in DNA Methylation, Histone Modification, and Other Domains of Epigenetics in LGGs

DNA demethylating agents, or DNA methyltransferase inhibitors (DNMTIs), were investigated early on [91], given the hypermethylated phenotype of IDHmt gliomas. Preclinical glioma models investigating long-term 5-azacitidine and decitabine demonstrated significant tumor growth inhibition [116,117], which another group of authors demonstrated to be enhanced by combination with temozolomide [118]. However, these results have not yet been translated to the clinical setting. In a clinical trial of 12 patients with IDHmt recurrent gliomas (astrocytic or oligodendroglial histology), 5-azacitidine demonstrated minimal activity [119]. Current ongoing trials include those testing 5-azacytidine, either as a single agent or in combination with IDHmt inhibitors (NCT03666559, NCT03684811), while another phase I trial is ongoing to evaluate ASTX727, a combination of decitabine and a cytidine deaminase inhibitor in recurrent or progressive IDHmt gliomas (NCT03922555) [91] (Table 2).

Despite prior knowledge of their presence, the role of histone modifications in LGG therapeutics has come to the fore only in recent years [45]. The clinical utility of histone modification in LGGs is best exemplified through the Histone Deacetylase (HDAC) inhibitors. Panobinostat achieved feasibility in Phase I trials using glioma cells, and FDA approval for off-label use for diffuse gliomas [89]. Its combinations with the proteasome inhibitor marizomib have also been explored in preclinical studies [89,120] (Cooney et al., 2020; Kilburn et al., 2018). Finally, it has also been demonstrated that valproate, the well-known antiepileptic, and Panabinostat both inhibit IDHmt glioma cell lines [91].

Finally, Bromodomain and Extra-Terminal Motif (BET) inhibitors are a target of promise. BET proteins are key in epigenetic regulation, and promote the expression of multiple oncogenes [91]. IDHmt glioma cells have been found to be sensitive to two BET inhibitors (JQ1 and GS-626510) [121].

8. Conclusions

Several prognostic biomarkers and potential therapeutic targets may be identified in cellular structures and processes associated with DNA methylation and histone modification in low-grade gliomas. Diagnostic and/or therapeutic targeting of MGMT promoter methylation, TET-hTDG-BER pathway, G-CIMP association, PARP inhibition, IDH and 2-HG-associated processes, TERT mutation and ARL9-associated pathways, DNA Methyltransferase (DNMT) inhibition, Histone Deacetylase (HDAC) inhibition, BET inhibition, and CpG site DNA methylation signature, along with others, present exciting avenues for translational research. However, much of the evidence remains restricted to preclinical studies, warranting further investigation to demonstrate true clinical utility.

Author Contributions: Conceptualization, A.O., M.S.A.; Writing—Original Draft Preparation, A.O., V.B.; Writing—Review and Editing, A.O., V.B., R.S.A., A.A.K., M.W.M.; Supervision, R.R.K., Y.O., M.W.M., M.S.A. All authors have read and agreed to the published version of the manuscript.

Funding: This research received no external funding.

Institutional Review Board Statement: Not applicable as this is a review of prior literature.

Informed Consent Statement: Not applicable as this is a review of prior literature.

Data Availability Statement: Not Applicable as no datasets generated in the work.

Conflicts of Interest: Rupesh Kotecha: Personal fees from Accuray Inc., Elekta AB, ViewRay Inc., Novocure Inc., Elsevier Inc., Brainlab, Kazia Therapeutics, Castle Biosciences, and institutional research funding from Medtronic Inc., Blue Earth Diagnostics Ltd., Novocure Inc., GT Medical Technologies, AstraZeneca, Exelixis, ViewRay Inc., Brainlab, Cantex Pharmaceuticals, and Kazia Therapeutics. Manmeet Singh Ahluwalia: Grants from AstraZeneca, BMS, Bayer, Incyte, Pharmacyclics, Novocure, MimiVax, Merck. Consultation fees from Bayer, Novocure, Kiyatec, Insightec, GSK, Xoft, Nuvation, Cellularity, SDP Oncology, Apollomics, Prelude, Janssen, Tocagen, Voyager Therapeutics, Viewray, Caris Lifesciences, Pyramid Biosciences, Varian Medical Systems, Cairn Therapeutics, Anheart Therapeutics, Theraguix. Scientific Advisory Board membership of Cairn Therapeutics, Pyramid Biosciences, Modifi Biosciences, Guardian Research Network. Stock shareholder of MimiVax, Cytodyn, MedInnovate Advisors LLC, The rest of the authors declare no conflict of interest relevant to the manuscript.

References

1. Schiff, D. Low-grade gliomas. *Continuum (Minneap Minn)* **2015**, *21*, 345–354. [CrossRef]
2. Jooma, R.; Waqas, M.; Khan, I. Diffuse Low-Grade Glioma—Changing Concepts in Diagnosis and Management: A Review. *Asian J. Neurosurg.* **2019**, *14*, 356–363. [CrossRef]
3. Ohgaki, H.; Kleihues, P. Epidemiology and etiology of gliomas. *Acta Neuropathol.* **2005**, *109*, 93–108. [CrossRef]
4. Ostrom, Q.T.; Price, M.; Neff, C.; Cioffi, G.; Waite, K.A.; Kruchko, C.; Barnholtz-Sloan, J.S. CBTRUS Statistical Report: Primary Brain and Other Central Nervous System Tumors Diagnosed in the United States in 2015–2019. *Neuro Oncol.* **2022**, *24*, v1–v95. [CrossRef]
5. Louis, D.N.; Perry, A.; Wesseling, P.; Brat, D.J.; Cree, I.A.; Figarella-Branger, D.; Hawkins, C.; Ng, H.K.; Pfister, S.M.; Reifenberger, G.; et al. The 2021 WHO Classification of Tumors of the Central Nervous System: A summary. *Neuro Oncol.* **2021**, *23*, 1231–1251. [CrossRef]
6. Forst, D.A.; Nahed, B.V.; Loeffler, J.S.; Batchelor, T.T. Low-grade gliomas. *Oncologist* **2014**, *19*, 403–413. [CrossRef]
7. Schiff, D.; Van den Bent, M.; Vogelbaum, M.A.; Wick, W.; Miller, C.R.; Taphoorn, M.; Pope, W.; Brown, P.D.; Platten, M.; Jalali, R.; et al. Recent developments and future directions in adult lower-grade gliomas: Society for Neuro-Oncology (SNO) and European Association of Neuro-Oncology (EANO) consensus. *Neuro Oncol.* **2019**, *21*, 837–853. [CrossRef]
8. Weller, M.; van den Bent, M.; Tonn, J.C.; Stupp, R.; Preusser, M.; Cohen-Jonathan-Moyal, E.; Henriksson, R.; Le Rhun, E.; Balana, C.; Chinot, O.; et al. European Association for Neuro-Oncology (EANO) guideline on the diagnosis and treatment of adult astrocytic and oligodendroglial gliomas. *Lancet Oncol.* **2017**, *18*, e315–e329. [CrossRef]
9. Weller, M.; van den Bent, M.; Preusser, M.; Le Rhun, E.; Tonn, J.C.; Minniti, G.; Bendszus, M.; Balana, C.; Chinot, O.; Dirven, L.; et al. EANO guidelines on the diagnosis and treatment of diffuse gliomas of adulthood. *Nat. Rev. Clin. Oncol.* **2021**, *18*, 170–186. [CrossRef]
10. Louis, D.N.; Ohgaki, H.; Wiestler, O.D.; Cavenee, W.K.; Burger, P.C.; Jouvet, A.; Scheithauer, B.W.; Kleihues, P. The 2007 WHO classification of tumours of the central nervous system. *Acta Neuropathol.* **2007**, *114*, 97–109. [CrossRef]
11. Hartmann, C.; Hentschel, B.; Tatagiba, M.; Schramm, J.; Schnell, O.; Seidel, C.; Stein, R.; Reifenberger, G.; Pietsch, T.; von Deimling, A.; et al. Molecular markers in low-grade gliomas: Predictive or prognostic? *Clin. Cancer Res.* **2011**, *17*, 4588–4599. [CrossRef]
12. Capper, D.; Jones, D.T.W.; Sill, M.; Hovestadt, V.; Schrimpf, D.; Sturm, D.; Koelsche, C.; Sahm, F.; Chavez, L.; Reuss, D.E.; et al. DNA methylation-based classification of central nervous system tumours. *Nature* **2018**, *555*, 469–474. [CrossRef]
13. Yan, H.; Parsons, D.W.; Jin, G.; McLendon, R.; Rasheed, B.A.; Yuan, W.; Kos, I.; Batinic-Haberle, I.; Jones, S.; Riggins, G.J.; et al. IDH1 and IDH2 mutations in gliomas. *N. Engl. J. Med.* **2009**, *360*, 765–773. [CrossRef]
14. Brat, D.J.; Aldape, K.; Colman, H.; Figarella-Branger, D.; Fuller, G.N.; Giannini, C.; Holland, E.C.; Jenkins, R.B.; Kleinschmidt-DeMasters, B.; Komori, T.; et al. cIMPACT-NOW update 5: Recommended grading criteria and terminologies for IDH-mutant astrocytomas. *Acta Neuropathol.* **2020**, *139*, 603–608. [CrossRef]
15. Wiestler, B.; Capper, D.; Sill, M.; Jones, D.T.; Hovestadt, V.; Sturm, D.; Koelsche, C.; Bertoni, A.; Schweizer, L.; Korshunov, A.; et al. Integrated DNA methylation and copy-number profiling identify three clinically and biologically relevant groups of anaplastic glioma. *Acta Neuropathol.* **2014**, *128*, 561–571. [CrossRef]
16. Suzuki, H.; Aoki, K.; Chiba, K.; Sato, Y.; Shiozawa, Y.; Shiraishi, Y.; Shimamura, T.; Niida, A.; Motomura, K.; Ohka, F.; et al. Mutational landscape and clonal architecture in grade II and III gliomas. *Nat. Genet.* **2015**, *47*, 458–468. [CrossRef]
17. Louis, D.N.; Perry, A.; Reifenberger, G.; von Deimling, A.; Figarella-Branger, D.; Cavenee, W.K.; Ohgaki, H.; Wiestler, O.D.; Kleihues, P.; Ellison, D.W. The 2016 World Health Organization Classification of Tumors of the Central Nervous System: A summary. *Acta Neuropathol.* **2016**, *131*, 803–820. [CrossRef]
18. Brat, D.J.; Verhaak, R.G.; Aldape, K.D.; Yung, W.K.; Salama, S.R.; Cooper, L.A.; Rheinbay, E.; Miller, C.R.; Vitucci, M.; Morozova, O.; et al. Comprehensive, Integrative Genomic Analysis of Diffuse Lower-Grade Gliomas. *N. Engl. J. Med.* **2015**, *372*, 2481–2498.
19. Louis, D.N.; Aldape, K.; Brat, D.J.; Capper, D.; Ellison, D.W.; Hawkins, C.; Paulus, W.; Perry, A.; Reifenberger, G.; Figarella-Branger, D.; et al. Announcing cIMPACT-NOW: The Consortium to Inform Molecular and Practical Approaches to CNS Tumor Taxonomy. *Acta Neuropathol.* **2017**, *133*, 1–3. [CrossRef]
20. Louis, D.N.; Wesseling, P.; Aldape, K.; Brat, D.J.; Capper, D.; Cree, I.A.; Eberhart, C.; Figarella-Branger, D.; Fouladi, M.; Fuller, G.N.; et al. cIMPACT-NOW update 6: New entity and diagnostic principle recommendations of the cIMPACT-Utrecht meeting on future CNS tumor classification and grading. *Brain Pathol.* **2020**, *30*, 844–856. [CrossRef]
21. Gonzalez Castro, L.N.; Wesseling, P. The cIMPACT-NOW updates and their significance to current neuro-oncology practice. *Neurooncol. Pract.* **2021**, *8*, 4–10. [CrossRef]
22. Ozair, A.; Khan, E.; Bhat, V.; Faruqi, A.; Nanda, A. Pediatric CNS Tumors: From Modern Classification System to Current Principles of Management. In *Central Nervous System Tumors*, 1st ed.; Turner, F., Ed.; InTechOpen: London, UK, 2021.
23. Mahajan, S.; Suri, V.; Sahu, S.; Sharma, M.C.; Sarkar, C. World Health Organization Classification of Tumors of the Central Nervous System 5(th) Edition (WHO CNS5): What's new? *Indian J. Pathol. Microbiol.* **2022**, *65*, S5–S13.
24. Wen, P.Y.; Packer, R.J. The 2021 WHO Classification of Tumors of the Central Nervous System: Clinical implications. *Neuro Oncol.* **2021**, *23*, 1215–1217. [CrossRef]
25. Komori, T. The 2021 WHO classification of tumors, 5th edition, central nervous system tumors: The 10 basic principles. *Brain Tumor Pathol.* **2022**, *39*, 47–50. [CrossRef]

26. Mandonnet, E.; Delattre, J.Y.; Tanguy, M.L.; Swanson, K.R.; Carpentier, A.F.; Duffau, H.; Cornu, P.; Van Effenterre, R.; Alvord, E.C., Jr.; Capelle, L. Continuous growth of mean tumor diameter in a subset of grade II gliomas. *Ann. Neurol.* **2003**, *53*, 524–528. [CrossRef]
27. Pallud, J.; Blonski, M.; Mandonnet, E.; Audureau, E.; Fontaine, D.; Sanai, N.; Bauchet, L.; Peruzzi, P.; Frénay, M.; Colin, P.; et al. Velocity of tumor spontaneous expansion predicts long-term outcomes for diffuse low-grade gliomas. *Neuro Oncol.* **2013**, *15*, 595–606. [CrossRef]
28. Esteller, M. Cancer epigenomics: DNA methylomes and histone-modification maps. *Nat. Rev. Genet.* **2007**, *8*, 286–298. [CrossRef]
29. Portela, A.; Esteller, M. Epigenetic modifications and human disease. *Nat. Biotechnol.* **2010**, *28*, 1057–1068. [CrossRef]
30. Dubuc, A.M.; Mack, S.; Unterberger, A.; Northcott, P.A.; Taylor, M.D. The epigenetics of brain tumors. *Methods Mol. Biol.* **2012**, *863*, 139–153.
31. Hanahan, D.; Weinberg, R.A. The hallmarks of cancer. *Cell* **2000**, *100*, 57–70. [CrossRef]
32. Hanahan, D.; Weinberg, R.A. Hallmarks of cancer: The next generation. *Cell* **2011**, *144*, 646–674. [CrossRef] [PubMed]
33. Esteller, M. Aberrant DNA methylation as a cancer-inducing mechanism. *Annu. Rev. Pharmacol. Toxicol.* **2005**, *45*, 629–656. [CrossRef] [PubMed]
34. Goll, M.G.; Bestor, T.H. Eukaryotic cytosine methyltransferases. *Annu. Rev. Biochem.* **2005**, *74*, 481–514. [CrossRef] [PubMed]
35. Gusyatiner, O.; Hegi, M.E. Glioma epigenetics: From subclassification to novel treatment options. *Semin. Cancer Biol.* **2018**, *51*, 50–58. [CrossRef] [PubMed]
36. Hermann, A.; Gowher, H.; Jeltsch, A. Biochemistry and biology of mammalian DNA methyltransferases. *Cell Mol. Life Sci.* **2004**, *61*, 2571–2587. [CrossRef] [PubMed]
37. Deaton, A.M.; Bird, A. CpG islands and the regulation of transcription. *Genes Dev.* **2011**, *25*, 1010–1022. [CrossRef] [PubMed]
38. Esteller, M.; Corn, P.G.; Baylin, S.B.; Herman, J.G. A gene hypermethylation profile of human cancer. *Cancer Res.* **2001**, *61*, 3225–3229.
39. Yin, Y.; Morgunova, E.; Jolma, A.; Kaasinen, E.; Sahu, B.; Khund-Sayeed, S.; Das, P.K.; Kivioja, T.; Dave, K.; Zhong, F.; et al. Impact of cytosine methylation on DNA binding specificities of human transcription factors. *Science* **2017**, *356*, eaaj2239. [CrossRef]
40. Quina, A.S.; Buschbeck, M.; Di Croce, L. Chromatin structure and epigenetics. *Biochem. Pharmacol.* **2006**, *72*, 1563–1569. [CrossRef]
41. Huang, Y.; Rao, A. Connections between TET proteins and aberrant DNA modification in cancer. *Trends Genet.* **2014**, *30*, 464–474. [CrossRef]
42. Scourzic, L.; Mouly, E.; Bernard, O.A. TET proteins and the control of cytosine demethylation in cancer. *Genome Med.* **2015**, *7*, 9. [CrossRef]
43. Maiti, A.; Drohat, A.C. Thymine DNA glycosylase can rapidly excise 5-formylcytosine and 5-carboxylcytosine: Potential implications for active demethylation of CpG sites. *J. Biol. Chem.* **2011**, *286*, 35334–35338. [CrossRef]
44. Zhang, L.; Lu, X.; Lu, J.; Liang, H.; Dai, Q.; Xu, G.L.; Luo, C.; Jiang, H.; He, C. Thymine DNA glycosylase specifically recognizes 5-carboxylcytosine-modified DNA. *Nat. Chem. Biol.* **2012**, *8*, 328–330. [CrossRef] [PubMed]
45. Dabrowski, M.J.; Wojtas, B. Global DNA Methylation Patterns in Human Gliomas and Their Interplay with Other Epigenetic Modifications. *Int. J. Mol. Sci.* **2019**, *20*, 3478. [CrossRef]
46. Cheishvili, D.; Boureau, L.; Szyf, M. DNA demethylation and invasive cancer: Implications for therapeutics. *Br. J. Pharmacol.* **2015**, *172*, 2705–2715. [CrossRef] [PubMed]
47. Cui, X.L.; Nie, J.; Ku, J.; Dougherty, U.; West-Szymanski, D.C.; Collin, F.; Ellison, C.K.; Sieh, L.; Ning, Y.; Deng, Z.; et al. A human tissue map of 5-hydroxymethylcytosines exhibits tissue specificity through gene and enhancer modulation. *Nat. Commun.* **2020**, *11*, 6161. [CrossRef] [PubMed]
48. Ravichandran, M.; Jurkowska, R.Z.; Jurkowski, T.P. Target specificity of mammalian DNA methylation and demethylation machinery. *Org. Biomol. Chem.* **2018**, *16*, 1419–1435. [CrossRef] [PubMed]
49. Papanicolau-Sengos, A.; Aldape, K. DNA Methylation Profiling: An Emerging Paradigm for Cancer Diagnosis. *Annu. Rev. Pathol.* **2022**, *17*, 295–321. [CrossRef] [PubMed]
50. Pan, Y.; Liu, G.; Zhou, F.; Su, B.; Li, Y. DNA methylation profiles in cancer diagnosis and therapeutics. *Clin. Exp. Med.* **2018**, *18*, 1–14. [CrossRef]
51. Kulis, M.; Esteller, M. DNA methylation and cancer. *Adv. Genet.* **2010**, *70*, 27–56. [PubMed]
52. Nguyen, C.T.; Gonzales, F.A.; Jones, P.A. Altered chromatin structure associated with methylation-induced gene silencing in cancer cells: Correlation of accessibility, methylation, MeCP2 binding and acetylation. *Nucleic Acids Res.* **2001**, *29*, 4598–4606. [CrossRef]
53. Fahrner, J.A.; Eguchi, S.; Herman, J.G.; Baylin, S.B. Dependence of histone modifications and gene expression on DNA hypermethylation in cancer. *Cancer Res.* **2002**, *62*, 7213–7218.
54. Ballestar, E.; Paz, M.F.; Valle, L.; Wei, S.; Fraga, M.F.; Espada, J.; Cigudosa, J.C.; Huang, T.H.; Esteller, M. Methyl-CpG binding proteins identify novel sites of epigenetic inactivation in human cancer. *Embo J.* **2003**, *22*, 6335–6345. [CrossRef] [PubMed]
55. Mellai, M.; Monzeglio, O.; Piazzi, A.; Caldera, V.; Annovazzi, L.; Cassoni, P.; Valente, G.; Cordera, S.; Mocellini, C.; Schiffer, D. MGMT promoter hypermethylation and its associations with genetic alterations in a series of 350 brain tumors. *J. Neurooncol.* **2012**, *107*, 617–631. [CrossRef]

56. Bady, P.; Kurscheid, S.; Delorenzi, M.; Gorlia, T.; van den Bent, M.J.; Hoang-Xuan, K.; Vauléon, É.; Gijtenbeek, A.; Enting, R.; Thiessen, B.; et al. The DNA methylome of DDR genes and benefit from RT or TMZ in IDH mutant low-grade glioma treated in EORTC 22033. *Acta Neuropathol.* **2018**, *135*, 601–615. [CrossRef]
57. van Thuijl, H.F.; Mazor, T.; Johnson, B.E.; Fouse, S.D.; Aihara, K.; Hong, C.; Malmström, A.; Hallbeck, M.; Heimans, J.J.; Kloezeman, J.J.; et al. Evolution of DNA repair defects during malignant progression of low-grade gliomas after temozolomide treatment. *Acta Neuropathol.* **2015**, *129*, 597–607. [CrossRef]
58. Mathur, R.; Zhang, Y.; Grimmer, M.R.; Hong, C.; Zhang, M.; Bollam, S.; Petrecca, K.; Clarke, J.; Berger, M.S.; Phillips, J.J.; et al. MGMT promoter methylation level in newly diagnosed low-grade glioma is a predictor of hypermutation at recurrence. *Neuro Oncol.* **2020**, *22*, 1580–1590. [CrossRef] [PubMed]
59. Houillier, C.; Wang, X.; Kaloshi, G.; Mokhtari, K.; Guillevin, R.; Laffaire, J.; Paris, S.; Boisselier, B.; Idbaih, A.; Laigle-Donadey, F.; et al. IDH1 or IDH2 mutations predict longer survival and response to temozolomide in low-grade gliomas. *Neurology* **2010**, *75*, 1560–1566. [CrossRef] [PubMed]
60. Ricard, D.; Idbaih, A.; Ducray, F.; Lahutte, M.; Hoang-Xuan, K.; Delattre, J.Y. Primary brain tumours in adults. *Lancet* **2012**, *379*, 1984–1996. [CrossRef]
61. Harutyunyan, A.S.; Krug, B.; Chen, H.; Papillon-Cavanagh, S.; Zeinieh, M.; De Jay, N.; Deshmukh, S.; Chen, C.C.L.; Belle, J.; Mikael, L.G.; et al. H3K27M induces defective chromatin spread of PRC2-mediated repressive H3K27me2/me3 and is essential for glioma tumorigenesis. *Nat. Commun.* **2019**, *10*, 1262. [CrossRef]
62. Voon, H.P.J.; Udugama, M.; Lin, W.; Hii, L.; Law, R.H.P.; Steer, D.L.; Das, P.P.; Mann, J.R.; Wong, L.H. Inhibition of a K9/K36 demethylase by an H3.3 point mutation found in paediatric glioblastoma. *Nat. Commun.* **2018**, *9*, 3142. [CrossRef] [PubMed]
63. Labussière, M.; Boisselier, B.; Mokhtari, K.; Di Stefano, A.L.; Rahimian, A.; Rossetto, M.; Ciccarino, P.; Saulnier, O.; Paterra, R.; Marie, Y.; et al. Combined analysis of TERT, EGFR, and IDH status defines distinct prognostic glioblastoma classes. *Neurology* **2014**, *83*, 1200–1206. [CrossRef]
64. Killela, P.J.; Reitman, Z.J.; Jiao, Y.; Bettegowda, C.; Agrawal, N.; Diaz, L.A., Jr.; Friedman, A.H.; Friedman, H.; Gallia, G.L.; Giovanella, B.C.; et al. TERT promoter mutations occur frequently in gliomas and a subset of tumors derived from cells with low rates of self-renewal. *Proc. Natl. Acad. Sci. USA* **2013**, *110*, 6021–6026. [CrossRef] [PubMed]
65. Chan, A.K.; Yao, Y.; Zhang, Z.; Chung, N.Y.; Liu, J.S.; Li, K.K.; Shi, Z.; Chan, D.T.; Poon, W.S.; Zhou, L.; et al. TERT promoter mutations contribute to subset prognostication of lower-grade gliomas. *Mod. Pathol.* **2015**, *28*, 177–186. [CrossRef]
66. Karsy, M.; Guan, J.; Cohen, A.L.; Jensen, R.L.; Colman, H. New Molecular Considerations for Glioma: IDH, ATRX, BRAF, TERT, H3 K27M. *Curr. Neurol. Neurosci. Rep.* **2017**, *17*, 19. [CrossRef]
67. Ohba, S.; Kuwahara, K.; Yamada, S.; Abe, M.; Hirose, Y. Correlation between IDH, ATRX, and TERT promoter mutations in glioma. *Brain Tumor Pathol.* **2020**, *37*, 33–40. [CrossRef]
68. Arita, H.; Narita, Y.; Fukushima, S.; Tateishi, K.; Matsushita, Y.; Yoshida, A.; Miyakita, Y.; Ohno, M.; Collins, V.P.; Kawahara, N.; et al. Upregulating mutations in the TERT promoter commonly occur in adult malignant gliomas and are strongly associated with total 1p19q loss. *Acta Neuropathol.* **2013**, *126*, 267–276. [CrossRef] [PubMed]
69. Chan, S.M.; Thomas, D.; Corces-Zimmerman, M.R.; Xavy, S.; Rastogi, S.; Hong, W.J.; Zhao, F.; Medeiros, B.C.; Tyvoll, D.A.; Majeti, R. Isocitrate dehydrogenase 1 and 2 mutations induce BCL-2 dependence in acute myeloid leukemia. *Nat. Med.* **2015**, *21*, 178–184. [CrossRef]
70. Chiba, K.; Johnson, J.Z.; Vogan, J.M.; Wagner, T.; Boyle, J.M.; Hockemeyer, D. Cancer-associated TERT promoter mutations abrogate telomerase silencing. *eLife* **2015**, *4*, e07918. [CrossRef]
71. Heidenreich, B.; Kumar, R. TERT promoter mutations in telomere biology. *Mutat. Res. Rev. Mutat. Res.* **2017**, *771*, 15–31. [CrossRef]
72. Guilleret, I.; Yan, P.; Grange, F.; Braunschweig, R.; Bosman, F.T.; Benhattar, J. Hypermethylation of the human telomerase catalytic subunit (hTERT) gene correlates with telomerase activity. *Int. J. Cancer* **2002**, *101*, 335–341. [CrossRef] [PubMed]
73. Zinn, R.L.; Pruitt, K.; Eguchi, S.; Baylin, S.B.; Herman, J.G. hTERT is expressed in cancer cell lines despite promoter DNA methylation by preservation of unmethylated DNA and active chromatin around the transcription start site. *Cancer Res.* **2007**, *67*, 194–201. [CrossRef]
74. Patel, B.; Taiwo, R.; Kim, A.H.; Dunn, G.P. TERT, a promoter of CNS malignancies. *Neurooncol. Adv.* **2020**, *2*, vdaa025. [CrossRef] [PubMed]
75. Castelo-Branco, P.; Choufani, S.; Mack, S.; Gallagher, D.; Zhang, C.; Lipman, T.; Zhukova, N.; Walker, E.J.; Martin, D.; Merino, D.; et al. Methylation of the TERT promoter and risk stratification of childhood brain tumours: An integrative genomic and molecular study. *Lancet Oncol.* **2013**, *14*, 534–542. [CrossRef]
76. Lindsey, J.C.; Schwalbe, E.C.; Potluri, S.; Bailey, S.; Williamson, D.; Clifford, S.C. TERT promoter mutation and aberrant hypermethylation are associated with elevated expression in medulloblastoma and characterise the majority of non-infant SHH subgroup tumours. *Acta Neuropathol.* **2014**, *127*, 307–309. [CrossRef] [PubMed]
77. Lalchungnunga, H.; Hao, W.; Maris, J.M.; Asgharzadeh, S.; Henrich, K.O.; Westermann, F.; Tweddle, D.A.; Schwalbe, E.C.; Strathdee, G. Genome wide DNA methylation analysis identifies novel molecular subgroups and predicts survival in neuroblastoma. *Br. J. Cancer* **2022**, *127*, 2006–2015. [CrossRef]
78. Yan, Y.; Jiang, Y. RACK1 affects glioma cell growth and differentiation through the CNTN2-mediated RTK/Ras/MAPK pathway. *Int. J. Mol. Med.* **2016**, *37*, 251–257. [CrossRef] [PubMed]

79. Wang, Y.; Guan, G.; Cheng, W.; Jiang, Y.; Shan, F.; Wu, A.; Cheng, P.; Guo, Z. ARL2 overexpression inhibits glioma proliferation and tumorigenicity via down-regulating AXL. *BMC Cancer* **2018**, *18*, 599. [CrossRef] [PubMed]
80. Wang, Y.; Zhao, W.; Liu, X.; Guan, G.; Zhuang, M. ARL3 is downregulated and acts as a prognostic biomarker in glioma. *J. Transl. Med.* **2019**, *17*, 210. [CrossRef]
81. Tan, Y.; Zhang, S.; Xiao, Q.; Wang, J.; Zhao, K.; Liu, W.; Huang, K.; Tian, W.; Niu, H.; Lei, T.; et al. Prognostic significance of ARL9 and its methylation in low-grade glioma. *Genomics* **2020**, *112*, 4808–4816. [CrossRef]
82. Guo, W.; Ma, S.; Zhang, Y.; Liu, H.; Li, Y.; Xu, J.T.; Yang, B.; Guan, F. Genome-wide methylomic analyses identify prognostic epigenetic signature in lower grade glioma. *J. Cell Mol. Med.* **2022**, *26*, 449–461. [CrossRef] [PubMed]
83. Guo, Y.; Li, Y.; Li, J.; Tao, W.; Dong, W. DNA Methylation-Driven Genes for Developing Survival Nomogram for Low-Grade Glioma. *Front. Oncol.* **2021**, *11*, 629521. [CrossRef] [PubMed]
84. Kornberg, R.D.; Lorch, Y. Twenty-five years of the nucleosome, fundamental particle of the eukaryote chromosome. *Cell* **1999**, *98*, 285–294. [CrossRef]
85. Kim, Y.Z. Altered histone modifications in gliomas. *Brain Tumor Res. Treat.* **2014**, *2*, 7–21. [CrossRef]
86. Ekwall, K. Genome-wide analysis of HDAC function. *Trends Genet.* **2005**, *21*, 608–615. [CrossRef] [PubMed]
87. Steger, D.J.; Workman, J.L. Remodeling chromatin structures for transcription: What happens to the histones? *Bioessays* **1996**, *18*, 875–884. [CrossRef]
88. Lewis, P.W.; Müller, M.M.; Koletsky, M.S.; Cordero, F.; Lin, S.; Banaszynski, L.A.; Garcia, B.A.; Muir, T.W.; Becher, O.J.; Allis, C.D. Inhibition of PRC2 activity by a gain-of-function H3 mutation found in pediatric glioblastoma. *Science* **2013**, *340*, 857–861. [CrossRef] [PubMed]
89. Cooney, T.M.; Lubanszky, E.; Prasad, R.; Hawkins, C.; Mueller, S. Diffuse midline glioma: Review of epigenetics. *J. Neurooncol.* **2020**, *150*, 27–34. [CrossRef] [PubMed]
90. Mackay, A.; Burford, A.; Carvalho, D.; Izquierdo, E.; Fazal-Salom, J.; Taylor, K.R.; Bjerke, L.; Clarke, M.; Vinci, M.; Nandhabalan, M.; et al. Integrated Molecular Meta-Analysis of 1,000 Pediatric High-Grade and Diffuse Intrinsic Pontine Glioma. *Cancer Cell* **2017**, *32*, 520–537.e525. [CrossRef]
91. Persico, P.; Lorenzi, E.; Losurdo, A.; Dipasquale, A.; Di Muzio, A.; Navarria, P.; Pessina, F.; Politi, L.S.; Lombardi, G.; Santoro, A.; et al. Precision Oncology in Lower-Grade Gliomas: Promises and Pitfalls of Therapeutic Strategies Targeting IDH-Mutations. *Cancers* **2022**, *14*, 1125. [CrossRef]
92. Yen, K.E.; Bittinger, M.A.; Su, S.M.; Fantin, V.R. Cancer-associated IDH mutations: Biomarker and therapeutic opportunities. *Oncogene* **2010**, *29*, 6409–6417. [CrossRef] [PubMed]
93. Sulkowski, P.L.; Corso, C.D.; Robinson, N.D.; Scanlon, S.E.; Purshouse, K.R.; Bai, H.; Liu, Y.; Sundaram, R.K.; Hegan, D.C.; Fons, N.R.; et al. 2-Hydroxyglutarate produced by neomorphic IDH mutations suppresses homologous recombination and induces PARP inhibitor sensitivity. *Sci. Transl. Med.* **2017**, *9*, eaal2463. [CrossRef]
94. Bready, D.; Placantonakis, D.G. Molecular Pathogenesis of Low-Grade Glioma. *Neurosurg. Clin. N. Am.* **2019**, *30*, 17–25. [CrossRef]
95. Liu, P.S.; Wang, H.; Li, X.; Chao, T.; Teav, T.; Christen, S.; Di Conza, G.; Cheng, W.C.; Chou, C.H.; Vavakova, M.; et al. α-ketoglutarate orchestrates macrophage activation through metabolic and epigenetic reprogramming. *Nat. Immunol.* **2017**, *18*, 985–994. [CrossRef]
96. McBrayer, S.K.; Mayers, J.R.; DiNatale, G.J.; Shi, D.D.; Khanal, J.; Chakraborty, A.A.; Sarosiek, K.A.; Briggs, K.J.; Robbins, A.K.; Sewastianik, T.; et al. Transaminase Inhibition by 2-Hydroxyglutarate Impairs Glutamate Biosynthesis and Redox Homeostasis in Glioma. *Cell* **2018**, *175*, 101–116.e124. [CrossRef]
97. Xu, W.; Yang, H.; Liu, Y.; Yang, Y.; Wang, P.; Kim, S.H.; Ito, S.; Yang, C.; Wang, P.; Xiao, M.T.; et al. Oncometabolite 2-hydroxyglutarate is a competitive inhibitor of α-ketoglutarate-dependent dioxygenases. *Cancer Cell* **2011**, *19*, 17–30. [CrossRef]
98. Williams, M.J.; Singleton, W.G.; Lowis, S.P.; Malik, K.; Kurian, K.M. Therapeutic Targeting of Histone Modifications in Adult and Pediatric High-Grade Glioma. *Front Oncol* **2017**, *7*, 45. [CrossRef]
99. Mellinghoff, I.K.; Ellingson, B.M.; Touat, M.; Maher, E.; De La Fuente, M.I.; Holdhoff, M.; Cote, G.M.; Burris, H.; Janku, F.; Young, R.J.; et al. Ivosidenib in Isocitrate Dehydrogenase 1-Mutated Advanced Glioma. *J. Clin. Oncol.* **2020**, *38*, 3398–3406. [CrossRef] [PubMed]
100. Mellinghoff, I.K.; Penas-Prado, M.; Peters, K.B.; Burris, H.A., 3rd; Maher, E.A.; Janku, F.; Cote, G.M.; de la Fuente, M.I.; Clarke, J.L.; Ellingson, B.M.; et al. Vorasidenib, a Dual Inhibitor of Mutant IDH1/2, in Recurrent or Progressive Glioma: Results of a First-in-Human Phase I Trial. *Clin. Cancer Res.* **2021**, *27*, 4491–4499. [CrossRef] [PubMed]
101. Mellinghoff, I.K.; Cloughesy, T.; Wen, P.; Taylor, J.; Maher, E.; Arrillaga-Romany, I.; Peters, K.; Choi, C.; Ellingson, B.; Lin, A.; et al. ACTR-66. A phase 1, open-label, perioperative study of Ivosidenib (AG-120) and Vorasidenib (AG-881) in recurrent IDH1 mutant, low-grade glioma: Updated results. *Neuro-Oncology* **2019**, *21*, vi28–vi29. [CrossRef]
102. Wick, A.; Bähr, O.; Schuler, M.; Rohrberg, K.; Chawla, S.P.; Janku, F.; Schiff, D.; Heinemann, V.; Narita, Y.; Lenz, H.J.; et al. Phase I Assessment of Safety and Therapeutic Activity of BAY1436032 in Patients with IDH1-Mutant Solid Tumors. *Clin. Cancer Res.* **2021**, *27*, 2723–2733. [CrossRef]
103. Natsume, A.; Arakawa, Y.; Narita, Y.; Sugiyama, K.; Hata, N.; Muragaki, Y.; Shinojima, N.; Kumabe, T.; Saito, R.; Motomura, K.; et al. The first-in-human phase I study of a brain penetrant mutant IDH1 inhibitor DS-1001 in patients with recurrent or progressive IDH1-mutant gliomas. *Neuro Oncol.* **2022**, *25*, 326–336. [CrossRef] [PubMed]

104. Platten, M.; Bunse, L.; Wick, A.; Bunse, T.; Le Cornet, L.; Harting, I.; Sahm, F.; Sanghvi, K.; Tan, C.L.; Poschke, I.; et al. A vaccine targeting mutant IDH1 in newly diagnosed glioma. *Nature* **2021**, *592*, 463–468. [CrossRef] [PubMed]
105. Rohle, D.; Popovici-Muller, J.; Palaskas, N.; Turcan, S.; Grommes, C.; Campos, C.; Tsoi, J.; Clark, O.; Oldrini, B.; Komisopoulou, E.; et al. An inhibitor of mutant IDH1 delays growth and promotes differentiation of glioma cells. *Science* **2013**, *340*, 626–630. [CrossRef] [PubMed]
106. Popovici-Muller, J.; Lemieux, R.M.; Artin, E.; Saunders, J.O.; Salituro, F.G.; Travins, J.; Cianchetta, G.; Cai, Z.; Zhou, D.; Cui, D.; et al. Discovery of AG-120 (Ivosidenib): A First-in-Class Mutant IDH1 Inhibitor for the Treatment of IDH1 Mutant Cancers. *ACS Med. Chem. Lett.* **2018**, *9*, 300–305. [CrossRef]
107. Kopinja, J.; Sevilla, R.S.; Levitan, D.; Dai, D.; Vanko, A.; Spooner, E.; Ware, C.; Forget, R.; Hu, K.; Kral, A.; et al. A Brain Penetrant Mutant IDH1 Inhibitor Provides In Vivo Survival Benefit. *Sci. Rep.* **2017**, *7*, 13853. [CrossRef]
108. Berghoff, A.S.; Kiesel, B.; Widhalm, G.; Wilhelm, D.; Rajky, O.; Kurscheid, S.; Kresl, P.; Wöhrer, A.; Marosi, C.; Hegi, M.E.; et al. Correlation of immune phenotype with IDH mutation in diffuse glioma. *Neuro Oncol.* **2017**, *19*, 1460–1468. [CrossRef]
109. Pellegatta, S.; Valletta, L.; Corbetta, C.; Patanè, M.; Zucca, I.; Riccardi Sirtori, F.; Bruzzone, M.G.; Fogliatto, G.; Isacchi, A.; Pollo, B.; et al. Effective immuno-targeting of the IDH1 mutation R132H in a murine model of intracranial glioma. *Acta Neuropathol. Commun.* **2015**, *3*, 4. [CrossRef]
110. Kadiyala, P.; Carney, S.V.; Gauss, J.C.; Garcia-Fabiani, M.B.; Haase, S.; Alghamri, M.S.; Núñez, F.J.; Liu, Y.; Yu, M.; Taher, A.; et al. Inhibition of 2-hydroxyglutarate elicits metabolic reprogramming and mutant IDH1 glioma immunity in mice. *J. Clin. Invest.* **2021**, *131*, e139542. [CrossRef]
111. Wang, Y.; Wild, A.T.; Turcan, S.; Wu, W.H.; Sigel, C.; Klimstra, D.S.; Ma, X.; Gong, Y.; Holland, E.C.; Huse, J.T.; et al. Targeting therapeutic vulnerabilities with PARP inhibition and radiation in IDH-mutant gliomas and cholangiocarcinomas. *Sci. Adv.* **2020**, *6*, eaaz3221. [CrossRef] [PubMed]
112. Higuchi, F.; Nagashima, H.; Ning, J.; Koerner, M.V.A.; Wakimoto, H.; Cahill, D.P. Restoration of Temozolomide Sensitivity by PARP Inhibitors in Mismatch Repair Deficient Glioblastoma is Independent of Base Excision Repair. *Clin. Cancer Res.* **2020**, *26*, 1690–1699. [CrossRef]
113. Tateishi, K.; Wakimoto, H.; Iafrate, A.J.; Tanaka, S.; Loebel, F.; Lelic, N.; Wiederschain, D.; Bedel, O.; Deng, G.; Zhang, B.; et al. Extreme Vulnerability of IDH1 Mutant Cancers to NAD+ Depletion. *Cancer Cell* **2015**, *28*, 773–784. [CrossRef]
114. Karpel-Massler, G.; Ishida, C.T.; Bianchetti, E.; Zhang, Y.; Shu, C.; Tsujiuchi, T.; Banu, M.A.; Garcia, F.; Roth, K.A.; Bruce, J.N.; et al. Induction of synthetic lethality in IDH1-mutated gliomas through inhibition of Bcl-xL. *Nat. Commun.* **2017**, *8*, 1067. [CrossRef] [PubMed]
115. Spino, M.; Kurz, S.C.; Chiriboga, L.; Serrano, J.; Zeck, B.; Sen, N.; Patel, S.; Shen, G.; Vasudevaraja, V.; Tsirigos, A.; et al. Cell Surface Notch Ligand DLL3 is a Therapeutic Target in Isocitrate Dehydrogenase-mutant Glioma. *Clin. Cancer Res.* **2019**, *25*, 1261–1271. [CrossRef] [PubMed]
116. Turcan, S.; Fabius, A.W.; Borodovsky, A.; Pedraza, A.; Brennan, C.; Huse, J.; Viale, A.; Riggins, G.J.; Chan, T.A. Efficient induction of differentiation and growth inhibition in IDH1 mutant glioma cells by the DNMT Inhibitor Decitabine. *Oncotarget* **2013**, *4*, 1729–1736. [CrossRef] [PubMed]
117. Borodovsky, A.; Salmasi, V.; Turcan, S.; Fabius, A.W.; Baia, G.S.; Eberhart, C.G.; Weingart, J.D.; Gallia, G.L.; Baylin, S.B.; Chan, T.A.; et al. 5-azacytidine reduces methylation, promotes differentiation and induces tumor regression in a patient-derived IDH1 mutant glioma xenograft. *Oncotarget* **2013**, *4*, 1737–1747. [CrossRef]
118. Yamashita, A.S.; da Costa Rosa, M.; Borodovsky, A.; Festuccia, W.T.; Chan, T.; Riggins, G.J. Demethylation and epigenetic modification with 5-azacytidine reduces IDH1 mutant glioma growth in combination with temozolomide. *Neuro Oncol.* **2019**, *21*, 189–200. [CrossRef]
119. Federici, L.; Capelle, L.; Annereau, M.; Bielle, F.; Willekens, C.; Dehais, C.; Laigle-Donadey, F.; Hoang-Xuan, K.; Delattre, J.Y.; Idbaih, A.; et al. 5-Azacitidine in patients with IDH1/2-mutant recurrent glioma. *Neuro Oncol.* **2020**, *22*, 1226–1228. [CrossRef]
120. Kilburn, L.B.; Kocak, M.; Baxter, P.; Poussaint, T.Y.; Paulino, A.C.; McIntyre, C.; Lemenuel-Diot, A.; Lopez-Diaz, C.; Kun, L.; Chintagumpala, M.; et al. A pediatric brain tumor consortium phase II trial of capecitabine rapidly disintegrating tablets with concomitant radiation therapy in children with newly diagnosed diffuse intrinsic pontine gliomas. *Pediatr. Blood Cancer* **2018**, *65*. [CrossRef]
121. Bai, H.; Harmancı, A.S.; Erson-Omay, E.Z.; Li, J.; Coşkun, S.; Simon, M.; Krischek, B.; Özduman, K.; Omay, S.B.; Sorensen, E.A.; et al. Integrated genomic characterization of IDH1-mutant glioma malignant progression. *Nat. Genet.* **2016**, *48*, 59–66. [CrossRef]

Disclaimer/Publisher's Note: The statements, opinions and data contained in all publications are solely those of the individual author(s) and contributor(s) and not of MDPI and/or the editor(s). MDPI and/or the editor(s) disclaim responsibility for any injury to people or property resulting from any ideas, methods, instructions or products referred to in the content.

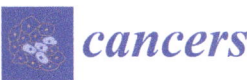

Article

GBM Cells Exhibit Susceptibility to Metformin Treatment According to TLR4 Pathway Activation and Metabolic and Antioxidant Status

Isabele Fattori Moretti [1,*], Antonio Marcondes Lerario [2], Paula Rodrigues Sola [1], Janaína Macedo-da-Silva [3], Mauricio da Silva Baptista [4], Giuseppe Palmisano [3], Sueli Mieko Oba-Shinjo [1] and Suely Kazue Nagahashi Marie [1,*]

[1] Laboratory of Molecular and Cellular Biology (LIM 15), Department of Neurology, Faculdade de Medicina FMUSP, Universidade de Sao Paulo, Sao Paulo 01246-903, SP, Brazil
[2] Department of Internal Medicine, Division of Metabolism, Endocrinology and Diabetes, University of Michigan, Ann Arbor, MI 48108, USA
[3] GlycoProteomics Laboratory, Department of Parasitology, ICB, University of Sao Paulo, São Paulo 05508-000, SP, Brazil
[4] Biochemistry Department, Institute of Chemistry, Universidade de Sao Paulo, São Paulo 05508-900, SP, Brazil
* Correspondence: imortetti@usp.br (I.F.M.); sknmarie@usp.br (S.K.N.M.); Tel.: +55-11-3061-7458 (S.K.N.M.)

Simple Summary: An analysis of metformin (MET) treatment in combination with temozolomide (TMZ) in two glioblastoma cell lines, U87MG and A172, stimulated with lipopolysaccharide (LPS), a TLR4 agonist was conducted. Both cells presented blunted mitochondrial respiration leading to oxidative stress after MET treatment, and decreased cell viability after MET + TMZ treatment. U87MG cells presented increased apoptosis after MET + LPS + TMZ treatment by increment of ER stress, and downregulation of BLC2. A172, with an upregulated antioxidant background, including *SOD1*, exhibited cell cycle arrest after MET + TMZ treatment. The observed differential response was associated with a distinct metabolic status: glycolytic/plurimetabolic (GPM) subtype in U87MG and mitochondrial (MTC) in A172. TCGA-GBM-RNASeq in silico analysis showed that GPM-GBM cases with an activated TLR4 pathway might respond to MET, but the concomitant *CXCL8*/IL8 upregulation may demand a combination treatment with an IL8 inhibitor. MET combined with an antioxidant inhibitor, such as anti-SOD1, may be indicated for MTC-GBM cases.

Abstract: Glioblastoma (GBM) is an aggressive brain cancer associated with poor overall survival. The metabolic status and tumor microenvironment of GBM cells have been targeted to improve therapeutic strategies. TLR4 is an important innate immune receptor capable of recognizing pathogens and danger-associated molecules. We have previously demonstrated the presence of TLR4 in GBM tumors and the decreased viability of the GBM tumor cell line after lipopolysaccharide (LPS) (TLR4 agonist) stimulation. In the present study, metformin (MET) treatment, used in combination with temozolomide (TMZ) in two GBM cell lines (U87MG and A172) and stimulated with LPS was analyzed. MET is a drug widely used for the treatment of diabetes and has been repurposed for cancer treatment owing to its anti-proliferative and anti-inflammatory actions. The aim of the study was to investigate MET and LPS treatment in two GBM cell lines with different metabolic statuses. MET treatment led to mitochondrial respiration blunting and oxidative stress with superoxide production in both cell lines, more markedly in U87MG cells. Decreased cell viability after MET + TMZ and MET + LPS + TMZ treatment was observed in both cell lines. U87MG cells exhibited apoptosis after MET + LPS + TMZ treatment, promoting increased ER stress, unfolded protein response, and BLC2 downregulation. LPS stimulation of U87MG cells led to upregulation of *SOD2* and genes related to the TLR4 signaling pathway, including *IL1B* and *CXCL8*. A172 cells attained upregulated antioxidant gene expression, particularly *SOD1*, *TXN* and *PRDX1-5*, while MET treatment led to cell-cycle arrest. In silico analysis of the TCGA-GBM-RNASeq dataset indicated that the glycolytic plurimetabolic (GPM)-GBM subtype had a transcriptomic profile which overlapped with U87MG cells, suggesting

Citation: Moretti, I.F.; Lerario, A.M.; Sola, P.R.; Macedo-da-Silva, J.; Baptista, M.d.S.; Palmisano, G.; Oba-Shinjo, S.M.; Marie, S.K.N. GBM Cells Exhibit Susceptibility to Metformin Treatment According to TLR4 Pathway Activation and Metabolic and Antioxidant Status. *Cancers* **2023**, *15*, 587. https://doi.org/10.3390/cancers15030587

Academic Editor: Edward Pan

Received: 20 December 2022
Revised: 10 January 2023
Accepted: 14 January 2023
Published: 18 January 2023

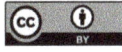

Copyright: © 2023 by the authors. Licensee MDPI, Basel, Switzerland. This article is an open access article distributed under the terms and conditions of the Creative Commons Attribution (CC BY) license (https:// creativecommons.org/licenses/by/ 4.0/).

GBM cases exhibiting this metabolic background with an activated inflammatory TLR4 pathway may respond to MET treatment. For cases with upregulated *CXCL8*, coding for IL8 (a pro-angiogenic factor), combination treatment with an IL8 inhibitor may improve tumor growth control. The A172 cell line corresponded to the mitochondrial (MTC)-GBM subtype, where MET plus an antioxidant inhibitor, such as anti-SOD1, may be indicated as a combinatory therapy.

Keywords: GBM; U87MG; A172; Metformin; LPS; antioxidant; cell cycle arrest; apoptosis

1. Introduction

Glioblastoma (GBM), a WHO grade 4 astrocytoma, is the most aggressive and malignant brain tumor [1], with an overall survival (OS) of 15 months [2], despite the current standard of care treatment consisting of surgical tumor macroresection followed by radiotherapy and chemotherapy with the alkylating agent temozolomide (TMZ) [3]. The limited effectiveness of therapeutic modalities available has been attributed to tumor invasiveness and high tumor heterogeneity [4]. Moreover, metabolic plasticity guarantees tumor fitness, where a blockade of metabolic pathways has been a focus of combination therapy strategies [5].

Metformin (MET), 1,1-dimethylbiguanide hydrochloride, known for its hypoglycemic action and widely used as the first-line medication for the treatment of type 2 diabetes [6], has been repurposed for cancer therapy. Known MET actions include regulation of AMPK pathway activity and mitochondria oxidative stress through inhibition of the oxidative phosphorylation (OXPHOS) complex I [7]. MET can also inhibit hexokinase activity and reduce cell glucose consumption, as well as act on the NFκB canonical pathway decreasing IL8 [8], IL6, and TNF expression [9]. Moreover, recent studies have shown the role of MET in inhibiting NLRP3 inflammasome activation and IL1β production in alveolar macrophages [10]; involving inhibition of NFκB-NLRP3-mediated endothelial cell pyroptosis [11]; and of fatty acid synthase (FASN) with suppression of the proinflammatory response through the FASN/AKT pathway [12]. Additionally, inhibition of tumor growth using MET treatment has been described for several types of cancer, including colon, breast, prostate, pancreatic, lung, endometrial carcinomas, melanoma, and leukemia [13–18]. In particular, MET is a promising therapeutic option for brain tumors, given its hydrophilic property and permeability across the blood–brain barrier, as demonstrated in animal models [19,20]. In fact, the effects of MET on GBM cell viability have been studied previously [21–23], and several clinical trials of combination treatment with MET for GBM patients have been conducted [24].

We have previously demonstrated activation of the TLR4 signaling pathway in GBM, mainly the mesenchymal subtype, and upregulation of IL1β and DNA repair genes through late activation of NFκB in GBM cells stimulated with lipopolysaccharide (LPS). The LPS-stimulated GBM cells had decreased tumor cell viability with the use of treatment combining DNA repair inhibitor and TMZ, which proved more effective than treatment with TMZ alone [25].

In the present study, MET treatment, used in combination with TMZ in two GBM cell lines (U87MG and A172) and stimulated using LPS, was analyzed. The aims were to analyze the signaling pathways activated by MET, LPS and TMZ treatment used alone and in combination, and to identify predictive markers of treatment response.

2. Materials and Methods

2.1. Cell Culture

GBM cellular lines U87MG and A172 were acquired from ATCC. Lineages authentication by short tandem repeats analysis was performed using the GenePrint 10 System (Promega, Madison, WI, USA). Cells were maintained in DMEM (Dulbecco's Modified Eagle's Medium) (Thermo Fisher Scientific, Waltham, MA, USA) with the addition of 10%

fetal bovine serum (FBS) (Cultilab, Campinas, Brazil), streptomycin (100 µg/mL), and penicillin (100 IU/mL) (Thermo Fisher Scientific). Cells were incubated at 37 °C with 5% CO_2 and were routinely tested for mycoplasma contamination.

2.2. Cell Treatment

The following reagents: LPS from *Escherichia coli* O55:B5, MET and TMZ (Merck, Readington Township, NJ, USA) were used in U87MG and A172 cell cultures in single or combination treatments. Controls consisted of non-treated cells or treated with DMSO when TMZ was used. Proliferation curves with PrestoBlue reagent (Thermo Fisher Scientific) were performed to determine the half maximal inhibitory concentration (IC50) dose of a single treatment. The IC50 was used for all assays. Assays before (time 0) and after 24 and/or 48 h of treatment were analyzed, according to Figure 1, which shows the schematic experimental design with the time points of the cellular functional analysis: cell viability, apoptosis, cell cycle, mitochondria respiration and superoxide measurements, and transcriptomic analysis.

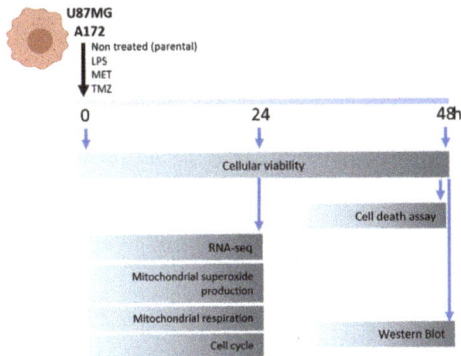

Figure 1. The schematic presentation of the experimental design.

2.3. Cell Viability and Apoptosis Assays

For the cell viability analyses, cells were plated in 96 wells plate (2×10^3 cells/well) and analyzed at different time points (24, 48 h). PrestoBlue Cell Viability Reagent was used according to the manufacturer's instructions (Thermo Fisher Scientific). Glomax equipment (Promega) was used to evaluate the fluorescence intensity after incubation (excitation at 540 nm, emission at 560 nm). Treatments were done in octuplicate, and two wells without the cell culture medium were used to access the background for each time point to be subtracted from each measurement value.

Cell-death assays of U87MG and A172 cell lines were analyzed after 48h of treatment. Cells were trypsinized, and the medium containing possible necrotic and late apoptotic cells was collected. The Dead Cell Apoptosis Kit (Thermo Fischer Scientific) containing Annexin V conjugated with FITC and propidium iodide (PI) was used following the instructions of the manufacturer. Cell death measurements were performed in the flow cytometry system BD FACSCanto (Beckton Dickinson, East Rutherford, NJ, USA). The analysis was done by FlowJo version 10 (Beckton Dickinson). For the analysis, a non-stained population of cells was used to set the percentage of alive cells. Positivity only for Annexin V was considered as early apoptosis, double positivity for Annexin V and PI was considered as late apoptosis, and positivity only for PI was considered as necrotic cells.

2.4. Mitochondrial Superoxide Assay

Production of superoxide by mitochondria after 24 h of treatment in U87MG and A172 cells was assessed by flow cytometry and compared to non-treated cells, in triplicate for each treatment. The MitoSOX Red Mitochondrial Superoxide Indicator kit was used following the instructions of the manufacturer (Thermo Fischer Scientific). MitoSOX fluorescence was assessed in the flow cytometer FACSCanto (Beckton Dickinson). MitoSOX positivity was analyzed by FlowJo version 10.

2.5. Mitochondrial Respiration Analysis

The Seahorse XFe24 Analyzer (Agilent Technology, Santa Clara, CA, USA) equipment was used for mitochondrial respiration analysis of U87MG and A172 cell lines after treatment. The Cell Mito Stress Test Kit was used to access mitochondria viability. Cells were plated in the Seahorse plate and treated with MET and LPS single and combined, in triplicate for each treatment, for 24 h, at 37 °C and 5% CO_2. Next, cells were washed, and the medium was changed to an un-buffered medium and maintained in a 37 °C incubator free of CO_2. The oxygen consumption rate (OCR) was measured following the Mito Stress program, and treatment was as follow: 2 µM oligomycin, for inhibiting ATP synthase (OXPHOS complex V), and decreasing OCR; 2 µM carbonyl cyanide 3-chlorophenylhydrazone (CCCP), for collapsing the proton gradient, disrupting the mitochondrial membrane, and maximizing OCR through OXPHOS complex IV; 5 µM antimycin A for inhibiting complex III and rotenone for inhibiting complex I, leading to a mitochondria shutdown.

2.6. Cell Cycle Analysis

Analyses of U87MG and A172 cell cycle phases were accessed by flow cytometry. Previously to treatment with LPS, MET, and TMZ, cells were synchronized by incubation with FBS-free DMEM with 0.5% bovine serum albumin for 24 h. Subsequently, cells were treated for 24 h in triplicate and fixed with cold ethanol in increasing concentrations (25, 50, 75, 90%). After fixation, cells were washed and incubated with PI. PI fluorescence was accessed by flow cytometry FACSCanto (Beckton Dickinson). Analysis was performed using FlowJo version 10, using the cell cycle interface.

2.7. High-Throughput Sequencing for Transcriptome Analysis

Total RNA of U87MG and A172 cells after 24 h of treatment with LPS and/or MET was extracted using the RNeasy mini kit (Qiagen, Hilden, Germany) for the transcriptomic analysis. Untreated cells were considered as the control. Two independent experiments in duplicate were performed for each condition. RNA integrity and concentration were accessed using RNA screentape in the 4200 Tapestation system (Agilent Technologies). The QuantSeq 3′ mRNA-Seq Library Prep kit FWD for Illumina (Lexogen, Vienna, Austria) was used for library construction from 500 ng of total RNA following the recommendations of the manufacturer. The library concentration was measured using the Qubit dsDNA HS Assay Kit (Thermo Fisher Scientific), and the size distribution was determined using the Agilent D1000 ScreenTape System on TapeStation 4200 (Agilent Technologies). Sequencing was performed using the NextSeq 500 platform (Illumina, San Diego, CA, USA) at the next-generation sequencing facility core (SELA) at Faculdade de Medicina da Universidade de São Paulo (FMUSP). Sequencing data were aligned to the GRCh38 version of the human genome and quantified using the R-Bioconductor package QuasR using HiSAT2 as the aligner [26]. The GFF file containing the gene models was obtained from ftp.ensembl.org (accessed on 20 November 2022). Sequencing quality and alignment metrics were assessed with FastQC and RNASEQC, respectively. Downstream analyses were performed in R using specific Bioconductor and CRAN tools, and briefly described. Normalization was performed with edgeR using the trimmed-mean (TMM) method. We used sva to remove occult/unwanted sources of variation from the data. The R-Bioconductor package limma was used to assess differential gene expression in each group, and to perform log2 counts per million reads mapped (CPM) in the transformation of the data. Principal component analysis was performed using the prcomp function from R-stats, and graphically depicted as biplots constructed using ggplot2. To identify modules of co-regulated genes among the differentially expressed genes, we used heatmap and cutree to perform hierarchical clustering and to build heatmaps displaying these modules. We used Pearson correlation as the similarity metric, and the ward D2 clustering algorithm. We used clusterProfiler to perform gene set enrichment analysis for each module of co-regulated genes. Expression data were centered on the mean of each gene. Additional gene set enrichment analyses were performed by online tools such as Gene Ontology [27–29] resources and String consortium [30,31]. The metabolic subtype for the cell lines was determined by the analysis of a combined score of marker gene expressions for glycolytic plurimetabolic (GPM) and mitochondrial (MTC subtypes described by Garofano et al. (2021) [32]. We used GSVA [33] to calculate these scores. For the heatmaps, the data were normalized by z-score. The logCPM for each gene was subtracted by the mean and divided by the standard deviation.

2.8. Western Blot

Protein extraction of U87MG and A172 cells was performed after 48 h of treatment using the lysis buffer (10 mM Hepes, 1% SDS, 1.5 mM $MgCl_2$, 1 mM KCl, 1 mM DTT, and 0.1% NP-40), protease and phosphatase inhibitors (Sigma-Aldrich, St. Louis, MO, USA). Samples were quantified by Qubit protein Assay kit platform (Thermo Fisher Scientific) and solubilized in sample buffer containing 60 mM Tris-HCl, 2% SDS, 10% glycerol, and 0.01% bromophenol blue. A total of 25 µg of proteins were separated by SDS-PAGE and electro-transferred to PVDF membranes, which were directly incubated with blocking buffer (5% bovine serum albumin (BSA) in Tris-buffered saline (TBS) and 0.05% Tween-20 (TBST)) for 1h. Subsequently, samples were incubated with primary antibodies: anti-BCL2 (2876, Cell signaling, Denver, MA, USA) and anti-β-actin (Sigma-Aldrich, A2228, 1:10,000) for loading control, followed by secondary antibody conjugated with horseradish peroxidase for anti-mouse diluted 1:4000 (Abcam, Cambridge, MA, USA) was used for detection of proteins. Immunoreactive bands were detected with the ChemiDoc XRS Imaging System equipment and protein quantification was performed using the ImageJ software (vesion 1.53t).

2.9. In Silico Analysis

The astrocytoma dataset from The Cancer Genome Atlas (TCGA) was downloaded from Genomics Data Commons Data Portal [34], and the data were normalized by DEseq software. GBM cases with clinical follow-up data were selected for the analysis. Data analysis was done by heatmap for visualization using z-score to normalize RPKM values.

2.10. Statistical Analysis

Statistical analysis was performed using the program SPSS version 23.0 (IBM Corporation, Armonk, NY, USA), Graph Pad Prism (GraphPad Software Inc., San Diego, CA, USA), and R studio [35]. The Kolmogorov–Smirnov test was applied to verify the normal distribution of the results. For non-parametric analysis, Kruskal-Wallis and post hoc Dunn test were used to assess the differences among three or more groups. For two groups comparison, the Mann–Whitney test was used. For parametric analysis, One-way ANOVA and Tukey post hoc test was used, and for multiple variables comparison, two-way ANOVA and Bonferroni or Tukey were used as post hoc tests. Correlation analysis was done by Pearson's test when parametric, and Spearman's when non-parametric. The Corrplot package was used for correlation visualization [36]. Statistical significance was considered when $p < 0.05$. The Kaplan–Meier estimator was applied for the TCGA-GPM-GBM subtype using *SOD2* and *CXCL8* expression ratio, where the cases were stratified as high and low according to the mean value for the ratio. Statistical analysis for the survival distribution was performed by Logrank test.

3. Results

3.1. Characterization of U87MG and A172 GBM Cell Lines

The effect of LPS and MET treatment, used alone and in combination, on U87MG and A172 GBM cell lines, was analyzed given that both present TLR4 expression [37] (Supplementary Figure S1A), and the fact that an increased apoptotic rate with the use of LPS and TMZ co-treatment in U87MG cells has been previously demonstrated by our group [24]. Also, U87MG and A172 cell lines were selected for an additional metabolic intervention with MET because U87MG cells exhibited upregulation of genes related to glycolytic process, while A172 cells showed a marked upregulation of genes related to complex I of OXPHOS, as evidenced by transcriptome analysis (Figure 2A). Moreover, the overall expression levels of genes attributed as markers for the glycolytic plurimetabolic (GPM) GBM subtype and mitochondrial (MTC) GBM subtype, according to Garofano et al. (2021) [32], were upregulated in U87MG and A172 cell lines, respectively (Supplementary Figure S1B).

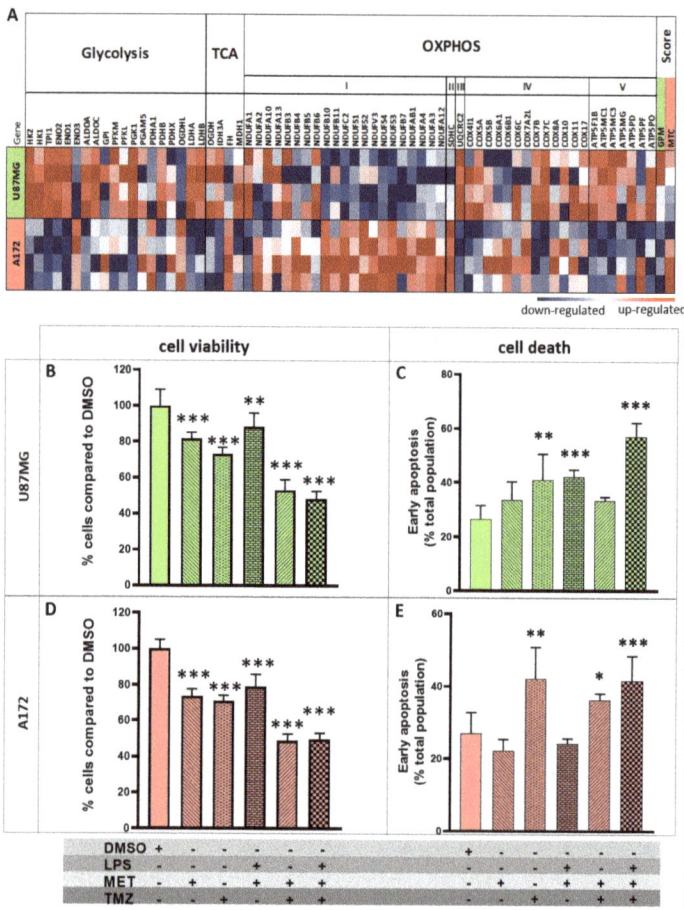

Figure 2. Cell viability and death assays for A172 and U87MG treatment with LPS, MET, and TMZ. (**A**) Heatmap presenting expression values for the genes related to glycolysis, TCA cycle and oxidative phosphorylation normalized by z−score. A score value for the expression of genes attributed as a marker for glycolytic plurimetabolic (GPM) and mitochondrial (MTC) GBM subtypes according to Garofano's (2021) classification [32]. Upregulated genes are presented in red and downregulated genes in blue. Graph bars representing the viability plotted for the single and combined treatments for LPS, MET, and TMZ in U87MG; (**B**) and A172 (**D**) after 48 h of treatment (**) $p < 0.01$, (***) $p < 0.001$ by one−way ANOVA post hoc Tukey test. Cellular death was analyzed by flow cytometry 48 h after treatments for U87MG; (**C**) and A172; and (**E**), and the results for initial apoptosis are presented. The graphs represent the percentage of the population in initial apoptosis through the positivity for annexin and PI negative in bars for each treatment condition. (*) $p < 0.05$, (**) $p < 0.01$, (***) $p < 0.001$ by two−way ANOVA post hoc Tukey test.

3.2. U87MG and A172 Cell Viability and Cell Death with LPS, MET and TMZ Treatment

Cell viability and cell death assays were performed to analyze U87MG and A172 cell proliferation after use of LPS, MET, and TMZ treatment alone and in combination. In a previous study, we described a decrease in U87MG cell viability following the use of LPS + TMZ treatment [25]. By comparison, MET + TMZ treatment after 48 h in the present study led to a more significant decrease in cell viability (53%) ($p < 0.001$, one-way ANOVA post hoc Tukey test, relative to parental cells treated with DMSO), while MET alone led to a decrease of 19%, TMZ alone 37% or LPS + MET 12% ($p < 0.05$, one-way ANOVA post hoc Tukey test, relative to parental cells with DMSO) (Figure 2B). Analyses were performed at 24 and 48 h, and higher differences for the treatments group was observed after 48 h (Supplementary Figure S2A). The cell death assay revealed a significant increase in initial apoptosis only with the use of the LPS + MET + TMZ treatment combination after 48 h (57%) ($p < 0.001$, two-way ANOVA post hoc Tukey test, relative to parental cells + vehicle DMSO) (Figure 2C and Supplementary Figure S2B).

A172 cells also showed a significant decrease in cell viability (48%, $p < 0.001$, one-way ANOVA post hoc Tukey test, after 48 h) for the MET + TMZ treatment combination (Figure 2D), yielding similar results to the LPS + MET + TMZ treatment (49%). Moreover, no difference in the cell death assay was observed for treatment alone or combined in A172 cells (Figure 2E). Interestingly, treatment with TMZ alone resulted in a 42% increase in initial apoptosis of A172 cells compared to control cells (A172 cells + vehicle DMSO) (Figure 2E). In both cell lines, no differences were observed in late apoptosis (Supplementary Figure S2C).

3.3. Altered Signaling Pathways in U87MG and A172 Cells after LPS and MET Treatment Alone and in Combination

The results of the cell viability assay and cell death for the signaling pathways involved were analyzed by high-throughput sequencing of the transcriptome of both cell lines treated with LPS and MET, alone and in combination.

The RNASeq of U87MG cells yielded 12,396 genes with 212 differentially expressed genes (DEGs) for LPS treatment, 362 DEGs for MET treatment and 1810 DEGs for combined LPS + MET treatment with an adjusted p (adj p) < 0.1 compared to non-treated cells. To identify the clusters of DEGs, a Pearson's correlation analysis was performed, which identified 6 different clusters for the comparison of the four groups (U87MG parental cells, LPS alone, MET alone and LPS + MET treated cells) (Figure 3A). The clusters included enrichment of DEGs associated with different signaling pathways (Figure 3B). Cluster 1 showed upregulated genes after combined treatment (LPS + MET), whereas cluster 2 included upregulated genes only after MET treatment, while both clusters were related to apoptotic signaling pathway on the gene ontology enrichment analysis. Additionally, Cluster 1 included genes related to endoplasmic reticulum (ER) stress response and Cluster 2 to a process of import into cell pathways. Clusters 3 and 6 included genes downregulated after MET treatment, where the genes in Cluster 3 were related to response to wound and regulation of ERK1 and ERK2 cascade pathways, while the genes in Cluster 6 were related to actin filament assembly with increment of downregulation after combined (LPS + MET) treatment. Cluster 4 included upregulated genes after LPS treatment with enrichment for regulation of inflammatory response and vasculature development, and Cluster 5 included downregulated genes after LPS treatment enriched for ion transport and regulation (Figure 3A,B).

The RNASeq of A172 cells detected 13,059 genes, with 1278 DEGs after MET treatment and 1204 DEGs after LPS + MET combined treatment compared to non-treated cells, with an adj $p < 0.1$. Interestingly, LPS stimulation promoted no alteration in DEG profile relative to non-treated cells. The Pearson's correlation analysis for the DEGs showed four clusters of correlation (Figure 3C). Cluster 1 included upregulated genes after MET treatment with enrichment of genes related to the amino acid metabolic process and import into the cell pathways, while Cluster 2 included downregulated genes after MET treatment related to chromosome segregation and mitotic nuclear division. Cluster 3 also included downregulated genes after MET treatment associated with the reactive oxygen metabolic process. Cluster 4 presented no significant enriched pathway (Figure 3C,D).

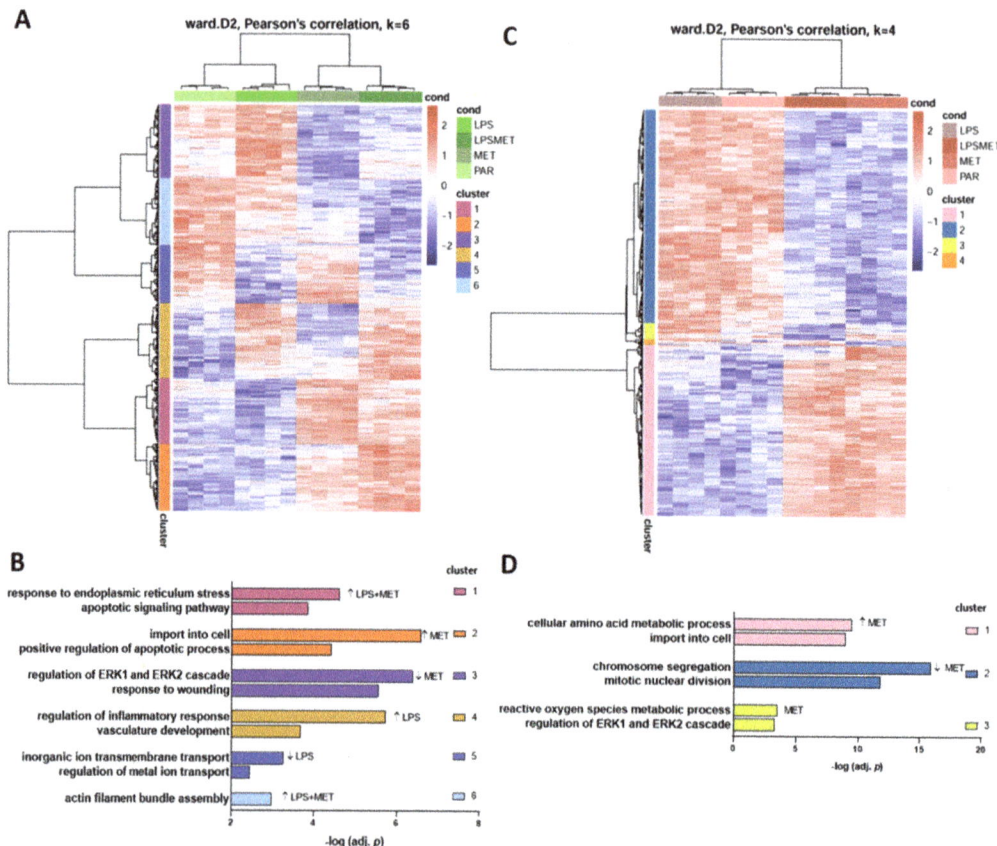

Figure 3. Transcriptome analysis for U87MG and A172 at 24 h after LPS and MET single and combined treatments compared to non−treated cells. A heatmap for the expression values after each treatment is presented and Pearson's correlation analysis for clusterization of the different groups showed six different clusters for U87MG (**A**) and four clusters for A172 (**C**). The top two gene ontology enrichment pathways identified in each cluster are shown in bars with the −log adj p for U87MG (**B**) and A172 (**D**).

3.4. U87MG Cells Were Prone to Mitochondrial Stress after MET Treatment

With regard to MET inhibition at the level of complex I of OXPHOS with consequent increase in reactive oxygen species (ROS) production, the MitoSOX assay was performed under the different treatment conditions.

An increase in mitochondrial superoxide production was observed in U87MG cells, as 100% of cells were positive for mitochondrial superoxide after MET treatment, a result replicated for the treatments combining TMZ or LPS ($p < 0.0001$ compared to non-treated condition, one-way ANOVA, post-hoc Tukey test) (Figure 4A and Supplementary Figure S3A). By contrast, A172 cells showed only 50% positivity when treated with MET, a rate unchanged by the treatment combination with TMZ or LPS ($p < 0.0001$ compared to non-treated cells, one-way ANOVA, post-hoc Tukey test) (Figure 4A and Supplementary Figure S3B).

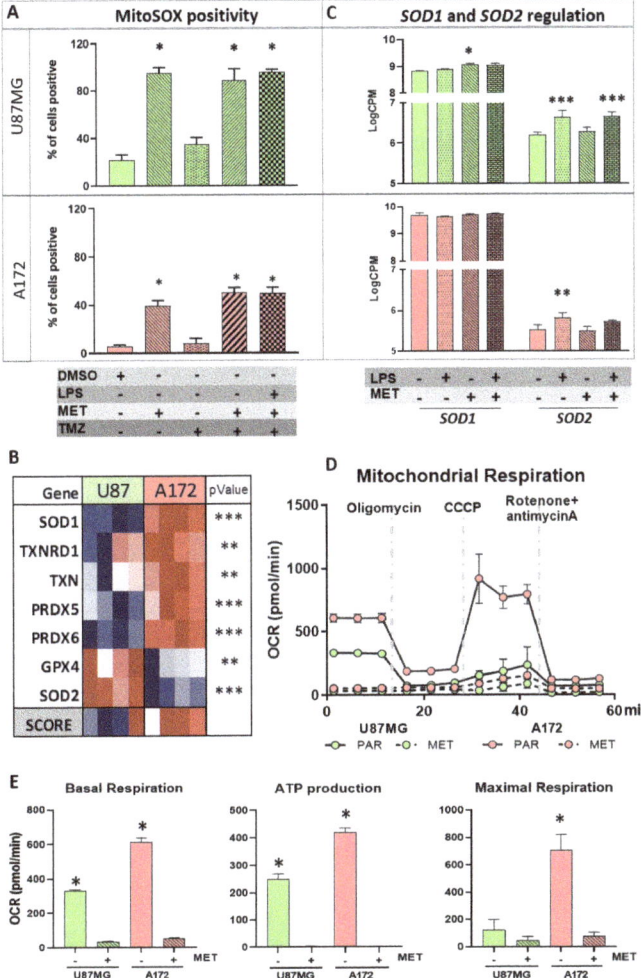

Figure 4. Mitochondrial stress. (**A**) The superoxide production in mitochondria after LPS, MET, and TMZ single and combined treatments for U87MG and A172. Graph bars represent the percentage of positive cells for MitoSOX. (*) $p < 0.0001$, One–wayANOVA post hoc Tukey test; (**B**) heatmap presenting the expression levels of antioxidant-related genes in U87MG and A172 cells. Presenting score values for the pathway for both cells (**) $p < 0.01$, and (***) $p < 0.001$, Limma t-test; (**C**) values for logCPM for *SOD1* and *SOD2* represented by the graph bars for U87MG and A172 after LPS, MET and LPS + MET treatment (*) $p < 0.05$, (**) $p < 0.01$, and $p < 0.001$, Limma t-test; (**D**) mitochondrial respiration by Seahorse, following the mitochondrial stress analysis. The oxygen consumption rate (OCR) curves along the time interval up to 60 min are presented according to applied drugs; and (**E**) histograms of basal respiration calculated by OCR before oligomycin incubation; ATP production evaluated by oligomycin–OCR subtracted from baseline cellular rate and maximal mitochondria respiration calculated as the value after CCCP–OCR subtracted from the value after rotenone- and antimycin A–OCR for U87MG and A172 in non-treated and MET treated. (*) $p < 0.0001$, one–way ANOVA followed by Tukey test. Red (parental-PAR), blue (MET treated) for U87MG and lilac (PAR), green (MET treated) for A172.

The antioxidant genes expressed in mitochondria were evaluated in U87MG and A172 parental cells to better understand the observed difference between the two cell lines.

Interestingly, significantly higher expression of an important enzyme responsible for converting superoxide in hydrogen peroxide [38] located in the mitochondrial intermembrane (*SOD1*) was observed in A172 cells at higher levels than in U87MG cells (logFC = 0.773 and adj $p < 0.0001$). Additionally, expressions of *TXNRD1*, *TXN*, *PRDX5* and *PRDX6* coding for thioredoxin reductase 1, thioredoxin, peroxiredoxin 5 and peroxiredoxin 6 proteins, respectively, located in mitochondria, were higher in A172 cells. In contrast, U87MG cells exhibited higher expression of SOD2 compared to A172 cells (logFC = 0.738, adj $p < 0.0001$). SOD2 encodes a mitochondrial protein that binds to the superoxide by products of OXPHOS and converts them into hydrogen peroxide and diatomic oxygen [39] (Figure 4B). *GPX4*, a member of glutathione peroxidase that is active in mitochondria, was the only other upregulated antioxidant gene in U87MG cells. Therefore, the number of upregulated genes coding for antioxidant enzymes located in mitochondria was greater in A172 than in U87MG cells, corroborating the results of the MitoSOX assay with massive production of superoxide in U87MG cells. Interestingly, *SOD1* was upregulated after MET treatment in U87MG cell, while upregulation of *SOD2* was observed with LPS stimulation, but not with MET treatment in the two cell lines (Figure 4C).

The mitochondrial respiration of U87MG and A172 cells was measured by a Seahorse metabolic analyzer (Figure 4D). Basal mitochondrial respiration was calculated based on the reduction of the extracellular OCR through the inhibition of ATP synthase by oligomycin. U87MG cells had lower basal respiration than A172 cells ($p < 0.0001$, one-way ANOVA followed by Tukey test), while MET treatment blunted mitochondrial respiration in both cell lines. U87MG cells also had lower ATP production in comparison to A172 cells, calculated by subtracting oligomycin rate from baseline OCR ($p < 0.0001$, one-way ANOVA followed by Tukey test), and no ATP production was observed after MET treatment because the basal respiration was blocked. The maximal mitochondrial respiration capacity was calculated by collapsing the mitochondrial inner membrane and disrupting the mitochondrial membrane potential with CCCP, and by blocking complexes I and III of OXPHOS with rotenone and antimycin A, respectively. A172 cells exhibited significantly higher maximal mitochondrial capacity compared to U87MG cells ($p < 0.0001$), corroborating the high mitochondrial metabolism observed in A172 cells. These results confirmed the effect of MET treatment in both cell lines (Figure 4E). Treatment with LPS alone, or in combination with MET, produced the same results observed after MET treatment in both cell lines (Supplementary Figure S3C).

3.5. A172 Cells Showed G2/M Cell Cycle Arrest after MET Treatment

Cluster 2 of the RNASeq analysis of A172 cells treated with MET showed a significant downregulation of genes related to chromosome segregation, in congruence with the results of the cell cycle assay. Interestingly, MET treatment alone of A172 cells did not lead to cell-cycle arrest. However, a significant increase in A172 cells (75%) at the G2/M phase, together with a shortened S-phase, was observed with the use of MET + TMZ combined treatment for 24 h ($p < 0.0001$, two-way ANOVA post-hoc Tukey test) (Figure 5A and Supplementary Figure S4A,B). In fact, a significant downregulation of 20 genes associated with chromosome segregation was detected in A172 cells after MET treatment, with a similar result after combined MET + LPS treatment in the RNASeq analysis (Figure 5B). These genes were related to different roles, such as chromosome condensation, kinetochore and microtubule organization and regulation, centromere separation and kinesin regulation. Among these genes, *NUP62*, *SKA2*, *TOP2A*, and *HJURP* were the most downregulated in MET-treated A172 cells compared to non-treated cells (logFC < −0.4, adj $p < 0.005$), while none had significant differential expression in U87MG cells under the same treatment conditions (Figure 5B).

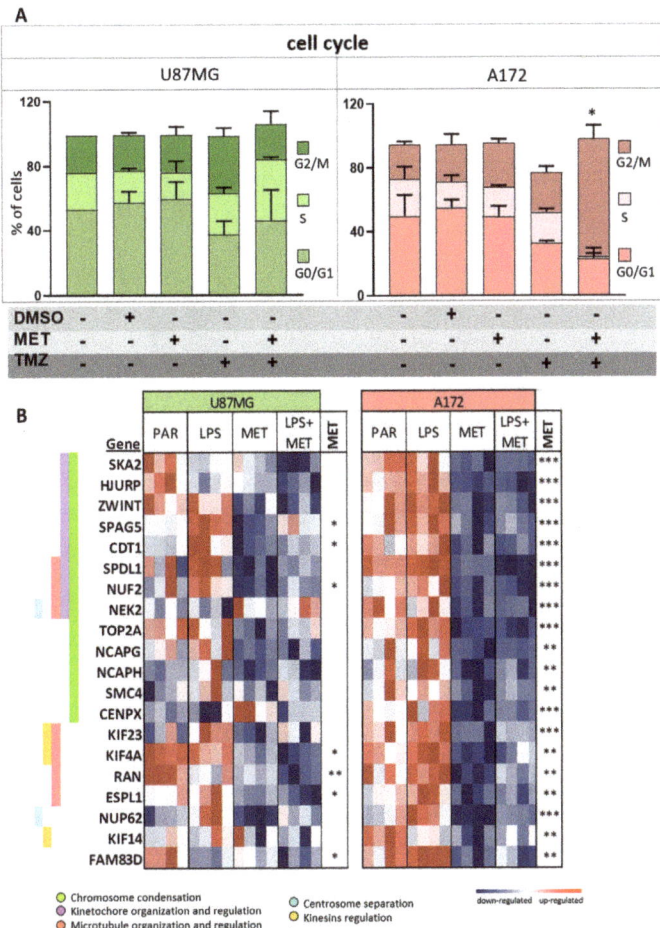

Figure 5. Cell cycle analysis and expression of genes related to chromosome segregation. (**A**) Cell cycle analysis for U87MG and A172 after MET and TMZ single and combined treatments. The bars represent each treatment condition. (*) $p < 0.0001$, two−way ANOVA post hoc Tukey test. G0/G1 phase (bottom bar), S phase (medium bar), G2/M phase (top bar); and (**B**) heatmap of chromosome segregation-related gene expressions after LPS and MET single and combined treatments in U87MG and A172 cells relative to non-treated controls. (*) $p < 0.05$, (**) $p < 0.01$, and (***) $p < 0.001$, Limma t-test for MET in comparison to PAR.

3.6. U87MG and A172 Cells Showed Upregulation of ER Stress and U87MG Cells Proved Prone to Apoptosis after MET Treatment

ER stress-related genes *ATF4*, *ATF6* and *DDIT3* (coding for CHOP), were upregulated in both cell lines after treatment with MET or LPS + MET. Additionally, pro-apoptotic genes *CHAC*, *TRIB3*, *PMAIP1*, *BBC3* and *BAX* were also upregulated in both cell lines, but more significantly in U87MG cells and after combined LPS + MET treatment ($3.2 \times 10^{-11} < p < 0.02$, compared to non-treated cells). Additionally, after MET or LPS + MET treatment, U87MG cells exhibited significant downregulation of anti-apoptotic genes, including *MCL1*, *PDK1* and *BCL2* ($p < 0.005$) (Figure 6A). Notably, the decrease in *BCL2* expression was confirmed at the protein level by Western blot in U87MG cells after MET + LPS treatment (Figure 6B, original Western blot is in Supplementary information original images). By contrast, none of these anti-apoptotic genes were downregulated in A172 cells after treatment with MET or LPS + MET.

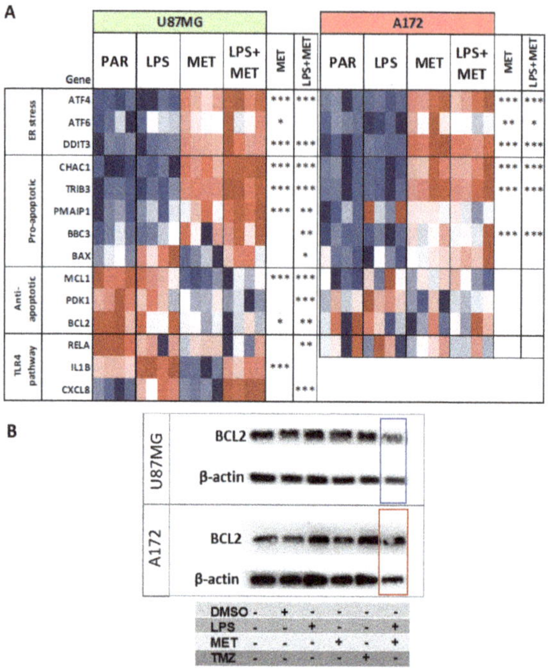

Figure 6. ER stress, pro- and anti-apoptotic and TLR4 pathway related gene expressions. (**A**) Heatmap for expression values of genes related to ER stress, pro−apoptotic, anti−apoptotic and TLR4 pathway in U87MG cells and A172 cells after LPS and MET single and combined treatments, (*) $p < 0.05$, (**) $p < 0.01$, and (***) $p < 0.001$, Limma t-test for LPS + MET combined and MET single treatment compared to non−treated cells; and (**B**) Western blot results for BCL2 of U87MG and A172 parental, DMSO, LPS, TMZ, MET single treated cells. β-actin was used for protein loading control.

Another difference between U87MG and A172 cells involved TLR4 signaling pathway activation. Expression of *RELA*, coding for p65 subunit of NFκB, and of *IL1B*, was downregulated in U87MG after MET treatment, most significantly for *IL1B* expression. However, higher upregulation of *CXCL8*, coding for IL8, was observed after LPS + MET treatment compared to LPS treatment alone. By contrast, A172 cells showed no differential expression for *RELA*, while no *CXCL8* and *IL1B* expression was detected for any of the treatment conditions (Figure 6A).

3.7. In Silico Validation of the Results in the TCGA-GBM-RNASeq Dataset

Of the 160 GBM cases in the TCGA-RNASeq dataset, 77 were stratified according to the metabolic classification proposed by Garofano et al. (2021) [32] into GPM ($n = 34$) subtype with similarities to the U87MG cell line, and MTC ($n = 43$) subtype with similarities to the A172 cell line. Interestingly, antioxidant genes, including *SOD1*, *TXN* and *PRDX1-5*, were upregulated in MTC cases (Figure 7A and Supplementary Figure S5), whereas *SOD2* (Figure 7A) and *TXNRD1* were upregulated in GPM ($p < 0.05$, Mann–Whitney test). Moreover, expression levels of antioxidant genes were significantly correlated to *SOD1* expression in MTC ($p < 0.05$, Spearman's test) (Figure 7B). In contrast, genes related to the TLR4 signaling pathway, including *TLR4*, *MYD88*, *TRAF6*, subunits of NFκB (*REL*, *RELA*, *RELB*, *NFKB1*) and *CXCL8*, were upregulated in GPM ($p < 0.05$, Mann-Whitney test) (Figure 7A and Supplementary Figure S5). More specifically, expression of *SOD2* and *CXCL8* was higher in GPM-GBM than in MTC-GBM (Figure 7C) and the analysis of the impact of upregulation of these two genes, according to the Kaplan–Meier estimator, showed that *CXCL8* upregulation was more negative than *SOD2* upregulation, as GPM-GBM cases with lower SOD2/CXCL8 ratio had an OS of 7.72 months compared to 22.26 months for cases with a higher ratio (p = 0.002, Logrank test) (Figure 7D). Taken together, this in silico analysis of the MTC-GBM subtype revealing upregulation of antioxidant genes, especially *SOD1*, and the GPM-GBM subtype showing upregulation of *SOD2* and TLR4 pathway-related genes, mirrors the findings observed for A172 and U87MG cells, respectively.

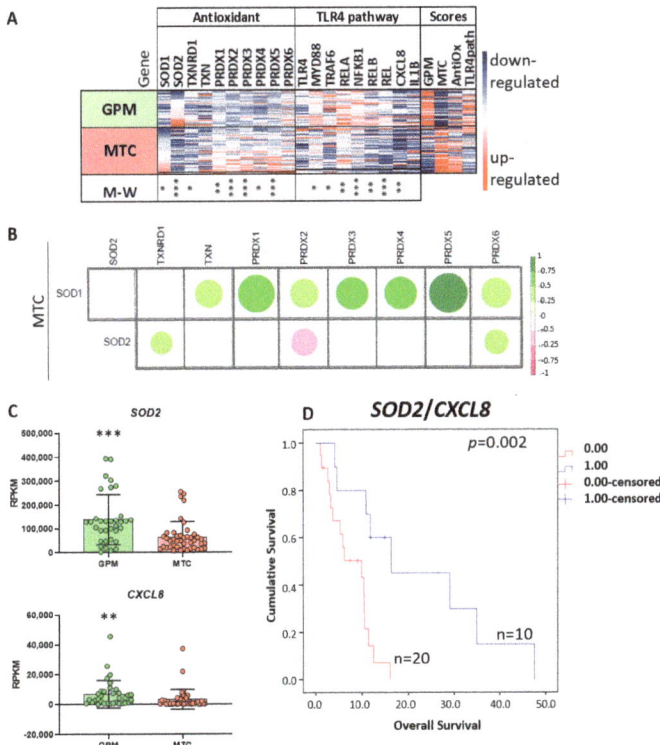

Figure 7. In silico validation of antioxidant and TLR4 pathway-related gene expressions in TCGA GBM-RNASeq dataset. (**A**) Heatmap of antioxidant and TLR4 pathway-related gene expressions normalized by z−score in 34 GPM and 43 MTC GBM subtypes according to Garofano's classification. The gene signatures for each case were calculated, and a score value was designated and normalized by z−score. (*) p < 0.05, (**) p < 0.01 (***), p < 0.001 (Mann–Whitney test); (**B**) in MTC, Spearman's correlation analysis showed strong correlation between the expression of *SOD1* and other antioxidant genes. The size of the circles is proportional to the p values, and positive (green) and negative (pink) correlations are presented according to the rho values in the bar scale at right. (**C**) RPKM values of *SOD2* and *CXCL8* for GPM− and MTC−GBM subtypes, graph bar presenting the mean values. Each circle represents a GBM case. (**) p < 0.01 (***), p < 0.001 (Mann–Whitney test); (**D**) in GPM, longer OS was presented by GBM cases with higher *SOD2/CXCL8* ratio in a Kaplan–Meier graph, p = 0.002 by log rank test (four cases were censored).

4. Discussion

GBM heterogeneity is a major factor limiting the effectiveness of therapeutic strategies available, creating the need to identify biomarkers to better stratify these tumors for specific combination therapies. We analyzed the response of two GBM cell lines to treatment with MET, LPS and TMZ, used alone and in combination. The U87MG cell line harboring the

NF1 mutation and A172 cell line with *RB1* mutation, classified as the mesenchymal GBM subtype with the worst prognosis, were selected to investigate the effects of these treatment conditions. These two specific cell lines were also chosen for their distinct metabolic profile, where U87MG has a GPM profile and A172 a MTC profile, according to Garofano's proposed GBM stratification based on metabolic pathways [32]. Differences of response to MET were already associated to mutational status of GBM cell lines [40]. Herein, we investigated MET response associated with the metabolic status of GBM cell lines.

Decreased cell viability was detected after MET + TMZ and MET + LPS + TMZ treatments in both cell lines, corroborating previous reports of anti-tumor effects of MET + TMZ [41,42]. Combined LPS + MET treatment has been previously tested in a mouse model of colon rectal cancer, with decreased tumor cell migration and longer OS in this animal model [13]. However, to our knowledge, this is the first study of LPS + MET treatment in gliomas.

A MET effect on mitochondrial respiration was confirmed in U87MG and A172 cells. Although A172 cells exhibited mostly oxidative respiration, with higher expression of genes coding for complex I of OXPHOS compared with U87MG cells, MET treatment reduced ATP production and oxygen consumption in both cell lines. The decoupling of electron transport induced by MET led to oxidative stress with superoxide production, ER stress and unfolded protein response (UPR) activation in both cell lines. Elevated superoxide after MET treatment was previously described in hepatocellular carcinoma [43], and pancreatic cancer cells, where superoxide accumulation in the mitochondrial matrix was associated with alteration of superoxide dismutase (SOD) expression [16]. SODs are antioxidant proteins responsible for converting superoxide radicals into hydrogen peroxide. SOD1 is localized in cytosol and mitochondrial intermembrane space and SOD2 in mitochondrial matrix [39,44]. Interestingly, A172 cells exhibited high expression of SOD1 and of several other antioxidant genes coding for proteins located in the organelle, possibly explaining the lower production of mitochondrial ROS detected after MET treatment. Moreover, A172 cells had upregulated expression of pro-apoptotic genes, with no change in expression of anti-apoptotic genes and, consequently, no increase in apoptosis after MET treatment. Nevertheless, in A172 cells, MET treatment promoted cell-cycle alteration with G2/M arrest due to downregulation of several genes related to chromosome segregation. In particular, genes related to kinetochore (*HJURP*, *ZWINT*), centromere (*NUF2*, *NEK2*, *CENPX*), mitotic spindle (*SPDL1*, *SPAG5*), chromatid separation (*TOP2A*, *NCAPG*), chromosome assembly (*NCAPH*, *SMC4*) and microtubule binding (*CDT1*, *FAM83D*), were downregulated. The kinetochore is built in the centromere and connects the chromosome to microtubules. The NDC80 complex (coded by *NUF2*), the kinetochore structural component, maintains microtubule attachment, and its blockage affects chromosome segregation stability [45]. *CDT1* is associated with the stable attachment of microtubule to kinetochore in the formation of the pre-DNA replication complex [46]. *RAN* [47], *NEK2* [48], *SPDL1* are related to microtubule positioning, where the latter plays this role by recruiting dynein for kinetochore [49]. Kinesins, *KIF4*, *KIF23* and *KIF14*, are important molecules responsible for microtubule transportation and positioning [50], which were also downregulated in A172 cells after MET treatment. Therefore, treatment with MET alone led to cell-cycle arrest, but this intervention proved insufficient to induce cell death of A172 cells. In a bid to identify an analogy of these findings with human GBM cases, the GBM-RNASeq dataset of the TCGA was analyzed. The MTC-GBM subtype, corresponding to the A172 cell line expression profile, showed upregulation of *SOD1* expression and significant correlation with antioxidant gene expressions, predominantly with the *PRDX* family, *PRDX1-5*, and with *TXNRD1*. Given this increased antioxidant state may blunt the apoptotic response, antioxidant inhibitors may represent an alternative combination therapy for the MTC-GBM subtype. Previous studies have demonstrated suppression of the ROS signaling pathway and triggering of apoptosis by a specific SOD1 inhibitor LD100 [51], an efficient copper-chelating agent [52]. Therefore, SOD1 inhibitors, or other antioxidant drugs, may be eligible for use in combination treatment with MET for the MTC-GBM subtype to induce cell-cycle arrest and activation of the apoptotic pathway. Under this condition, SOD1 expression level may be used as an eligibility parameter for this combination therapy.

By contrast, U87MG cells showed upregulation of *SOD2*, with increased expression following LPS stimulation. However, the upregulation of this antioxidant proved insufficient to buffer the massive production of superoxide after MET treatment, exacerbated by the low expression of other mitochondrial antioxidant genes. ER response and UPR activation due to this oxidative stress resulted in increased apoptosis after MET treatment (33%), an increase which was significantly higher with MET + LPS + TMZ treatment (57%). The upregulation of pro-apoptotic genes and downregulation of anti-apoptotic genes, mainly *MCL1*, *PDK1* and *BCL2*, after MET and MET + LPS treatments contributed to the tumor cell death observed. In fact, a previous U87MG in vivo study showed delayed tumor growth with daily MET treatment [40], and better OS with MET + TMZ combined treatment [41]. MET treatment also induced TMZ sensitivity to a resistant GBM cell line [53]. In U251 and T98G GBM cell lines, a decrease of BCL2 and an increase of pro-apoptotic proteins were observed after MET treatment with enhancement of TMZ effect [54].

Additionally, unlike A172 cells, U87MG cells showed activation of the NFκB pathway leading to increased *IL1B* expression after LPS stimulation, confirming our previous evidence [25]. Notably, *IL1B* upregulation persisted after LSP + MET treatment, a phenomenon that might also control tumor growth, as a pyroptotic type of cell death via the cGAS-STING pathway was triggered by persistent stimulation of IL1β [55]. However, LPS treatment also increased *CXCL8*, coding for IL8, a known pro-angiogenic factor in the tumor microenvironment [56], where neovascularization is one of the main characteristics of GBM responsible for its aggressiveness. Moreover, SOD2 upregulation has been associated with poor prognosis in several tumors [57] and was associated with TMZ resistance in GBM cells and in xenograft models [58]. In fact, the transcriptomic analysis of the human GBM cases of the TGCA RNASeq dataset showed the GPM-GBM subtype had upregulation of *SOD2* and genes related to the TLR4 signaling pathway, including *CXCL8*, in comparison to the MTC-GBM subtype. The analysis of the impact of the two pro-tumoral genes, *SOD2* and *CXCL8*, showed a shorter OS for the GPM-GBM cases with lower *SOD2/CXCL8*, indicating that increased *CXCL8* expression may be more deleterious. Increased CXCL8 (IL8) expression may be addressed by a neutralizing IL8 monoclonal antibody, which has been tested in a phase I clinical trial for metastatic or unresectable solid tumors and in ongoing studies evaluating its effect in reducing mesenchymal features in tumor cells, rendering them less resistant to treatment [59]. To date, no SOD2 pharmacological inhibitors have been tested. Further in vivo studies are needed to determine the efficacy of the suggested combination therapies for GBM treatment.

5. Conclusions

In conclusion, U87MG, a mesenchymal GBM cell line with GPM metabolic background, responded with increased apoptosis after MET + LPS + TMZ treatment via increased ER stress and UPR response and downregulation of BCL2. A172; however, a mesenchymal GBM cell line with an MTC metabolic background, also attained an upregulated antioxidant status and MET treatment led to cell-cycle arrest. The present in vitro findings suggest that the GPM-GBM subtype with activated inflammatory TLR4 pathway may respond to MET treatment and that combination treatment with CXCL8/IL8-inhibitor may improve tumor growth control. The use of MET treatment, in combination with an antioxidant inhibitor such as anti-SOD1, may be an eligible approach for cases with the MTC-GBM subtype. The efficacy of the suggested combination therapies needs to be tested in vivo studies.

Supplementary Materials: The following supporting information can be downloaded at: https://www.mdpi.com/article/10.3390/cancers15030587/s1. Figure S1:(A) Immunofluorescence analysis exhibiting the presence of TLR4 (in red) in U87MG and A172 cells; (B) Heatmap showing the differential expression in U87MG and A172 cell lines for marker genes for glycolytic plurimetabolic (GPM) and mitochondrial (MTC) according to Garofano's classification (2021). Figure S2: U87MG and A172 cell death analyzed by flow cytometry. Figure S3: Superoxide production in mitochondria after LPS, MET, and TMZ single and combined treatments for U87MG. Figure S4: Cell cycle analysis for U87MG and A172 after LPS, MET and TMZ single and combined treatments. Figure S5: Heatmap of antioxidant genes, TLR4 pathway-related genes, marker genes for glycolytic plurimetabolic (GPM) and mitochondrial (MTC) subtypes. Original images: Western blot original figure. See Ref. [60].

Author Contributions: Conceptualization, I.F.M. and S.K.N.M.; methodology, I.F.M., A.M.L., P.R.S., J.M.-d.-S. and G.P.; validation, I.F.M., J.M.-d.-S. and A.M.L.; formal analysis, I.F.M. and S.K.N.M.; investigation, I.F.M. and S.K.N.M.; writing—original draft preparation, I.F.M. and S.K.N.M.; writing—review and editing, I.F.M., S.M.O.-S. and S.K.N.M.; supervision, S.K.N.M.; funding acquisition, S.M.O.-S., S.K.N.M., M.d.S.B. and G.P. All authors have read and agreed to the published version of the manuscript.

Funding: This research was supported by Conselho Nacional de Pesquisa (CNPq) "Bolsa de Produtividade": #304541/2020-6 (S.K.N.M.), #307854/2018-3 (G.P.), #317214/2021-7 (S.M.O.-S.); Sao Paulo Research Foundation (FAPESP, grants #04/12133-6 (S.K.N.M.), #2013/07937-8 (M.S.B.), #2020/02988-7 (S.K.N.M., S.M.O.-S.), #2018/18257-1 (G.P.), #2020/04923-0 (G.P.), #2021/00140-3 (J.M.-d.-S.); Coordenação de Aperfeiçoamento de Pessoal de Nível Superior—Brasil (CAPES/PROEX) grants #23038.018285/2019-21 (S.K.N.M., S.M.O.-S.), #88887.600107/2021-00 (I.F.M.) and (CAPES/NUFFIC) grants #062/15, 9999.001625 (S.K.N.M.), 88887.351607/2019-00 (I.F.M.); Fundação Faculdade de Medicina (FFM); and Faculdade de Medicina da USP (FMUSP).

Institutional Review Board Statement: The present study was approved by the HCFMUSP (process number: 059/15) and the FMUSP, ethical committee (process number: 278/15).

Informed Consent Statement: Not applicable.

Data Availability Statement: Not applicable.

Acknowledgments: We are grateful to Esper Kallas, coordinator of the FMUSP flow cytometry facility, for the use of the equipment and excellent assistance provided by their staff. We also would like to thank Marisa Passarelli for Metformin reagent donation. We thank Alicia J Kowaltowski for the Seahorse equipment use and the technical support of Camille C. Caldeira da Silva. We also thank the SELA Facility Core of School of Medicine, University of Sao Paulo (Fapesp grant #2014/50137-5), for assistance with sequencing.

Conflicts of Interest: The authors declare no conflict of interest.

References

1. Louis, D.N.; Perry, A.; Wesseling, P.; Brat, D.J.; Cree, I.A.; Figarella-Branger, D.; Hawkins, C.; Ng, H.K.; Pfister, S.M.; Reifenberger, G.; et al. The 2021 WHO Classification of Tumors of the Central Nervous System: A summary. *Neuro Oncol.* **2021**, *23*, 1231–1251. [CrossRef]
2. Villano, J.L.; Seery, T.E.; Bressler, L.R. Temozolomide in malignant gliomas: Current use and future targets. *Cancer Chemother. Pharmacol.* **2009**, *64*, 647–655. [CrossRef]
3. Stupp, R.; Mason, W.P.; van den Bent, M.J.; Weller, M.; Fisher, B.; Taphoorn, M.J.; Belanger, K.; Brandes, A.A.; Marosi, C.; Bogdahn, U.; et al. Radiotherapy plus concomitant and adjuvant temozolomide for newly diagnosed glioblastoma. *N. Engl. J. Med.* **2005**, *352*, 987–996. [CrossRef]
4. Louis, D.N.; Ohgaki, H.; Wiestler, O.D.; Cavenee, W.K.; Burger, P.C.; Jouvet, A.; Scheithauer, B.W.; Kleihues, P. The 2007 WHO Classification of Tumours of the Central Nervous System. *Acta Neuropathol.* **2007**, *114*, 97–109. [CrossRef]
5. Mazurek, M.; Litak, J.; Kamieniak, P.; Kulesza, B.; Jonak, K.; Baj, J.; Grochowski, C. Metformin as Potential Therapy for High-Grade Glioma. *Cancers.* **2020**, *12*, 210. [CrossRef]
6. Fujita, Y.; Inagaki, N. Metformin: New Preparations and Nonglycemic Benefits. *Curr. Diabetes Rep.* **2017**, *17*, 5. [CrossRef]
7. Wang, Y.; An, H.; Liu, T.; Qin, C.; Sesaki, H.; Guo, S.; Radovick, S.; Hussain, M.; Maheshwari, A.; Wondisford, F.E.; et al. Metformin Improves Mitochondrial Respiratory Activity through Activation of AMPK. *Cell Rep.* **2019**, *29*, 1511–1523.e5. [CrossRef]
8. Xiao, Z.; Wu, W.; Poltoratsky, V. Metformin Suppressed CXCL8 Expression and Cell Migration in HEK293/TLR4 Cell Line. *Mediat. Inflamm.* **2017**, *2017*, 6589423. [CrossRef]
9. Kim, J.; Kwak, H.J.; Cha, J.Y.; Sesaki, H.; Guo, S.; Radovick, S.; Hussain, M.; Maheshwari, A.; Wondisford, F.E.; O'Rourke, B.; et al. Metformin suppresses lipopolysaccharide (LPS)-induced inflammatory response in murine macrophages via activating transcription factor-3 (ATF-3) induction. *J. Biol. Chem.* **2014**, *289*, 23246–23255. [CrossRef]
10. Xian, H.; Liu, Y.; Nilsson, A.R.; Gatchalian, R.; Crother, T.R.; Tourtellotte, W.G.; Zhang, Y.; Aleman-Muench, G.R.; Lewis, G.; Chen, W.; et al. Metformin inhibition of mitochondrial ATP and DNA synthesis abrogates NLRP3 inflammasome activation and pulmonary inflammation. *Immunity* **2021**, *54*, 1463–1477.e11. [CrossRef]
11. Zhang, Y.; Zhang, H.; Li, S.; Huang, K.; Jiang, L.; Wang, Y. Metformin Alleviates LPS-Induced Acute Lung Injury by Regulating the SIRT1/NF-κB/NLRP3 Pathway and Inhibiting Endothelial Cell Pyroptosis. *Front. Pharmacol.* **2022**, *13*, 801337. [CrossRef]

12. Xiong, W.; Sun, K.-Y.; Zhu, Y.; Zhang, X.; Zhou, Y.-H.; Zou, X. Metformin alleviates inflammation through suppressing FASN-dependent palmitoylation of Akt. *Cell Death Dis.* **2021**, *12*, 934. [CrossRef]
13. Wu, X.; Qian, S.; Zhang, J.; Feng, J.; Luo, K.; Sun, L.; Zhao, L.; Ran, Y.; Sun, L.; Wang, J.; et al. Lipopolysaccharide promotes metastasis via acceleration of glycolysis by the nuclear factor-κB/snail/hexokinase3 signaling axis in colorectal cancer. *Cancer Metab.* **2021**, *9*, 23. [CrossRef]
14. Xue, C.; Wang, C.; Sun, Y.; Meng, Q.; Liu, Z.; Huo, X.; Sun, P.; Sun, H.; Ma, X.; Ma, X.; et al. Targeting P-glycoprotein function, p53 and energy metabolism: Combination of metformin and 2-deoxyglucose reverses the multidrug resistance of MCF-7/Dox cells to doxorubicin. *Oncotarget* **2017**, *8*, 8622–8632. [CrossRef]
15. Khan, A.S.; Frigo, D.E. A spatiotemporal hypothesis for the regulation; role; and targeting of AMPK in prostate cancer. *Nat. Rev. Urol.* **2017**, *14*, 164–180. [CrossRef]
16. Warkad, M.S.; Kim, C.H.; Kang, B.G.; Park, S.H.; Jung, J.S.; Feng, J.H.; Inci, G.; Kim, S.C.; Suh, H.W.; Lim, S.S.; et al. Metformin-induced ROS upregulation as amplified by apigenin causes profound anticancer activity while sparing normal cells. *Sci. Rep.* **2021**, *11*, 14002. [CrossRef]
17. Takahashi, A.; Kimura, F.; Yamanaka, A.; Takebayashi, A.; Kita, N.; Takahashi, K.; Murakami, T. Metformin impairs growth of endometrial cancer cells via cell cycle arrest and concomitant autophagy and apoptosis. *Cancer Cell Int.* **2014**, *14*, 53. [CrossRef]
18. Tseng, H.-W.; Li, S.-C.; Tsai, K.-W. Metformin Treatment Suppresses Melanoma Cell Growth and Motility Through Modulation of microRNA Expression. *Cancers* **2019**, *11*, 209. [CrossRef]
19. Markowicz-Piasecka, M.; Sikora, J.; Szydłowska, A.; Skupień, A.; Mikiciuk-Olasik, E.; Huttunen, K.M. Metformin–A Future Therapy for Neurodegenerative Diseases. *Pharm. Res.* **2017**, *34*, 2614–2627. [CrossRef]
20. Łabuzek, K.; Suchy, D.; Gabryel, B.; Bielecka, A.; Liber, S.; Okopień, B. Quantification of metformin by the HPLC method in brain regions; cerebrospinal fluid and plasma of rats treated with lipopolysaccharide. *Pharmacol. Rep.* **2010**, *62*, 956–965. [CrossRef]
21. Albayrak, G.; Konac, E.; Akin Dere, U.; Emmez, H. Targeting Cancer Cell Metabolism with Metformin; Dichloroacetate and Memantine in Glioblastoma (GBM). *Turk. Neurosurg.* **2021**, *31*, 233–237. [CrossRef]
22. Soraya, H.; Sani, N.A.; Jabbari, N.; Rezaie, J. Metformin Increases Exosome Biogenesis and Secretion in U87 MG Human Glioblastoma Cells: A Possible Mechanism of Therapeutic Resistance. *Arch. Med. Res.* **2021**, *52*, 151–162. [CrossRef]
23. Rezaei, N.; Neshasteh-Riz, A.; Mazaheri, Z.; Koosha, F.; Hoormand, M. The Combination of Metformin and Disulfiram-Cu for Effective Radiosensitization on Glioblastoma Cells. *Cell J.* **2020**, *22*, 263–272. [CrossRef]
24. Ohno, M.; Kitanaka, C.; Miyakita, Y.; Tanaka, S.; Sonoda, Y.; Mishima, K.; Ishikawa, E.; Takahashi, M.; Yanagisawa, S.; Ohashi, K.; et al. Metformin with Temozolomide for Newly Diagnosed Glioblastoma: Results of Phase I Study and a Brief Review of Relevant Studies. *Cancers* **2022**, *14*, 4222. [CrossRef]
25. Moretti, I.F.; Lerario, A.M.; Trombetta-Lima, M.; Sola, P.R.; da Silva Soares, R.; Oba-Shinjo, S.M.; Marie, S.K.N. Late p65 nuclear translocation in glioblastoma cells indicates non-canonical TLR4 signaling and activation of DNA repair genes. *Sci. Rep.* **2021**, *11*, 1333. [CrossRef]
26. Kim, D.; Langmead, B.; Salzberg, S.L. HISAT: A fast spliced aligner with low memory requirements. *Nat. Methods* **2015**, *12*, 357–360. [CrossRef]
27. The Gene Ontology Consortium. The Gene Ontology Resource: 20 years and still GOing strong. *Nucleic Acids Res.* **2019**, *47*, D330–D338. [CrossRef]
28. The Gene Ontology Consortium. The Gene Ontology resource: Enriching a GOld mine. *Nucleic Acids Res.* **2021**, *49*, D325–D334. [CrossRef]
29. Carbon, S.; Ireland, A.; Mungall, C.J.; Shu, S.; Marshall, B.; Lewis, S.; AmiGO Hub; Web Presence Working Group. AmiGO: Online access to ontology and annotation data. *Bioinformatics* **2009**, *25*, 288–289. [CrossRef]
30. Snel, B.; Lehmann, G.; Bork, P.; Huynen, M.A. STRING: A web-server to retrieve and display the repeatedly occurring neighbourhood of a gene. *Nucleic Acids Res.* **2000**, *28*, 3442–3444. [CrossRef]
31. Szklarczyk, D.; Gable, A.L.; Nastou, K.C.; Lyon, D.; Kirsch, R.; Pyysalo, S.; Doncheva, N.T.; Legeay, M.; Fang, T.; Bork, P.; et al. The STRING database in 2021: Customizable protein-protein networks; and functional characterization of user-uploaded gene/measurement sets. *Nucleic Acids Res.* **2021**, *49*, D605–D612. [CrossRef]
32. Garofano, L.; Migliozzi, S.; Oh, Y.T.; D'Angelo, F.; Najac, R.D.; Ko, A.; Frangaj, B.; Caruso, F.P.; Yu, K.; Yuan, J.; et al. Pathway-based classification of glioblastoma uncovers a mitochondrial subtype with therapeutic vulnerabilities. *Nat. Cancer* **2021**, *2*, 141–156. [CrossRef]
33. Hänzelmann, S.; Castelo, R.; Guinney, J. GSVA: Gene set variation analysis for microarray and RNA-seq data. *BMC Bioinform.* **2013**, *14*, 7. [CrossRef]
34. Cerami, E.; Gao, J.; Dogrusoz, U.; Gross, B.E.; Sumer, S.O.; Aksoy, B.A.; Jacobsen, A.; Byrne, C.J.; Heuer, M.L.; Larsson, E.; et al. The cBio cancer genomics portal: An open platform for exploring multidimensional cancer genomics data. *Cancer Discov.* **2012**, *2*, 401–404. [CrossRef]
35. R Studio Team. *RStudio: Integrated Development Environment for R*; RStudio, PBC: Boston, MA, USA, 2020. Available online: http://www.rstudio.com/ (accessed on 3 November 2022).
36. Wei, T.; Simko, V.; Levy, M.; Xie, Y.; Jin, Y.; Zemla, J. Package 'corrplot'. *Statistician* **2017**, *56*, 316–324.
37. Moretti, I.F.; Franco, D.G.; de Almeida Galatro, T.F.; Oba-Shinjo, S.M.; Marie, S.K.N. Plasmatic membrane toll-like receptor expressions in human astrocytomas. *PLoS ONE* **2018**, *13*, e0199211. [CrossRef]

38. Baek, Y.; Woo, T.-G.; Ahn, J.; Lee, D.; Kwon, Y.; Park, B.J.; Ha, N.C. Structural analysis of the overoxidized Cu/Zn-superoxide dismutase in ROS-induced ALS filament formation. *Commun. Biol.* **2022**, *5*, 1085. [CrossRef]
39. Candas, D.; Li, J.J. MnSOD in oxidative stress response-potential regulation via mitochondrial protein influx. *Antioxid. Redox Signal.* **2014**, *20*, 1599–1617. [CrossRef]
40. Sesen, J.; Dahan, P.; Scotland, S.J.; Saland, E.; Dang, V.T.; Lemarié, A.; Tyler, B.M.; Brem, H.; Toulas, C.; Cohen-Jonathan Moyal, E.; et al. Metformin Inhibits Growth of Human Glioblastoma Cells and Enhances Therapeutic Response. *PLoS ONE* **2015**, *10*, e0123721. [CrossRef]
41. Xiong, Z.S.; Gong, S.F.; Si, W.; Jiang, T.; Li, Q.L.; Wang, T.J.; Wang, W.J.; Wu, R.Y.; Jiang, K. Effect of metformin on cell proliferation, apoptosis, migration and invasion in A172 glioma cells and its mechanisms. *Mol. Med. Rep.* **2019**, *20*, 887–894. [CrossRef]
42. Lee, J.E.; Lim, J.H.; Hong, Y.K.; Yang, S.H. High-Dose Metformin Plus Temozolomide Shows Increased Anti-tumor Effects in Glioblastoma In Vitro and In Vivo Compared with Monotherapy. *Cancer Res. Treat.* **2018**, *50*, 1331–1342. [CrossRef]
43. Gou, S.; Qiu, L.; Yang, Q.; Li, P.; Zhou, X.; Sun, Y.; Zhou, X.; Zhao, W.; Zhai, W.; Li, G.; et al. Metformin leads to accumulation of reactive oxygen species by inhibiting the NFE2L1 expression in human hepatocellular carcinoma cells. *Toxicol. Appl. Pharmacol.* **2021**, *420*, 115523. [CrossRef]
44. Okado-Matsumoto, A.; Fridovich, I. Subcellular Distribution of Superoxide Dismutases (SOD) in Rat Liver: Cu;Zn-SOD in mitochondria. *J. Biol. Chem.* **2001**, *276*, 38388–38393. [CrossRef]
45. Vorozhko, V.V.; Emanuele, M.J.; Kallio, M.J.; Stukenberg, P.T.; Gorbsky, G.J. Multiple mechanisms of chromosome movement in vertebrate cells mediated through the Ndc80 complex and dynein/dynactin. *Chromosoma* **2008**, *117*, 169–179. [CrossRef]
46. Varma, D.; Chandrasekaran, S.; Sundin, L.J.; Reidy, K.T.; Wan, X.; Chasse, D.A.; Nevis, K.R.; DeLuca, J.G.; Salmon, E.D.; Cook, J.G. Recruitment of the human Cdt1 replication licensing protein by the loop domain of Hec1 is required for stable kinetochore-microtubule attachment. *Nat. Cell Biol.* **2012**, *14*, 593–603. [CrossRef]
47. Oh, D.; Yu, C.-H.; Needleman, D.J. Spatial organization of the Ran pathway by microtubules in mitosis. *Proc. Natl. Acad. Sci. USA* **2016**, *113*, 8729–8734. [CrossRef]
48. Fry, A.M.; O'Regan, L.; Sabir, S.R.; Bayliss, R. Cell cycle regulation by the NEK family of protein kinases. *J. Cell Sci.* **2012**, *125*, 4423–4433. [CrossRef]
49. Griffis, E.R.; Stuurman, N.; Vale, R.D. Spindly, a novel protein essential for silencing the spindle assembly checkpoint; recruits dynein to the kinetochore. *J. Cell Biol.* **2007**, *177*, 1005–1015. [CrossRef]
50. Liang, Y.J.; Yang, W.X. Kinesins in MAPK cascade: How kinesin motors are involved in the MAPK pathway? *Gene* **2019**, *684*, 1–9. [CrossRef]
51. Li, X.; Chen, Y.; Zhao, J.; Shi, J.; Wang, M.; Qiu, S.; Hu, Y.; Xu, Y.; Cui, Y.; Liu, C.; et al. The Specific Inhibition of SOD1 Selectively Promotes Apoptosis of Cancer Cells via Regulation of the ROS Signaling Network. *Oxidative Med. Cell. Longev.* **2019**, *2019*, 9706792. [CrossRef]
52. Dong, X.; Zhang, Z.; Zhao, J.; Lei, J.; Chen, Y.; Li, X.; Chen, H.; Tian, J.; Zhang, D.; Liu, C.; et al. The rational design of specific SOD1 inhibitors via copper coordination and their application in ROS signaling research. *Chem. Sci.* **2016**, *7*, 6251–6262. [CrossRef]
53. Yang, S.H.; Li, S.; Lu, G.; Xue, H.; Kim, D.H.; Zhu, J.J.; Liu, Y. Metformin treatment reduces temozolomide resistance of glioblastoma cells. *Oncotarget* **2016**, *7*, 78787–78803. [CrossRef] [PubMed]
54. Valtorta, S.; Dico, A.L.; Raccagni, I.; Gaglio, D.; Belloli, S.; Politi, L.S.; Martelli, C.; Diceglie, C.; Bonanomi, M.; Ercoli, G.; et al. Metformin and temozolomide, a synergic option to overcome resistance in glioblastoma multiforme models. *Oncotarget* **2017**, *8*, 113090–113104. [CrossRef] [PubMed]
55. Aarreberg, L.D.; Esser-Nobis, K.; Driscoll, C.; Shuvarikov, A.; Roby, J.A.; Gale, M., Jr. Interleukin-1β Induces mtDNA Release to Activate Innate Immune Signaling via cGAS-STING. *Mol Cell* **2019**, *74*, 801–815.e6. [CrossRef]
56. De Palma, M.; Biziato, D.; Petrova, T.V. Microenvironmental regulation of tumour angiogenesis. *Nat. Rev. Cancer* **2017**, *17*, 457–474. [CrossRef] [PubMed]
57. Miar, A.; Hevia, D.; Muñoz-Cimadevilla, H.; Astudillo, A.; Velasco, J.; Sainz, R.M.; Mayo, J.C. Manganese superoxide dismutase (SOD2/MnSOD)/catalase and SOD2/GPx1 ratios as biomarkers for tumor progression and metastasis in prostate, colon, and lung cancer. *Free Radic. Biol. Med.* **2015**, *85*, 45–55. [CrossRef]
58. Chang, K.Y.; Hsu, T.I.; Hsu, C.C.; Tsai, S.Y.; Liu, J.J.; Chou, S.W.; Liu, M.S.; Liou, J.P.; Ko, C.Y.; Chen, K.Y.; et al. Specificity protein 1-modulated superoxide dismutase 2 enhances temozolomide resistance in glioblastoma; which is independent of O(6)-methylguanine-DNA methyltransferase. *Redox Biol.* **2017**, *13*, 655–664. [CrossRef]
59. Bilusic, M.; Heery, C.R.; Collins, J.M.; Donahue, R.N.; Palena, C.; Madan, R.A.; Karzai, F.; Marté, J.L.; Strauss, J.; Gatti-Mays, M.E.; et al. Phase I trial of HuMax-IL8 (BMS-986253), an anti-IL-8 monoclonal antibody; in patients with metastatic or unresectable solid tumors. *J. Immunother. Cancer* **2019**, *7*, 240. [CrossRef]
60. Verhaak, R.G.W.; Hoadley, K.A.; Purdom, E.; Wang, V.; Qi, Y.; Wilkerson, M.D.; Miller, C.R.; Ding, L.; Golub, T.; Mesirov, J.P.; et al. Integrated Genomic Analysis Identifies Clinically Relevant Subtypes of Glioblastoma Characterized by Abnormalities in PDGFRA, IDH1, EGFR, and NF1. *Cancer Cell* **2010**, *17*, 98–110. [CrossRef]

Disclaimer/Publisher's Note: The statements, opinions and data contained in all publications are solely those of the individual author(s) and contributor(s) and not of MDPI and/or the editor(s). MDPI and/or the editor(s) disclaim responsibility for any injury to people or property resulting from any ideas, methods, instructions or products referred to in the content.

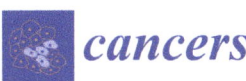

Review

Preclinical Models of Low-Grade Gliomas

Pushan Dasgupta [1], Veerakumar Balasubramanyian [2], John F. de Groot [3,*] and Nazanin K. Majd [2,*]

1. Department of Neurology, Dell Medical School, University of Texas at Austin, Austin, TX 78712, USA
2. Department of Neuro-Oncology, UT MD Anderson Cancer Center, Houston, TX 77030, USA
3. Department of Neurosurgery, University of California San Francisco, San Francisco, CA 94143, USA
* Correspondence: john.degroot@ucsf.edu (J.F.d.G.); nkmajd@mdanderson.org (N.K.M.)

Simple Summary: Preclinical models are essential for the advancement of our understanding of glioma biology and the development of novel therapeutics. Much of our progress in the treatment of low-grade glioma has been hampered by our limited ability to develop ideal preclinical models. This has proven to be a formidable task given the complex factors one must account for, such as genetic background, intratumoral heterogeneity, intact blood–brain barrier, and the tumor microenvironment. As new knowledge is acquired regarding low-grade glioma, preclinical models must be refined and adjusted to reflect the actual biology of human glioma as closely as possible. In this review, we delve into in vitro and in vivo models of low-grade glioma with particular attention to illuminating the multifaceted task of developing the most optimal models.

Abstract: Diffuse infiltrating low-grade glioma (LGG) is classified as WHO grade 2 astrocytoma with isocitrate dehydrogenase (IDH) mutation and oligodendroglioma with IDH1 mutation and 1p/19q codeletion. Despite their better prognosis compared with glioblastoma, LGGs invariably recur, leading to disability and premature death. There is an unmet need to discover new therapeutics for LGG, which necessitates preclinical models that closely resemble the human disease. Basic scientific efforts in the field of neuro-oncology are mostly focused on high-grade glioma, due to the ease of maintaining rapidly growing cell cultures and highly reproducible murine tumors. Development of preclinical models of LGG, on the other hand, has been difficult due to the slow-growing nature of these tumors as well as challenges involved in recapitulating the widespread genomic and epigenomic effects of IDH mutation. The most recent WHO classification of CNS tumors emphasizes the importance of the role of IDH mutation in the classification of gliomas, yet there are relatively few IDH-mutant preclinical models available. Here, we review the in vitro and in vivo preclinical models of LGG and discuss the mechanistic challenges involved in generating such models and potential strategies to overcome these hurdles.

Keywords: glioma; low-grade glioma; preclinical models; IDH-mutant glioma; patient avatars

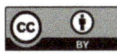

1. Introduction

Diffuse gliomas are the most common malignant tumors of the central nervous system (CNS) in adults [1]. They make up about 30% of all brain and 80% of all malignant brain tumors [2,3]. Diffuse low-grade gliomas account for approximately 15% of all gliomas in the United States and have a 5-year survival rate ranging from 30% to 80% [1]. Glioblastoma (WHO grade IV) is the most common adult glioma, accounting for 15% of all primary brain and central nervous system tumors and has a 2-year survival rate of 26.5% [1,4].

Diffuse gliomas are heterogenous groups of tumors that are universally incurable despite multimodality standard-of-care treatments, which include surgery, radiation therapy, and chemotherapy. There is an unmet need to develop novel therapeutics to improve patient outcomes. To achieve this goal, it is imperative to improve our understanding of glioma biology and to establish preclinical models that resemble the clinical and molecular characteristics of human glioma as closely as possible. Creating effective models for low-grade glioma has revealed unique challenges, as these tumors are slow growing, unlike their higher-grade counterpart, glioblastoma. Many researchers have contributed to our current ability to create effective models; however, there remains much more to do.

In this review, we will discuss the grading, classification, and molecular pathology of low-grade gliomas, the knowledge of which is important in understanding preclinical models of gliomas. We also explain properties of an ideal preclinical model and existing in vitro and in vivo models of low-grade gliomas.

1.1. Diffuse Low-Grade Gliomas

In the WHO 2021 classification, there are three primary categories of adult-type diffuse gliomas: isocitrate dehydrogenase (*IDH*)-mutant, 1p/19q codeleted oligodendroglioma; IDH-mutant, non-codeleted astrocytoma; and IDH-wildtype glioblastoma [5]. Diffuse low-grade glioma is classified as WHO grade 1 and 2 astrocytoma with *IDH* mutation or oligodendroglioma with *IDH* mutation and 1p/19q codeletion.

1.2. Grading and Classification of Gliomas

The grading and classification of gliomas have gone through several changes throughout the years. The first grading system was developed by Albert Broders at the Mayo Clinic and employed a numerical grading system dividing tumors into four histological grades of malignancy [6]. This system did not take into account clinical history. The histological grading system uses the "AMEN" score, which consists of nuclear atypia (A), mitosis (M), microvascular/endothelial proliferation (E), and necrosis (N) to evaluate malignancy [7]. In this system, grade 3 tumors required a significant mitotic count, while grade 4 tumors required microvascular proliferation or necrosis. However, this histological grading system was intrinsically subjective, with inter- and intra-observer variabilities [8]. The WHO grading system strived to provide a biology-oriented grade which was based more on estimated clinical outcome. The 2016 WHO classification of CNS tumors introduced integrated molecular and histological diagnoses to classify CNS tumors, and the 2021 WHO classification further expanded upon molecular features [9].

1.3. Molecular Pathology of Low-Grade Gliomas

The presence of the *IDH1* mutation has become a defining factor for adult diffuse low-grade glioma. Roughly 70% of grade 2–3 gliomas harbor mutations in either *IDH1* or its mitochondrial counterpart *IDH2* [10]. Often, these tumors are seen in younger patients and carry a better prognosis [11].

The normal function of IDH is to convert isocitrate to alpha-ketoglutarate (α-KG) [12]. Mutations in *IDH1* or *IDH2* are exclusively missense mutations of the arginine residues in the active site of the enzyme, which is R132 for IDH1 and R172 for IDH2 [10,13]. These mutations lead to neomorphic enzymatic activity, resulting in the production of the oncometabolite D-2-hydroxyglutarate (2-HG) from alpha-ketoglutarate (α-KG) [12]. The oncometabolite 2-HG inhibits a large number of α-KG-dependent enzymes involved in fatty acid synthesis and maintenance of redox potential and results in metabolic stress in IDH-mutant tumors [14,15]. In addition, 2-HG also inhibits DNA and histone demethylation, which results in a hypermethylated epigenetic state (G-CIMP phenotype) leading to impaired cell differentiation and dysregulation of oncogenes and tumor suppressor genes [16–18].

1.4. IDH-Mutant Astrocytoma

IDH-mutant astrocytoma encompasses grade 2 and grade 3 tumors that have *IDH1* or *IDH2* mutations without 1p/19q codeletion. Morphologically, these tumors are hypercellular and composed of diffusely infiltrative fibrillary glial cells [9,19]. The WHO does not provide a firm definition for a significant mitotic rate that would characterize a grade 3 tumor. However, in general grade 3 tumors will have a higher mitotic rate than grade 2 tumors and also display histologic features of anaplasia. Grade 4 IDH-mutant astrocytomas are defined by the presence of microvascular proliferation, necrosis, and/or homozygous deletion of cyclin-dependent kinase inhibitor 2A/B (*CDKN2A/B*) in IDH-mutant astrocytoma.

Beyond *IDH1* and *IDH2* mutations, adult-type IDH-mutant low-grade astrocytomas commonly harbor inactivating mutations in *TP53* and *ATRX*. *TP53* is the most frequently mutated gene in cancer. Its product, p53, is a tumor suppressor with roles as a regulator of cell cycle arrest and apoptosis [20,21]. ATRX is a regulator of chromatin remodeling and transcription and is known to form a chromatin remodeling complex with death domain-associated protein (DAXX), leading to the deposition of H3.3 in telomeric regions, pericentric heterochromatin, and various regions of repeat DNA [22,23]. One explanation for the co-occurrence of *TP53* and *ATRX* mutations is that cells deficient in ATRX undergo p53-dependent cell death [24,25]. ATRX-deficient tumors exhibit a pathological form of telomere maintenance whereby telomeres are lengthened in a telomerase-independent process called alternative lengthening of telomeres [26]. Intriguingly, there are rare infratentorial variants of IDH-mutant astrocytoma that have distinct molecular and clinical characteristics with relatively worse prognosis [9].

1.5. IDH-Mutant Oligodendroglioma

IDH-mutant oligodendroglioma is defined by the presence of 1p19q codeletion in the context of either *IDH1* or *IDH2* mutation and are either grade 2 or 3. Compared with grade 2 tumors, grade 3 tumors have histological features such as increased cellularity, marked atypia, greater mitotic activity, microvascular proliferation, and necrosis [27]. Genetically, the presence of homozygous *CDKN2A* and/or *CDKN2B* deletion classifies an oligodendroglioma as grade 3 [28]. Mutations in the TERT promoter occur frequently in these tumors. The catalytic subunit of telomerase is encoded by *TERT*, and point mutations in the promoter lead to TERT overexpression and thus telomere elongation [29,30]. Abnormal telomere maintenance seems to be a central process in gliomagenesis, which is implied by the mutual exclusivity of *TERT* promoter and *ATRX* mutations in IDH-mutant adult gliomas. *CIC* gene mutations are seen in up to 70% of oligodendrogliomas and have been linked to worse survival [31,32]. Such mutations interrupt the CIC protein's repressor functions by rendering the protein truncated, degraded, or non-functional [32]. This leads to upregulation of the ETS-Pea3 family of transcription factors, ETV1, ETV4, and ETV5, which are known oncoproteins and have been shown to induce cell proliferation in melanoma, prostate cancer, and gastrointestinal stromal tumors [33–35]. Transcriptomic analysis of CIC-mutant gliomas demonstrated an upregulation of the ETS/Pea3 family of proteins, which are normally repressed by the wildtype CIC protein [32,36]. Together, these findings suggest that the aggressiveness of CIC-mutant subsets of oligodendroglioma may be due to the inactivation of the repressor effects of CIC and increased expression of the ETS family of oncoproteins, which are involved in cell proliferation and invasion.

Inactivating *FUBP1* mutations also occur in 15% to 30% of oligodendrogliomas [31]. FUBP1 loss has been shown to cause widespread changes in both RNA splicing and expression of aberrant driver isoforms [37], but its precise role in gliomagenesis is not clear. Oligodendrogliomas with both *CIC* and *FUBP1* mutations are exceedingly rare. Further studies are needed to establish the relationship, if any, between these inactivating mutations and chemosensitivity in these tumors. Understanding the molecular genetics of IDH-mutant gliomas and their association with prognostic risk stratification is crucial in our interpretation of data generated from preclinical models.

1.6. Ideal Preclinical Model of Low-Grade Gliomas

In order to make new biologic discoveries of low-grade gliomas and to make progress in developing novel therapeutics, it is imperative to have preclinical models that accurately recapitulate the human disease. Beyond the fundamentals of reproducibility and stability, an ideal preclinical model should demonstrate genetic background, intratumoral heterogeneity, and a microenvironment that closely resemble those of human diffuse glioma.

However, developing an ideal model that captures all these elements in vivo has been challenging. In vitro generation of murine IDH-mutant cell lines or creating stable patient-derived IDH-mutant lines that retain the IDH-mutant status have proven to be elusive.

2. Cell Culture Models

2.1. Murine Cell Lines

An early model of diffuse glioma from the 1970s relied on carcinogen-induced gliomagenesis, where N-ethyl-nitrosourea (ENU) was injected into pregnant rats [38]. It is thought that the in utero exposure of embryos to ENU induces brain tumors, as injection of ENU in adult animals does not lead to the generation of brain tumors [39]. There are several key mutations that drive the ENU-induced glioma formation in rats, including *Braf*, *Tp53*, and *Pdgfrα* mutations; *Cdkn2a* deletion; and *Egfr* amplification [40]. Even though these molecular aberrations are also commonly seen in human diffuse gliomas, the ENU-induced model of gliomagenesis has poorly reproducible characteristics of glioma formation [41]. Several researchers took advantage of the heterogeneity derived from the use of alkylating agents to generate diverse glioma models. This led to the creation of many different murine glioma cell lines. Among the more commonly used are C6 glioma, 9L gliosarcoma, T9 glioma, RG2 glioma, F98 glioma, CNS-1 glioma, and BT4C glioma [42]. These lines do not harbor IDH mutations and are considered high-grade glioma models, which demonstrates that this method is not suitable for generating IDH-mutant murine cell lines.

Another method used to generate glioma murine lines is the CRE/LOX system. Bardella et al. created a murine glioma model that had conditional, inducible expression of the mutant Idh1 in the subventricular zone (SVZ) stem cell niche in the adult mouse. Since previous researchers had noticed that mutant *Idh1* knock-in mice under the control of nestin died perinatally and exhibited brain hemorrhages [43], the researchers created a tamoxifen-inducible system and initiated the tamoxifen at 5 to 6 weeks of age [44]. In this manner, the mice survived, and the resulting cells were more proliferative and displayed invasive characteristics. However, attempts to culture IDH1-mutant neurospheres from the SVZ of these mice were not successful. The authors therefore grew primary SVZ cells dissected from IDH-wildtype mouse pups and stably expressed mutant IDH1.

2.2. Patient-Derived Cell Lines

Patient-derived cell lines are a common tool used across cancers including glioblastoma, which are commonly grown in culture as tumor spheres. There has been a great need for human patient-derived cell lines that endogenously express mutant *IDH1* with the ability to initiate tumors in mice that also retain low-grade genetic characteristics. Far fewer *IDH*-mutant than *IDH*-wildtype lines are available, as it has been more challenging to develop such lines. Luchman et al. took a resected tumor from a patient with grade 3 IDH-mutant astrocytoma and generated a stable cell line that retained the IDH1 mutation and exhibited self-renewal and multipotency [45]. The authors named this neurosphere line BT142. These cells were injected into the striata of NOD/SCID mice, which formed tumors with cells that were poorly differentiated with enlarged hyperchromatic irregularly round to angulated nuclei and scant cytoplasm. The researchers found that growth was much faster in vivo than in vitro. In fact, they performed serial xenografts using cells from the xenografted tumor and were able to propagate the line while retaining the mutant IDH1 status. The 2-HG to 2-KG ratio in conditioned medium of this line demonstrated that this model recapitulated metabolic alterations expected in IDH-mutant cells. Another notable IDH-mutant line is TS603, which was generated from a patient with grade 3 IDH-mutant oligodendroglioma harboring a codeletion of 1p and 19q [46].

3. Murine Models

3.1. Murine-Derived Genetically Engineered Mouse Models

Our growing knowledge of driver mutations involved in gliomagenesis has led to the development of genetically engineered mouse models and murine cell lines from them.

One prominent method for developing these genetically engineered mouse models uses viral vectors to initiate tumor formation through the delivery of cancer-initiating genes. This system allows for glia-specific gene transfer in vivo using replication-competent ALV splice acceptor (RCAS) viral vectors and a transgenic mouse line (Gtv-a) that produces the receptor for ALV-A (TVA) from the astrocyte-specific promoter for the gene encoding glial fibrillary acidic protein (*Gfap*) [47]. Philip et al. used an RCAS/TVA mouse glioma model to demonstrate in vivo that *IDH* R132H promotes gliomagenesis [48]. However, Idh1 mutation alone was not sufficient to drive tumor development. Glioma development did not occur when mutant Idh1 was expressed in a genetic background with loss of *Cdkn2a*, *Atrx*, and *Pten* in vivo. However, the addition of PDGFA expression in this combination resulted in glioma development in 88% of injected mice. When wildtype Idh1 was expressed instead of mutant Idh1 in the same background, only 20% of the injected mice developed glioma. These data support a context-specific role of mutant IDH1 as a promoter of gliomagenesis when it is able to work with PDGFA in a genetic background of *Cdkn2a*, *Atrx*, and *Pten* loss.

3.2. Patient-Derived Xenograft Models

Another approach for developing murine models of low-grade glioma is to use tissue from patients. In this xenograft approach, the idea is to take glioma cells from patient tumors and then grow them in mice. In order to create a more context-specific model, orthotopic xenograft systems are created where patient-derived tumor cells are grown in the brains of mice. Klink et al. took tumor tissue from a patient with recurrent grade 3 oligodendroglioma, enzymatically dissociated it, and then grew cell aggregates in serum-free medium with epidermal growth factor and fibroblast growth factor [49]. They subsequently injected these cells intracranially into eGFP NOD/SCID mice. Tumors that grew in the mice demonstrated a diffusely infiltrating tumor pathology with round tumor nuclei and clear cytoplasm, which were consistent with oligodendroglioma histology. Genetic comparisons between the patient's tumor and the xenograft tumor showed maintenance of the 1p and 19q losses in addition to maintenance of losses on chromosomes 6, 11, and 14. Exome sequencing of the patient tumor and the xenograft revealed that they both had mutations in *IDH*, *FUBP1*, and *CIC*. However, the xenograft did not perfectly match the patient's tumor, as there were gains on chromosomes 11 and 4q. This work represented the first model in which a human oligodendroglioma could maintain its histological and molecular features in an intracranial mouse xenograft over serial passages.

Zeng et al. looked at the differences in generating patient-derived xenograft models in mice using tissue from patients with different grades of glioma. They took tumor tissues from 16 patient tumors of various grades and implanted them in mice, from which they established 11 glioma xenograft models. Not surprisingly, the researchers found that higher grades were associated with greater success in generating xenografts, with success rates of 33.33% for grade 2, 60.0% for grade 3, and 87.50% for grade 4 [50]. IDH-wildtype status and high Ki67 expression correlated with greater success in generating xenografts. These xenografts recapitulated the major histologic and molecular characteristics and key immunophenotypic features of the original tumors.

Navis et al. generated a mutant IDH1 oligodendroglioma xenograft line, which they characterized from a histological and metabolic standpoint. Though this line was established before the role of mutant IDH1 was discovered, the xenograft tumors were found to produce elevated levels of the oncometabolite D-2HG [51], as would be expected in an IDH-mutant line.

4. Emerging Models
4.1. Patient Avatars of Low-Grade Gliomas

An alternative model to cancer cell lines or mouse models is organoid models. They consist of tissue spheroids derived from progenitor cells or processed from tumor resections [52,53]. Unlike relatively homogeneous 3D spheroids, organoids are composed of multiple cell types, allow for self-organization, differentiation, mixed heterogeneity, and recapitulate features of in vivo cell growth all within the culture environment [54]. Thus, organoid models have the attractive combination of both supporting higher throughput studies and also maintaining diverse cell populations [55]. Recently, Abdullah et al. established a patient-derived LGG organoid model [55]. They collected specimens from brain tumor resections in 15 LGG patients which were then parcellated and placed in specialized media and cultured under 5% oxygen for 4-24 weeks before processing and analysis. The LGG organoid model recapitulated the histological features, molecular markers of stemness, proliferation, and vascular composition of the primary tumor. Moreover, they were also capable of maintaining parental tumor cellular heterogeneity, proliferative capacity, and distinctive genomic alterations [55]. Thus, patient-derived LGG organoids represent a unique patient avatar of LGG.

4.2. The Promise of In Silico Models

Despite the best preclinical biological models, the issues of cost, human effort, and time all limit the ease of advancements. In silico approaches offer another means of modeling LGG that circumvent these issues. There is tremendous promise in this area that some studies are beginning to unearth. A proof of concept has been shown in a recent study where a mathematical model of LGG response to temozolomide (TMZ) and radiation therapy (RT) was constructed to carry out in silico experiments to explore different treatment regimens [56]. They used longitudinal imaging data from LGG patients to obtain patient-specific parameters. Using their models, computer simulations showed that concurrent cycles of TMZ and RT could provide better therapeutic efficacy than concomitant radio-chemotherapy [56]. The authors found clinical trial validation of their in silico results in the clinical trial by Van den Bent et al., where it was found that deferring RT in LGGs did not alter survival time [56,57]. This study provides evidence that in silico models can be useful in the study of low-grade gliomas. It also underscores the potential that these in silico preclinical models can provide.

5. Challenges and Strategies in the Development of Low-Grade Glioma Models

Developing models of low-grade glioma has been a challenging endeavor. One major challenge has been in modeling the appropriate genetic background. Different types of vectors for gene delivery have been utilized by different groups to accomplish this (Table 1). Another challenge has been in the incorporation of the immune microenvironment. Various strategies have been employed to address these difficulties resulting in multiple LGG models (Table 2).

Table 1. Vectors used for gene delivery in LGG models [58].

Viral or Nonviral	Vector Type	Advantage	Limitations	Example
Viral	Retrovirus	Cell-specific infection	Safety concerns when transducing oncogenes	[48,59,60]
Viral	Lentivirus	Infects both dividing and nondividing cells	Safety concerns when transducing oncogenes	[61,62]
Viral	Adenovirus	No genome integration	High immunogenicity	[63]
Nonviral	Nonviral transposon (Sleeping Beauty)	Suitable for discovery of tumor drivers	Genome integration may disrupt gene expression	[64]

Table 2. LGG models.

Model Category	Specific Model	Genes Involved	Genetic Heterogeneity	Immunocompetent	Brain Micro-Environment	Blood–Brain Barrier	Reproducible
Murine cell line	ENU-induced murine tumor cells	BRAF, TP53, PDGFRα, CDKN2a, EGFR, and no IDH	yes	no	no	no	no
Murine cell line	IDH1 mutant expression in SVC cells	IDH	no	no	no	no	yes
Patient-derived cell line	BT142	IDH	no	no	no	no	yes
Patient-derived cell line	TS603	IDH, 1p/19q codeletion	no	no	no	no	yes
Murine-derived GEMMs	Sleeping Beauty transposase system	IDH, TP53, and ATRX	no	yes	yes	yes	yes
Murine-derived GEMMs	RCAS-mutIDH-PDGFA-CDKN2A-ATRX-PTEN	IDH, CDKN2a, ATRX, PTEN, and PDGFA	no	yes	yes	yes	yes
Murine derived GEMMs	RCAS-mutIDH-PDGF driven-p53 knockdown	IDH, PDGF, and TP53	no	yes	yes	yes	yes
Patient-derived murine model	Various LGG orthotopic xenografts	IDH, FUBP1, and CIC	partially	no	partially	yes	yes
Genetically modified neurosphere	hESCs with lentiviral modification	IDH, TP53, and ATRX	no	no	no	no	yes
Mouse to mouse xenograft	PDGF-B overexpressing mouse NSC into mouse brain	PDGF-B	partially	yes	yes	yes	yes
iPSC	human LGG iPSC	IDH	partially	no	no	no	yes

5.1. IDH Status

In order to study the role of IDH in low-grade glioma in vivo, Sasaki et al. generated Nes-$Idh1^{R132H/wt}$ (Nes-KI) mice and control Nes-$Idh1^{wt/wt}$ (Nes-WT) mice using Cre Lox technology with the *Nestin* promoter as the driver for expression of mutant IDH [43]. Their work was the first in vivo study to demonstrate that the metabolite D2HG, which is associated with the *Idh1* R132H mutation that inhibits mouse embryonic brain development. Notably, brain-specific expression of this *Idh1* mutation caused brain hemorrhage and perinatal death. Intracellular ROS levels were dramatically reduced in *Idh1*-KI brain cells, which also had an elevated $NADP^+$/NADPH ratio and catalase activity. D2HG was found to impair collagen maturation, disrupting basement membrane structure and prompting a stress response in the endoplasmic reticulum. The authors concluded that D2HG associated with the Idh1-mutant enzyme may function as an oncometabolite that induces HIF target gene transactivation, disrupts collagen maturation, and impairs basement membrane structure [43].

The same researchers wanted to develop an IDH-mutant glioma mouse model. Since the $Idh1^{R132H/wt}$ (Nes-KI) line was lethal, they crossed $Idh1^{LSL/wt}$ mice with *GFAP-Cre* mice to generate *GFAP-KI* mutants. In contrast to *Nes-KI* mice, which could not survive to adulthood, some of the *GFAP-KI* mice did. This created an opportunity to establish a model for low-grade IDH R132-mutant glioma. However, the GFAP-KI mice had a much shorter lifespan than their controls and did not develop glioma. The authors interpreted this to indicate that either mutated IDH alone is insufficient for gliomagenesis or that the mice did not live long enough to develop gliomas. The authors attempted to cross GFAP-KI mice with mice harboring deletion of the tumor suppressor *Trp53* to enhance glioma formation, but these mice displayed a broad spectrum of systemic tumors due to the leaky expression of CRE. This demonstrated the challenge of generating *Idh1*-KI mice that express mutant IDH1 protein exclusively in the brain and can be crossed with tumor-prone mice.

To circumvent the issue of embryonal lethality, Pirozzi et al. generated a mutant *Idh1* conditional knock-in model that produced mice heterozygous for the mutant *Idh1* [63]. This was conducted using a targeting vector containing a stop cassette flanked by LoxP sites and the *Idh1*- 132H mutation. The preceding LoxP-flanked stop sequence blocks the expression of the modified allele, resulting in a knocked-out allele that is restored through Cre-recombinase-mediated excision of the stop cassette. Neural stem cells (NSCs), which are found in the SVZ of the lateral ventricles, are a purported cell of origin for glioma and are known to produce other NSCs as well as differentiated cells. In order to induce excision of the stop cassette and expression of mutant *Idh1*, NSC lines isolated from embryonic day 14.5 mice were transduced with adenoviral-Cre-recombinase (ad-Cre) or adenoviral-GFP (ad-GFP) as control. When mutant *Idh1* was expressed, the NSCs had a reduced ability to undergo neuronal differentiation and reduced proliferation because of p53-mediated cell cycle arrest. It was also noted in vivo that *Idh1* R132H expression reduced proliferation of cells within the germinal zone of the SVZ [63]. The authors interpreted the results to suggest that mutant IDH1 is detrimental to the glioma cell of origin and the microenvironment.

In order to better understand the mutations involved in gliomagenesis of low-grade glioma, Modrek et al. modeled mutant-IDH1 low-grade glioma formation in NSCs derived from human embryonic stem cells [61]. They sought to investigate glioma progression by introducing the core genetic changes found in low-grade glioma. This consisted of lentiviral expression of R132H-mutant IDH1 and short hairpin RNA (shRNA)-mediated knockdown of p53 and ATRX. Loss of ATRX as the second hit resulted in nonviable cells. They focused on conditions that were most biologically relevant: vector only, mutant IDH1 alone ("1-hit"), mutant IDH1 with p53 knockdown ("2-hit"), and mutant IDH1 with P53 and ATRX knockdown ("3-hit"). Their data supported that gliomagenesis occurs in the order of IDH mutation, then p53 loss, and finally ATRX loss.

To characterize their NSCs as proper models of low-grade glioma, the same researchers profiled NSCs' DNA methylomes and transcriptomes. All conditions with mutant IDH had elevated levels of global methylation, and when the DNA methylation data of the NSCs with mutant IDH were compared with human low-grade glioma from TCGA [65], there was clustering of IDH1-mutant gliomas with IDH-mutant NSCs. In an analysis of transcriptomic data from RNA-seq, the various IDH-mutant NSCs also clustered with different groups of IDH-mutant low-grade glioma patients from TCGA data sets. Karyotypic analysis revealed that the 3-hit NSCs had significantly elevated numbers of chromosomal fragments, consistent with the genomic instability seen in low-grade gliomas [65,66]. Altogether, these IDH-mutant NSCs had DNA methylome, transcriptome, and karyotype similar to those of low-grade gliomas.

The researchers next found that combined IDH mutation and p53/ATRX loss blocked NSC differentiation. On flow cytometric analysis, 1-hit and 3-hit NSCs had low levels of NSC surface marker CD133 and high levels of restricted glial progenitor marker CD44 compared with vector-only and 2-hit NSCs. Similarly, 1-hit and 3-hit NSCs had near-complete differentiation block when they were directed to differentiate to neurons and astrocytes, while control vector and 2-hit NSCs were able to differentiate. The researchers also identified transcriptional downregulation of SOX2 as a central mechanism underlying the differentiation block [61].

In order to understand the impact of *Idh1* R132H in the context of *Atrx* and *Trp53* loss, Nunez et al. generated an *Idh1*-mutant mouse glioma model using the Sleeping Beauty transposase system [64]. The Sleeping Beauty (SB) transposon system is a nonviral DNA transfer tool that takes advantage of transposable elements (TEs), which are DNA sequences with the ability to move from one genomic location to another. SB takes advantage of the nonreplicative cut-and-paste mechanism that TEs employ in nature. TEs are comprised of a gene encoding the transposase, which is the enzyme that catalyzes the transposition reaction flanked by transposon-specific terminal inverted repeat (TIR) sequences containing binding sites for the transposase. The transposase excises the TE by binding to sequences at the TIRs and inducing double-stranded breaks (DSBs) at both ends. The excised TE then integrates into a different location when the transposase finds a suitable target site and performs the reinsertion of its own genetic code [67]. SB takes advantage of this mechanism by having an expression cassette for the SB transposase and an artificial TE (gene of interest flanked by TIRs) sitting on two separate plasmids such that the transposase is able to stably integrate the gene of interest into the cell's genome, enabling sustained transgene expression [68].

Nunez et al. used the combination of sh*Trp53*, sh*ATRX*, and mutant *Idh1* with RTK/RAS/PI3K activation to induce gliomas. Increased DNA damage response (DDR) from epigenetic reprogramming of the tumor cells' transcriptome mediated genomic stability in their IDH1-mutant glioma model in the context of *Atrx* and *p53* knockdown. Furthermore, the researchers found that IDH1 R132H induced transcriptional activation of ataxia-telangiectasia mutated (*Atm*), which resulted in efficient DNA repair activity through homologous recombination DNA repair. This was a clinically relevant finding, as radiation therapy failed to prolong survival in the IDH1-mutant tumor-bearing mice, but pharmacological inhibition of DDR prolonged survival due to radiosensitivity. Taken together, these findings opened up the potential that DDR inhibition combined with radiation therapy could be a novel therapeutic approach for IDH1 R132H glioma patients harboring *ATRX* and *TP53* inactivating mutations.

5.2. Immune Microenvironment

Some in vivo models have shed light on the unique role of the tumor microenvironment in the development of low-grade glioma. To study the progressive change in the actions of immune cells and glioma cells, Appolloni et al. used a glioma mouse model driven by the overexpression of the *Pdgfb* oncogene [59]. In their model, multifocal gliomas were first generated by injecting E14 embryos with replication-incompetent retroviral vectors expressing PDGFB in the lateral ventricles. Early-onset tumors displayed histological features of low-grade tumors, while late-onset tumors showed those of high-grade tumors. Orthotopic transplantation of early-onset gliomas did not produce secondary tumors, while injection of late-onset tumors did. However, injection of early-onset tumors in NOD/SCID immunocompromised mice did result in tumors demonstrating a role of the adaptive immune system. When secondary tumors from early-onset tumors were injected in NOD/SCID immunocompetent mice, they were able to generate tumors. The authors interpreted this to indicate that the residual immune system components in NOD/SCID mice enabled tumors to progress toward higher grades. Genetic analysis showed a downregulation of immune response and inflammation genes in the late-onset tumors compared to the early-onset tumors. Furthermore, they found greater infiltration by CD8-positive lymphocytes in the brains of mice with low-grade tumors, suggesting that low-grade, but not high-grade, gliomas stimulate such infiltration. Overall, their work showed the important role of the immune system on patterns of progression to malignancy over time.

Further work on mutant IDH focused on investigating the effect of this mutation on the immunologic tumor microenvironment. Amankulor et al. employed a strategy using mutant IDH1 and wildtype IDH1 mouse glioma models whose initiating events were identical, with the exception of *Idh1* mutation status. This was conducted using the RCAS/TVA system to ectopically express mutant IDH1 (R132H) in PDGF-driven gliomas [60]. In this system, RCAS retroviral vectors transfer genes into cells that express the Tva receptor. Three different mouse strains were used in which the Tva receptor was expressed from the *Nestin* promoter (Ntva): Ntva_$Ink4a/Arf^{-/-}$, Ntva_$Ink4a/Arf^{+/-}$, and Ntva_$Ink4a/Arf^{+/+}$. In this fashion, RCAS would transfer genes to CNS progenitors. RCAS–PDGF-producing DF1 cells were injected with either DF1 cells producing RCAS–wildtype *Idh1*-sh*Trp53* (wtIdh1) or RCAS–mutant Idh1-shTrp53 (muIdh1) in mice. Thus, the researchers were able to generate tumors that had the same genetic background and differed only in *Idh1* mutation status. When the RNA expression patterns were compared between mutant *Idh1* mouse glioma and wildtype *Idh1* mouse glioma, a differential association with gene expression of immune system processes was found, with wildtype *Idh1* mouse gliomas having strong associations with the positive regulation of immune responses. Genes related to leukocyte and neutrophil migration were relatively downregulated in muIdh1 mouse gliomas. Furthermore, flow cytometric analysis of single-cell suspensions from brain tissue of mice with IDH1-mutant gliomas displayed significantly fewer CD45+ immune cells compared with brain tissue of mice with wildtype *Idh1* gliomas. To investigate the extent of neutrophil chemotaxis in mutant IDH1 gliomas, the researchers conducted migration experiments on neutrophils in the presence of muIdh1 cells. Their data indicated that chemotaxis to muIdh1 gliomas was repressed, as tissue homogenates of wtIdh1 mouse gliomas had roughly double the migration index of muIdh1 mouse gliomas. Conditioned medium experiments further suggested that tissue homogenates from IDH1-mutant mouse gliomas may contain lower levels of neutrophil chemoattractants. Genetic and proteomic analysis of muIdh1 mouse glioma tissues demonstrated the downregulation of cytokine protein expression.

In the same study, the researchers assessed whether differences in the immune microenvironment were the biological cause of survival differences between mice with muIdh1 versus wtIdh1 gliomas. Intriguingly, treatment of wtIdh1 and muIdh1 tumor-bearing mice with an anti-Ly6g (1A8) or isotype control (2A3) antibody to deplete neutrophil populations demonstrated a significant survival benefit for mice with wtIdh1 tumors with neutrophil depletion, but no significant effect was seen on mice with muIdh1 tumors. Taken together, these findings demonstrated that muIdh1 has unique effects on the immune microenvironment, which may have a role in the survival differences between muIdh1 and wtIdh1 tumors.

Liu et al. went further in trying to understand the role of mutant IDH1 in gliomagenesis using a preclinical model of low-grade glioma. They used two samples of freshly resected low-grade gliomas, with one being an astrocytoma with mutant IDH1 R132C and another being an oligodendroglioma with mutant IDH1 R132H [62]. They generated induced pluripotent stem cells (iPSCs) from these lines by transducing them with the reprogramming factors *OCT4*, *SOX2*, *KLF4*, and *c-MYC*. The resultant low-grade glioma iPSCs (LGG-iPSCs) were confirmed to be reprogrammed, as they had pluripotency markers and were capable of differentiating into tissues from all three embryonic germ layers. Intriguingly, these reprogrammed cells no longer contained *IDH1* mutations, indicating that *IDH1* mutations inhibit somatic reprogramming. Array-based comparative genomic hybridization analysis on primary low-grade glioma cells and the derived LGG-iPSCs demonstrated regional amplifications on chromosome Xq23 on astrocytoma LGG-iPSCs and 7q31 on oligodendroglioma LGG-iPSCs. These regional amplifications were not seen in the genomes of healthy individuals but were seen in higher frequency in low-grade gliomas [62]. The researchers reasoned that these regional amplifications are early genetic lesions that occur before *IDH1* mutations and that the mutation in *IDH1* is likely not the initiating factor in gliomagenesis.

6. Conclusions

Continuous progress is being made on the important endeavor of creating ideal preclinical models of low-grade glioma. This effort has been more challenging than creating models of high-grade gliomas, which often have greater success rates. However, adequate models are crucial for the advancement of our understanding of low-grade glioma. The attempts to circumvent many of the challenges in developing these models have shed light on our understanding of the fundamental biology that drives gliomagenesis. Those studies have also highlighted the importance of factors beyond genetics, such as the immune microenvironment of the tumor. Further research is needed to yield models that will more closely parallel human gliomas, creating the ideal system to develop and test novel therapeutics for the future.

Author Contributions: P.D. contributed to the conceptualization, writing of the manuscript, original draft preparation, subsequent review and editing, and writing of the revised manuscript. V.B. contributed to the conceptualization and subsequent review of the manuscript. J.F.d.G. contributed to the conceptualization, original draft preparation, and subsequent review and editing. N.K.M. contributed to the conceptualization, original draft preparation, and subsequent review and editing. All authors have read and agreed to the published version of the manuscript.

Funding: APC was provided by the Faculty Fund of N.K.M., Department of Neuro-Oncology, MD Anderson Cancer Center, Houston, TX 77030, USA.

Data Availability Statement: Data sharing is not applicable to this article.

Acknowledgments: Editorial support was provided by Bryan Tutt, Scientific Editor, Research Medical Library, MD Anderson Cancer Center.

Conflicts of Interest: The authors declare no conflict of interest.

References

1. Ostrom, Q.T.; Cioffi, G.; Gittleman, H.; Patil, N.; Waite, K.; Kruchko, C.; Barnholtz-Sloan, J.S. CBTRUS Statistical Report: Primary Brain and Other Central Nervous System Tumors Diagnosed in the United States in 2012-2016. *Neuro. Oncol.* **2019**, *21* (Suppl. 5), v1–v100. [CrossRef] [PubMed]
2. Goodenberger, M.L.; Jenkins, R.B. Genetics of adult glioma. *Cancer Genet.* **2012**, *205*, 613–621. [CrossRef]
3. Louis, D.N.; Ohgaki, H.; Wiestler, O.D.; Cavenee, W.K.; Burger, P.C.; Jouvet, A.; Scheithauer, B.W.; Kleihues, P. The 2007 WHO classification of tumours of the central nervous system. *Acta Neuropathol.* **2007**, *114*, 97–109. [CrossRef] [PubMed]
4. Stupp, R.; Mason, W.P.; van den Bent, M.J.; Weller, M.; Fisher, B.; Taphoorn, M.J.; Belanger, K.; Brandes, A.A.; Marosi, C.; Bogdahn, U.; et al. Radiotherapy plus concomitant and adjuvant temozolomide for glioblastoma. *N. Engl. J. Med.* **2005**, *352*, 987–996. [CrossRef] [PubMed]
5. Louis, D.N.; Perry, A.; Wesseling, P.; Brat, D.J.; Cree, I.A.; Figarella-Branger, D.; Hawkins, C.; Ng, H.K.; Pfister, S.M.; Reifenberger, G.; et al. The 2021 WHO Classification of Tumors of the Central Nervous System: A summary. *Neuro. Oncol.* **2021**, *23*, 1231–1251. [CrossRef]
6. Wright, J.R.; Albert, C. Broders' paradigm shifts involving the prognostication and definition of cancer. *Arch. Pathol. Lab. Med.* **2012**, *136*, 1437–1446. [CrossRef]
7. Perry, A.; Brat, D.J. *Practical Surgical Neuropathology: A Diagnostic Approach*; Elsevier: Amsterdam, The Netherlands, 2018.
8. Komori, T. Grading of adult diffuse gliomas according to the 2021 WHO Classification of Tumors of the Central Nervous System. *Lab. Invest.* **2022**, *102*, 126–133. [CrossRef]
9. Whitfield, B.T.; Huse, J.T. Classification of adult-type diffuse gliomas: Impact of the World Health Organization 2021 update. *Brain Pathol.* **2022**, *32*, e13062. [CrossRef]
10. Yan, H.; Parsons, D.W.; Jin, G.; McLendon, R.; Rasheed, B.A.; Yuan, W.; Kos, I.; Batinic-Haberle, I.; Jones, S.; Riggins, G.J.; et al. IDH1 and IDH2 mutations in gliomas. *N. Engl. J. Med.* **2009**, *360*, 765–773. [CrossRef]
11. Sanson, M.; Marie, Y.; Paris, S.; Idbaih, A.; Laffaire, J.; Ducray, F.; El Hallani, S.; Boisselier, B.; Mokhtari, K.; Hoang-Xuan, K.; et al. Isocitrate dehydrogenase 1 codon 132 mutation is an important prognostic biomarker in gliomas. *J. Clin. Oncol.* **2009**, *27*, 4150–4154. [CrossRef]
12. Dang, L.; White, D.W.; Gross, S.; Bennett, B.D.; Bittinger, M.A.; Driggers, E.M.; Fantin, V.R.; Jang, H.G.; Jin, S.; Keenan, M.C.; et al. Cancer-associated IDH1 mutations produce 2-hydroxyglutarate. *Nature* **2009**, *462*, 739–744. [CrossRef]
13. Hartmann, C.; Meyer, J.; Balss, J.; Capper, D.; Mueller, W.; Christians, A.; Felsberg, J.; Wolter, M.; Mawrin, C.; Wick, W.; et al. Type and frequency of IDH1 and IDH2 mutations are related to astrocytic and oligodendroglial differentiation and age: A study of 1,010 diffuse gliomas. *Acta Neuropathol.* **2009**, *118*, 469–474. [CrossRef]
14. Duncan, C.G.; Barwick, B.G.; Jin, G.; Rago, C.; Kapoor-Vazirani, P.; Powell, D.R.; Chi, J.T.; Bigner, D.D.; Vertino, P.M.; Yan, H. A heterozygous IDH1R132H/WT mutation induces genome-wide alterations in DNA methylation. *Genome. Res.* **2012**, *22*, 2339–2355. [CrossRef]
15. van Lith, S.A.; Molenaar, R.; van Noorden, C.J.; Leenders, W.P. Tumor cells in search for glutamate: An alternative explanation for increased invasiveness of IDH1 mutant gliomas. *Neuro. Oncol.* **2014**, *16*, 1669–1670. [CrossRef]
16. Flavahan, W.A.; Drier, Y.; Liau, B.B.; Gillespie, S.M.; Venteicher, A.S.; Stemmer-Rachamimov, A.O.; Suvà, M.L.; Bernstein, B.E. Insulator dysfunction and oncogene activation in IDH mutant gliomas. *Nature* **2016**, *529*, 110–114. [CrossRef] [PubMed]
17. Lu, C.; Ward, P.S.; Kapoor, G.S.; Rohle, D.; Turcan, S.; Abdel-Wahab, O.; Edwards, C.R.; Khanin, R.; Figueroa, M.E.; Melnick, A.; et al. IDH mutation impairs histone demethylation and results in a block to cell differentiation. *Nature* **2012**, *483*, 474–478. [CrossRef]
18. Turcan, S.; Rohle, D.; Goenka, A.; Walsh, L.A.; Fang, F.; Yilmaz, E.; Campos, C.; Fabius, A.W.; Lu, C.; Ward, P.S.; et al. IDH1 mutation is sufficient to establish the glioma hypermethylator phenotype. *Nature* **2012**, *483*, 479–483. [CrossRef]
19. Perez, A.; Huse, J.T. The Evolving Classification of Diffuse Gliomas: World Health Organization Updates for 2021. *Curr. Neurol. Neurosci. Rep.* **2021**, *21*, 67. [CrossRef]
20. Kandoth, C.; McLellan, M.D.; Vandin, F.; Ye, K.; Niu, B.; Lu, C.; Xie, M.; Zhang, Q.; McMichael, J.F.; Wyczalkowski, M.A.; et al. Mutational landscape and significance across 12 major cancer types. *Nature* **2013**, *502*, 333–339. [CrossRef]
21. Bykov, V.J.N.; Eriksson, S.E.; Bianchi, J.; Wiman, K.G. Targeting mutant p53 for efficient cancer therapy. *Nat. Rev. Cancer* **2018**, *18*, 89–102. [CrossRef]
22. Lewis, P.W.; Elsaesser, S.J.; Noh, K.M.; Stadler, S.C.; Allis, C.D. Daxx is an H3.3-specific histone chaperone and cooperates with ATRX in replication-independent chromatin assembly at telomeres. *Proc. Natl. Acad. Sci. USA* **2010**, *107*, 14075–14080. [CrossRef] [PubMed]
23. Goldberg, A.D.; Banaszynski, L.A.; Noh, K.M.; Lewis, P.W.; Elsaesser, S.J.; Stadler, S.; Dewell, S.; Law, M.; Guo, X.; Li, X.; et al. Distinct factors control histone variant H3.3 localization at specific genomic regions. *Cell* **2010**, *140*, 678–691. [CrossRef] [PubMed]
24. Conte, D.; Huh, M.; Goodall, E.; Delorme, M.; Parks, R.J.; Picketts, D.J. Loss of Atrx sensitizes cells to DNA damaging agents through p53-mediated death pathways. *PLoS ONE* **2012**, *7*, e52167. [CrossRef] [PubMed]
25. Bérubé, N.G.; Mangelsdorf, M.; Jagla, M.; Vanderluit, J.; Garrick, D.; Gibbons, R.J.; Higgs, D.R.; Slack, R.S.; Picketts, D.J. The chromatin-remodeling protein ATRX is critical for neuronal survival during corticogenesis. *J. Clin. Invest.* **2005**, *115*, 258–267. [CrossRef]

26. Heaphy, C.M.; de Wilde, R.F.; Jiao, Y.; Klein, A.P.; Edil, B.H.; Shi, C.; Bettegowda, C.; Rodriguez, F.J.; Eberhart, C.G.; Hebbar, S.; et al. Altered telomeres in tumors with ATRX and DAXX mutations. *Science* **2011**, *333*, 425. [CrossRef]
27. Figarella-Branger, D.; Mokhtari, K.; Dehais, C.; Jouvet, A.; Uro-Coste, E.; Colin, C.; Carpentier, C.; Forest, F.; Maurage, C.A.; Vignaud, J.M.; et al. Mitotic index, microvascular proliferation, and necrosis define 3 groups of 1p/19q codeleted anaplastic oligodendrogliomas associated with different genomic alterations. *Neuro. Oncol.* **2014**, *16*, 1244–1254. [CrossRef]
28. Appay, R.; Dehais, C.; Maurage, C.A.; Alentorn, A.; Carpentier, C.; Colin, C.; Ducray, F.; Escande, F.; Idbaih, A.; Kamoun, A.; et al. CDKN2A homozygous deletion is a strong adverse prognosis factor in diffuse malignant IDH-mutant gliomas. *Neuro. Oncol.* **2019**, *21*, 1519–1528. [CrossRef]
29. Bell, R.J.; Rube, H.T.; Xavier-Magalhães, A.; Costa, B.M.; Mancini, A.; Song, J.S.; Costello, J.F. Understanding TERT Promoter Mutations: A Common Path to Immortality. *Mol. Cancer Res.* **2016**, *14*, 315–323. [CrossRef]
30. Horn, S.; Figl, A.; Rachakonda, P.S.; Fischer, C.; Sucker, A.; Gast, A.; Kadel, S.; Moll, I.; Nagore, E.; Hemminki, K.; et al. TERT promoter mutations in familial and sporadic melanoma. *Science* **2013**, *339*, 959–961. [CrossRef] [PubMed]
31. Bettegowda, C.; Agrawal, N.; Jiao, Y.; Sausen, M.; Wood, L.D.; Hruban, R.H.; Rodriguez, F.J.; Cahill, D.P.; McLendon, R.; Riggins, G.; et al. Mutations in CIC and FUBP1 contribute to human oligodendroglioma. *Science* **2011**, *333*, 1453–1455. [CrossRef]
32. Gleize, V.; Alentorn, A.; Connen de Kérillis, L.; Labussière, M.; Nadaradjane, A.A.; Mundwiller, E.; Ottolenghi, C.; Mangesius, S.; Rahimian, A.; Ducray, F.; et al. CIC inactivating mutations identify aggressive subset of 1p19q codeleted gliomas. *Ann. Neurol.* **2015**, *78*, 355–374. [CrossRef] [PubMed]
33. Baena, E.; Shao, Z.; Linn, D.E.; Glass, K.; Hamblen, M.J.; Fujiwara, Y.; Kim, J.; Nguyen, M.; Zhang, X.; Godinho, F.J.; et al. ETV1 directs androgen metabolism and confers aggressive prostate cancer in targeted mice and patients. *Genes Dev.* **2013**, *27*, 683–698. [CrossRef] [PubMed]
34. Jang, B.G.; Lee, H.E.; Kim, W.H. ETV1 mRNA is specifically expressed in gastrointestinal stromal tumors. *Virchows Arch.* **2015**, *467*, 393–403. [CrossRef] [PubMed]
35. Padul, V.; Epari, S.; Moiyadi, A.; Shetty, P.; Shirsat, N.V. ETV/Pea3 family transcription factor-encoding genes are overexpressed in CIC-mutant oligodendrogliomas. *Genes Chromosomes Cancer* **2015**, *54*, 725–733. [CrossRef]
36. Dissanayake, K.; Toth, R.; Blakey, J.; Olsson, O.; Campbell, D.G.; Prescott, A.R.; MacKintosh, C. ERK/p90(RSK)/14-3-3 signalling has an impact on expression of PEA3 Ets transcription factors via the transcriptional repressor capicúa. *Biochem. J.* **2011**, *433*, 515–525. [CrossRef]
37. Elman, J.S.; Ni, T.K.; Mengwasser, K.E.; Jin, D.; Wronski, A.; Elledge, S.J.; Kuperwasser, C. Identification of FUBP1 as a Long Tail Cancer Driver and Widespread Regulator of Tumor Suppressor and Oncogene Alternative Splicing. *Cell Rep.* **2019**, *28*, 3435–3449.e5. [CrossRef]
38. Russell, W.L.; Kelly, E.M.; Hunsicker, P.R.; Bangham, J.W.; Maddux, S.C.; Phipps, E.L. Specific-locus test shows ethylnitrosourea to be the most potent mutagen in the mouse. *Proc. Natl. Acad. Sci. USA* **1979**, *76*, 5818–5819. [CrossRef]
39. Slikker, W.; Mei, N.; Chen, T. N-ethyl-N-nitrosourea (ENU) increased brain mutations in prenatal and neonatal mice but not in the adults. *Toxicol. Sci.* **2004**, *81*, 112–120. [CrossRef]
40. Wang, Q.; Satomi, K.; Oh, J.E.; Hutter, B.; Brors, B.; Diessl, N.; Liu, H.K.; Wolf, S.; Wiestler, O.; Kleihues, P.; et al. Braf Mutations Initiate the Development of Rat Gliomas Induced by Postnatal Exposure to N-Ethyl-N-Nitrosourea. *Am. J. Pathol.* **2016**, *186*, 2569–2576. [CrossRef]
41. Lenting, K.; Verhaak, R.; Ter Laan, M.; Wesseling, P.; Leenders, W. Glioma: Experimental models and reality. *Acta Neuropathol.* **2017**, *133*, 263–282. [CrossRef]
42. Barth, R.F.; Kaur, B. Rat brain tumor models in experimental neuro-oncology: The C6, 9L, T9, RG2, F98, BT4C, RT-2 and CNS-1 gliomas. *J. Neurooncol.* **2009**, *94*, 299–312. [CrossRef]
43. Sasaki, M.; Knobbe, C.B.; Itsumi, M.; Elia, A.J.; Harris, I.S.; Chio, I.I.; Cairns, R.A.; McCracken, S.; Wakeham, A.; Haight, J.; et al. D-2-hydroxyglutarate produced by mutant IDH1 perturbs collagen maturation and basement membrane function. *Genes Dev.* **2012**, *26*, 2038–2049. [CrossRef]
44. Bardella, C.; Al-Dalahmah, O.; Krell, D.; Brazauskas, P.; Al-Qahtani, K.; Tomkova, M.; Adam, J.; Serres, S.; Lockstone, H.; Freeman-Mills, L.; et al. Expression of Idh1. *Cancer Cell* **2016**, *30*, 578–594. [CrossRef]
45. Luchman, H.A.; Stechishin, O.D.; Dang, N.H.; Blough, M.D.; Chesnelong, C.; Kelly, J.J.; Nguyen, S.A.; Chan, J.A.; Weljie, A.M.; Cairncross, J.G.; et al. An in vivo patient-derived model of endogenous IDH1-mutant glioma. *Neuro. Oncol.* **2012**, *14*, 184–191. [CrossRef]
46. Rohle, D.; Popovici-Muller, J.; Palaskas, N.; Turcan, S.; Grommes, C.; Campos, C.; Tsoi, J.; Clark, O.; Oldrini, B.; Komisopoulou, E.; et al. An inhibitor of mutant IDH1 delays growth and promotes differentiation of glioma cells. *Science* **2013**, *340*, 626–630. [CrossRef]
47. Holland, E.C.; Celestino, J.; Dai, C.; Schaefer, L.; Sawaya, R.E.; Fuller, G.N. Combined activation of Ras and Akt in neural progenitors induces glioblastoma formation in mice. *Nat. Genet.* **2000**, *25*, 55–57. [CrossRef]
48. Philip, B.; Yu, D.X.; Silvis, M.R.; Shin, C.H.; Robinson, J.P.; Robinson, G.L.; Welker, A.E.; Angel, S.N.; Tripp, S.R.; Sonnen, J.A.; et al. Mutant IDH1 Promotes Glioma Formation In Vivo. *Cell Rep.* **2018**, *23*, 1553–1564. [CrossRef]
49. Klink, B.; Miletic, H.; Stieber, D.; Huszthy, P.C.; Campos Valenzuela, J.A.; Valenzuela, J.A.; Balss, J.; Wang, J.; Schubert, M.; Sakariassen, P.; et al. A novel, diffusely infiltrative xenograft model of human anaplastic oligodendroglioma with mutations in FUBP1, CIC, and IDH1. *PLoS ONE* **2013**, *8*, e59773. [CrossRef]

50. Zeng, W.; Tang, Z.; Li, Y.; Yin, G.; Liu, Z.; Gao, J.; Chen, Y.; Chen, F. Patient-derived xenografts of different grade gliomas retain the heterogeneous histological and genetic features of human gliomas. *Cancer Cell Int.* **2020**, *20*, 1. [CrossRef]
51. Navis, A.C.; Niclou, S.P.; Fack, F.; Stieber, D.; van Lith, S.; Verrijp, K.; Wright, A.; Stauber, J.; Tops, B.; Otte-Holler, I.; et al. Increased mitochondrial activity in a novel IDH1-R132H mutant human oligodendroglioma xenograft model: In situ detection of 2-HG and α-KG. *Acta Neuropathol. Commun.* **2013**, *1*, 18. [CrossRef]
52. Rosenbluth, J.M.; Schackmann, R.C.J.; Gray, G.K.; Selfors, L.M.; Li, C.M.; Boedicker, M.; Kuiken, H.J.; Richardson, A.; Brock, J.; Garber, J.; et al. Organoid cultures from normal and cancer-prone human breast tissues preserve complex epithelial lineages. *Nat. Commun.* **2020**, *11*, 1711. [CrossRef] [PubMed]
53. Walsh, A.J.; Cook, R.S.; Skala, M.C. Functional Optical Imaging of Primary Human Tumor Organoids: Development of a Personalized Drug Screen. *J. Nucl. Med.* **2017**, *58*, 1367–1372. [CrossRef] [PubMed]
54. Hubert, C.G.; Rivera, M.; Spangler, L.C.; Wu, Q.; Mack, S.C.; Prager, B.C.; Couce, M.; McLendon, R.E.; Sloan, A.E.; Rich, J.N. A Three-Dimensional Organoid Culture System Derived from Human Glioblastomas Recapitulates the Hypoxic Gradients and Cancer Stem Cell Heterogeneity of Tumors Found In Vivo. *Cancer Res.* **2016**, *76*, 2465–2477. [CrossRef] [PubMed]
55. Abdullah, K.G.; Bird, C.E.; Buehler, J.D.; Gattie, L.C.; Savani, M.R.; Sternisha, A.C.; Xiao, Y.; Levitt, M.M.; Hicks, W.H.; Li, W.; et al. Establishment of patient-derived organoid models of lower-grade glioma. *Neuro. Oncol.* **2022**, *24*, 612–623. [CrossRef]
56. Ayala-Hernández, L.E.; Gallegos, A.; Schucht, P.; Murek, M.; Pérez-Romasanta, L.; Belmonte-Beitia, J.; Pérez-García, V.M. Optimal Combinations of Chemotherapy and Radiotherapy in Low-Grade Gliomas: A Mathematical Approach. *J. Pers. Med.* **2021**, *11*, 1036. [CrossRef]
57. van den Bent, M.J.; Afra, D.; de Witte, O.; Ben Hassel, M.; Schraub, S.; Hoang-Xuan, K.; Malmström, P.O.; Collette, L.; Piérart, M.; Mirimanoff, R.; et al. Long-term efficacy of early versus delayed radiotherapy for low-grade astrocytoma and oligodendroglioma in adults: The EORTC 22845 randomised trial. *Lancet* **2005**, *366*, 985–990. [CrossRef]
58. Seano, G. Brain Tumors. In *Mouse Models of Diffuse Lower-Grade Gliomas of the Adult*; Archontidi, S., Joppé, S., Khenniche, Y., Bardella, C., Huillard, E., Eds.; Humana Press: Totowa, NJ, USA, 2021; Volume 158, pp. 3–39.
59. Appolloni, I.; Alessandrini, F.; Ceresa, D.; Marubbi, D.; Gambini, E.; Reverberi, D.; Loiacono, F.; Malatesta, P. Progression from low- to high-grade in a glioblastoma model reveals the pivotal role of immunoediting. *Cancer Lett.* **2019**, *442*, 213–221. [CrossRef]
60. Amankulor, N.M.; Kim, Y.; Arora, S.; Kargl, J.; Szulzewsky, F.; Hanke, M.; Margineantu, D.H.; Rao, A.; Bolouri, H.; Delrow, J.; et al. Mutant IDH1 regulates the tumor-associated immune system in gliomas. *Genes Dev.* **2017**, *31*, 774–786. [CrossRef]
61. Modrek, A.S.; Golub, D.; Khan, T.; Bready, D.; Prado, J.; Bowman, C.; Deng, J.; Zhang, G.; Rocha, P.P.; Raviram, R.; et al. Low-Grade Astrocytoma Mutations in IDH1, P53, and ATRX Cooperate to Block Differentiation of Human Neural Stem Cells via Repression of SOX2. *Cell Rep.* **2017**, *21*, 1267–1280. [CrossRef]
62. Liu, Z.; Che, P.; Mercado, J.J.; Hackney, J.R.; Friedman, G.K.; Zhang, C.; You, Z.; Zhao, X.; Ding, Q.; Kim, K.; et al. Characterization of iPSCs derived from low grade gliomas revealed early regional chromosomal amplifications during gliomagenesis. *J. Neurooncol.* **2019**, *141*, 289–301. [CrossRef]
63. Pirozzi, C.J.; Carpenter, A.B.; Waitkus, M.S.; Wang, C.Y.; Zhu, H.; Hansen, L.J.; Chen, L.H.; Greer, P.K.; Feng, J.; Wang, Y.; et al. Mutant IDH1 Disrupts the Mouse Subventricular Zone and Alters Brain Tumor Progression. *Mol. Cancer Res.* **2017**, *15*, 507–520. [CrossRef]
64. Núñez, F.J.; Mendez, F.M.; Kadiyala, P.; Alghamri, M.S.; Savelieff, M.G.; Garcia-Fabiani, M.B.; Haase, S.; Koschmann, C.; Calinescu, A.A.; Kamran, N.; et al. IDH1-R132H acts as a tumor suppressor in glioma via epigenetic up-regulation of the DNA damage response. *Sci. Transl. Med.* **2019**, *11*, 1427. [CrossRef]
65. Brat, D.J.; Verhaak, R.G.; Aldape, K.D.; Yung, W.K.; Salama, S.R.; Cooper, L.A.; Rheinbay, E.; Miller, C.R.; Vitucci, M.; Morozova, O.; et al. Comprehensive, Integrative Genomic Analysis of Diffuse Lower-Grade Gliomas. *N. Engl. J. Med.* **2015**, *372*, 2481–2498. [CrossRef]
66. Cohen, A.L.; Colman, H. Glioma biology and molecular markers. *Cancer Treat. Res.* **2015**, *163*, 15–30. [CrossRef]
67. Vigdal, T.J.; Kaufman, C.D.; Izsvák, Z.; Voytas, D.F.; Ivics, Z. Common physical properties of DNA affecting target site selection of sleeping beauty and other Tc1/mariner transposable elements. *J. Mol. Biol.* **2002**, *323*, 441–452. [CrossRef]
68. Amberger, M.; Ivics, Z. Latest Advances for the Sleeping Beauty Transposon System: 23 Years of Insomnia but Prettier than Ever: Refinement and Recent Innovations of the Sleeping Beauty Transposon System Enabling Novel, Nonviral Genetic Engineering Applications. *Bioessays* **2020**, *42*, e2000136. [CrossRef]

Disclaimer/Publisher's Note: The statements, opinions and data contained in all publications are solely those of the individual author(s) and contributor(s) and not of MDPI and/or the editor(s). MDPI and/or the editor(s) disclaim responsibility for any injury to people or property resulting from any ideas, methods, instructions or products referred to in the content.

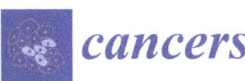

Review

Novel Therapeutic Approaches in Neoplastic Meningitis

Atulya Aman Khosla [1], Shreya Saxena [1], Ahmad Ozair [1,2], Vyshak Alva Venur [3,4], David M. Peereboom [5] and Manmeet S. Ahluwalia [1,*]

1. Miami Cancer Institute, Baptist Health South Florida, Miami, FL 33176, USA
2. Faculty of Medicine, King George's Medical University, Lucknow 226003, India
3. Fred Hutchinson Cancer Center, University of Washington, Seattle, WA 98109, USA
4. University of Washington Cancer Consortium, Seattle, WA 98195, USA
5. Cleveland Clinic Lerner College of Medicine, Cleveland Clinic Main Campus, Cleveland, OH 44195, USA
* Correspondence: manmeeta@baptisthealth.net

Simple Summary: Neoplastic meningitis (NM) is a frequent complication of cancer and is associated with a poor prognosis. The currently available therapies aim to alleviate symptoms and preserve the quality of life. It comprises a multimodal approach, including surgery, intrathecal and systemic chemotherapy, and radiotherapy. The specific treatment is individualized, based on clinical practice guidelines and expert opinion. There are multiple clinical trials undertaken to evaluate the efficacy of novel therapies, including targeted and immunotherapies. This article presents an updated review of treatment approaches in NM.

Abstract: Central nervous system (CNS) metastasis from systemic cancers can involve the brain parenchyma, leptomeninges, or the dura. Neoplastic meningitis (NM), also known by different terms, including leptomeningeal carcinomatosis and carcinomatous meningitis, occurs due to solid tumors and hematologic malignancies and is associated with a poor prognosis. The current management paradigm entails a multimodal approach focused on palliation with surgery, radiation, and chemotherapy, which may be administered systemically or directly into the cerebrospinal fluid (CSF). This review focuses on novel therapeutic approaches, including targeted and immunotherapeutic agents under investigation, that have shown promise in NM arising from solid tumors.

Keywords: neoplastic; meningitis; leptomeningeal; chemotherapy; radiotherapy; intrathecal; immunotherapy

Citation: Khosla, A.A.; Saxena, S.; Ozair, A.; Venur, V.A.; Peereboom, D.M.; Ahluwalia, M.S. Novel Therapeutic Approaches in Neoplastic Meningitis. *Cancers* 2023, 15, 119. https://doi.org/10.3390/cancers15010119

Academic Editor: Edward Pan

Received: 25 October 2022
Revised: 18 December 2022
Accepted: 23 December 2022
Published: 25 December 2022

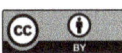

Copyright: © 2022 by the authors. Licensee MDPI, Basel, Switzerland. This article is an open access article distributed under the terms and conditions of the Creative Commons Attribution (CC BY) license (https:// creativecommons.org/licenses/by/ 4.0/).

1. Introduction

Neoplastic meningitis (NM), also known as leptomeningeal metastasis or leptomeningeal carcinomatosis, refers to the involvement of the subarachnoid space and leptomeninges-arachnoid and pia mater by primary tumor spread. The incidence of NM ranges from 5–8% in patients with solid tumors to 15% in patients with hematologic malignant spread, and it often accompanies metastases to the brain (BMs) [1]. NM has historically been associated with a dismal prognosis of 2–4 months, and it continues to remain poor, with patients presenting with a wide range of clinical features from simultaneous involvement of multiple locations throughout the neuraxis [1,2]. The diagnosis of NM requires a high index of clinical suspicion and is made by imaging with cerebrospinal fluid (CSF) studies. The management of patients with NM has evolved tremendously over the past decade, improving both the quality of life and survival. This narrative review highlights these advancements in management, focusing on new therapeutic modalities, including targeted and immunotherapies.

2. Epidemiology

The incidence of NM is around 5% in patients with metastatic cancer, with most patients being diagnosed late in the disease course [3]. Brain metastases frequently accompany NM in as much as 50–80% of patients with NM [4]. The most common solid tumors resulting in NM include breast cancer, followed by lung cancer, melanoma, gastrointestinal malignancies, and metastases from an unknown primary [5]. Among patients with lung cancer, NM occurs most frequently with epidermal growth factor receptor (EGFR) positive non-small cell lung cancer (NSCLC). Similarly, in breast cancer, tumors harboring the human epidermal growth factor receptor 2 (HER2) are more likely to spread to the leptomeninges [6,7]. Primary parenchymal brain tumors also have the potential to spread through the leptomeninges or via the CSF [8]. Surgical resection and stereotactic radiosurgery inpatients with brain metastases have rarely been associated with consequent NM due to spillage and consequent seeding of malignant cells. A multi-institutional analysis studying radiographic NM subtypes showed a greater risk of neurologic death among the classical NM pattern, as compared to nodular NM [9–11]. The risk of leptomeningeal seeding has been greater with the omission of whole-brain radiation therapy (WBRT) and reported more with piecemeal rather than en-bloc resections [12,13]. Finally, with the development of targeted therapies and associated improvements in survival, the incidence of NM with or without BM has increased [14].

3. Pathogenesis

The pathophysiology of NM involves a multifactorial process in which tumor cells spread from the primary tumor, traverse the vasculature, and seed at a location where they can enter the CSF. A key process in the pathway is the breakdown of the brain barrier (Figure 1).

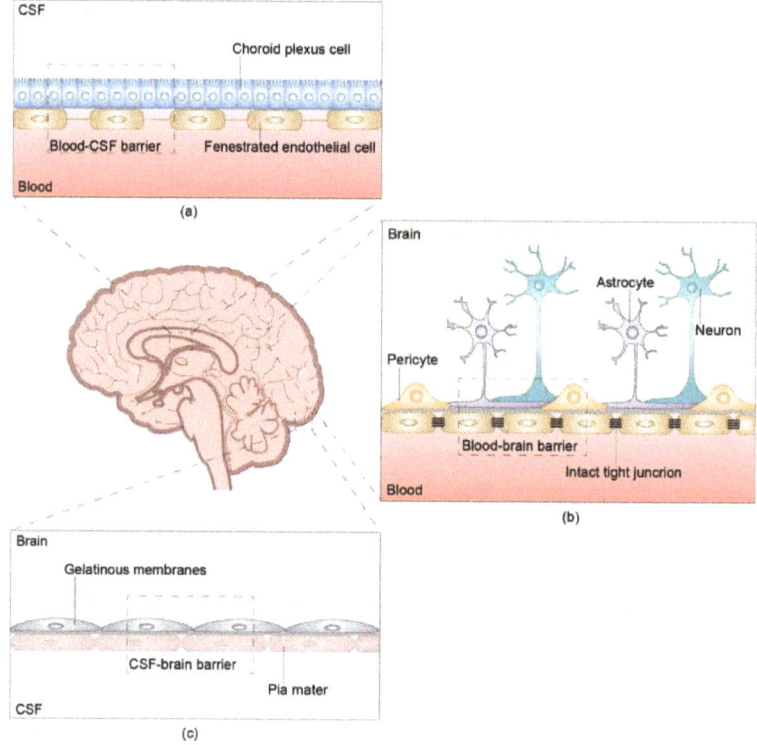

Figure 1. The structure and composition of the brain barrier The brain barrier consists of three parts: the blood- cerebrospinal fluid (CSF) barrier, blood–brain barrier, and CSF-brain barrier. (**a**) The blood-CSF barrier is located between the blood and CSF in the ventricular choroid plexus. (**b**) The

blood–brain barrier (BBB) is located between microvascular endothelial cells and the nerve cells of the brain and spinal cord. There are intact tight junctions between capillary endothelial cells that prevent the passage of macromolecules other than water and certain ions. The intact and continuous capillary basement membrane is surrounded by a glial membrane of protruding astrocytes. The BBB, main barrier that protects the CNS, prevents many macromolecules from entering the brain and selectively pumps harmful substances out of the brain. (**c**) The CSF-brain barrier is located between the CSF in the ventricles and subarachnoid space and the nerve cells of the brain and spinal cord. Reproduced with Permission from Wang, Y., Yang, X., Li, N.J., Xue, J.X. Leptomeningeal metastases in non-small cell lung cancer: Diagnosis and treatment. Lung Cancer. 2022;174:1–13. doi:10.1016/j.lungcan.2022.09.013 [15].

Involvement of the leptomeninges, which comprise the arachnoid and pia mater, allows the malignant cells to grow and reach throughout the subarachnoid space via the CSF [16]. While present inside the CSF, the tumor cells are preserved from immune surveillance and attack, which aids in their further proliferation, referred to as the CSF sanctuary phenomenon [17].

There exist various means via which the tumor cells reach the CSF, with hematogenous dissemination being the most common. Other routes include a direct extension from pachymeningeal or dural metastases, infiltration along nerve sheaths, spread from choroid plexus metastases, and rarely, from tumors arising within the meninges itself [18]. Cranial nerve involvement by tumors comes in several shapes or forms, many of which give rise to the cranial neuropathies in neoplastic meningitis and some of which contribute to the causation of neoplastic meningitis as well (Table 1).

Table 1. Mechanisms of nerve invasion: several mechanisms of nerve involvement are known and vary from mechanical lesions to different oncological patterns. Abbreviations: NGF, Nerve growth factor; NCAM, Neural Cell Adhesion Molecule. Reproduced with Permission from Grisold W, Grisold A. Cancer around the brain. Neurooncol Pract. 2014; 1(1): 13–21. doi:10.1093/nop/npt002 [19].

Type of Nerve Growth	Subgroups	Remarks
Mechanical causes	Compression	
	Engulfing	
	Pushing and stretching of the nerve by mass lesion	
Invasion	Direct invasion (local infiltration)	
	Perineural	
	Endoneurial	
	Intravascular spread	
Metastasis	Isolated intranerval (rare)	
Perineurial spread	Anterograde	
	Retrograde	
	Particular patterns:	
	Spread via nerve scaffolds	
	Dermatomal spread	
	Anastomotic spread from one nerve region into another	
Tumor invasion—nerve growth	Peripheral nerve sprouting	Observed experimentally
Growth factors	NGF, NCAM, other local factors promoting nerve growth	
Angiosoma vs. common anatomical distribution	Concept of metastatic distribution	The angiosoma concept divides the skull into 13 different angiosomas

The causation of a multitude of symptoms is attributed to various pathophysiological mechanisms, like cerebral edema, due to BBB disruption or direct tumor involvement, leading to cranial nerve and spinal root dysfunction. Invasion of the brain parenchyma can interfere with circulation and cause diffuse cerebral dysfunction. Finally, increased intracranial pressure, due to either mass effect or flow obstruction, leads to hydrocephalus and associated symptoms.

4. Clinical Features

NM classically has a multifocal involvement, and despite presenting with a single symptom, a thorough neurologic evaluation reveals further sites of CNS affection. The specific clinical symptoms are attributable to sites of invasion by leptomeningeal disease itself, or to sequela like hydrocephalus. Headache is the most common symptom of NM, the presenting symptom in 30–50% of patients, and can be due to either meningeal irritation or increased intracranial pressure (ICP) [20]. An association with neck stiffness suggests headache due to meningeal irritation, whereas accompanying symptoms of nausea with vomiting and signs including papilledema point towards increased ICP. Various presentations of encephalopathy are also common in NM due to hydrocephalus, seizures, or diffuse cerebral dysfunction. This can present as disorientation, personality changes, confusion, and forgetfulness. Seizures are observed in up to 25% of patients with NM due to parenchymal irritation from invasion, edema, or adjacent leptomeningeal deposits [21]. The occurrence of epileptiform activity is frequently confused with plateau waves, which occur during positional changes and are a marker of increased ICP. These can be associated with positional headache, dizziness, presyncope, or episodes of frank syncope, and their presence should follow a workup for increased ICP [22]. Cerebellar dysfunction is reported in 20% of patients at presentation and can cause midline and lateral cerebellar symptoms [4].

Invasion of cranial nerves in the subarachnoid symptoms leads to a multitude of symptoms due to cranial neuropathies. Diplopia is the most common symptom and can be caused by the involvement of either cranial nerves III, IV, or VI [23]. Trigeminal nerve involvement leads to sensory changes over the face, with a classic presentation of facial numbness known as the "numb chin syndrome." [24]. Facial and vestibulocochlear nerve involvement leads to weakness of facial muscles and sensorineural hearing loss, respectively, and lower cranial nerve dysfunction causes dysphagia, dysarthria, and hoarseness, due to laryngopharyngeal involvement. Spinal nerve root involvement has also been reported, with resultant radiculopathy and cauda equina syndrome, with lower spinal roots more frequently involved than the cervical roots. Finally, cortical signs are rarely seen and suggest an accompanying parenchymal invasion.

5. Diagnosis

A thorough evaluation, including a complete history and physical examination, is pertinent to identify clues of NM's multifocal involvement. Neuroimaging studies include a gadolinium-enhanced magnetic resonance imaging (MRI) scan of the brain and cervical, thoracic and lumbar spine, or computed tomography (CT) scan with contrast, with the former having greater sensitivity. However, an MRI is less specific than a CSF cytology examination and depicts enhancing foci within the sulci, cisterns, and subarachnoid space in the spine [25]. These findings can be accompanied by ventriculomegaly, and fluid-attenuated inversion recovery (FLAIR) images depict hyperintensity due to increased protein content in the CSF [26].

The lumbar puncture could show an elevated opening pressure, and CSF examination typically reveals elevated protein and low glucose concentrations, lymphocytic pleocytosis. The derangement in all the parameters is uncommon; however, a completely normal CSF examination is rare [27]. Xanthochromia may be seen with hemorrhage from the leptomeningeal deposits, primarily originating from melanoma [28]. The definitive diagnostic finding by identifying malignant cells within the CSF carries a high specificity, but the sensitivity is low due to sampling issues and may necessitate repeat lumbar punctures. Immunohistochemical studies in the CSF yield may assist in diagnosing patients with NM due to unknown primary [29].

The concentration of tumor markers may also carry relevance, as an increase with respect to serum concentration is strongly suggestive of NM. A rise in the concentration of

CSF tumor makers more than 2–3% of serum values is unlikely due to simple diffusion or serum contamination unless an increased CSF albumin concentration is also present- which indicates disruption of the BBB [30]. Novel techniques, including identifying circulating tumor cells and cell-free DNA in CSF, carry high sensitivity and specificity and have been increasingly used in the last few years [31]. Evaluation of CSF by flow cytometry accords importance in the assessment of patients with suspected NM due to primary central nervous system lymphoma or other subtypes of non-Hodgkin lymphoma with a propensity for CNS involvement. The CSF examination reveals an elevated protein concentration, lymphocyte-predominant pleocytosis, and decreased glucose levels, with flow cytometry confirming the presence of malignant lymphoid cells [32].

6. Management

The management strategies for patients with neoplastic meningitis (NM) aim to improve neurologic function, prolong survival and prevent further neurologic deterioration. A multidisciplinary tumor board is essential to deciding individual treatment strategies, with inputs from a team of neurosurgeons, radiation oncologists, neuro-oncologists, and medical oncologists. The treatment options are broadly categorized into systemic therapies, radiation therapies (RT), and therapies instilled directly into the CSF: intrathecal therapies (IT).

6.1. Symptomatic Management

The development of increased intracranial pressure (ICP) is a frequent consequence of NM, owing to the hindrance of CSF outflow via the arachnoid granulations. Medical therapies exploited to curb the increasing ICP consist of acetazolamide to decrease the CSF production from choroid plexus and, occasionally, hyperosmotic agents such as mannitol and hypertonic saline to treat acute symptomatic raised ICP. Mechanical means of ICP reduction may need to be employed in refractory cases, with the ventriculoperitoneal shunt leading to improvements in both acute decompensation and overall survival [33,34]. Theoretical risks of seeding the tumor cells from CSF to the peritoneum exist, but the overall benefit far outweighs the benefits of CSF redirection [35]. Seizures can be managed with various antiepileptic drugs, with levetiracetam being an excellent first-line option, considering its low risk of drug interactions [36]. Similar to patients with BMs, routine prophylaxis with anti-seizure drugs is not advised, as it leads to unnecessary adverse effects associated with these drugs.

6.2. Radiotherapy

Radiotherapy in NM serves the role of symptom palliation in managing bulky disease and may improve subsequent penetration of systemic therapies by disturbing the blood–brain barrier (BBB) [37]. It, however, has not demonstrated an improvement in survival. The extent of RT is tailored according to the extent of neuraxis affected, with focal RT preferred to ablate localized bulky metastases while limiting dose-related toxicity. Whole-brain RT (WBRT) is employed more often, especially in the setting of concomitant brain metastases (BMs), but is associated with significant cognitive decline and toxicity, when combined with systemic therapies. The typical regimen of WBRT delivers a radiation dose of 30 Gy in 10 fractions, but an attenuated course is preferred for patients unable to tolerate an increased dose or duration of treatment, commonly with 20 Gy being delivered in 4 Gy fractions [38].

Based on disease distribution, RT can improve function rapidly in symptomatic patients with or without radiographic evidence of disease. NM leading to radiculopathies or cauda equina syndrome causes varying pain levels, weakness, and bowel and bladder involvement and can be effectively treated with prompt lumbosacral RT [39]. Focused skull-base RT can manage different cranial neuropathies, with the routine dose delivered being 30 Gy in 10 fractions. Avoiding radiation to the temporal lobe can avoid subsequent memory deficits and is primarily pursued in patients having received WBRT in the past [40].

Patients with diffuse cerebral involvement present with encephalopathy, and WBRT is utilized to treat NM and concomitant BMs. The subset of patients experiencing symptomatic improvement with radiotherapy is those with a lower radiographic bulk and a shorter duration of symptoms, with those suffering from prolonged symptoms deriving little to no benefit [41].

The use of memantine and hippocampal avoidance techniques has shown promise in reducing the rate of cognitive deterioration in BMs, but its role in NM remains unclear. Finally, the use of an even more extensive approach, craniospinal irradiation (CSI), targets a broader area theoretically but is infrequently employed in clinical practice. Other than its significant radiation exposure to the abdominal organs, CSI destroys a considerable amount of marrow in the vertebral bodies, making future use of immunosuppressive chemotherapy difficult [35]. Irradiation with a proton beam instead may avoid these toxicities. A phase II trial comparing craniospinal proton irradiation with photon-involved-field radiotherapy recently reported favorable outcomes with the use of proton therapy in patients with solid tumor NM. A significant improvement was noted in CNS PFS (7.5 mths vs. 6.6 mths) and OS (9.9 mths vs. 6.0 mths) with no difference in toxicity outcomes with the use of proton irradiation [42].

6.3. Intrathecal Chemotherapy

Intrathecal (IT) chemotherapy has the theoretical advantage of delivering anticancer agents directly to the site of solid metastases and allowing sufficient concentration to be administered throughout the CSF in case of diffuse metastases. However, since the diffusion beyond the CSF is limited only to a few millimeters, IT chemotherapy is employed in non-bulky disease and to treat bulky metastases post-radiation. By avoiding the route through BBB, IT chemotherapy allows a lower dose of cytotoxic agents to be delivered, thereby lowering the risks of systemic toxicity. The IT chemotherapy regimens involve three phases: high-dose induction, intermediate-dose consolidation, and low-dose maintenance [43].

The two main routes for the administration of IT chemotherapies include a lumbar puncture (LP) or via a ventricular reservoir (e.g., Ommaya reservoir). The advantages associated with using the Ommaya reservoir include a better distribution throughout the CSF compartment, avoidance of repeated LPs, and thus greater ease of administration. Ideally, A CSF flow study is conducted prior to administering IT chemotherapy to ensure an unobstructed CSF path and optimal drug distribution. The CSF flow studies described by Chamberlain utilized the isotopes Technetium-99 or Indium-111, and if the reports suggested an obstruction, IT chemotherapy was not opted for [44].

The procedural risks associated with both these approaches constitute the main drawback of this treatment route. These include, but are not limited to, CNS infection, cerebral herniation, and CSF leak [45]. The ventricular reservoirs carry additional risks, including catheter misplacement, tip occlusion, and aseptic, chemical, or septic meningitis. Cessation of therapy with the removal of the reservoir may be required to manage these complications. Besides, the drugs administered intrathecally have short half-lives, with concentrations declining to subtherapeutic levels in matter of hours, and complete elimination in 1–2 days [46].

Other serious complications associated with IT chemotherapy include the occurrence of progressive leukoencephalopathy. It typically occurs with intrathecal methotrexate and has a chronic presentation with cognitive symptoms, incontinence, seizures, and gait alterations. The incidence further increases upon the combination with RT, which forms the basis of the recommendation of administering RT and IT methotrexate at least 2–3 weeks apart. Liposomal cytarabine is a sustained-release form of the drug, which requires a biweekly administration, and may achieve more homogenous CSF distribution than the non-liposomal form [47]. However, it did not demonstrate increased survival or response rates compared to IT methotrexate across a clinical trial or retrospective case review [48,49]. In 1998, Glantz and colleagues reported findings from a classic trial comparing liposomal cytarabine versus methotrexate, both injected intrathecally. They found that while median survival was not significantly different, the time elapsed without symptoms or toxicity (TWIST) was significantly higher, being 99 days for cytarabine and 28 days for methotrexate (Table 2).

Table 2. Comparison of key results associated with liposomal cytarabine versus methotrexate, both injected intrathecally. TWIST = time elapsed without symptoms or toxicity. n = number of patients. Reproduced with permission from Beauchesne P. Intrathecal chemotherapy for treatment of leptomeningeal dissemination of metastatic tumors. Lancet Oncol. 2010; 11(9): 871–879. doi:10.1016/S1470-2045(10)70034-6 [1].

	Liposomal Cytarabine (n = 31)	Methotrexate (n = 30)	p Value
Response (cytology rendered negative and clinical condition stable or improved)	8	6	0.76
Median duration of response	39 days	26 days	0.31
Time before neurological progression	58 days	30 days	0.0068
Survival directly linked to the meningitis	343 days	98 days	0.074
Median survival	105 days	78 days	0.15
Survival > 6 months	13	5	0.15
Survival > 1 year	5	2	0.43
Grade 3 toxicity	24	20	
Duration of Grade 3 toxicity	18 days	11 days	0.2
TWIST	99 days	28 days	<0.05

Besides, conus medullaris syndrome with arachnoiditis occurs with liposomal cytarabine, which may be prevented to some extent by spacing IT and systemic chemotherapy and administering corticosteroids. The occurrence of bone marrow suppression is common with the use of various cytotoxic agents, with folinic acid rescue recommended after the administration of methotrexate [50]. Finally, acute myelopathy, a disastrous complication classically associated with methotrexate use, can present as quadriparesis or locked-in syndrome. A diagnostic spinal MRI study can reveal normal findings or T2-hyperintense lesions in the posterior columns. It may also be caused by the use of thiotepa or cytarabine and can be differentiated from myelopathy due to tumor progression by measurement of myelin basic protein in the CSF, which rises in case of drug-induced myelopathy.

Commonly used drugs included as part of IT chemotherapy are methotrexate, thiotepa, topotecan, cytarabine, and sustained-release liposomal cytarabine, and thus the number of available options is limited compared to those which can be administered systematically. Owing to the dearth of clinical trials conducted to date, it has been difficult to conclude a definite superiority of one agent over another. Moreover, most of the studies have been single-arm studies, using different endpoints and not taking into account the multiple subtypes or histologies of the primary tumor [35].

IT therapy was shown to increase survival up to 7.5 months in a cohort of patients with NM from breast cancer upon being treated with a combinatorial regimen of RT with IT methotrexate, cytarabine, or thiotepa [51]. In another subset of patients with NM due to NSCLC studied by Chamberlain et al., the median survival was 5.0 months, with the same combinatorial regimen utilized [52]. However, the results of the only randomized clinical trial conducted to date comparing the efficacy of IT chemotherapy with systemic chemotherapy revealed no difference in patient survival or neurologic response amongst the groups. Boogerd et al. conducted this study on 35 patients with NM due to breast cancer and noted an increased risk of neurotoxicity with IT chemotherapy. Finally, a retrospective analysis by Bokstein et al. involving 104 patients with NM revealed no benefit and an increased risk of complications with IT chemotherapy when combined with RT and systemic chemotherapy, compared to a regimen excluding IT chemotherapy [53]. Recent results from a phase I/II study of intrathecal trastuzumab in HER-2 positive cancer with NM showed an OS of 8.3 months for patients with any HER-2 positive histology and

10.5 months in HER-2 positive breast cancer [54]. Pharmacokinetic studies depicted a stable CSF concentration of trastuzumab, suggesting promising future studies on the subject [54].

6.4. Systemic Therapy

6.4.1. Chemotherapy

The utilization of systemic chemotherapy assumes importance in treating associated systemically active disease while avoiding cognitive decline and procedural complications linked to WBRT and IT therapies, respectively. Systemic agents have shown some activity due to the BBB breakdown in the NM setting, although efficacy depends heavily on tumor subtype and histology. Some commonly used systemic chemotherapy agents utilized are described in Table 3.

Table 3. Standard and experimental systemic chemotherapy drugs for treatment of neoplastic meningitis. Reproduced with permission from Beauchesne P. Intrathecal chemotherapy for treatment of leptomeningeal dissemination of metastatic tumors. Lancet Oncol. 2010; 11(9): 871–879. doi:10.1016/S1470-2045(10)70034-6 [1].

	Available for Routine Use	Induction	Consolidation	Maintenance
Methotrexate	Yes	10–15 mg twice weekly (for 4 weeks)	10–15 mg once weekly (for 4 weeks)	10–15 mg once a month
Thiotepa	Yes	10 mg twice weekly (for 4 weeks)	10 mg once weekly (for 4 weeks)	10 mg once a month
Cytarabine	Yes	25–100 mg twice weekly (for 4 weeks)	25–100 mg once weekly (for 4 weeks)	25–100 mg once a month
Liposomal cytarabine	Yes	50 mg every 2 weeks (for 8 weeks)	50 mg every 4 weeks (for 24 weeks)	
Topotecan	Yes	0.4 mg twice weekly (for 6 weeks)	0.4 mg once per week (for 6 weeks)	0.4 mg twice monthly for 4 months, then monthly thereafter
Mafosfamide	No	20 mg once or twice weekly until CSF remission	20 mg weekly	20 mg every 2–6 weeks
Etoposide	Yes	0.5 mg/day for 5 days every other week (for 8 weeks)	0.5 mg/day for 5 days every other week (for 4 weeks)	0.5 mg/day for 5 days once a month
Floxuridine	No	1 mg/day continued for as long as possible		
Diaziquone	No	1–2 mg twice weekly for few weeks		
Mercaptopurine	No	10 mg twice weekly for 4 weeks		
Busulfan	No	5–17 mg twice weekly for 2 weeks		

Non-targeted agents like methotrexate, a dihydrofolate reductase inhibitor, have historically been used to treat primary central nervous system lymphoma. It has also demonstrated efficacy in treating NM originating from solid tumors like squamous cell carcinoma (SCC) of the head and neck. The use of high-dose intravenous methotrexate demonstrated a significant increase in survival compared to IT methotrexate, when used as a sole treatment for managing NM, with a median survival of 13.8 mths (vs. 2.3 mths) [55]. Thiotepa, a DNA alkylating agent, does cross the BBB, but its use remains limited as an IT agent. Systemic temozolomide, a current standard of care in treating gliomas, has not demonstrated appreciable efficacy in managing NM. The pyrimidine analog, cytarabine, has shown efficacy in treating CNS leukemia, especially in patients with isolated CNS involvement [56].

6.4.2. Targeted Therapies

With an ever-increasing knowledge of driver mutations and molecular targets, the development of targeted therapies has been progressing at a rapid pace. Non-squamous cell lung carcinoma harboring a mutation in epidermal growth factor receptor (EGFR) has been successfully targeted by erlotinib, which has led to extended survival in patients with NM [57]. Another study reported a median survival of 14 months among patients treated with erlotinib for NM associated with NSCLC [58]. Newer EGFR tyrosine kinase inhibitors (TKIs) such as afatinib and osimertinib have demonstrated better CNS penetration and have a critical established role in the management of BMs from EGFR-mutated NSCLC [59,60]. A case reported the efficacy of a combination of afatinib and cetuximab in a patient with NM due to NSCLC, leading to the resolution of NM lesions [61]. The BLOOM study, a recently concluded phase I clinical trial, demonstrated considerable efficacy with osimertinib, a 3rd generation TKI, in NM arising from NSCLC. Among 18 patients with NM, five patients (28%) had a confirmed response, and 14 patients (78%) achieved disease control upon being evaluated by MRI imaging [62].

Regarding NM arising from NSCLC harboring mutations involving the anaplastic lymphoma kinase (ALK) gene, new-generation ALK inhibitor alectinib has shown considerable CSF penetration and activity in NM [63,64]. The efficacy of ceritinib, another 2nd generation ALK inhibitor, has been reported recently in NM caused by ALK-mutated NSCLC as part of the ASCEND-7 trial. In a cohort of 18 patients with NM, the whole-body ORR was 16.7%, with the median PFS and OS being 5.2 and 7.2 months, respectively [65]. Lorlatinib, one of the newer ALK inhibitors, has CNS penetration, as seen by adverse effects, and case reports show initial efficacy [66].

Mutations in human epidermal growth factor receptor 2 (HER2) have been shown to be associated with an increased risk of CNS spread [67]. Trials involving trastuzumab, a HER2 inhibitor, have shown good CNS response in metastatic breast cancer with spread to the brain, but separate results with respect to response in NM are unavailable [68]. Ongoing trials evaluating the efficacy of lapatinib, a dual EGFR, and HER2 inhibitor, in treating NM have completed recruitment, and results are awaited (NCT02650752). In combination with capecitabine, a 5-fluorouracil prodrug, lapatinib has also demonstrated an encouraging CNS response in the LANDSCAPE trial studying efficacy in patients with BMs [69]. Neratinib, a HER2-targeting tyrosine kinase inhibitor combined with capecitabine, demonstrated promising intracranial activity in patients with HER2 overexpressing breast cancer [70]. There are case series of efficacy in leptomeningeal metastases [71]. Preliminary results from a phase II trial evaluating the effectiveness of the combination of tucatinib-trastuzumab-capecitabine in the treatment of NM from HER2+ breast cancer have reported a median OS of 11.9 months in a cohort of 17 patients (NCT03501979) [72]. Retrospective studies of an antibody-drug conjugate, trastuzumab deruxtecan, in patients with HER2 breast cancer and NM showed initial evidence of activity, and more recently, the DEBBRAH trial included patients with both BM and NM, and the published data showed excellent responses in patients with BM while the data for NM is awaited [73].

Mutations in v-Raf murine sarcoma viral oncogene homolog B (BRAF) are prevalent in melanoma, with its subtype BRAFv600E being the most common subtype [74]. Three separate case reports have described the efficacy of BRAFv600E inhibitors, dabrafenib, and vemurafenib, in treating NM arising from melanoma. The clinical trials published so far have focused on BMs from melanoma, but trials evaluating the efficacy of immunotherapies in NM due to melanoma are underway (NCT02939300) (Table 4).

Table 4. Overview of clinical trials evaluating targeted therapy in neoplastic meningitis. Original table, updated till October 2022. Abbreviations: OS: Overall survival, PFS: Progression-free survival, DCR: Disease control rate, DOR: Duration of response, A/E: Adverse Effects, QoL: Quality of Life.

Study	Targeted Therapy	Primary Site	Estimated Completion	N	Primary Endpoint (s)	Secondary Endpoint (s)
NCT04833205	EGFR-TKI + Nimotuzumab	Lung	April 2023	30	PFS	OS, A/E
NCT04425681	Osimertinib + Bevacizumab	Lung	June 2021	20	PFS, ORR	OS, A/E
NCT04944069	Almonertinib + Bevacizumab	Lung	March 2025	69	OS	PFS, ORR, DCR, DOR
NCT04778800	Almonertinib	Lung	February 2024	60	iPFS	DCR, PFS, OS
NCT02616393	Tesevatinib	Lung	April 2018	36	ORR	PFS, OS, TTP, QoL
NCT05146219	TY-9591	Lung	December 2014	60	ORR	DCR, OS, DOR, PFS
NCT04233021	Osimertinib	Lung	July 2022	113	ORR	OS, PFS, A/E, QoL
NCT03257124	AZD-9291	Lung	December 2021	80	ORR, OS	DCR, OS, DOR, PFS, A/E
NCT03711422	Afatinib	Lung	September 2021	25	PFS, OS, ORR	A/E

6.4.3. Immunotherapies

A myriad of immunotherapies, ranging from immune checkpoint inhibitors (ICIs) to CAR T cell therapies, have been incorporated into the management of multiple types of tumors. Immune checkpoint blockade, with the use of antibodies targeted against programmed death-1 (PD1), its ligand (PD-L1), or cytotoxic T lymphocyte-associated protein-4 (CTLA-4), leads to disinhibition of T-cells, allowing them to target tumor cells effectively. All three categories of drugs, anti-PD1, anti-PD-L1, and anti-CTLA-4, have demonstrated efficacy against BMs from NSCLC and melanoma [75–77].

A limited number of studies have evaluated the impact of ICIs on managing NM. A phase II study evaluated the combination of nivolumab and ipilimumab in 18 patients with NM and reported an OS of 44% at three months. In addition, a complete response was observed in one patient (5.6%), with stable and progressive disease in 7 (38.9%) and 4 (22.2%) patients, respectively [78]. Multiple phase II trials are underway, and the results depicting the efficacy of PD-1 inhibitors pembrolizumab and nivolumab are keenly awaited (NCT02886525, NCT04729348). Meanwhile, studies involving PD-L1 inhibitors durvalumab and avelumab have been started to demonstrate safety and a tolerable dose for treating NM to inspire future studies involving variable combinations of ICIs (NCT03719768, NCT04356222). Hendriks et al. evaluated a cohort of 1288 patients of NSCLC treated with ICIs, among which 19 patients were observed to have NM. A PFS of 2.0 and a median OS of 3.7 months were reported in that cohort. [79]. Finally, Geukes Foppen et al. evaluated a series of 39 patients with NM due to melanoma and reported an abysmal prognosis even after using ipilimumab at 15.8 weeks [80].

Other clinical trials currently ongoing related to NM due to breast cancer are evaluating the efficacy of CAR T cell therapy (HER2 CAR) and a bi-specific antibody (HER2Bi) (NCT03696030, NCT03661424). Preliminary results from the NM cohort of patients receiving abemaciclib, a cyclin-dependent kinase 4/6 (CDK 4/6) inhibitor, in breast cancer revealed a PFS of 5.9 months and an OS of 8.4 months [81]. Regarding the utilization of immunotherapies to treat NM due to melanoma, two separate cohort studies have demonstrated the use of IT interleukin-2 (IL-2) with varying chemotherapy combinations and reported a similar survival of 7.8–7.9 months, respectively. [82,83]. Finally, intrathecal administration of the immunotherapeutic agent nivolumab has also been attempted in a single-arm phase I/Ib trial (NCT03025256) in patients with NM due to melanoma. Preliminary results include a median OS of 42% at six months, 30% at 12 months, and a tolerable side effect profile, with no grade 4 or 5 toxicities [84] (Table 5).

Table 5. Overview of clinical trials evaluating immunotherapy in neoplastic meningitis. Original table, updated till October 2022. Abbreviations: OS: Overall survival, PFS: Progression-free survival, DLT: Dose Limiting Toxicity, ORR: Objective Response Rate, A/E: Adverse Effects, IT: Intrathecal, CAR-T: Chimeric Antigen Receptor T-cell, N: Number of patients. NSCLC: Non-Small Cell Lung Cancer.

Study	Type of Immunotherapy	Type of Study	Primary Site	N	Therapy	Outcome
NCT02886525	Immune checkpoint inhibitor	Phase II	Multiple	102	Pembrolizumab	ORR, OS, Extracranial ORR
NCT04729348	Immune checkpoint inhibitor	Phase II	Multiple	19	Pembrolizumab + lenvatinib	% alive at 6 mth
NCT03719768	Immune checkpoint inhibitor	Phase I	Multiple	16	Avelumab	Safety, DLT
NCT04356222	Immune checkpoint inhibitor	Phase I	NSCLC	30	Durvalumab	OS, PFS, AEs
NCT03696030	CAR T cells	Phase I	Breast	39	HER-2 CAR-T cells	DLT, AEs
NCT03661424	Immunomodulator	Phase I	Breast	16	Bi-specific antibody (HER2Bi)	AEs: frequency/type/severity/duration
NCT02308020 [81]	Immunomodulator	Phase II	Breast	7 *	Abemaciclib	PFS: 5.9 mth OS: 8.4 mth
Hendriks et al. [79]	Immune checkpoint inhibitor	Retrospective cohort	Lung	19	Pembrolizumab or nivolumab	PFS: 2.0 mth OS: 3.7 mth
Ferguson et al. [82]	Immunomodulator	Retrospective cohort	Melanoma	178	IT IL-2, other combinations with chemo	OS: 7.9 mth
Glitza et al. [83]	Immunomodulator	Retrospective cohort	Melanoma	43	IT IL – 2 ± chemoradiotherapy	OS: 7.8 mth
Geukes Foppen et al. [80]	Immune checkpoint inhibitor	Retrospective cohort	Melanoma	10 **	Ipilimumab	OS: 15.8 wks

* 7 patients in cohort with NM, 58 patients analyzed in total. ** 6 patients received ipilimumab, 39 patients analyzed in total.

6.4.4. Other Novel Therapies

Clinical trials evaluating ANG1005, or paclitaxel trevatide, are underway among newly diagnosed NM from breast cancer (NCT03613181). It is a taxane derivative designed to cross the BBB and is made from three paclitaxel molecules covalently linked to Angiopep-2 [85]. IT-delivered monoclonal antibodies have been used to deliver selected radiation or therapeutic agents. This approach of targeted radioimmunotherapy has been used in a phase I study evaluating iodine-131 labeled monoclonal antibody 3F8, targeting GD2-positive NM. A sufficient intra-CSF concentration was achieved, without significant toxicity, with three out of thirteen patients with a radiographic response [86]. A phase II study utilizing this agent is currently underway (NCT00445965). The glycoprotein 4Ig-B7H3 is present on various tumors, targeted by iodine-131 labeled 8H9 monoclonal antibody, and is currently being evaluated in phase I clinical trial (NCT00089245) (Table 6).

Table 6. Overview of Clinical trials evaluating intrathecal therapies in neoplastic meningitis. Original table, updated till October 2022. Abbreviations: OS: Overall survival, PFS: Progression-free survival, DLT, ORR: Objective Response Rate, RR: Response Rate, N: Number of patients, NSCLC: Non-Small Cell Lung Cancer, SCLC: Small Cell Lung Cancer.

Study	Treatment Arms	Primary Site	N	Outcome
Hitchins [87]	IT methotrexate	SCLC (29%), Breast (25%), 1° brain (9%), NSCLC (7%), lymphoma (7%)	44	ORR: 61%
	IT methotrexate+ IT cytosine arabinoside			ORR: 45%
Grossman [88]	IT methotrexate	Breast (48%), lung (23%), lymphoma (19%)	52	OS: 15.9 weeks
	IT thiotepa			OS: 14.1 weeks

Table 6. *Cont.*

Study	Treatment Arms	Primary Site	N	Outcome
Glantz [49]	IT methotrexate	Breast (36%), NSCLC (10%), 1° brain (23%), melanoma (8%), SCLC (7%)	61	RR: 20%, OS: 78 days
	IT liposomal cytarabine			RR: 26%, OS: 105 days
Glantz [89]	IT cytosine arabinoside	Lymphoma (100%)	28	RR: 15%, OS: 63 days
	IT liposomal cytarabine			RR: 71%, OS: 99 days
Shapiro [90]	IT liposomal cytarabine	Solid tumors (80%), lymphoma (20%)	128	PFS: 34 days
	IT cytosine arabinoside			PFS: 50 days

7. Conclusions

Neoplastic meningitis remains a disease process with poor survival outcomes due to the tumor microenvironment, the inherently aggressive nature of the neoplasm, and the restricted delivery of therapeutic drugs due to the blood–brain barrier. Its management remains a challenge due to limited evidence from a small number of clinical trials. This results in various non-standardized treatment regimens, which are personalized according to patient and source tumor characteristics. There is a need for prospective studies focusing on selected histological tumor types and gauging the efficacy of novel therapeutics which have become available within the last few years. The utilization of improved diagnostic biomarkers and an understanding of the molecular differences between the primary site and metastatic disease will lead to the development of targeted therapies. Assessment of these drugs within clinical trials, including patients with NM as sub-groups, will help define better therapeutic management of patients affected by leptomeningeal tumor dissemination.

Author Contributions: Conceptualization, A.A.K., S.S., A.O., V.A.V., D.M.P. and M.S.A.; methodology, A.A.K., A.O. and V.A.V.; writing—original draft preparation, A.A.K., A.O., V.A.V., D.M.P. and M.S.A.; writing—review and editing, A.A.K., A.O., V.A.V., D.M.P. and M.S.A.; visualization, A.A.K., A.O. and V.A.V.; supervision, D.M.P. and M.S.A.; project administration, N/A; funding acquisition, N/A. All authors have read and agreed to the published version of the manuscript.

Funding: This research received no external funding.

Conflicts of Interest: Manmeet Singh Ahluwalia Disclosures: Grants: Astrazeneca, BMS, Bayer, Incyte, Pharmacyclics, Novocure, Mimivax, Merck. Consultation: Bayer, Novocure, Kiyatec, Insightec, GSK, Xoft, Nuvation, Cellularity, SDP Oncology, Apollomics, Prelude, Janssen, Tocagen, Voyager Therapeutics, Viewray, Caris Lifesciences, Pyramid Biosciences, Varian Medical Systems, Cairn Therapeutics, Anheart Therapeutics, Theraguix. Scientific Advisory Board: Cairn Therapeutics, Pyramid Biosciences, Modifi Biosciences. Stock shareholder: Mimivax, Cytodyn, MedInnovate Advisors LLC. David M. Peereboom Disclosures: Consulting or Advisory Role: Orbus Therapeutics, Sumitomo Dainippon Pharma Oncology Inc, Stemline Therapeutics, Novocure. Research Funding: Pfizer (Inst), Novartis (Inst), Neonc Technologies (Inst), Orbus Therapeutics (Inst), Bristol Myers Squibb (Inst), Genentech/Roche (Inst), Pharmacyclics (Inst), Bayer (Inst), Karyopharm Therapeutics (Inst), Apollomics (Inst), Vigeo Therapeutics (Inst), Global Coalition for Adaptive Research (Inst), MimiVax (Inst), Ono Pharmaceutical (Inst), Mylan (Inst).

References

1. Beauchesne, P. Intrathecal chemotherapy for treatment of leptomeningeal dissemination of metastatic tumours. *Lancet Oncol.* **2010**, *11*, 871–879. [CrossRef]
2. Chorti, E.; Kebir, S.; Ahmed, M.S.; Keyvani, K.; Umutlu, L.; Kanaki, T.; Zaremba, A.; Reinboldt-Jockenhoefer, F.; Knispel, S.; Gratsias, E.; et al. Leptomeningeal disease from melanoma-Poor prognosis despite new therapeutic modalities. *Eur. J. Cancer* **2021**, *148*, 395–404. [CrossRef] [PubMed]
3. DeAngelis, L.M. Current diagnosis and treatment of leptomeningeal metastasis. *J. Neurooncol.* **1998**, *38*, 245–252. [CrossRef] [PubMed]
4. Clarke, J.L.; Perez, H.R.; Jacks, L.M.; Panageas, K.S.; Deangelis, L.M. Leptomeningeal metastases in the MRI era. *Neurology* **2010**, *74*, 1449–1454. [CrossRef] [PubMed]

5. Balestrino, R.; Rudà, R.; Soffietti, R. Brain Metastasis from Unknown Primary Tumour: Moving from Old Retrospective Studies to Clinical Trials on Targeted Agents. *Cancers* **2020**, *12*, 3350. [CrossRef]
6. Li, Y.S.; Jiang, B.Y.; Yang, J.J.; Tu, H.Y.; Zhou, Q.; Guo, W.B.; Yan, H.H.; Wu, Y.L. Leptomeningeal Metastases in Patients with NSCLC with EGFR Mutations. *J. Thorac. Oncol.* **2016**, *11*, 1962–1969. [CrossRef]
7. Altundag, K.; Bondy, M.L.; Mirza, N.Q.; Kau, S.W.; Broglio, K.; Hortobagyi, G.N.; Rivera, E. Clinicopathologic characteristics and prognostic factors in 420 metastatic breast cancer patients with central nervous system metastasis. *Cancer* **2007**, *110*, 2640–2647. [CrossRef]
8. Andersen, B.M.; Miranda, C.; Hatzoglou, V.; DeAngelis, L.M.; Miller, A.M. Leptomeningeal metastases in glioma: The Memorial Sloan Kettering Cancer Center experience. *Neurology* **2019**, *92*, e2483–e2491. [CrossRef]
9. Norris, L.K.; Grossman, S.A.; Olivi, A. Neoplastic meningitis following surgical resection of isolated cerebellar metastasis: A potentially preventable complication. *J. Neurooncol.* **1997**, *32*, 215–223. [CrossRef]
10. Trifiletti, D.M.; Romano, K.D.; Xu, Z.; Reardon, K.A.; Sheehan, J. Leptomeningeal disease following stereotactic radiosurgery for brain metastases from breast cancer. *J. Neurooncol.* **2015**, *124*, 421–427. [CrossRef]
11. Prabhu, R.S.; Turner, B.E.; Asher, A.L.; Marcrom, S.R.; Fiveash, J.B.; Foreman, P.M.; Press, R.H.; Buchwald, Z.S.; Curran, W.J., Jr.; Patel, K.R.; et al. Leptomeningeal disease and neurologic death after surgical resection and radiosurgery for brain metastases: A multi-institutional analysis. *Adv. Radiat. Oncol.* **2021**, *6*, 100644. [CrossRef] [PubMed]
12. Ahn, J.H.; Lee, S.H.; Kim, S.; Joo, J.; Yoo, H.; Lee, S.H.; Shin, S.H.; Gwak, H.S. Risk for leptomeningeal seeding after resection for brain metastases: Implication of tumor location with mode of resection. *J. Neurosurg.* **2012**, *116*, 984–993. [CrossRef] [PubMed]
13. Cagney, D.N.; Lamba, N.; Sinha, S.; Catalano, P.J.; Bi, W.L.; Alexander, B.M.; Aizer, A.A. Association of Neurosurgical Resection With Development of Pachymeningeal Seeding in Patients With Brain Metastases. *JAMA Oncol.* **2019**, *5*, 703–709. [CrossRef] [PubMed]
14. Omuro, A.M.; Kris, M.G.; Miller, V.A.; Franceschi, E.; Shah, N.; Milton, D.T.; Abrey, L.E. High incidence of disease recurrence in the brain and leptomeninges in patients with nonsmall cell lung carcinoma after response to gefitinib. *Cancer* **2005**, *103*, 2344–2348. [CrossRef]
15. Wang, Y.; Yang, X.; Li, N.J.; Xue, J.X. Leptomeningeal metastases in non-small cell lung cancer: Diagnosis and treatment. *Lung Cancer.* **2022**, *174*, 1–13. [CrossRef] [PubMed]
16. Fidler, I.J.; Yano, S.; Zhang, R.D.; Fujimaki, T.; Bucana, C.D. The seed and soil hypothesis: Vascularisation and brain metastases. *Lancet Oncol.* **2002**, *3*, 53–57. [CrossRef]
17. Leal, T.; Chang, J.E.; Mehta, M.; Robins, H.I. Leptomeningeal Metastasis: Challenges in Diagnosis and Treatment. *Curr. Cancer Ther. Rev.* **2011**, *7*, 319–327. [CrossRef]
18. Chang, E.L.; Lo, S. Diagnosis and management of central nervous system metastases from breast cancer. *Oncologist* **2003**, *8*, 398–410. [CrossRef]
19. Grisold, W.; Grisold, A. Cancer around the brain. *Neurooncol Pract.* **2014**, *1*, 13–21. [CrossRef]
20. Kaplan, J.G.; DeSouza, T.G.; Farkash, A.; Shafran, B.; Pack, D.; Rehman, F.; Fuks, J.; Portenoy, R. Leptomeningeal metastases: Comparison of clinical features and laboratory data of solid tumors, lymphomas and leukemias. *J. Neurooncol.* **1990**, *9*, 225–229. [CrossRef]
21. Lara-Medina, F.; Crismatt, A.; Villarreal-Garza, C.; Alvarado-Miranda, A.; Flores-Hernández, L.; González-Pinedo, M.; Gamboa-Vignolle, C.; Ruiz-González, J.D.; Arrieta, O. Clinical features and prognostic factors in patients with carcinomatous meningitis secondary to breast cancer. *Breast J.* **2012**, *18*, 233–241. [CrossRef] [PubMed]
22. Laas, R.; Arnold, H. Compression of the outlets of the leptomeningeal veins–the cause of intracranial plateau waves. *Acta Neurochir (Wien)* **1981**, *58*, 187–201. [CrossRef] [PubMed]
23. Clarke, J.L. Leptomeningeal metastasis from systemic cancer. *Continuum. (Minneap. Minn.)* **2012**, *18*, 328–342. [CrossRef] [PubMed]
24. Lossos, A.; Siegal, T. Numb chin syndrome in cancer patients: Etiology, response to treatment, and prognostic significance. *Neurology* **1992**, *42*, 1181–1184. [CrossRef] [PubMed]
25. Straathof, C.S.; de Bruin, H.G.; Dippel, D.W.; Vecht, C.J. The diagnostic accuracy of magnetic resonance imaging and cerebrospinal fluid cytology in leptomeningeal metastasis. *J. Neurol.* **1999**, *246*, 810–814. [CrossRef]
26. Singh, S.K.; Leeds, N.E.; Ginsberg, L.E. MR imaging of leptomeningeal metastases: Comparison of three sequences. *AJNR Am. J. Neuroradiol.* **2002**, *23*, 817–821.
27. Glantz, M.J.; Cole, B.F.; Glantz, L.K.; Cobb, J.; Mills, P.; Lekos, A.; Walters, B.C.; Recht, L.D. Cerebrospinal fluid cytology in patients with cancer: Minimizing false-negative results. *Cancer* **1998**, *82*, 733–739. [CrossRef]
28. Lossos, A.; Siegal, T. Spinal subarachnoid hemorrhage associated with leptomeningeal metastases. *J. Neurooncol.* **1992**, *12*, 167–171. [CrossRef]
29. Bigner, S.H. Cerebrospinal fluid (CSF) cytology: Current status and diagnostic applications. *J. Neuropathol. Exp. Neurol.* **1992**, *51*, 235–245. [CrossRef]
30. Malkin, M.G.; Posner, J.B. Cerebrospinal fluid tumor markers for the diagnosis and management of leptomeningeal metastases. *Eur. J. Cancer Clin. Oncol.* **1987**, *23*, 1–4. [CrossRef]

31. Boire, A.; Brandsma, D.; Brastianos, P.K.; Le Rhun, E.; Ahluwalia, M.; Junck, L.; Glantz, M.; Groves, M.D.; Lee, E.Q.; Lin, N.; et al. Liquid biopsy in central nervous system metastases: A RANO review and proposals for clinical applications. *Neuro Oncol.* **2019**, *21*, 571–584. [CrossRef] [PubMed]
32. Wilson, W.H.; Bromberg, J.E.; Stetler-Stevenson, M.; Steinberg, S.M.; Martin-Martin, L.; Muñiz, C.; Sancho, J.M.; Caballero, M.D.; Davidis, M.A.; Brooimans, R.A.; et al. Detection and outcome of occult leptomeningeal disease in diffuse large B-cell lymphoma and Burkitt lymphoma. *Haematologica* **2014**, *99*, 1228–1235. [CrossRef] [PubMed]
33. Lee, S.H.; Kong, D.S.; Seol, H.J.; Nam, D.H.; Lee, J.I. Ventriculoperitoneal shunt for hydrocephalus caused by central nervous system metastasis. *J. Neurooncol.* **2011**, *104*, 545–551. [CrossRef] [PubMed]
34. Jung, T.Y.; Chung, W.K.; Oh, I.J. The prognostic significance of surgically treated hydrocephalus in leptomeningeal metastases. *Clin. Neurol. Neurosurg.* **2014**, *119*, 80–83. [CrossRef]
35. Lukas, R.V.; Thakkar, J.P.; Cristofanilli, M.; Chandra, S.; Sosman, J.A.; Patel, J.D.; Kumthekar, P.; Stupp, R.; Lesniak, M.S. Leptomeningeal metastases: The future is now. *J. Neurooncol.* **2022**, *156*, 443–452. [CrossRef]
36. Zima, L.A.; Tulpule, S.; Samson, K.; Shonka, N. Seizure prevalence, contributing factors, and prognostic factors in patients with leptomeningeal disease. *J. Neurol. Sci.* **2019**, *403*, 19–23. [CrossRef]
37. Lumniczky, K.; Szatmári, T.; Sáfrány, G. Ionizing Radiation-Induced Immune and Inflammatory Reactions in the Brain. *Front. Immunol.* **2017**, *8*, 517. [CrossRef]
38. Graham, P.H.; Bucci, J.; Browne, L. Randomized comparison of whole brain radiotherapy, 20 Gy in four daily fractions versus 40 Gy in 20 twice-daily fractions, for brain metastases. *Int. J. Radiat. Oncol. Biol. Phys.* **2010**, *77*, 648–654. [CrossRef]
39. Le Rhun, E.; Weller, M.; Brandsma, D.; Van den Bent, M.; de Azambuja, E.; Henriksson, R.; Boulanger, T.; Peters, S.; Watts, C.; Wick, W.; et al. EANO-ESMO Clinical Practice Guidelines for diagnosis, treatment and follow-up of patients with leptomeningeal metastasis from solid tumours. *Ann. Oncol.* **2017**, *28* (Suppl. 4), iv84–iv99. [CrossRef]
40. Le Rhun, E.; Preusser, M.; van den Bent, M.; Andratschke, N.; Weller, M. How we treat patients with leptomeningeal metastases. *ESMO Open* **2019**, *4* (Suppl. 2), e000507. [CrossRef]
41. Zhen, J.; Wen, L.; Lai, M.; Zhou, Z.; Shan, C.; Li, S.; Lin, T.; Wu, J.; Wang, W.; Xu, S.; et al. Whole brain radiotherapy (WBRT) for leptomeningeal metastasis from NSCLC in the era of targeted therapy: A retrospective study. *Radiat. Oncol.* **2020**, *15*, 185. [CrossRef] [PubMed]
42. Yang, J.T.; Wijetunga, N.A.; Pentsova, E.; Wolden, S.; Young, R.J.; Correa, D.; Zhang, Z.; Zheng, J.; Steckler, A.; Bucwinska, W.; et al. Randomized Phase II Trial of Proton Craniospinal Irradiation Versus Photon Involved-Field Radiotherapy for Patients With Solid Tumor Leptomeningeal Metastasis. *J. Clin. Oncol.* **2022**, *40*, Jco2201148. [CrossRef] [PubMed]
43. Chamberlain, M.C. Neoplastic meningitis. *Neurologist* **2006**, *12*, 179–187. [CrossRef] [PubMed]
44. Chamberlain, M.C. Radioisotope CSF flow studies in leptomeningeal metastases. *J. Neurooncol.* **1998**, *38*, 135–140. [CrossRef]
45. Groves, M.D. Leptomeningeal disease. *Neurosurg. Clin. N. Am.* **2011**, *22*, 67–78. [CrossRef]
46. Esteva, F.J.; Soh, L.T.; Holmes, F.A.; Plunkett, W.; Meyers, C.A.; Forman, A.D.; Hortobagyi, G.N. Phase II trial and pharmacokinetic evaluation of cytosine arabinoside for leptomeningeal metastases from breast cancer. *Cancer Chemother. Pharmacol.* **2000**, *46*, 382–386. [CrossRef]
47. Phuphanich, S.; Maria, B.; Braeckman, R.; Chamberlain, M. A pharmacokinetic study of intra-CSF administered encapsulated cytarabine (DepoCyt) for the treatment of neoplastic meningitis in patients with leukemia, lymphoma, or solid tumors as part of a phase III study. *J. Neurooncol.* **2007**, *81*, 201–208. [CrossRef]
48. Le Rhun, E.; Taillibert, S.; Zairi, F.; Kotecki, N.; Devos, P.; Mailliez, A.; Servent, V.; Vanlemmens, L.; Vennin, P.; Boulanger, T.; et al. A retrospective case series of 103 consecutive patients with leptomeningeal metastasis and breast cancer. *J. Neurooncol.* **2013**, *113*, 83–92. [CrossRef]
49. Glantz, M.J.; Jaeckle, K.A.; Chamberlain, M.C.; Phuphanich, S.; Recht, L.; Swinnen, L.J.; Maria, B.; LaFollette, S.; Schumann, G.B.; Cole, B.F.; et al. A randomized controlled trial comparing intrathecal sustained-release cytarabine (DepoCyt) to intrathecal methotrexate in patients with neoplastic meningitis from solid tumors. *Clin. Cancer Res.* **1999**, *5*, 3394–3402.
50. Chamberlain, M.C. Neoplastic meningitis. *Oncologist* **2008**, *13*, 967–977. [CrossRef]
51. Chamberlain, M.C.; Kormanik, P.R. Carcinomatous meningitis secondary to breast cancer: Predictors of response to combined modality therapy. *J. Neurooncol.* **1997**, *35*, 55–64. [CrossRef]
52. Chamberlain, M.C.; Kormanik, P. Carcinoma meningitis secondary to non-small cell lung cancer: Combined modality therapy. *Arch. Neurol.* **1998**, *55*, 506–512. [CrossRef] [PubMed]
53. Bokstein, F.; Lossos, A.; Siegal, T. Leptomeningeal metastases from solid tumors: A comparison of two prospective series treated with and without intra-cerebrospinal fluid chemotherapy. *Cancer* **1998**, *82*, 1756–1763. [CrossRef]
54. Kumthekar, P.U.; Avram, M.J.; Lassman, A.B.; Lin, N.U.; Lee, E.; Grimm, S.A.; Schwartz, M.; Bell Burdett, K.L.; Lukas, R.V.; Dixit, K.; et al. A Phase I/II Study of Intrathecal Trastuzumab in HER-2 Positive Cancer with Leptomeningeal Metastases: Safety, Efficacy, and Cerebrospinal Fluid Pharmacokinetics. *Neuro Oncol.* **2022**, *1*, noac195. [CrossRef]
55. Glantz, M.J.; Cole, B.F.; Recht, L.; Akerley, W.; Mills, P.; Saris, S.; Hochberg, F.; Calabresi, P.; Egorin, M.J. High-dose intravenous methotrexate for patients with nonleukemic leptomeningeal cancer: Is intrathecal chemotherapy necessary? *J. Clin. Oncol.* **1998**, *16*, 1561–1567. [CrossRef] [PubMed]

56. Morra, E.; Lazzarino, M.; Brusamolino, E.; Pagnucco, G.; Castagnola, C.; Bernasconi, P.; Orlandi, E.; Corso, A.; Santagostino, A.; Bernasconi, C. The role of systemic high-dose cytarabine in the treatment of central nervous system leukemia. Clinical results in 46 patients. *Cancer* **1993**, *72*, 439–445. [CrossRef] [PubMed]
57. Liao, B.C.; Lee, J.H.; Lin, C.C.; Chen, Y.F.; Chang, C.H.; Ho, C.C.; Shih, J.Y.; Yu, C.J.; Yang, J.C. Epidermal Growth Factor Receptor Tyrosine Kinase Inhibitors for Non-Small-Cell Lung Cancer Patients with Leptomeningeal Carcinomatosis. *J. Thorac. Oncol.* **2015**, *10*, 1754–1761. [CrossRef] [PubMed]
58. Morris, P.G.; Reiner, A.S.; Szenberg, O.R.; Clarke, J.L.; Panageas, K.S.; Perez, H.R.; Kris, M.G.; Chan, T.A.; DeAngelis, L.M.; Omuro, A.M. Leptomeningeal metastasis from non-small cell lung cancer: Survival and the impact of whole brain radiotherapy. *J. Thorac. Oncol.* **2012**, *7*, 382–385. [CrossRef] [PubMed]
59. Hochmair, M. Medical Treatment Options for Patients with Epidermal Growth Factor Receptor Mutation-Positive Non-Small Cell Lung Cancer Suffering from Brain Metastases and/or Leptomeningeal Disease. *Target. Oncol.* **2018**, *13*, 269–285. [CrossRef]
60. Park, K.; Tan, E.H.; O'Byrne, K.; Zhang, L.; Boyer, M.; Mok, T.; Hirsh, V.; Yang, J.C.; Lee, K.H.; Lu, S.; et al. Afatinib versus gefitinib as first-line treatment of patients with EGFR mutation-positive non-small-cell lung cancer (LUX-Lung 7): A phase 2B, open-label, randomised controlled trial. *Lancet Oncol.* **2016**, *17*, 577–589. [CrossRef]
61. Lin, C.H.; Lin, M.T.; Kuo, Y.W.; Ho, C.C. Afatinib combined with cetuximab for lung adenocarcinoma with leptomeningeal carcinomatosis. *Lung Cancer* **2014**, *85*, 479–480. [CrossRef] [PubMed]
62. Yang, J.C.H.; Kim, S.W.; Kim, D.W.; Lee, J.S.; Cho, B.C.; Ahn, J.S.; Lee, D.H.; Kim, T.M.; Goldman, J.W.; Natale, R.B.; et al. Osimertinib in Patients With Epidermal Growth Factor Receptor Mutation-Positive Non-Small-Cell Lung Cancer and Leptomeningeal Metastases: The BLOOM Study. *J. Clin. Oncol.* **2020**, *38*, 538–547. [CrossRef] [PubMed]
63. Gadgeel, S.M.; Gandhi, L.; Riely, G.J.; Chiappori, A.A.; West, H.L.; Azada, M.C.; Morcos, P.N.; Lee, R.M.; Garcia, L.; Yu, L.; et al. Safety and activity of alectinib against systemic disease and brain metastases in patients with crizotinib-resistant ALK-rearranged non-small-cell lung cancer (AF-002JG): Results from the dose-finding portion of a phase 1/2 study. *Lancet Oncol.* **2014**, *15*, 1119–1128. [CrossRef] [PubMed]
64. Arrondeau, J.; Ammari, S.; Besse, B.; Soria, J.C. LDK378 compassionate use for treating carcinomatous meningitis in an ALK translocated non-small-cell lung cancer. *J. Thorac. Oncol.* **2014**, *9*, e62–e63. [CrossRef]
65. Chow, L.Q.M.; Barlesi, F.; Bertino, E.M.; van den Bent, M.J.; Wakelee, H.A.; Wen, P.Y.; Chiu, C.H.; Orlov, S.; Chiari, R.; Majem, M.; et al. ASCEND-7: Efficacy and Safety of Ceritinib Treatment in Patients with ALK-Positive Non-Small Cell Lung Cancer Metastatic to the Brain and/or Leptomeninges. *Clin. Cancer Res.* **2022**, *28*, 2506–2516. [CrossRef]
66. Sun, M.G.; Kim, I.Y.; Kim, Y.J.; Jung, T.Y.; Moon, K.S.; Jung, S.; Oh, I.J.; Kim, Y.C.; Choi, Y.D. Lorlatinib Therapy for Rapid and Dramatic Control of Brain and Spinal Leptomeningeal Metastases From ALK-Positive Lung Adenocarcinoma. *Brain Tumor Res. Treat.* **2021**, *9*, 100–105. [CrossRef]
67. Barnholtz-Sloan, J.S.; Sloan, A.E.; Davis, F.G.; Vigneau, F.D.; Lai, P.; Sawaya, R.E. Incidence proportions of brain metastases in patients diagnosed (1973 to 2001) in the Metropolitan Detroit Cancer Surveillance System. *J. Clin. Oncol.* **2004**, *22*, 2865–2872. [CrossRef]
68. Murthy, R.K.; Loi, S.; Okines, A.; Paplomata, E.; Hamilton, E.; Hurvitz, S.A.; Lin, N.U.; Borges, V.; Abramson, V.; Anders, C.; et al. Tucatinib, Trastuzumab, and Capecitabine for HER2-Positive Metastatic Breast Cancer. *N. Engl. J. Med.* **2020**, *382*, 597–609. [CrossRef]
69. Bachelot, T.; Romieu, G.; Campone, M.; Diéras, V.; Cropet, C.; Dalenc, F.; Jimenez, M.; Le Rhun, E.; Pierga, J.Y.; Gonçalves, A.; et al. Lapatinib plus capecitabine in patients with previously untreated brain metastases from HER2-positive metastatic breast cancer (LANDSCAPE): A single-group phase 2 study. *Lancet Oncol.* **2013**, *14*, 64–71. [CrossRef]
70. Freedman, R.A.; Gelman, R.S.; Anders, C.K.; Melisko, M.E.; Parsons, H.A.; Cropp, A.M.; Silvestri, K.; Cotter, C.M.; Componeschi, K.P.; Marte, J.M.; et al. TBCRC 022: A Phase II Trial of Neratinib and Capecitabine for Patients With Human Epidermal Growth Factor Receptor 2-Positive Breast Cancer and Brain Metastases. *J. Clin. Oncol.* **2019**, *37*, 1081–1089. [CrossRef]
71. Pellerino, A.; Soffietti, R.; Bruno, F.; Manna, R.; Muscolino, E.; Botta, P.; Palmiero, R.; Rudà, R. Neratinib and Capecitabine for the Treatment of Leptomeningeal Metastases from HER2-Positive Breast Cancer: A Series in the Setting of a Compassionate Program. *Cancers* **2022**, *14*, 1192. [CrossRef] [PubMed]
72. OncLive. Safety and Efficacy of Tucatinib–Trastuzumab-Capecitabine Regimen for Treatment of Leptomeningeal Metastasis in HER2+ Breast Cancer: Results from TBCRC049, A Phase 2 Non-Randomized Study: OncLive; 2022 [updated 11 March 2022]. Available online: https://www.onclive.com/view/safety-efficacy-of-tucatinib-trastuzumab-capecitabine-regimen-for-treatment-of-lm-in-her2-breast-cancer (accessed on 22 October 2022).
73. Pérez-García, J.M.; Batista, M.V.; Cortez, P.; Ruiz-Borrego, M.; Cejalvo, J.M.; de la Haba-Rodriguez, J.; Garrigós, L.; Racca, F.; Servitja, S.; Blanch, S.; et al. Trastuzumab Deruxtecan in Patients with Central Nervous System Involvement from HER2-Positive Breast Cancer: The DEBBRAH Trial. *Neuro Oncol.* **2022**, noac144. [CrossRef] [PubMed]
74. Hill, M.V.; Vidri, R.J.; Deng, M.; Handorf, E.; Olszanski, A.J.; Farma, J.M. Real-world frequency of BRAF testing and utilization of therapies in patients with advanced melanoma. *Melanoma Res.* **2022**, *32*, 79–87. [CrossRef] [PubMed]
75. Rounis, K.; Skribek, M.; Makrakis, D.; De Petris, L.; Agelaki, S.; Ekman, S.; Tsakonas, G. Correlation of Clinical Parameters with Intracranial Outcome in Non-Small Cell Lung Cancer Patients with Brain Metastases Treated with Pd-1/Pd-L1 Inhibitors as Monotherapy. *Cancers* **2021**, *13*, 1562. [CrossRef]

76. Gauvain, C.; Vauléon, E.; Chouaid, C.; Le Rhun, E.; Jabot, L.; Scherpereel, A.; Vinas, F.; Cortot, A.B.; Monnet, I. Intracerebral efficacy and tolerance of nivolumab in non-small-cell lung cancer patients with brain metastases. *Lung Cancer* **2018**, *116*, 62–66. [CrossRef]
77. Hodi, F.S.; O'Day, S.J.; McDermott, D.F.; Weber, R.W.; Sosman, J.A.; Haanen, J.B.; Gonzalez, R.; Robert, C.; Schadendorf, D.; Hassel, J.C.; et al. Improved survival with ipilimumab in patients with metastatic melanoma. *N. Engl. J. Med.* **2010**, *363*, 711–723. [CrossRef]
78. Brastianos, P.K.; Strickland, M.R.; Lee, E.Q.; Wang, N.; Cohen, J.V.; Chukwueke, U.; Forst, D.A.; Eichler, A.; Overmoyer, B.; Lin, N.U.; et al. Phase II study of ipilimumab and nivolumab in leptomeningeal carcinomatosis. *Nat. Commun.* **2021**, *12*, 5954. [CrossRef]
79. Hendriks, L.E.L.; Bootsma, G.; Mourlanette, J.; Henon, C.; Mezquita, L.; Ferrara, R.; Audigier-Valette, C.; Mazieres, J.; Lefebvre, C.; Duchemann, B.; et al. Survival of patients with non-small cell lung cancer having leptomeningeal metastases treated with immune checkpoint inhibitors. *Eur. J. Cancer* **2019**, *116*, 182–189. [CrossRef]
80. Geukes Foppen, M.H.; Brandsma, D.; Blank, C.U.; van Thienen, J.V.; Haanen, J.B.; Boogerd, W. Targeted treatment and immunotherapy in leptomeningeal metastases from melanoma. *Ann. Oncol.* **2016**, *27*, 1138–1142. [CrossRef]
81. Tolaney, S.M.; Sahebjam, S.; Le Rhun, E.; Bachelot, T.; Kabos, P.; Awada, A.; Yardley, D.; Chan, A.; Conte, P.; Diéras, V.; et al. A Phase II Study of Abemaciclib in Patients with Brain Metastases Secondary to Hormone Receptor-Positive Breast Cancer. *Clin Cancer Res.* **2020**, *26*, 5310–5319. [CrossRef]
82. Ferguson, S.D.; Bindal, S.; Bassett, R.L., Jr.; Haydu, L.E.; McCutcheon, I.E.; Heimberger, A.B.; Li, J.; O'Brien, B.J.; Guha-Thakurta, N.; Tetzlaff, M.T.; et al. Predictors of survival in metastatic melanoma patients with leptomeningeal disease (LMD). *J. Neurooncol.* **2019**, *142*, 499–509. [CrossRef] [PubMed]
83. Glitza, I.C.; Rohlfs, M.; Guha-Thakurta, N.; Bassett, R.L., Jr.; Bernatchez, C.; Diab, A.; Woodman, S.E.; Yee, C.; Amaria, R.N.; Patel, S.P.; et al. Retrospective review of metastatic melanoma patients with leptomeningeal disease treated with intrathecal interleukin-2. *ESMO Open* **2018**, *3*, e000283. [CrossRef] [PubMed]
84. John, I.; Foster, A.P.; Haymaker, C.L.; Bassett, R.L.; Lee, J.J.; Rohlfs, M.L.; Richard, J.; Iqbal, M.; McCutcheon, I.E.; Ferguson, S.D.; et al. Intrathecal (IT) and intravenous (IV) nivolumab (N) for metastatic melanoma (MM) patients (pts) with leptomeningeal disease (LMD). *J. Clin. Oncol.* **2021**, *39* (Suppl. 15), 9519. [CrossRef]
85. Kumthekar, P.; Tang, S.C.; Brenner, A.J.; Kesari, S.; Piccioni, D.E.; Anders, C.; Carrillo, J.; Chalasani, P.; Kabos, P.; Puhalla, S.; et al. ANG1005, a Brain-Penetrating Peptide-Drug Conjugate, Shows Activity in Patients with Breast Cancer with Leptomeningeal Carcinomatosis and Recurrent Brain Metastases. *Clin. Cancer Res.* **2020**, *26*, 2789–2799. [CrossRef]
86. Kramer, K.; Humm, J.L.; Souweidane, M.M.; Zanzonico, P.B.; Dunkel, I.J.; Gerald, W.L.; Khakoo, Y.; Yeh, S.D.; Yeung, H.W.; Finn, R.D.; et al. Phase I study of targeted radioimmunotherapy for leptomeningeal cancers using intra-Ommaya 131-I-3F8. *J. Clin. Oncol.* **2007**, *25*, 5465–5470. [CrossRef] [PubMed]
87. Hitchins, R.N.; Bell, D.R.; Woods, R.L.; Levi, J.A. A prospective randomized trial of single-agent versus combination chemotherapy in meningeal carcinomatosis. *J. Clin. Oncol.* **1987**, *5*, 1655–1662. [CrossRef]
88. Grossman, S.A.; Finkelstein, D.M.; Ruckdeschel, J.C.; Trump, D.L.; Moynihan, T.; Ettinger, D.S. Randomized prospective comparison of intraventricular methotrexate and thiotepa in patients with previously untreated neoplastic meningitis. Eastern Cooperative Oncology Group. *J. Clin. Oncol.* **1993**, *11*, 561–569. [CrossRef]
89. Glantz, M.J.; LaFollette, S.; Jaeckle, K.A.; Shapiro, W.; Swinnen, L.; Rozental, J.R.; Phuphanich, S.; Rogers, L.R.; Gutheil, J.C.; Batchelor, T.; et al. Randomized trial of a slow-release versus a standard formulation of cytarabine for the intrathecal treatment of lymphomatous meningitis. *J. Clin. Oncol.* **1999**, *17*, 3110–3116. [CrossRef]
90. Shapiro, W.R.; Schmid, M.; Glantz, M.; Miller, J.J. A randomized phase III/IV study to determine benefit and safety of cytarabine liposome injection for treatment of neoplastic meningitis. *J. Clin. Oncol.* **2006**, *24* (Suppl. 18), 1528. [CrossRef]

Disclaimer/Publisher's Note: The statements, opinions and data contained in all publications are solely those of the individual author(s) and contributor(s) and not of MDPI and/or the editor(s). MDPI and/or the editor(s) disclaim responsibility for any injury to people or property resulting from any ideas, methods, instructions or products referred to in the content.

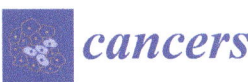

Article

Bevacizumab beyond Progression for Newly Diagnosed Glioblastoma (BIOMARK): Phase II Safety, Efficacy and Biomarker Study

Motoo Nagane [1,*], Koichi Ichimura [2], Ritsuko Onuki [3], Daichi Narushima [3], Mai Honda-Kitahara [4], Kaishi Satomi [5], Arata Tomiyama [6], Yasuhito Arai [7], Tatsuhiro Shibata [7], Yoshitaka Narita [8], Takeo Uzuka [9], Hideo Nakamura [10], Mitsutoshi Nakada [11], Yoshiki Arakawa [12], Takanori Ohnishi [13], Akitake Mukasa [14], Shota Tanaka [14], Toshihiko Wakabayashi [15], Tomokazu Aoki [16], Shigeki Aoki [17], Soichiro Shibui [18], Masao Matsutani [19], Keisuke Ishizawa [20], Hideaki Yokoo [21], Hiroyoshi Suzuki [22], Satoshi Morita [23], Mamoru Kato [3] and Ryo Nishikawa [24]

1. Department of Neurosurgery, Kyorin University Faculty of Medicine, Tokyo 181-8611, Japan
2. Department of Brain Disease Translational Research, Juntendo University Graduate School of Medicine, Tokyo 113-8421, Japan
3. Division of Bioinformatics, National Cancer Center Research Institute, Tokyo 104-0045, Japan
4. Division of Brain Tumor Translational Research, National Cancer Center Research Institute, Tokyo 104-0045, Japan
5. Department of Diagnostic Pathology, National Cancer Center Hospital, Tokyo 104-0045, Japan
6. Department of Brain Disease Translational Research, Juntendo University Faculty of Medicine, Tokyo 113-8421, Japan
7. Division of Cancer Genomics, National Cancer Center Research Institute, Tokyo 104-0045, Japan
8. Department of Neurosurgery and Neuro-Oncology, National Cancer Center Hospital, Tokyo 104-0045, Japan
9. Department of Neurosurgery, Dokkyo Medical University, Tochigi 321-0293, Japan
10. Department of Neurosurgery, Faculty of Life Sciences, Kumamoto University, Kumamoto 860-8555, Japan
11. Department of Neurosurgery, Graduate School of Medical Sciences, Kanazawa University, Kanazawa 920-1192, Japan
12. Department of Neurosurgery, Graduate School of Medicine, Kyoto University, Kyoto 606-8501, Japan
13. Department of Neurosurgery, Graduate School of Medicine, Ehime University, Ehime 790-0052, Japan
14. Department of Neurosurgery, Graduate School of Medicine, The University of Tokyo, Tokyo 113-8654, Japan
15. Department of Neurosurgery, Graduate School of Medicine, Nagoya University, Aichi 464-8601, Japan
16. Department of Neurosurgery, Kyoto Medical Center, Kyoto 612-8555, Japan
17. Department of Radiology, Graduate School of Medicine, Juntendo University, Tokyo 113-8421, Japan
18. Department of Neurosurgery, Teikyo University Hospital, Kawasaki 213-8507, Japan
19. Department of Neurosurgery, Kurosawa Hospital, Gunma 370-1203, Japan
20. Department of Pathology, Saitama Medical University, Saitama 350-0495, Japan
21. Department of Human Pathology, Graduate School of Medicine, Gunma University, Gunma 371-8511, Japan
22. Department of Pathology and Laboratory Medicine, National Hospital Organization Sendai Medical Center, Miyagi 983-8520, Japan
23. Department of Biomedical Statistics and Bioinformatics, Graduate School of Medicine, Kyoto University, Kyoto 606-8501, Japan
24. Department of Neuro-Oncology/Neurosurgery, Saitama Medical University International Medical Center, Saitama 350-1298, Japan

* Correspondence: mnagane@ks.kyorin-u.ac.jp; Tel.: +81-422-47-5511

Simple Summary: This was a multicenter, single-arm, phase II study comprising two protocol treatments. Patients were enrolled after craniotomy or biopsy and initiated the concurrent phase; oral daily temozolomide concomitant with radiation therapy during the first 6 weeks of treatment. Bevacizumab was intravenously administered every other week. The protocol-defined secondary therapy (i.e., BBP regimen) was given as bevacizumab monotherapy or in combination with other chemotherapeutic agents upon first progression or recurrence until further progression or unacceptable toxicity developed. The primary endpoint, the 2-year survival rate of the BBP group, was 27.0% and was unmet. Expression profiling using RNA sequencing identified that Cluster 2, enriched with the genes involved in macrophage or microglia activation, was associated with longer OS and PFS independent of the *MGMT* methylation status.

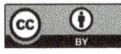

Abstract: We evaluated the efficacy and safety of bevacizumab beyond progression (BBP) in Japanese patients with newly diagnosed glioblastoma and explored predictors of response to bevacizumab. This phase II study evaluated a protocol-defined primary therapy by radiotherapy with concurrent and adjuvant temozolomide plus bevacizumab, followed by bevacizumab monotherapy, and secondary therapy (BBP: bevacizumab upon progression). Ninety patients received the protocol-defined primary therapy (BBP group, $n = 25$). Median overall survival (mOS) and median progression-free survival (mPFS) were 25.0 and 14.9 months, respectively. In the BBP group, in which O^6-methylguanine-DNA methyltransferase (*MGMT*)-unmethylated tumors predominated, mOS and mPFS were 5.8 and 1.9 months from BBP initiation and 16.8 and 11.4 months from the initial diagnosis, respectively. The primary endpoint, the 2-year survival rate of the BBP group, was 27.0% and was unmet. No unexpected adverse events occurred. Expression profiling using RNA sequencing identified that Cluster 2, which was enriched with the genes involved in macrophage or microglia activation, was associated with longer OS and PFS independent of the *MGMT* methylation status. Cluster 2 was identified as a significantly favorable independent predictor for PFS, along with younger age and methylated *MGMT*. The novel expression classifier may predict the prognosis of glioblastoma patients treated with bevacizumab.

Keywords: bevacizumab; glioblastoma; temozolomide; progression; biomarker

1. Introduction

Glioblastoma (GBM), the most common primary brain tumor among adults, is an aggressive glioma with a poor prognosis [1] and recurrence in most patients [2]. Although the current standard of care for GBM involves surgical resection followed by radiotherapy with concurrent and adjuvant temozolomide (Stupp regimen) [3], the median progression-free survival (mPFS) is only 6.9 months, and median overall survival (mOS), 14.6 months [3]. $O6$-methylguanine-DNA methyltransferase (*MGMT*) promoter methylation is a strong prognosis factor and temozolomide response predictor for GBM [4–6].

Bevacizumab is a humanized monoclonal antibody against vascular endothelial growth factor A (VEGFA). VEGFA (known as VEGF) is the major angiogenic factor for tumor angiogenesis [7]. Therefore, an anti-VEGF antibody is expected to benefit patients with highly angiogenetic tumors, such as GBM [8–10]. Although several bevacizumab studies have been conducted in patients with newly diagnosed and recurrent GBM [11–14], evidence supporting an effective bevacizumab GBM regimen has been insufficient. Prolonged PFS without prolonged OS has been reported in patients with both newly diagnosed and recurrent GBM [11,12,15,16].

A new regimen, bevacizumab beyond progression (BBP), comprises the extended use of bevacizumab, added to second-line chemotherapy upon progression in unresectable, advanced, recurrent cancer, leading to OS prolongation in colorectal and breast cancers [17,18]. In highly angiogenic GBM, tumor cells may continuously produce VEGF even at recurrence and promote further angiogenesis. Bevacizumab discontinuation at disease progression may therefore result in acute tumor progression [19], which is considered to be one of the reasons for the extremely poor prognosis of patients, given that no effective second-line standard therapies have been developed yet. A retrospective pooled analysis of phase II studies suggested that PFS and OS were significantly improved in the BBP group compared with the non-BBP group [20]. However, two prospective phase II studies of BBP (TAMIGA and CABARET Part 2) did not show clear survival improvements [21,22].

Two previous phase III studies reported clinically inconsistent results [11,12]. This suggests there may be a subgroup in the GBM population in which bevacizumab could be more effective than others [11,21,22]. However, biomarkers to predict bevacizumab efficacy have not been thoroughly investigated. A retrospective analysis of the AVAglio study showed OS benefits for patients with isocitrate dehydrogenase 1 (*IDH1*) WT proneural

GBM when bevacizumab was combined with the standard regimen [23]. This observation suggested that there may be a subset of patients with GBM who could benefit from continuous administration of bevacizumab beyond progression.

This study (BIOMARK) evaluated the efficacy and safety of BBP in patients with newly diagnosed GBM after surgery. We conducted a thorough genomic analysis to investigate potential biomarkers to identify the subpopulations that may benefit most from BBP or bevacizumab first-line treatment.

2. Materials and Methods

2.1. Study Design

This was a multicenter, single-arm, phase II study comprising two protocol treatments: protocol-defined primary therapy (comprising concurrent, maintenance and monotherapy phases) and protocol-defined secondary therapy. Patients were enrolled within 7 to 21 days after craniotomy or biopsy and initiated the concurrent phase within the next 3 weeks; oral daily temozolomide (75 mg/m^2 per day) concomitant with radiation therapy (60 Gy: 2-Gy fractions 5 days/week) during the first 6 weeks of treatment. Bevacizumab was intravenously administered on Day 1 of Weeks 4, 6, and 8 at 10 mg/kg per dose (Figure S1).

In the maintenance phase, combination therapy with oral temozolomide (150 to 200 mg/m^2 per day on Days 1–5 every 4 weeks) and intravenous bevacizumab (10 mg/kg, on Days 1 and 15 of each cycle) was provided for up to twelve 4-week cycles (48 weeks), unless exacerbation or recurrence was observed. If temozolomide was discontinued during the concurrent or maintenance phase, the monotherapy phase was started from discontinuation. In the monotherapy phase, intravenous bevacizumab was administered at 10 mg/kg per dose in 2-week cycles or 15 mg/kg per dose in 3-week cycles until progression or recurrence was observed.

The protocol-defined secondary therapy (i.e., BBP regimen) was given as bevacizumab monotherapy or in combination with other chemotherapeutic agents upon first progression or recurrence. Bevacizumab was administered in 2-week or 3-week cycles until further progression or unacceptable toxicity developed, using the same bevacizumab dose as in the monotherapy phase.

2.2. Patients

Patients were eligible if they were aged 20–75 years; had newly diagnosed, histologically confirmed supratentorial GBM, Grade IV, by World Health Organization Classification of Tumours of the Central Nervous System, revised 4th Ed (the diagnosis was based on the WHO Classification at the time when the study was designed, see Results), without dissemination or gliomatosis cerebri; had an available surgical specimen (including fresh frozen specimen); had a Karnofsky Performance Status (KPS) $\geq$ 60; had adequate hematologic, hepatic, and renal function after surgery, and could provide informed consent. Patients with MRI-confirmed new bleeding after cranial surgery; history of chemotherapy, radiotherapy, or immunotherapy (including vaccines); or uncontrolled hypertension, history of stroke or unstable angina, myocardial infarction, intracranial abscess within 6 months before randomization, or a serious nonhealing wound were excluded.

2.3. Study Endpoint

The primary outcome (BBP efficacy) was the 2-year survival rate in patients who received at least one protocol-defined secondary therapy (defined as the BBP group). This endpoint was adopted from the 2-year survival rate in AVAglio, which was approximately 30% in both arms, providing an adequate margin for evaluation of the add-on effect of BBP. Secondary outcomes included the 2-year survival rate and OS among patients who received at least one protocol-defined therapy (full analysis set [FAS]), PFS, objective response rate (FAS), and safety. Quality of life and neurocognitive functions were also evaluated. Adverse event (AE) data were collected and reported using Common Terminology Criteria for Adverse Events version 4.0. Patients who did not have a confirmed cytological or histopathological GBM by central pathological review and had any efficacy data after starting protocol-defined therapies were excluded from the evaluations.

2.4. Biomarker Analysis

2.4.1. Biomarker Analysis Cohort

The entire FAS cohort except for one case for which tumor tissue was unavailable (89 cases) and 19 cases from the placebo-controlled group of the AVAglio study were subjected to the biomarker analysis. Fresh frozen surgical tumor specimens were available for all biomarker analysis cohort patients. Mutation analysis for *IDH1*/*IDH2* and the *TERT* promoter by pyrosequencing, targeted sequencing by Ion Proton, *MGMT* methylation analysis by pyrosequencing, and the genome-wide DNA methylation analysis by the EPIC array were performed in all cases. RNA sequencing and the NanoString analysis were performed in the cases where the quality of RNA was sufficient for each analysis (Table S1). Six patients had *IDH1* R132H mutation (three patients in the FAS and three in AVAglio). These cases were excluded from further biomarker analysis.

2.4.2. Histopathological Review and Tumor Cell Content Estimation

The histopathological diagnoses of all patients were reviewed according to the revised 4th edition of the WHO Classification of Tumours of the Central Nervous System by consensus of three board-certified pathologists (KI, HY, HS) [24]. For tumor cell content estimation, a portion of the fresh frozen tumor specimen subjected to the biomarker analysis was formalin-fixed and paraffin-embedded. The entire area of hematoxylin–eosin stained slides was visually inspected by a single board-certified pathologist (KS), and the percentage of tumor cell contents and necrotic fractions were estimated in each case by microscope.

2.4.3. DNA/RNA Extraction

DNA was extracted from the frozen tumor tissues using a DNeasy Blood & Tissue Kit (Qiagen, Tokyo, Japan). Total RNA was extracted from the frozen tumor tissues using an miRNeasy Micro Kit (Qiagen, Tokyo, Japan).

2.4.4. IDH1/2 Mutation/TERT Promoter Mutation/MGMT Promoter Methylation Analysis

The presence of the hotspot mutations in *IDH1*, *IDH2*, and the *TERT* promoter was assessed by pyrosequencing for all cases enrolled in the study as previously described [25]. The methylation status of the *MGMT* promoter was analyzed by pyrosequencing after bisulfite modification of genomic DNA extracted from tumor specimens as described [25]. Based on an outcome-based study to determine an optimal cutoff to judge *MGMT* promoter methylation in a series of 276 newly diagnosed GBMs, we used a cutoff of $\geq 16\%$ for *MGMT* methylation. The details of this study will be described elsewhere (Ichimura, manuscript in preparation).

2.4.5. Targeted Sequence by Ion Proton

Target sequencing for all coding exons of 93 genes known to be frequently mutated in brain tumors was performed using an Ion Proton Sequencer and the Ion Chef System (Thermo Fisher Scientific, Tokyo, Japan) according to the manufacturer's instruction as previously described [26]. Reads were mapped onto the hg19 human reference genome sequence, and variant call was performed using Ion Reporter software (Thermo Fisher Scientific, https://ionreporter.thermofisher.com/ir/ (accessed on 10 April 2019)). UCSC Common SNPs were excluded.

2.4.6. RNA Sequencing

RNA sequencing was essentially performed as described previously [27]. Briefly, total RNA was quantified using Qubit RNA Assay Kit (Thermo Fisher Scientific) and quality-controlled using Agilent RNA6000 Nano Kit on an Agilent 2100 Bioanalyzer (Agilent Technologies Japan, Ltd., Tokyo, Japan). PolyA-RNA was selected from 300 ng of total

RNA, and cDNA was generated, followed by PCR amplification. cDNA Library for RNA sequencing was prepared using a NEBnext Ultra II Directional RNA Library prep with Beads (New England Biolabs Japan, Inc.). The library was quality-controlled using the Agilent 2100 Bioanalyzer and quantified using a Kapa Library Quantification Kit (NIPPON Genetics CO., Ltd.) and subjected to paired-end sequencing of 101-bp fragments using a TruSeq PE Cluster Kit v3HS (FC401-3001) on HiSeq2500 DNA sequencer (Illumina).

2.4.7. Clustering and GSEA of RNAseq

First, we removed poly-A tail from 3′end and low-quality bases (quality < 30) from 5′ and 3′ end of RNA-seq reads. We also removed RNA-seq reads whose lengths are less than 30 bp. All preprocessing was performed by PRINSEQ (version 0.20.4). After preprocessing, we calculated TPM from RNA-seq data with RSEM (version 1.2.28). RSEM internally mapped RNA-seq reads to the human reference genome GRCh38 by STAR (version 2.7.1a). Then, we constructed TPM matrix where each column shows each patient, and each row shows each gene. By using TPM matrix as input, we finally performed Ward's hierarchical clustering using Euclidean distance. Each TPM score was log2 transformed before clustering. R software (version 4.0.0) was used to perform all the statistical analyses. After the patients were clustered into two groups, the TPM matrix and the cluster labels were used to perform GSEA by GSEA software (version 4.1.0, https://www.gsea-msigdb.org/gsea/index.jsp (accessed on 1 July 2021), https://www.gsea-msigdb.org/gsea/index.jsp (accessed on 1 July 2021)).

2.4.8. Genome-Wide Methylation Analysis and DKFZ Methylation Classification

For DNA methylation analysis, 500 ng of DNA extracted from frozen tumor specimen was bisulfite-modified using an EZ DNA Methylation Kit (Zymo Research, Cat.D-5002). The Infinium Methylation EPIC BeadChip Kit (Illumina, San Diego, CA, USA, hereafter EPIC array) was used to obtain genome-wide DNA methylation profiles according to the manufacturer's instructions as previously described [28]. The raw IDAT files were uploaded to the MolecularNeuropathology website developed by the German Cancer Research Center (DKFZ)/University Hospital Heidelberg/German Consortium for Translational Cancer Research (DKTK) (the DKFZ classifier v11b4, https://www.molecularneuropathology.org/mnp? (accessed on 14 August 2021)) to obtain methylation profile-based classification and subtype scores (Table S1).

2.4.9. Copy Number Alteration Analysis

Raw IDAT files from EPIC were processed using the minfi package (version 1.34.0) in R statistical environment (version 4.0.4), and quality control was performed. Mset objects generated from the raw IDAT files were used as the input data for copy number variation analysis using the conumee package (version 1.22.0). Using the genome annotations, 843,349 probes were used for further analysis. Unprocessed IDAT files of nine normal control samples were downloaded from the NCBI Gene Expression Omnibus (GEO) under the accession number GSE119776 [29]. Copy number loci proceeded by conumee package were taken as the average of each gene using R. A widely used heuristic to identify gain or loss of each gene is determined to use a symmetrical absolute cutoff of ±0.1 for conumee processed data [30].

2.4.10. NanoString

The same set of genes as used by Sandmann et al. [23] for Gene Expression Subtype Classification according to Phillips et al. [31] was used for the NanoString analysis in this study (Table S2). nCounter Custom CodeSet for 31 target genes and 9 control genes was designed by NanoString. nCounter assay was performed according to the manufacturer's instruction using 300 ng of total RNA.

2.4.11. Phillips' Classification by NanoString

We downloaded NanoString gene expression data of GSE84010 from the GEO database as a reference. The downloaded NanoString gene expressions were labeled by three subtypes, proneural, mesenchymal, and proliferative. For each subtype, we calculated centroids of NanoString gene expression. Then, we evaluated Pearson's correlation coefficient between the centroids of each subtype and normalized gene expressions of each patient in our BIOMARK cohort. Each patient was assigned to the subtype showing the highest correlation. Patients showing no positive correlation with any subtype were labeled as unclassified.

2.4.12. Clustering of DNA Methylation Data

Beta-values of MethylationEPIC data were used for the clustering analysis of Priority 1. The EPIC probe annotations for hg38 were obtained from Zhou et al. [32]. (https://zwdzwd.github.io/InfiniumAnnotation (accessed on 7 October 2018)). Annotations excluded probes filtered out by the recommended general purpose masking, probes targeting sex chromosomes, and probes with SNPs within 5 bp from their 3′-ends. Subsequently, probes including missing values in the data of Priority 1 samples were excluded. Furthermore, the standard deviations (SDs) were calculated among the samples, and probes within the top 1% SDs were extracted. These processes left 5787 probes, which were used for the clustering analysis. The analysis was performed using R software (version 4.1.1) and gplots package (version 3.1.1). Priority 1 samples were clustered on Euclidean distances using Ward hierarchical clustering method ("ward.D2" method from hclust function).

2.5. Data Collection and Assessments

2.5.1. Efficacy Evaluation

Efficacy was evaluated in the FAS and BBP groups, according to the Response Assessment in Neuro-Oncology Criteria for high-grade glioma [33]. A gadolinium-enhancing measurable lesion was one with a maximum perpendicular diameter of 10 mm (slice thickness of $\leq$5 mm). Measurements were made within 3 days after surgery and then at every 12 weeks during the maintenance phase.

2.5.2. Definitions of OS (BBP Cohort, FAS) and PFS

OS in the BBP cohort and FAS was defined as the time (months) from the day of enrollment to death from any cause. Patients lost to follow-up were censored on the day when survival was last confirmed. PFS was defined as the time from the day of enrollment to the date of disease progression or death due to any cause.

2.5.3. Response Rate

Among patients with measurable lesions included in the efficacy analysis, the response rate was determined as the proportion of patients with a complete response (CR) or partial response (PR) after treatment.

2.6. Statistical Analysis

Assuming the expected 2-year survival rate of 50% and the threshold 2-year survival rate of 30%, which were derived from the AVAglio study of the Japanese patients and the entire patients in the bevacizumab arm, respectively [11], 45 patients were required in the BBP group to maintain a power $\geq$80% with a one-sided significance level of 5% for the 24-month registration and 24-month observation periods. Considering the ratio of patients who could start the protocol-defined secondary therapy and patient withdrawals, the total target sample size was 90 patients. Efficacy analyses were performed on the FAS and BBP groups. The Kaplan–Meier method was used to analyze survival, and the Greenwood formula was used to calculate 90% confidence intervals (CIs). Statistical methods for biomarker analysis are described in Section 2.4. The significance level was set at 5% (one-sided). Analyses of clinical data were performed using SAS version 9.4 (SAS Institute Japan Ltd., Tokyo, Japan).

3. Results

3.1. Patients

From June 2015 to December 2016, 94 patients were enrolled from 39 sites in Japan. Data cutoff was 17 January 2019, when all outcome surveys were completed, corresponding with the protocol-specified follow-up. In total, 83 patients discontinued. The major reasons were: AEs (34.0%), progression/recurrence during the second-line treatment (24.5%), and patient decline (18.1%). All 94 patients received protocol-defined primary therapy (Safety Analysis Set). Of these, 90 were diagnosed with GBM by central pathological review and were included in the FAS (Figure S2). Twenty-seven patients received protocol-defined secondary therapy (BBP), and of these, 25 without protocol deviations were included in the BBP group. Of these, 13 received either temozolomide (n = 12) or nimustine (n = 2) in combination with bevacizumab (one patient was treated with both sequentially), while the remaining 12 continued bevacizumab alone as BBP (Table S3).

The median age was 60.5 years (range, 22–75 years). Approximately half of patients (52%) had a KPS of 50–80. Most (79%) were not receiving corticosteroids at baseline. *MGMT* gene promoter methylation was observed in 33% of patients. The percentage of patients with WT *IDH1* was 93%, whereas 5% had *IDH1* mutations. Those diffuse gliomas with histological features of GBM, which were diagnosed as GBM according to the WHO Classification, 4th Ed., at the time of enrollment, have been re-classified as Astrocytoma, IDH-mutant, CNS WHO grade 4 in the latest WHO Classification, 5th Ed. (reference WHO CNS5). As such, survival analyses primarily focused on the IDH-wildtype tumors. *TERT* gene promoter mutation was observed in 66% of patients (Table 1).

Table 1. Patients' characteristics.

Patients (%)	XXXXX	BIOMARK (n = 94)	AVAglio * (BEV) (n = 464)
Age	Median	60.5	57
	(Range)	(22–75)	(20–84)
Sex	Male	57	62
RPA class	III	17	17
	IV	7	57
	V	14	26
	Data missing	62	
KPS	50–80	52	33
	90–100	48	67
MMSE score	<27	45	24
	≥27	49	76
	Data missing	6	
Corticosteroids	On	79	41
	Off	21	59
GBM Histology	Confirmed	94	95
	Unconfirmed	6	5
MGMT status	Methylated	33	26
	Non-methylated	65	49
	Data missing	2	25
IDH status	IDH wildtype	93	nd
	IDH mutated	5	nd
	Data missing	2	nd
TERT promoter status	TERT wildtype	32	nd
	TERT mutated	66	nd
	Data missing	2	nd

(* Selected characteristics only, modified from Chinot, 2014 NEJM). Abbreviations: BEV: bevacizumab; GBM: glioblastoma; *IDH*: isocitrate dehydrogenase; KPS Karnofsky performance status; *MGMT*: O^6-methylguanine-DNA methyltransferase; MMSE: mini-mental state examination; nd: not determined; RPA: recursive partitioning analysis.

3.2. Primary Endpoint

3.2.1. Survival: 2-Year Survival Rate

In the FAS ($n = 90$), mOS was 25.0 months (95% CI: 21.7–26.3) and mPFS was 14.9 months (95% CI: 11.8–18.3). The 2-year survival rate was 52.4% (90% CI: 43.3%–60.8%), and the 2-year PFS rate was 25.7% (90% CI: 18.3%–33.7%) (Figure 1A). In patients in the FAS solely with *IDH1*-WT GBM ($n = 85$), the mOS was 24.8 months (95% CI: 19.7–26.3) and the mPFS was 14.8 months (95% CI: 11.7–17.2) (Figure S3). In the BBP group ($n = 25$, all *IDH1*-WT), the mOS and mPFS from the initial diagnosis were 16.8 months (95% CI: 14.0–23.2) and 11.4 months (95% CI: 9.0–17.1), respectively. The 2-year survival rate was 27.0% (90% CI: 13.6%–42.4%), which did not meet the prespecified target value (50%) (primary endpoint). The 2-year PFS rate was 8.0% (90% CI: 2.0%–19.7%). In the BBP group, mOS and mPFS from the initiation of BBP were 5.8 months (95% CI: 3.9–6.9) and 1.9 months (95% CI: 1.1–2.9), respectively (Figure 1B,C). The patient background was similar between the patients in this study and those in AVAglio (Table 1) [11].

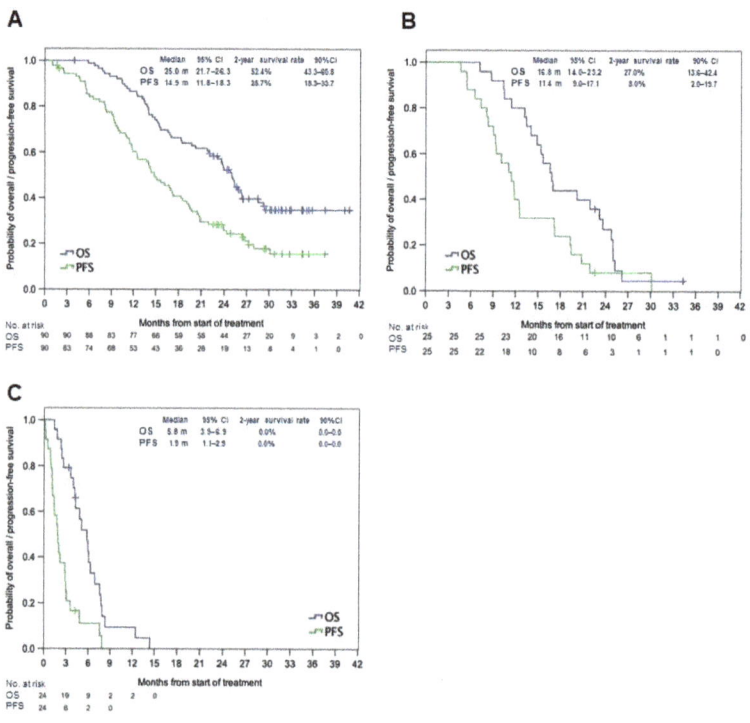

Figure 1. Median OS and PFS in the full analysis set (**A**), in the BBP group after initial treatment (**B**), and the BBP group after the first recurrence (**C**). Abbreviations: BBP: bevacizumab beyond progression; CI: confidence interval; mo: months; OS: overall survival; PFS: progression-free survival.

3.2.2. Subgroup Analysis of the Primary Endpoint: Survival and MGMT Methylation Status

Subgroup analysis using *MGMT* methylation status as a stratification factor was performed on the survival data. In the FAS, *MGMT* gene promoter was methylated in 29 patients (32%) and unmethylated in 59 patients (66%) (unknown in two patients). Patients with methylated *MGMT* had a significantly longer OS (mOS not reached vs. 22.6 months, hazard ratio [HR]: 0.27 [95% CI: 0.13–0.55], $p = 0.0003$) and PFS (mPFS 21.9 months vs. 11.8 months, HR: 0.34 [95% CI: 0.19–0.59], $p = 0.0001$) than those with unmethylated *MGMT* (Figure 2A,B). In the BBP group ($n = 25$), the *MGMT* promoter was methylated only in four (16%) patients, and it was unmethylated in 21 (84%) patients; the BBP group had a considerably higher proportion of patients with unmethylated *MGMT*. In contrast, surviving patients without progression for more than 2 years [Alive for more than 2 years with No Progression (ANP)] (*n* = 16) comprised 11 (69%) with methylated *MGMT* promoter and 5 (31%) with unmethylated *MGMT* promoter. *MGMT* methylation in the BBP group was significantly lower than in the ANP cohort (*p* = 0.001, Fisher's exact test) (Table S4).

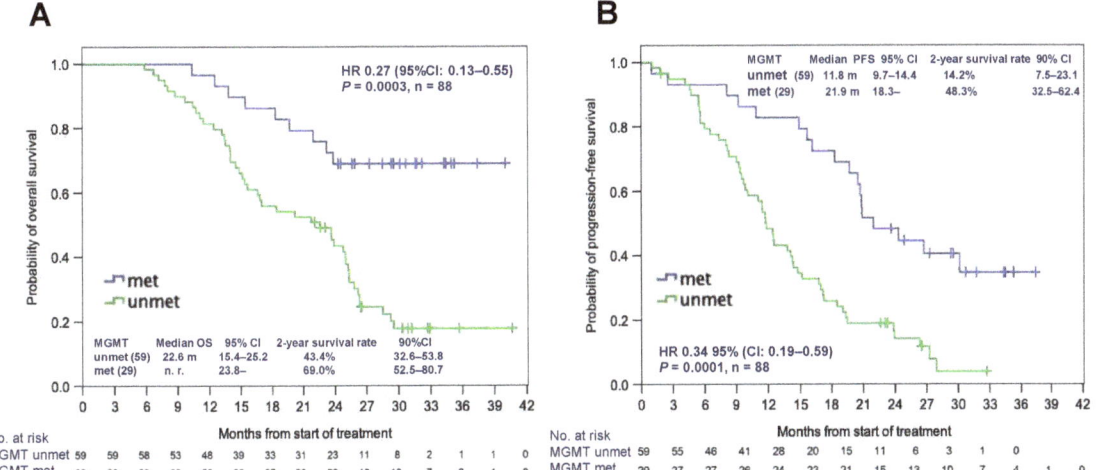

Figure 2. Median OS (**A**) and PFS (**B**) according to the *MGMT* methylation status in the full analysis set. Abbreviations: HR: hazard ratio; met: methylated; *MGMT*: O^6-methylguanine-DNA methyltransferase; mo: months; unmet: unmethylated; OS: overall survival; PFS: progression-free survival.

3.3. Secondary Endpoints: Objective Response Rate, Safety

Regarding the objective response, in the FAS (*n* = 90), 39 patients who had a measurable lesion were evaluable for response; six had CR, nine had PR (i.e., overall response rate of 38.5%), twenty had stable disease (SD), and four had PD. In the BBP group (*n* = 25; 12 were evaluable), two had CR, three had PR, and seven had SD; none had PD.

Regarding safety, the protocol-defined therapies were generally well tolerated. Frequently observed AEs of special interest for bevacizumab (all grades) included hypertension (42.6%), proteinuria (29.8%), and mucocutaneous bleeding (10.6%) (Table S5). Other common AEs including myelosuppression (all grades) were lymphopenia (50%), neutropenia (27.7%), thrombocytopenia (19.1%), anemia (5.3%), appetite loss (30.9%), constipation (30.9%), nausea (18.1%), and fatigue (13.8%).

Common Grade 3 or 4 AEs were hypertension (29.8%), wound healing complications and cerebral hemorrhage (2.1%, each), and lymphopenia (41.5%). The occurrence of Grade ≥ 3 arterial thromboembolic events was 1.1% (Table S5). No new unknown toxicities were encountered.

3.4. Biomarker Analysis

3.4.1. Methylation Classifier

When the German Cancer Research Center (DKFZ) methylation classifier was applied using methylation array data, eight patients (seven patients in the FAS and one in AVAglio) were classified as non-GBM (Priority 2, Table S1). The remaining 93 patients (78 in the FAS and 15 in AVAglio) of histologically verified *IDH1*-WT GBM were considered the biomarker cohort (Priority 1, Table S1). Among these 93 patients, nine tumors (seven in the FAS and two in AVAglio) were classified as non-neoplastic tissues, and two tumors (FAS) were unclassifiable by the DKFZ methylation classifier. These 11 tumors were diagnosed as GBM by pathology review and had mutations typically found in GBM.

3.4.2. No Survival Benefit in the Proneural Subtype

To validate the findings of Sandmann et al. [23], in which *IDH1* WT proneural glioblastoma may derive an OS benefit from first-line bevacizumab treatment, we applied the gene expression classification with mesenchymal, proliferative, and proneural subtypes proposed by Phillips et al. [31] using NanoString technology [3]. All Priority 1 cases, except two cases, were successfully classified by NanoString analysis (Table S1). There were no significant differences in OS or PFS from the initial treatment among Phillips expression subtypes (Figure S4) [31]. Compared with Japanese patients with *IDH1* WT GBM enrolled in the AVAglio control arm (no bevacizumab, hereafter the "control cohort"), there were no significant differences in OS or PFS in any expression subtypes, including the proneural subtype (Figure S5).

3.4.3. Novel Expression Cluster Predicted Longer Survival

Next, clustering analysis using the 1000 most differentially expressed genes (Top 1000 Coefficient Variance) from the RNA sequencing data of the biomarker cohort (Priority 1 including 59 BIOMARK and eight control samples) was performed. As a result, 59 patients in the BIOMARK cohort were classified into two clusters (30 in Cluster 1 and 29 in Cluster 2) (Figure 3A). Using the same condition, eight patients in the control cohort were classified in Cluster 1 and five in Cluster 2. In the BIOMARK cohort, significantly prolonged OS was observed in Cluster 2 by the Wilcoxon test ($p = 0.032$, Figure 3B). PFS tended to be longer in Cluster 2 (Wilcoxon test, $p = 0.065$) (Figure 3C). In the control cohort ($n = 13$), no difference in survival between the two clusters was observed (Figure 3D,E). When comparing survival in BIOMARK and control by cluster, OS tended to be longer (log-rank test $p = 0.050$) in Cluster 2 of BIOMARK compared with Cluster 2 of control (Figure 3F), while there were no differences in PFS (Figure 3G).

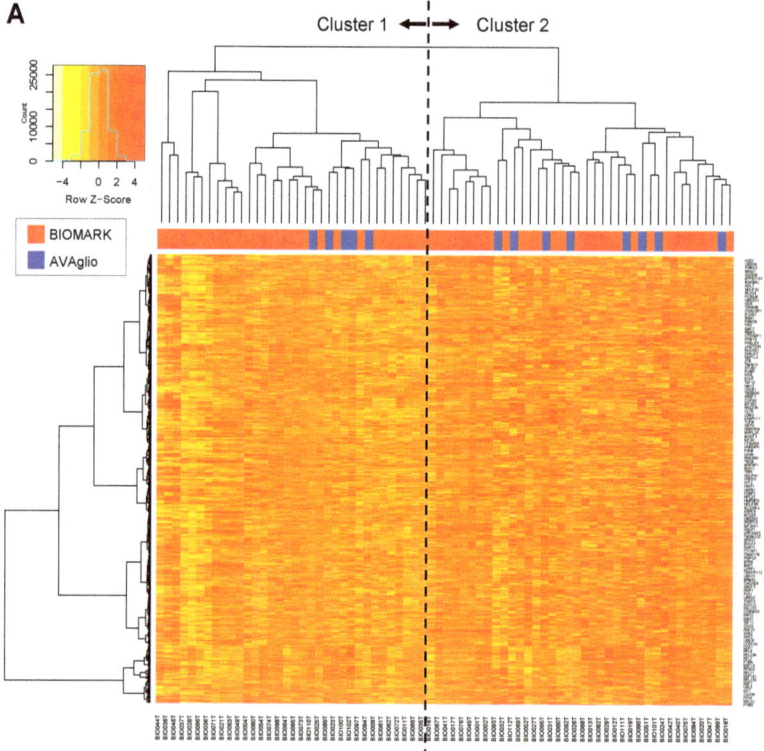

Figure 3. *Cont.*

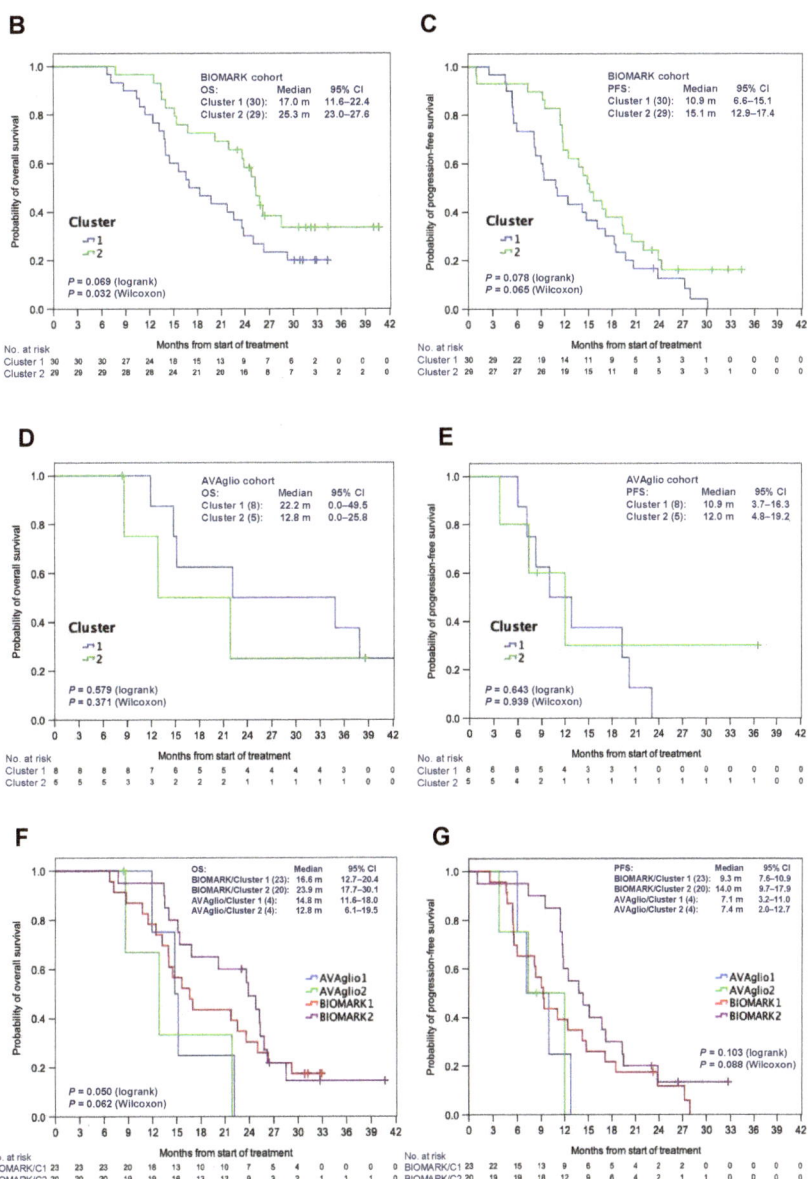

Figure 3. Heatmap of the 1000 genes that are most differentially expressed across the BIOMARK and AVAglio control cohorts (**A**). OS (**B**) and PFS (**C**) in the BIOMARK cohort and OS (**D**) and PFS (**E**) in the control cohort using the RNAseq Classifier. OS (**F**) and PFS (**G**) by Cluster in the BIOMARK and control cohorts with unmethylated *MGMT*.

3.4.4. Gene Set Enrichment Analysis Identified Distinct Expression Signatures

Gene Set Enrichment Analysis for the differentially expressed genes showed that Cluster 1 was enriched with genes involved in the processing and biogenesis of non-coding RNA and ribosomes, as well as telomere organization defined by Molecular Signatures Database v7.4 (http://www.gsea-msigdb.org/gsea/msigdb/index.jsp (accessed on 1 July 2021)) (Figure 4A, Figures S6 and S7, Table S6). Cluster 1 was also enriched with genes that represent signatures of the RB1 pathway (Table S7). Cluster 2 was enriched with genes involved in macrophage or microglia activation (Figure 4B, Figures S6 and S7, Table S8) and genes representing signatures of the p53 pathway or *KRAS* (Table S9). Notably, Cluster 1 was enriched with genes downregulated in endothelial cells by treatment with VEGFA, whereas Cluster 2 was enriched with genes upregulated in endothelial cells by treatment with VEGFA (Figure 4A,B; Tables S10 and S11).

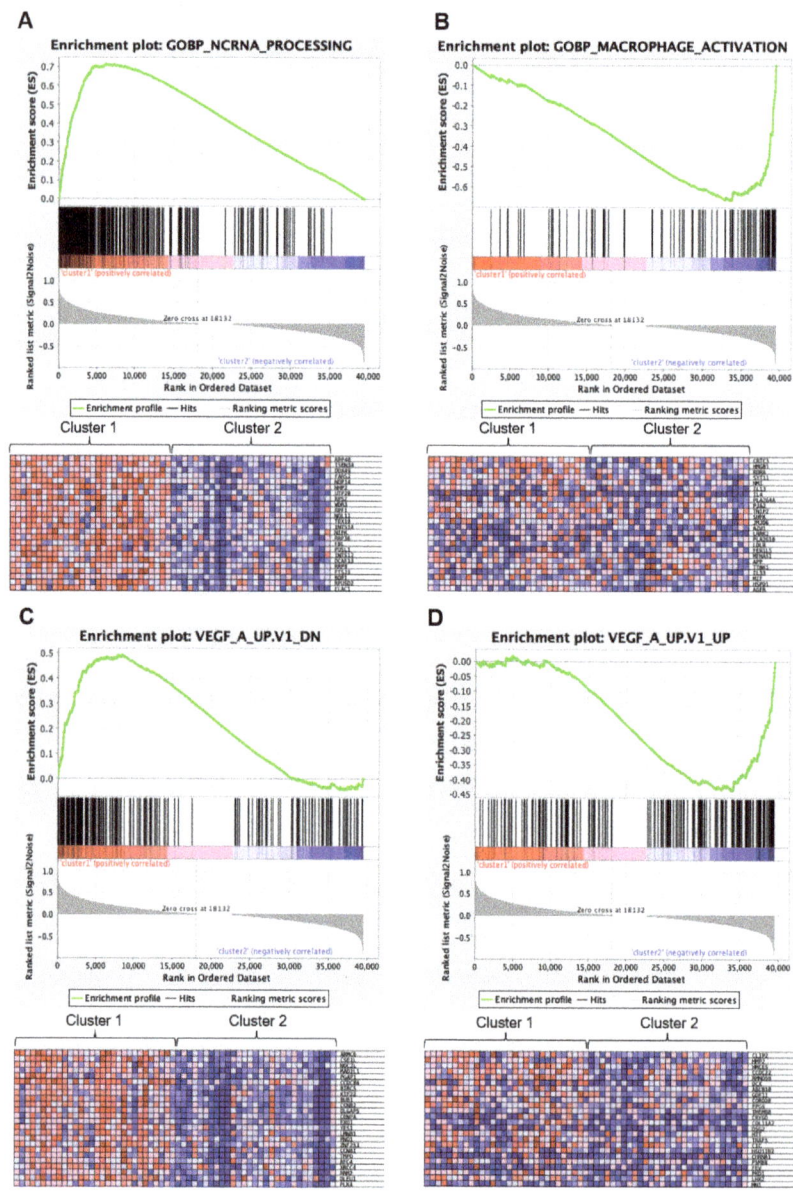

Figure 4. Gene Set Enrichment Analysis (Obtained through Gene Set Enrichment Analysis, https://www.gsea-msigdb.org/gsea/index.jsp (accessed on 1 July 2021)). (**A**) Top panel, enrichment plot

for the Gene Set GOBP_NCRNA_PROCESSING (genes involved in any process that results in the conversion of primary non-coding RNA transcripts), enriched in Cluster 1. Bottom panel, a heat map of the clustering result using the GOBP_NCRNA_PROCESSING gene set. Only the top 24 most differentially expressed genes between Cluster 1 and 2 are shown. (**B**) Top panel, enrichment plot for the Gene Set GOBP_MACROPHAGE_ACTIVATION (genes involved in a change in morphology and behavior of a macrophage upon cytokine stimulation), enriched in Cluster 2. Bottom panel, a heatmap of the clustering result using the GOBP_MACROPHAGE_ACTIVATION gene set. Only the top 24 most differentially expressed genes between Cluster 1 and 2 are shown. (**C**) Top panel, enrichment plot for the Gene Set VEGF_A_UP.V1_DN (genes downregulated by treatment with VEGFA), enriched in Cluster 1. Bottom panel, a heatmap of the clustering result using the VEGF_A_UP.V1_DN gene set. Only the top 24 most differentially expressed genes between Cluster 1 and 2 are shown. (**D**) Top panel, enrichment plot for the Gene Set VEGF_A_UP.V1_UP (genes upregulated by treatment with VEGFA), enriched in Cluster 2. Bottom panel, a heatmap of the clustering result using the VEGF_A_UP.V1_UP gene set. Only the top 24 most differentially expressed genes between Cluster 1 and 2 are shown.

3.4.5. Genetic and Epigenetic Profiles

CDKN2A homozygous deletion was significantly more frequent in Cluster 1 (p = 0.037, Fisher's exact test, Table S12). Alterations of the RB1 pathway (either *CDKN2A* homozygous deletion, *CDK4* amplification, or *RB1* mutation) and trisomy 20 were also significantly more common in Cluster 1 (p = 0.0251 and p = 0.0048). Frequencies of other molecular features examined, including *TERT* promoter mutations, *MGMT* methylation, Trisomy 7, Monosomy 10, or *EGFR* amplification, all of which are characteristic of GBM [34], were not significantly different between the two clusters (Table S12).

Using the Cox hazard model, we performed a multivariate analysis adjusted by sex, age, and *MGMT* methylation status. Cluster 2, younger age, and methylated *MGMT* status were identified as significantly favorable independent prognostic factors for PFS. Regarding OS, methylated *MGMT* status was the only favorable independent prognostic factor (Table 2).

Table 2. Multivariate analysis using Cox hazard model.

Overall Survival				
Factors	Hazard Ratio	95% CI	*p*-Value	c-Index
Sex: M/F	1.159	0.610–2.200	0.6524	0.669
Age	1.025	0.997–1.054	0.0860	0.669
MGMT: met/unmet	2.46	1.083–5.599	0.0316	0.669
Cluster: 1/2	0.582	0.310–1.092	0.0920	0.669
Progression-free survival				
Sex: M/F	1.281	0.705–2.329	0.417	0.67
Age	1.032	1.006–1.058	0.0143	0.67
MGMT: met/unmet	1.893	1.013–3.536	0.0455	0.67
Cluster: 1/2	0.562	0.322–0.982	0.0431	0.67

Abbreviations: CI: confidence interval; met: methylated; MGMT: O^6-methylguanine-DNA methyltransferase; unmet: unmethylated.

We also attempted to identify a novel methylation class that may predict prognosis or response to bevacizumab using the genome-wide DNA methylation array data. Clustering analysis of Priority 1 using 5624 probes (top 1% standard deviation) yielded three methylation clusters (Stratum 1–3, Figure S8). However, none of the DNA methylation strata were significantly associated with OS, PFS, or 2-year survival rates (Figure S9A,B).

4. Discussion

The 2-year survival rate of patients who proceeded to BBP (bevacizumab beyond progression) upon progression after initial bevacizumab-based treatment (27.0%) did not meet the prespecified criteria (50%) in this study. However, patients in the BBP group (patients who underwent BBP) were the population with early recurrence. The BBP group was enriched with patients with unmethylated *MGMT*, a well-established unfavorable prognosis factor, compared with the ANP group (patients who survived without progression) in which those with methylated *MGMT* were predominant. Patients with unmethylated *MGMT* were prone to progress earlier than those with methylated *MGMT*, explaining the low survival rate in the BBP group. Nonetheless, BBP is not recommended for use beyond the steroid-sparing effect in patients with recurrent GBM, based on the failure to demonstrate survival benefits in studies such as this [21,22].

Regarding safety, the frequency and severity of bevacizumab-related AEs and other events in the AVAglio study were comparable with those observed in this study (Table S5). No unexpected AEs were observed. The reason for the more frequent occurrence of Grade 3 or 4 hypertension in this study than in AVAglio is unclear, but these events did not result in other complications.

One of the objectives was to explore biomarkers associated with the subpopulation that may respond to bevacizumab using prospectively collected fresh frozen tumor specimens to perform detailed genomic analysis. In the sub-analysis of AVAglio, patients with a proneural subtype with WT *IDH* in the bevacizumab group showed a significant improvement in OS [23]. In this study, no improvements in PFS or OS were observed in patients with the proneural subtype treated with bevacizumab. Thus, the result reported by Phillips et al. [31] was not reproduced in this study population [23]. The number of patients, especially in the control group, was considerably smaller in the current study compared with that of Sandmann et al. [23], which may explain the lack of reproducibility.

Through genome-wide gene expression profiling, we identified two novel expression classes. Significantly longer OS and a tendency for longer PFS were observed in Cluster 2 of the BIOMARK cohort. No difference was observed between the two clusters in the control cohort. This suggests that Cluster 2 may be predictive for patients who can benefit from first-line bevacizumab treatment. Cluster 1 was enriched with genes involved in ribosome biogenesis, most likely reflecting their high translational activity associated with the accelerated cell cycle. Concordantly, RB1 pathway gene alterations were significantly more common in Cluster 1, and RB1 pathway signatures were enriched in Cluster 1. Cluster 2 was enriched with genes involved in macrophage/microglial activation, presumably reflecting the increased infiltration of macrophage/microglia. Infiltrating tumor-associated macrophages and resident brain microglia (TAM) may promote the growth of GBM [35,36]. That there was no difference in the frequencies of molecular alterations characterizing GBM between the two clusters indicated that both clusters represent quintessential GBM [34]. Thus, our study identified a novel subset of bevacizumab-responsive GBM.

The most notable finding was that Cluster 1 was enriched with genes downregulated in endothelial cells by treatment with VEGFA, whereas Cluster 2 was enriched with the genes upregulated by VEGFA (https://www.gsea-msigdb.org/gsea/msigdb/ (accessed on 1 July 2021)). This suggests that Cluster 2 tumors may have been dependent on VEGFA signaling and, therefore, responsive to bevacizumab. The expression of VEGFA or VEGFR has not previously been associated with responsiveness to bevacizumab [37]. VEGFR is expressed in TAMs [38]. Considering that the expression signatures of Cluster 2 were predominantly genes associated with macrophage activation, it is likely that Cluster 2 contains high degrees of TAM infiltration. If TAMs are dependent on VEGF signaling, inhibition of VEGF signaling by bevacizumab may lead to repressing TAM-mediated promotion of GBM growth [35]. These findings should be further confirmed by histopathological investigation of the tumor specimen. For instance, the more translational activity and faster progression through the cell cycle in Cluster 1 might be reflected in more intact mitochondria per cell, more Ki-67 positive cells, or more mitotic figures in DNA/nuclear staining. Similarly, Cluster 2 might have a higher surface expression of the VEGFR and higher TAM infiltration. An extended biomarker analysis using histological specimens of the study is being planned. Although the biological basis of each cluster needs further exploration, our results may have introduced the possibility of predicting which patients could benefit from first-line bevacizumab treatment.

This study had several limitations. It was a single-arm, uncontrolled, unrandomized study with a small number of patients and limited follow-up period, with possible bias associated with using data from another study (placebo group in AVAglio) as control data. Although the number of patients in this cohort was small, it was the only available control cohort (those GBM patients who did not receive bevacizumab) at the time. Additionally, although the study was initially aimed at evaluating the efficacy and safety of BBP, the number of patients who experienced progression after first-line radiotherapy/temozolomide/bevacizumab treatment and were enrolled in the BBP group was unexpectedly low, making the primary endpoint analysis under-powered. The number of tumors subjected to RNA sequencing was limited because of suboptimal RNA quality in some samples. The small dataset means our study should be interpreted with caution, even if collected from a prospective clinical trial. Nonetheless, we believe that the study provides a new venue to explore the true efficacy of bevacizumab in GBMs.

5. Conclusions

The primary endpoint of BIOMARK was not met (the 2-year survival rate in the BBP group was 27.0% vs. the target of 50%). BBP was initiated in only a small subset (27/90 patients) of the entire cohort, where *MGMT*-unmethylated tumors were predominant. We identified a novel expression cluster that may predict the prognosis of GBM patients treated with bevacizumab. Further validation of the predictive value of the novel expression classifier is warranted.

Supplementary Materials: The following supporting information can be downloaded at: https://www.mdpi.com/article/10.3390/cancers14225522/s1, Doc S1: List of participating institutions and principal investigators.; Figure S1. BIOMARK study schema.; Figure S2: CONSORT diagram of the study.; Figure S3: Median overall survival and progression-free survival in the full analysis set solely with isocitrate dehydrogenase 1 WT glioblastoma.; Figure S4: Overall survival (OS) (A) and progression-free survival (PFS) (B) stratified by Phillips et al. subtypes: (MES) mesenchymal, (PRO) proliferative, and (PN) proneural; Figure S5: Overall survival (OS) (A, C, E) and progression-free survival (PFS) (B,D,F) of patients enrolled in BIOMARK and AVAglio (placebo group) studies stratified by Phillips et al. subtypes: mesenchymal (A,B), proliferative (C,D), and proneural (E,F).; Figure S6: Heatmap of the top 50 features for each phenotype in Cluster 1 and Cluster 2.; Figure S7: Gene Set Enrichment Analysis for genes up- or downregulated in various Gene Ontology Biological Processes.; Figure S8: Hierarchical clustering and heatmap of DNA methylation beta-values from Priority 1 samples.; Figure S9: Overall survival (OS) (A) and progression-free survival (PFS) (B) stratified by methylome stratum (1, 2, and 3).; Table S1: Biomarker analysis summary.; Table S2: Target and control genes for the NanoString analysis.; Table S3: Chemotherapeutic agent combined with BBP.; Table S4: *MGMT* promoter methylation status.; Table S5: Adverse events of special interest in patients treated with bevacizumab.; Table S6: Top 50 genes from the Gene Ontology Biological Process Gene sets enriched in Cluster 1.; Table S7: Top 50 genes from the Oncogenic Signature Gene sets enriched in Cluster 1.; Table S8: Top 50 genes from the Gene Ontology Biological Process Gene sets enriched in Cluster 2.; Table S9: Top 50 genes from the Oncogenic Signature Gene sets enriched in Cluster 2.; Table S10: Details of Gene Set Enrichment Analysis for Genes downregulated in HUVEC cells by treatment with VEGFA.; Table S11: Details of Gene Set Enrichment Analysis for Genes upregulated in HUVEC cells by treatment with VEGFA.; Table S12; Frequency of mutations and copy number alterations.

Author Contributions: Conceptualization, M.N. (Motoo Nagane), K.I. (Koichi Ichimura), Y.N., A.M., S.T., T.W., T.A. and R.N.; data curation, M.N. (Motoo Nagane), K.I. (Koichi Ichimura), R.O., D.N., M.K., K.S., A.T. and S.M.; formal analysis, M.N. (Motoo Nagane), K.I. (Koichi Ichimura), R.O., D.N., M.H.-K., Y.A. (Yasuhito Arai), T.S., S.M. and M.K.; funding acquisition, R.N.; investigation, M.N. (Motoo Nagane), K.I. (Koichi Ichimura), Y.N., T.U., H.N., M.N. (Mitsutoshi Nakada), Y.A. (Yoshiki Arakawa), T.O., A.M., S.T., T.W., T.A. and R.N.; methodology, R.O., D.N., Y.A. (Yasuhito Arai), T.S., S.M. and M.K.; project administration, R.N.; resources, M.N. (Motoo Nagane), K.I. (Koichi Ichimura), R.O., D.N., M.H.-K., K.S., A.T., Y.A. (Yasuhito Arai), T.S., Y.N., T.U., H.N., M.N. (Mitsutoshi Nakada), Y.A. (Yoshiki Arakawa), T.O., A.M., S.T., T.W., T.A., S.A., K.I. (Keisuke Ishizawa), H.Y., H.S., S.M., M.K. and R.N.; software, R.O., D.N., S.M. and M.K.; supervision, S.S., M.M. and R.N.; visualization, M.N. (Motoo Nagane), K.I. (Koichi Ichimura), R.O., D.N., S.M. and M.K.; writing—original draft, M.N. (Motoo Nagane), K.I. (Koichi Ichimura), and R.N.; writing—review and editing, all authors. All authors have read and agreed to the published version of the manuscript.

Funding: This research was funded by Chugai Pharmaceutical Co. Ltd.

Institutional Review Board Statement: The study was conducted in accordance with the Declaration of Helsinki and the Japanese Ethical Guidelines for Medical and Health Research Involving Human Subjects. The protocol was reviewed and approved by the institutional review board of each site.

Informed Consent Statement: Informed consent was obtained from all subjects involved in the study.

Data Availability Statement: All raw data including FASTQ files of RNA sequences, IDAT files from the DNA methylation arrays, and BAM files from target sequencing are available from the authors upon request.

Acknowledgments: The authors wish to thank Keyra Martinez Dunn. The authors thank Yuko Hibiya and Hiroshi Chikuta for the excellent technical assistance, and Josep Garcia of Hoffmann-La Roche AG for sharing information for the NanoString probes. Finally, we would like to thank the investigators and institutions listed in Doc. S1 for their participation and contributions to this trial.

Conflicts of Interest: M.N. (Motoo Nagane), Grants: AbbVie, Eisai, MSD, Chugai Pharma, Daiichi-Sankyo, Pfizer, Kyowa Kirin, Nippon Kayaku, Tsumura, Shionogi, Otsuka, Astellas, Teijin Pharma, Bayer, Ono Pharma, Sanofi, Toray, Takeda, Asahi Kasei Pharma, Mitsubishi Tanabe Pharma. Consulting: AbbVie, Bristol Myers Squibb, Daiichi-Sankyo, RIEMSER, Ono Pharma, Novartis, Novocure, Chugai Pharma, Sumitomo Dainippon Pharma. Honoraria: Chugai Pharma, Novocure, MSD, Daiichi-Sankyo, AbbVie, Ono Pharma, Nippon Kayaku, Sumitomo, Dainippon Pharma, Eisai, Kyowa Kirin, Otsuka, Bayer, UCB Japan. Travel: Ono Pharma, Chugai Pharma, Daiichi Sankyo, Bristol Myers Squibb, Eisai. K.I. (Koichi Ichimura), Grants: Daiichi Sankyo, Eisai, Therabiopharma, Riken Genesis, SRL. Consulting: Daiichi Sankyo. Honoraria: Chugai Pharmaceuticals, Astellas, Daiichi Sankyo, Meiji Seika Pharma, Eisai, Kyowa Kirin, Leica Microsystems. Travel: Chugai Pharmaceuticals, Kyowa Kirin, Daiichi Sankyo. Equipment: Blueprint Medicines. Y.N., Grants: Eisai, Dainippon-Sumitomo, AbbVie, Ono Pharmaceutical, Taiho Pharmaceutical, Daiichi-Sankyo, Bayer. Consulting: AbbVie, Dainippon-Sumitomo. Honoraria: Ono Pharmaceutical, Daiichi-Sankyo, Chugai Pharmaceutical. H.N., Consulting: Daiichi Sankyo Co. LTD., Honoraria: Eisai Co. LTD, Ono Pharmaceutical Co. LTD, MSD Co. LTD, Daiichi Sankyo Co. LTD, Novocure Co., Chugai Pharmaceutical Co. LTD. M.Nakada, Grants: Chugai Pharmaceutical Co., Eisai Japan co., Otsuka Pharmaceutical Co., MSD Co., Daiichi Sankyo Co., Ltd., Nippon Kayaku Co. Consulting: Novocure. Honoraria: Chugai Pharmaceutical Co., Daiichi Sankyo Co., Ltd., MSD Co., Novocure, Eisai Japan Co., Nippon Kayaku Co., Otsuka Pharmaceutical Co., Astellas Pharmaceutical Co. Y.Arakawa, Grants: Siemens, Philips, Sanofi, Nihon Medi-Physics, Mitsubishi Tanabe, Takeda, Stryker, Astellas Pharma, Taiho Pharma, Pfizer, Ono Pharmaceutical, Brainlab, Merck, Chugai, Eisai, Meiji Seika, Daiichi Sankyo, Zeiss, CLS Behring. Honoraria: Nippon Kayaku, AbbVie, Novocure, UCB Japan, Otsuka, CLS Behring, Ono Pharmaceutical, Brainlab, Merck, Chugai, Eisai, Meiji Seika, Daiichi Sankyo, Zeiss. A.M., Grants: Chugai Pharmaceutical, Eisai, Daiichi Sankyo, Otsuka Pharmaceutical, Teijin Pharma., Honoraria: Chugai Pharmaceutical, Eisai, Daiichi Sankyo, Otsuka Pharmaceutical, Ono Pharmaceutical, Novartis Pharmaceuticals, Novocure, Nippon Kayaku, Astellas Pharma, Boehringer Ingelheim. S.T., Grants: Ono Pharmaceutical Co., Ltd., Sumitomo Dainippon Pharma Co., Ltd., Eisai Co., Ltd., Takeda Science Foundation. Royalties: Goryo Chemical Inc. Honoraria: Daiichi-Sankyo Co., Ltd., Eisai Co., Ltd., Chugai Pharmaceutical Co., Ltd., Novocure Ltd. S.S., Honoraria: Chugai Pharmaceutical. Safety monitoring board membership: Chugai Pharmaceutical. R.N., Grants: Chugai Pharm, Eisai, AbbVie,

Toray, MSD. Consulting: Novocure. Honoraria: Chugai Pharm, MSD, Nippon Kayaku, Ono Pharma, Eisai, Daiichi-Sankyo. The remaining authors declare no conflicts of interest. The funders had no role in the design of the study; in the collection, analyses, or interpretation of data; in the writing of the manuscript; or in the decision to publish the results.

References

1. Thakkar, J.P.; Dolecek, T.A.; Horbinski, C.; Ostrom, Q.T.; Lightner, D.D.; Barnholtz-Sloan, J.S.; Villano, J.L. Epidemiologic and molecular prognostic review of glioblastoma. *Cancer Epidemiol. Biomark. Prev.* **2014**, *23*, 1985–1996. [CrossRef] [PubMed]
2. Li, Y.; Ali, S.; Clarke, J.; Cha, S. Bevacizumab in recurrent glioma: Patterns of treatment failure and implications. *Brain Tumor Res. Treat.* **2017**, *5*, 1–9. [CrossRef] [PubMed]
3. Stupp, R.; Mason, W.P.; van den Bent, M.J.; Weller, M.; Fisher, B.; Taphoorn, M.J.; Belanger, K.; Brandes, A.A.; Marosi, C.; Bogdahn, U.; et al. Radiotherapy plus concomitant and adjuvant temozolomide for glioblastoma. *N. Engl. J. Med.* **2005**, *352*, 987–996. [CrossRef] [PubMed]
4. Hegi, M.E.; Diserens, A.C.; Gorlia, T.; Hamou, M.F.; de Tribolet, N.; Weller, M.; Kros, J.M.; Hainfellner, J.A.; Mason, W.; Mariani, L.; et al. MGMT gene silencing and benefit from temozolomide in glioblastoma. *N. Engl. J. Med.* **2005**, *352*, 997–1003. [CrossRef] [PubMed]
5. Stupp, R.; Hegi, M.E.; Mason, W.P.; van den Bent, M.J.; Taphoorn, M.J.; Janzer, R.C.; Ludwin, S.K.; Allgeier, A.; Fisher, B.; Belanger, K.; et al. Effects of radiotherapy with concomitant and adjuvant temozolomide versus radiotherapy alone on survival in glioblastoma in a randomised phase III study: 5-year analysis of the EORTC-NCIC trial. *Lancet Oncol.* **2009**, *10*, 459–466. [CrossRef]
6. Esteller, M.; Garcia-Foncillas, J.; Andion, E.; Goodman, S.N.; Hidalgo, O.F.; Vanaclocha, V.; Baylin, S.B.; Herman, J.G. Inactivation of the DNA-repair gene MGMT and the clinical response of gliomas to alkylating agents. *N. Engl. J. Med.* **2000**, *343*, 1350–1354. [CrossRef]
7. Ferrara, N. VEGF-A: A critical regulator of blood vessel growth. *Eur. Cytokine Netw.* **2009**, *20*, 158–163. [CrossRef]
8. Ahir, B.K.; Engelhard, H.H.; Lakka, S.S. Tumor development and angiogenesis in adult brain tumor: Glioblastoma. *Mol. Neurobiol.* **2020**, *57*, 2461–2478. [CrossRef]
9. D'Alessio, A.; Proietti, G.; Lama, G.; Biamonte, F.; Lauriola, L.; Moscato, U.; Vescovi, A.; Mangiola, A.; Angelucci, C.; Sica, G. Analysis of angiogenesis related factors in glioblastoma, peritumoral tissue and their derived cancer stem cells. *Oncotarget* **2016**, *7*, 78541–78556. [CrossRef]
10. D'Alessio, A.; Proietti, G.; Sica, G.; Scicchitano, B.M. Pathological and molecular features of glioblastoma and its peritumoral tissue. *Cancers* **2019**, *11*, 469. [CrossRef]
11. Chinot, O.L.; Wick, W.; Mason, W.; Henriksson, R.; Saran, F.; Nishikawa, R.; Carpentier, A.F.; Hoang-Xuan, K.; Kavan, P.; Cernea, D.; et al. Bevacizumab plus radiotherapy-temozolomide for newly diagnosed glioblastoma. *N. Engl. J. Med.* **2014**, *370*, 709–722. [CrossRef]
12. Gilbert, M.R.; Dignam, J.J.; Armstrong, T.S.; Wefel, J.S.; Blumenthal, D.T.; Vogelbaum, M.A.; Colman, H.; Chakravarti, A.; Pugh, S.; Won, M.; et al. A randomized trial of bevacizumab for newly diagnosed glioblastoma. *N. Engl. J. Med.* **2014**, *370*, 699–708. [CrossRef] [PubMed]
13. Kreisl, T.N.; Kim, L.; Moore, K.; Duic, P.; Royce, C.; Stroud, I.; Garren, N.; Mackey, M.; Butman, J.A.; Camphausen, K.; et al. Phase II trial of single-agent bevacizumab followed by bevacizumab plus irinotecan at tumor progression in recurrent glioblastoma. *J. Clin. Oncol.* **2009**, *27*, 740–745. [CrossRef] [PubMed]
14. Nagane, M.; Nishikawa, R.; Narita, Y.; Kobayashi, H.; Takano, S.; Shinoura, N.; Aoki, T.; Sugiyama, K.; Kuratsu, J.; Muragaki, Y.; et al. Phase II study of single-agent bevacizumab in Japanese patients with recurrent malignant glioma. *Jpn. J. Clin. Oncol.* **2012**, *42*, 887–895. [CrossRef] [PubMed]
15. Friedman, H.S.; Prados, M.D.; Wen, P.Y.; Mikkelsen, T.; Schiff, D.; Abrey, L.E.; Yung, W.K.; Paleologos, N.; Nicholas, M.K.; Jensen, R.; et al. Bevacizumab alone and in combination with irinotecan in recurrent glioblastoma. *J. Clin. Oncol.* **2009**, *27*, 4733–4740. [CrossRef]
16. Weathers, S.P.; Han, X.; Liu, D.D.; Conrad, C.A.; Gilbert, M.R.; Loghin, M.E.; O'Brien, B.J.; Penas-Prado, M.; Puduvalli, V.K.; Tremont-Lukats, I.; et al. A randomized phase II trial of standard dose bevacizumab versus low dose bevacizumab plus lomustine (CCNU) in adults with recurrent glioblastoma. *J. Neurooncol.* **2016**, *129*, 487–494. [CrossRef]
17. Bennouna, J.; Sastre, J.; Arnold, D.; Österlund, P.; Greil, R.; Van Cutsem, E.; von Moos, R.; Viéitez, J.M.; Bouché, O.; Borg, C.; et al. Continuation of bevacizumab after first progression in metastatic colorectal cancer (ML18147): A randomised phase 3 trial. *Lancet Oncol.* **2013**, *14*, 29–37. [CrossRef]
18. von Minckwitz, G.; Puglisi, F.; Cortes, J.; Vrdoljak, E.; Marschner, N.; Zielinski, C.; Villanueva, C.; Romieu, G.; Lang, I.; Ciruelos, E.; et al. Bevacizumab plus chemotherapy versus chemotherapy alone as second-line treatment for patients with HER2-negative locally recurrent or metastatic breast cancer after first-line treatment with bevacizumab plus chemotherapy (TANIA): An open-label, randomised phase 3 trial. *Lancet Oncol.* **2014**, *15*, 1269–1278.
19. Okamoto, S.; Nitta, M.; Maruyama, T.; Sawada, T.; Komori, T.; Okada, Y.; Muragaki, Y. Bevacizumab changes vascular structure and modulates the expression of angiogenic factors in recurrent malignant gliomas. *Brain Tumor Pathol.* **2016**, *33*, 129–136. [CrossRef]

20. Reardon, D.A.; Herndon, J.E., 2nd; Peters, K.B.; Desjardins, A.; Coan, A.; Lou, E.; Sumrall, A.L.; Turner, S.; Lipp, E.S.; Sathornsumetee, S.; et al. Bevacizumab continuation beyond initial bevacizumab progression among recurrent glioblastoma patients. *Br. J. Cancer.* **2012**, *107*, 1481–1487. [CrossRef]
21. Brandes, A.A.; Gil-Gil, M.; Saran, F.; Carpentier, A.F.; Nowak, A.K.; Mason, W.; Zagonel, V.; Duboois, F.; Finocchiaro, G.; Fountzilas, G.; et al. A randomized phase ii trial (TAMIGA) evaluating the efficacy and safety of continuous bevacizumab through multiple lines of treatment for recurrent glioblastoma. *Oncologist* **2019**, *24*, 521–528. [CrossRef] [PubMed]
22. Hovey, E.J.; Field, K.M.; Rosenthal, M.A.; Barnes, E.H.; Cher, L.; Nowak, A.K.; Wheeler, H.; Sawkins, K.; Livingstone, A.; Phal, P.; et al. Continuing or ceasing bevacizumab beyond progression in recurrent glioblastoma: An exploratory randomized phase II trial. *Neurooncol. Pract.* **2017**, *4*, 171–181. [CrossRef] [PubMed]
23. Sandmann, T.; Bourgon, R.; Garcia, J.; Li, C.; Cloughesy, T.; Chinot, L.L.; Wick, W.; Nishikawa, R.; Mason, W.; Henriksson, R.; et al. Patients with proneural glioblastoma may derive overall survival benefit from the addition of bevacizumab to first-line radiotherapy and temozolomide: Retrospective analysis of the AVAglio trial. *J. Clin. Oncol.* **2015**, *33*, 2735–2744. [CrossRef]
24. Louis, D.N.; Ohgaki, H.; Wiestler, O.D.; Cavenee, W.K.; Ellison, D.W.; Figarella-Branger, D.; Perry, A.; Reifenberger, G.; von Deimling, A. *WHO Classification of Tumours of the Central Nervous System, Revised*, 4th ed.; Bosman, F.T., Jaffe, E.S., Lakhani, S.R., Ohgaki, H., Eds.; IARC: Lyon, France, 2016.
25. Arita, H.; Yamasaki, K.; Matsushita, Y.; Nakamura, T.; Shimokawa, A.; Takami, H.; Tanaka, S.; Mukasa, A.; Shirahata, M.; Shimizu, S.; et al. A combination of TERT promoter mutation and MGMT methylation status predicts clinically relevant subgroups of newly diagnosed glioblastomas. *Acta Neuropathol. Commun.* **2016**, *4*, 79. [CrossRef] [PubMed]
26. Nakano, Y.; Hasegawa, D.; Stewart, D.R.; Schultz, K.A.P.; Harris, A.K.; Hirato, J.; Uemura, S.; Tamura, A.; Saito, A.; Kawamura, A.; et al. Presacral malignant teratoid neoplasm in association with pathogenic DICER1 variation. *Mod. Pathol.* **2019**, *32*, 1744–1750. [CrossRef] [PubMed]
27. Takami, H.; Fukushima, S.; Aoki, K.; Satomi, K.; Narumi, K.; Hama, N.; Matsushita, Y.; Fukuoka, K.; Yamasaki, K.; Nakamura, T.; et al. Intratumoural immune cell landscape in germinoma reveals multipotent lineages and exhibits prognostic significance. *Neuropathol. Appl. Neurobiol.* **2020**, *46*, 111–124. [CrossRef]
28. Fukuoka, K.; Kanemura, Y.; Shofuda, T.; Fukushima, S.; Yamashita, S.; Narushima, D.; Kato, M.; Honda-Kitahara, M.; Ichikawa, H.; Kohno, T.; et al. Significance of molecular classification of ependymomas: C11orf95-RELA fusion-negative supratentorial ependymomas are a heterogeneous group of tumors. *Acta Neuropathol. Commun.* **2018**, *6*, 134. [CrossRef]
29. Mack, S.C.; Singh, I.; Wang, X.; Hirsch, R.; Wu, Q.; Villagomez, R.; Bernatchez, J.A.; Zhu, Z.; Gimple, R.C.; Kim, L.J.Y.; et al. Chromatin landscapes reveal developmentally encoded transcriptional states that define human glioblastoma. *J. Exp. Med.* **2019**, *216*, 1071–1090. [CrossRef]
30. Knoll, M.; Debus, J.; Abdollahi, A. cnAnalysis450k: An R package for comparative analysis of 450k/EPIC Illumina methylation array derived copy number data. *Bioinformatics* **2017**, *33*, 2266–2272. [CrossRef]
31. Phillips, H.S.; Kharbanda, S.; Chen, R.; Forrest, W.F.; Soriano, R.H.; Wu, T.D.; Misra, A.; Nigro, J.M.; Colman, H.; Soroceanu, L.; et al. Molecular subclasses of high-grade glioma predict prognosis, delineate a pattern of disease progression, and resemble stages in neurogenesis. *Cancer Cell* **2006**, *9*, 157–173. [CrossRef]
32. Zhou, W.; Laird, P.W.; Shen, H. Comprehensive characterization, annotation and innovative use of Infinium DNA methylation BeadChip probes. *Nucleic Acids Res.* **2017**, *45*, e22. [CrossRef] [PubMed]
33. Wen, P.Y.; Macdonald, D.R.; Reardon, D.A.; Cloughesy, T.F.; Sorensen, A.G.; Galanis, E.; Degroot, J.; Wick, W.; Gilbert, M.R.; Lassman, A.B.; et al. Updated response assessment criteria for high-grade gliomas: Response assessment in neuro-oncology working group. *J. Clin. Oncol.* **2010**, *28*, 1963–1972. [CrossRef] [PubMed]
34. Brat, D.J.; Aldape, K.; Colman, H.; Holland, E.C.; Louis, D.N.; Jenkins, R.B.; Kleinschmidt-DeMasters, B.K.; Perry, A.; Reifenberger, G.; Stupp, R.; et al. cIMPACT-NOW update 3: Recommended diagnostic criteria for "Diffuse astrocytic glioma, IDH-wildtype, with molecular features of glioblastoma, WHO grade IV". *Acta Neuropathol.* **2018**, *136*, 805–810. [CrossRef] [PubMed]
35. Chen, Z.; Feng, X.; Herting, C.J.; Garcia, V.A.; Nie, K.; Pong, W.W.; Rasmussen, R.; Dwivedi, B.; Seby, S.; Wolf, S.A.; et al. Cellular and molecular identity of tumor-associated macrophages in glioblastoma. *Cancer Res.* **2017**, *77*, 2266–2278. [CrossRef]
36. Dumas, A.A.; Pomella, N.; Rosser, G.; Guglielmi, L.; Vinel, C.; Millner, T.O.; Rees, J.; Aley, N.; Sheer, D.; Wei, J.; et al. Microglia promote glioblastoma via mTOR-mediated immunosuppression of the tumour microenvironment. *EMBO J.* **2020**, *39*, e103790. [CrossRef]
37. Lambrechts, D.; Lenz, H.J.; de Haas, S.; Carmeliet, P.; Scherer, S.J. Markers of response for the antiangiogenic agent bevacizumab. *J. Clin. Oncol.* **2013**, *31*, 1219–1230. [CrossRef]
38. Lisi, L.; Pia Ciotti, G.M.; Chiavari, M.; Ruffini, F.; Lacal, P.M.; Graziani, G.; Navarra, P. Vascular endothelial growth factor receptor 1 in glioblastoma-associated microglia/macrophages. *Oncol. Rep.* **2020**, *43*, 2083–2092. [CrossRef]

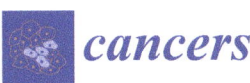

Review

Adenosine Targeting as a New Strategy to Decrease Glioblastoma Aggressiveness

Valentina Bova [1,†], Alessia Filippone [1,†], Giovanna Casili [1], Marika Lanza [1], Michela Campolo [1], Anna Paola Capra [1], Alberto Repici [1], Lelio Crupi [1], Gianmarco Motta [2], Cristina Colarossi [2], Giulia Chisari [2], Salvatore Cuzzocrea [1], Emanuela Esposito [1,*] and Irene Paterniti [1]

1 Department of Chemical, Biological, Pharmaceutical and Environmental Sciences, University of Messina, Viale Ferdinando Stagno D'Alcontres, 31-98166 Messina, Italy
2 Istituto Oncologico del Mediterraneo, Via Penninazzo 7, 95029 Viagrande, Italy
* Correspondence: eesposito@unime.it; Tel.: +39-090-676-5208
† These authors contributed equally to this work.

Simple Summary: Given the rising mortality rate caused by GBM, current therapies do not appear to be effective in counteracting tumor progression. The role of adenosine and its interaction with specific receptor subtypes in various physiological functions has been studied for years. Only recently, adenosine has been defined as a tumor-protective target because of its accumulation in the tumor microenvironment. Current knowledge of the adenosine pathway and its involvement in brain tumors would support research in the development of adenosine receptor antagonists that could represent alternative treatments for glioblastoma, used either alone and/or in combination with chemotherapy, immunotherapy, or both.

Abstract: Glioblastoma is the most commonly malignant and aggressive brain tumor, with a high mortality rate. The role of the purine nucleotide adenosine and its interaction with its four subtypes receptors coupled to the different G proteins, A1, A2A, A2B, and A3, and its different physiological functions in different systems and organs, depending on the active receptor subtype, has been studied for years. Recently, several works have defined extracellular adenosine as a tumoral protector because of its accumulation in the tumor microenvironment. Its presence is due to both the interaction with the A2A receptor subtype and the increase in CD39 and CD73 gene expression induced by the hypoxic state. This fact has fueled preclinical and clinical research into the development of efficacious molecules acting on the adenosine pathway and blocking its accumulation. Given the success of anti-cancer immunotherapy, the new strategy is to develop selective A2A receptor antagonists that could competitively inhibit binding to its endogenous ligand, making them reliable candidates for the therapeutic management of brain tumors. Here, we focused on the efficacy of adenosine receptor antagonists and their enhancement in anti-cancer immunotherapy.

Keywords: glioblastoma; adenosine; tumor microenvironment; A2AAR antagonist; immune evasion; adenosine receptors

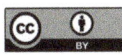

1. Introduction

Brain tumors affect different areas of the brain, including the cerebellum, and portions of the central nervous system (CNS), such as the spinal cord, that normally control voluntary and involuntary functions [1]. Physiologically and anatomically, the brain is separated from the blood by the blood–brain barrier (BBB), made up of tightly junctioned endothelial cells, astrocytes, and pericytes, which selectively control the exchange of substances between the two compartments [2]. Being intracranial, tumor cell growth causes an increase in the tumor mass that compresses the blood vessels, initiating a tumor-associated cerebral edema process that compromises the integrity of the BBB itself, and causes an active outflow of molecules [3]. It has been reported that the tumor mass increases the intracranial pressure that disrupts the homeostasis of the brain-affected area surrounding the tumor site and generates secondary effects [4].

Although clinical symptoms depend on the location and size of the tumor mass, the most common symptoms of all brain tumors include headache, seizures, nausea and vomiting, confusion and disorientation, loss of balance or dizziness, and memory loss (Figure 1B) [5]. The specific causes of brain tumors are unclear, but a set of risk factors should be considered in the tumor development and progression: age, exposure to ionizing radiation, decrease in immune defenses, and genetic predisposition of proto-oncogenes [6].

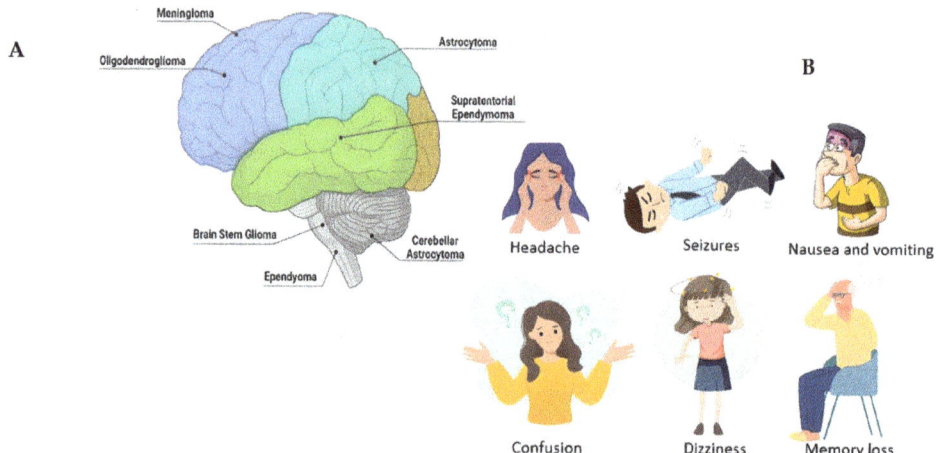

Figure 1. Figure created with Biorender.com. Classification of brain tumors (**A**). Main symptoms of brain tumors (**B**).

Still, CNS tumors are rare; they represent 1.6% of all tumors, especially in the last three decades, during which a progressive increase in the incidence of brain tumors development has been reported, particularly in adults over 65 years of age [7].

Brain tumors are classified into primary tumors, which originate in the brain, and can be benign and malignant tumors, and secondary tumors, which represent metastatic tumors [8]. A second classification is based on the origin of the cells from which brain tumors derive, such as glial cells, responsible for myelin production and represent 40% of all primary tumors and 78% of all malignant tumors [9]. One of the most common gliomas is astrocytoma, which originates from astrocyte cells and is distinguished by pilocytic tumors, very rare tumors that account for about 5% of gliomas and are more common in children [10]. Unlike other gliomas, these rarely develop into more aggressive tumors and can be cured with surgery [11]. There are also diffuse and anaplastic astrocytomas consisting mainly of immature cells, which, over time, tend to transform into more aggressive forms [12]. Oligodendroglioma originates from oligodendroglia cells and includes tumors with different grades and aggressivity, and ependymoma originates from ependymal cells that line the ventricular system and represent 2–3% of all brain tumors (Figure 1A) [13]. Finally, glioblastoma multiforme (GBM) is the most common, invasive, and malignant of all brain tumors, characterized by rapid growth and the invasion of adjacent regions of the brain, such as the meninges or cerebrospinal fluid [14].

According to the World Health Organization (WHO), GBM accounts for 75% of aggressive malignant brain tumors in adults [15] and has been classified as a grade IV tumor. Moreover, a further classification divides GBM into a primary tumor [16] that is aggressive and invasive whose are not derived from other diseases, and which represents the most common form (about 95%), affecting the elderly population. It is also classified as a secondary tumor [16], which derives instead from low-grade astrocytomas, with an incidence rate in young people [17]. Human GBM is a heterogeneous tumor consisting of tumor cells and a small portion of cancer stem cells (CSCs), which have a high tumorigenic potential and are characterized by excessive proliferation, invasiveness, and metastasis [18], and by high resistance to standard therapy, in which case the patient's estimated time of survival is about 15 months from the first diagnosis [19].

It was initially thought that GBM derived exclusively from glial cells, but scientific evidence has shown that there are other native cell types, similar to neuronal stem cells, from which GBM originates [20]. Glia, neurons, and stem cells show alterations in their functions that contribute to the development and progression of the tumor. There are two forms of heterogeneity in GBM: the intertumor and the intratumor. First, intertumoral heterogeneity refers to the genetic alterations that occur in individual tumors [21]. Secondly, intratumoral heterogeneity refers to the diversity of the phenotypes of the tumor cells that make up the tumor mass and other cellular entities recruited into TME, such as microglia and/or macrophages and endothelial cells [22]. However, it is difficult to identify their cell of origin [23] and remains a subject of debate to this day. Initially, considering the ability of astrocytes to replicate in the adult brain, it was hypothesized that an oncogenic alteration of astrocytes could give rise to GBM [23]; later, other hypotheses were developed, such as derivation from precursors such as oligodendrocytic or neuronal cells [24]. Recent studies have focused on glioma stem cells, which have the ability to self-renew and form tumors in vivo with the same characteristics as the primary tumor [25], offering greater resistance to chemotherapy, thus associating their presence with tumor heterogeneity [25,26]. Moreover, various pathways and molecular mechanisms are involved in the development and progression of GBM [27], including the microenvironment of GBM, characterized by hypoxic regions [18] whose oxygen deficiency determines the activation of the transcription factor; the hypoxia-inducible factor (HIF) [28], inducing gene transcription that promotes the production of various pro-angiogenic factors including vascular endothelial growth factor (VEGF) [29], which leads to the formation of new blood vessels; fibroblast growth factor (FGF) [30], which promotes the proliferation and differentiation of endothelial, smooth muscle, and fibroblast cells; and finally platelet growth factor (PDGF) [31], released by platelets and stimulating the proliferation and migration cancer cells, all factors that promote the progression of GBM.

The immune system is also an essential component for tumor development and progression, especially in GBM [32]. Activation of the immune system contributes to creating an immunosuppressive microenvironment in GBM [33], which consists of the production and release of immunosuppressive cytokines and chemokines, such as transforming growth factor-β (TGF-β), interleukin 10 (IL-10), prostaglandin E2 (PGE2), and many immune cells, such as immunosuppressive natural killer (NKT) cells, regulatory T/B cells (T/B-reg), tumor-associated macrophages (TAMs), and myeloid-derived suppressor cells (MDSC) [34,35].

The hypoxic state of the GBM microenvironment results in an increase in the concentration of adenosine, a small nucleoside and key mediator of several biological functions, thus defining it as tumor-derived adenosine [36]. In fact, adenosine through interaction with its four G protein-coupled receptors (GPCRs), A1, A2A, A2B, and A3, is involved in the blocking of anti-tumor immunity. Confirming what has been written, Hoskin et al. showed that adenosine, present in the GBM microenvironment, can inhibit the function of natural killer cells, as well as the ability of cytotoxic T cells to adhere to tumor cell targets [36]. In particular, it is thought that it is GBM itself, through activation of the A2A receptor, above all, which causes adenosine to carry out an activity opposite to the biological one. In fact, in this regard, almost 20% of human cancers contain mutations in genes that code for GPCRs [37]. By exploring the sequencing data from the Genomic Data Commons data portal (GDC), cancer-associated mutations of the A2A receptor affecting its activity were identified, further confirming the involvement of adenosine and its receptor in GBM development [38].

Treatment of GBM requires a multidisciplinary approach and consists of surgical excision, followed by radiation treatment with concomitant temozolomide (TMZ), and finally chemotherapy with TMZ [39], although, an unfavorable condition of combined treatment of radiotherapy and high-dose TMZ is lymphopenia, defined as a reduction in peripheral blood lymphocytes [40]. Where surgical excision is not possible, other therapeutic approaches are used, some of which have already been approved by regulatory agencies in the United States and consist of the use of monoclonal antibodies (mAb), such as Bevacizumab [41], a humanized mAb that blocks VEGF, blocking angiogenesis. Regorafenib is involved in GBM relapse, which acts on the processes of angiogenesis, with the modification of TME [42]. Tumor treatment field therapy (TTF) is a non-invasive anti-cancer treatment [43] that uses alternating electric fields tuned to low intensity (1–3V/cm) and intermediate frequency (100–300 kHz) to stop the splitting of solid tumor cells. This therapy has limitations due to its mechanism of action, which blocks biological processes, such as DNA repair mechanisms, and its cost [43,44]. Finally, gene therapy represents the recourse in the therapeutic approach for the treatment of GBM, which consists of the use of genetic fragments in association with viral vectors [45,46] capable of replicating within tumor cells, causing their death and also releasing viral particles capable of infecting and killing adjacent cancer cells [47]. In the context of GBM, considering the presence of immune cells with immunosuppressive action, an immune checkpoint has recently been identified, represented by BACE1; although BACE1 is a beta-secretase involved in the cleavage of the amyloid precursor protein [48] and used in the treatment of Alzheimer's disease (AD), its inhibition was effective for GBM. This approach represents an opportunity to safeguard depleted T lymphocytes, while also inducing increased infiltration of CD8$^+$ T lymphocytes into the GBM [49]. In addition, the use of chimeric antigen receptor T cells (CAT-T), which produce T cells capable of acting in TME, has been shown to be effective. Several antigens have been targeted with this technique, optimizing the anti-tumor activity [50]. A last therapeutic strategy recently discovered and still under development concerns the use of adenosine receptor antagonists [51], which have been shown to prevent the effects related to extracellular adenosine.

2. Adenosine and Adenosine Receptors (ARs)

Adenosine is a small molecule present throughout the human body, capable of performing various physiological functions following interaction with its receptor subtypes (A1, A2A, A2B, and A3). It is present in the cardiovascular system, where it modulates the vasoconstriction and vasodilation of arteries and veins [52]; in the metabolic context, adenosine inhibits lipolysis and induces bronchoconstriction [53,54], and regulates diuresis, muscle tone, and locomotion. At the level of the CNS, it exerts neuroprotective activity against ischemic events [55], hypoxia, and oxidative stress, and modulates the release of neurotransmitters; it is also involved in the regulation of cytokines and the production of T lymphocytes by the immune system [56,57]. There are two forms of adenosine: intracellular and extracellular [58], widely expressed in all tissues, and obtained by the dephosphorylation of its precursors, adenosine triphosphate (ATP), adenosine diphosphate (ADP), and adenosine monophosphate (AMP), or by hydrolysis of S-adenosylhomocysteine (SAH) [59]. Physiologically, the intracellular concentration of adenosine is regulated by an important enzyme known as adenosine kinase (ADK), and by two transporters: the equilibrative nucleoside transporters (ENT) and the bidirectional passive transporters, which play a critical role, as they allow free movement of adenosine across the cell membrane [60], and nucleoside concentrative transporters (CNTs), Na-dependent transporters that coordinate the adenosine gradient transport [61]. The direction of this nucleoside, absorbed or released by cells, is determined by the difference in concentration between the two forms, intracellular and extracellular, across the membrane [58]. Adenosine is defined as a "helper" in protecting cells such as neurons and cardiomyocytes against stressful conditions, allowing them to regulate their activity to reduce ATP requirements and ensure cell survival [58]. This is possible because adenosine can be released into the extracellular environment, where it acts as a specific modulator through cell surface receptors [56]; these receptors, called "ado receptors" (Ars), are GPCRs and are classified into four subtypes: A1, A2A, A2B, and A3 [62], which differ in the number of amino acids (Figure 2) and in their affinity towards adenosine. In fact, A1 and A2A possess a high affinity for adenosine compared to A2B and A3, which have a low affinity for the nucleoside [63].

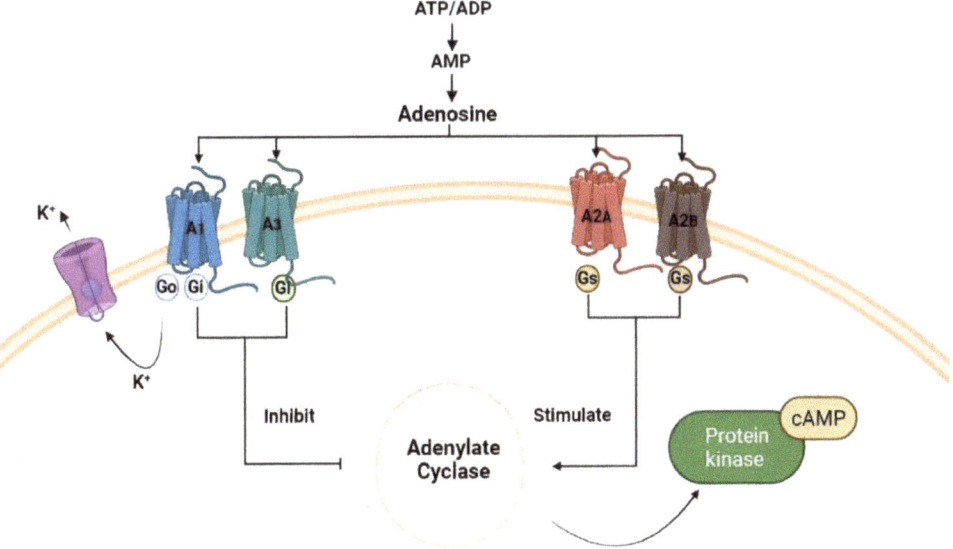

Figure 2. Figure created with Biorender.com. Production of adenosine starts from its precursors ATP, ADP, and AMP and subsequent binding of the nucleoside with the respective receptors A1, A2$_A$, A2$_B$, and A3.

Among them, A1A and A3A receptors are coupled to Gi and Go proteins that inhibit adenylate cyclase activity and reduce intracellular cAMP levels. This will result in the activation of phospholipase C(PLC)-β, thereby increasing inositol-1,4,5-triphosphate (IP$_3$) [64] and intracellular calcium levels, which in turn stimulate activation of the Ca-dependent protein kinase (PKC) and all calcium-binding proteins [64]. In the CNS, A1AR is expressed in microglia/macrophages and neurons, and plays a crucial role in their activation [65]; peripherally, it is also highly expressed in cardiac, renal, and adipose tissue. As demonstrated by Synowitz M. et al. in A1AR knockout mice, there is an increase in neuroinflammation and microglia activity [66], and this suggests that, in pathological conditions, A1AR activation produces a neuroprotective effect [67]. In physiological conditions, adenosine, through A1AR, determined a decrease in the proliferation of astrocytes, inducing the release of neurotrophic growth factor (NGF) [68]. A3AR, however, has a low expression in the CNS, but it is highly expressed in immune cells [59], cardiac cells, epithelial cells, colon mucosa, lung parenchyma, and bronchi. It is demonstrated that A3AR is expressed in cells involved in inflammatory processes, suggesting its potential involvement in inflammatory pathologies, such as lung injury, autoimmune diseases, and eye diseases [69]. Moreover, A3AR is present in many types of tumor cells, including astrocytomas, lymphoma, GBM, and other types of cancers [70].

A2AA and A2BA receptors are coupled to the Gs proteins, activating adenylate cyclase and increasing intracellular cAMP levels [71]; moreover, A2AAR activation can promote Protein kinase C (PKC) activation into cyclic AMP-dependent or independent mechanisms [72]. A2BAR activation, however, can stimulate PKC activity by coupling with the Gq protein [73]. They are mainly expressed in the CNS, especially in pre-synaptic regions of the hippocampus, where the release of neurotransmitters such as glutamate, acetylcholine, GABA, and noradrenaline is modulated [74,75], and in post-synaptic regions of the basal ganglia, where they modulate neuronal plasticity. They are also expressed in the astrocytes and oligodendrocytes [76,77] and on the cell surfaces of the immune system [78], such as regulatory T cells, macrophages, and natural killer cells (NKCs) [79], suggesting that they could be valid candidates for cancer immunotherapy. All subtypes of adenosine receptors are expressed on the surface of immune cells, such as macrophages and monocytes, and their expression is regulated by pro-inflammatory cytokines, especially IL-1B and the tumor necrosis factor (TNF) [80], which determined an increase in A2AAR levels on human monocytes [81]. The same pro-inflammatory stimuli regulate the expression of the A2BAR of the macrophages [82]. In physiological conditions, central A2AAR increases NGF and brain-derived neurotrophic factor (BDNF) levels from the hippocampus and cortical neurons [83]. Therefore, given both the prevalence of A2AAR in the CNS and its expression regulated by pro-inflammatory cytokines, this receptor plays a crucial role in inflammatory processes involving microglia, determining the release of IL-1β and IL-18 [84]. In fact, an antagonistic action against A2AAR prevents hippocampal neuroinflammation and IL-1β-induced exacerbation of neuronal toxicity [85]. Evidence showed that, in spinal intermediate neurons of the striatum, this receptor is related to the dopaminergic D2 receptor, where direct and indirect interactions with cholinergic, GABAergic, dopaminergic, and glutamatergic systems have been described, both in the basal ganglia and in other brain structures [86]. In the periphery, A2AAR is localized in the vascular smooth muscle and, together with A1AR, exerts a vasodilatory action. In this context, at the coronary levels, vasodilation mediated by the activation of A2AAR and A1AR is induced by the endothelial enzyme nitric oxidase synthase [87], producing large quantities of nitric oxide and inducing an increase in coronary flow, thus exerting a cardio-protective role [87], and this action depends on an increase in the intracellular cAMP levels [87]. Depending on the location of its receptors by which it interacts, adenosine exerts multiple physiological actions, including the protection of normal tissues and organs from the autoimmune response of immune cells, following binding with A2AAR [88]. In this regard, following damage to the cell, such as hypoxia, inflammation, and tissue injury, ADK activity is reduced, leading to increased levels of extracellular adenosine [59] in the extracellular space, which modulates the immune response, thus containing the inflammatory damage tissue. However, chronic exposure to extracellular adenosine can be harmful in some conditions, as adenosine itself can create an immunosuppressed niche, which is necessary for the development of neoplasia and infections [89,90]. In this context, it has been observed that T_{reg} cells can release ATP, convert it to adenosine, and cause cytotoxic T cell suppression in the local tumor environment [91].

3. The Role of Adenosine in Glioblastoma Multiforme

Studies report that extracellular adenosine is an important regulator of several aspects of tumorigenesis, angiogenesis, tumor cell growth, and metastasis [92]. Kezemi et al. provide an interesting review of the expression of adenosine receptors in different tumor cell lines and their effect, including proliferative and tumor-protective expressions, following their activation [93].

It is hypothesized that in the brain, ATP released from the pre- and post-synaptic terminals of neurons and glial cells is the source of extracellular adenosine [94]. In the extracellular area, adenosine is produced from ATP after dephosphorylation by specific ectoenzymes, in this case, CD39 and CD73, expressed in microglial cells [90]. In physiological conditions, CD39 and CD73 exert an important role in the purinergic signals delivered to immune cells through the conversion of ADP/ATP to AMP to adenosine [95]. The CD39/CD73 pathway changes with the pathophysiological context in which it is embedded [89]. It has been demonstrated in vivo study that mice deprived of CD73 presented a lower level of extracellular adenosine, suggesting that ATP degradation is the main source of extracellular adenosine [96]. CD39 is expressed on the surface of the regulatory T cells, and it is the dominant ectoenzyme that controls extracellular nucleoside concentration [90]. Considering that angiogenesis is an important process for the growth of the tumor cells, it has been demonstrated that in mice deprived of CD39, angiogenesis is blocked, causing a slowdown in tumor growth [95].

High concentrations of adenosine and its receptors have also been found in the interstitial fluid tumor, modulating tumor growth [97]. Since the TME contains high levels of extracellular adenosine, it is hypothesized that tumor-derived adenosine is a mechanism by which tumors evade the immune response [98,99]. This evasion strategy is due not so much to the inability of immune cells to recognize the tumor, but the failure of the immune system to activate in the presence of the antigen [100] due to the inhibition of T cells by adenosine itself [100].

It is known that the immune system, through antigen-presenting cells (APC), is able to recognize a specific antigen [101], subsequently allowing the binding with B and T lymphocytes through their receptors, B-cell receptor (BCR) and T-cell receptor (TCR), respectively, thus initiating the immune response. In this tumor context, the activation of the immune system will lead to the secretion of anti-cancer cytokines [102], such as Interferon-gamma (INF-γ), TNF-α, and IL-6, and cell phagocytosis to eliminate the tumor, thus becoming a tool for the development of new treatments in cancer therapy [103]. Nevertheless, most tumors are able to implement various mechanisms to evade the immune response, such as inhibiting tumor-specific immune cells [104]. As is often the case, a particular tumor may express an antigen that, if presented by resting cells or by unprofessional APCs, recognition of the TCR will not lead to tumor destruction, but to inactivation of the tumor-specific T cell [105] (Figure 3).

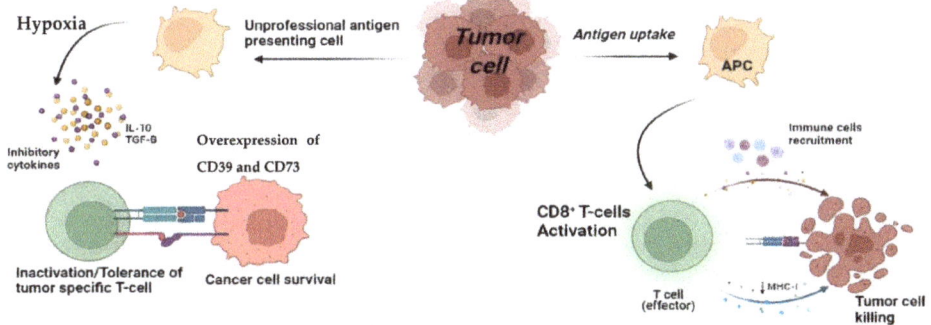

Figure 3. Figure created with Biorender.com. **Right:** induction of the immune response by antigen presenting by APC, with consequent activation of effector CD8⁺ T cells and recruitment of immune cells, with the elimination of the tumor cell. **Left:** lack of immune response, following antigen presentation by non-professional APC cells. The tumor microenvironment, characterized by hypoxia and the presence of inhibitory cytokines and cytokines such as IL-10 and TGF-β, leads to inactivation and/or tolerance of effector T cells with the consequent escape of the tumor from the immune response.

An important aspect of the mechanism of escape by the tumor from the immune system is the TME [106], which is characterized by a hypoxic state and is rich in inhibitory ligands and cytokines, such as IL-10 and TGF-β, which lead to tolerance by the immune cells towards the tumor [107,108] (Figure 3). These conditions determine the increase in the expression of CD39 and CD73 [89], present on the surface of the tumor by stimulating the production of extracellular adenosine, by activating A2AAR. Moreover, at the same time, there is a reduction in the activity of the adenosine metabolizing enzyme, ADK [109].

In addition, it has been reported that the deletion of functional adenosine receptors, in particular A1AR, results in increased GBM growth [66]. However, subsequent studies have found that the interaction of adenosine with A2AAR induces inhibition of the adaptive immune response, inhibiting the function of CD4[+] and CD8[+] T cells and NKCs and IL-2/Nkp46-activated NK cells specifically via A2AAR [110], thus promoting tumor escape from the immune system and metastasis [111,112]. Several in vitro and in vivo studies report that genetic deletion of the A2AAR enhances the anti-tumor responses, confirming adenosine's role in evading the tumor from the immune system [113]. Second, adenosine appears to block both the generation and effector phases of anti-tumor responses. In vitro studies have been conducted on GBM cell lines U87MG, U373MG [59], and ASB19, which were subjected to hypoxia [59] for 24 and 72 hrs using ATB702 dichloride hydrate (15uM), an ADK inhibitor, and resulted in an accumulation of adenosine [114]. Subsequently, the cells were treated with TMZ (100 μM), which resulted in a decrease in the vitality of the tumor cells compared with the control GBM cells, thus demonstrating the tumor-protective role of endogenous adenosine against TMZ [115].

It has been shown that extracellular adenosine, defined as an immunosuppressive factor through interaction with its receptor, exploiting the hypoxic condition of the TME [116], is able to lead to an increase in intracellular cAMP, inhibiting lymphocyte-mediated cytolysis and, consequently, functional inhibition of immune cells, thus acting as a protective shield against the tumor, helping it to evade the immune system [99]. Therefore, if GBM cells contribute to immunosuppression, the immune cells recruited into the tumor may also participate in its immune escape [32]. Indeed, most of the anti-tumor immune cells recruited to the TME adopt an immunosuppressive phenotype due to the cytokines secreted by GBM [32].

In this context, a large number of experiments have shown that the concentration of adenosine in the TME is much higher than in normal tissues [117].

Hypoxia and tissue damage are not the only factors determining the release of extracellular adenosine; it is also generated from extracellular nucleotides by ectonucleotidases [95] CD39 and CD73 [89]. Through clinical studies, CD73, rather than CD39, was found to be a critical component in adenosine accumulation and tumor immunosuppression. Indeed, overexpression of CD73 was reported to be a component of glioma cell adhesion and tumor cell–extracellular matrix interactions [118].

Moreover, high adenosine concentrations also induce receptor-independent reactions by reversing the reaction catalyzed by S-adenosylhomocysteine hydrolase (SAH-hydrolase), leading to an accumulation of SAH-inhibiting methyltransferases [119], as was shown in a recent study in which adenosine induced DNA hypomethylation in the brain by inhibiting trans-methylation reactions [120]. This connection between adenosine and methyl group metabolism is important for diagnostic purposes because an alteration in methyl group metabolism has been shown to be a risk factor in brain diseases such as GBM and neurodegenerative diseases [121,122].

In vitro and in vivo studies have shown that the presence of adenosine receptors in microglia is well established [123]. Cell cultures of rat microglia specifically express the A2AAR and were treated with the specific agonist CGS21680, inducing the expression of K[+] channels, which are linked to microglia activation [124]. Again, there is conflicting evidence regarding the role of this receptor: stimulation of the A2AAR in rat microglia induces the expression of nerve growth factor and its release, thus exerting a neuroprotective effect [125], and at the same time induces the expression of Cyclooxygenase-2 (COX-2) in rat microglia by releasing prostaglandin [126].

To confirm the involvement of adenosine and its receptors in tumorigenesis and its tumor-protective role, in vivo studies were conducted using the adenosine receptor agonists or antagonists [127]. A2AAR blocking using SCH58261, an A2AAR antagonist, inhibited the tumor growth, reducing CD4[+] and regulatory T cells, and improving the anti-tumor response by T cells [127].

There is conflicting evidence regarding adenosine-mediated receptor actions on GBM proliferation. In glioblastoma stem cells, activation of A1AR and A2BAR appears to have reduced tumor proliferation and induced apoptosis [119], whereas in non-glioblastoma stem cell lines, activation of A1, A2B and/or A3 receptors induced an increase in proliferation. Liu et al. reported a pro-proliferative action of adenosine mediated by activation of the A2B receptor on glioblastoma cell lines subjected to hypoxia [128].

4. Adenosine Receptor Antagonists

The A2R-mediated adenosine pathway and its immunosuppressive role has allowed research to focus on novel therapeutic approaches to provide prolonged life expectancy in patients with tumors refractory to other therapies. One such approach that has proved effective in enhancing immunotherapy involves the development of selective adenosine receptor antagonists [129], which are able to prevent the effects of extracellular adenosine produced by both tissue and T cells [127]. Given that the first clinical trials of A2AAR antagonists date back to 2020, further clinical studies are underway regarding the antitumor activity, as well as the efficacy, of these new therapeutic candidates.

Adenosine receptor antagonists belong to a variety of chemical classes and are divided into two groups: xanthine derivates, of which the best known are Istradefylline (KW-6002) [130] and 3,7-dimethyl-1-propargylxanthine derivates (DMPX), and non-xanthine derivates, the Polyheterocyclic nitrogen system, especially Ciforadenant (CPI-444) and Imaradenant (AZD4635) [131] (Figure 4).

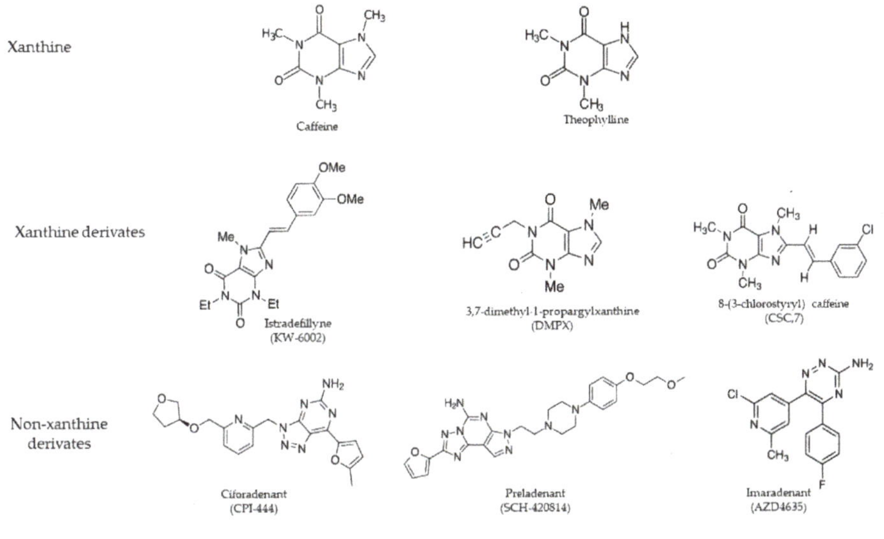

Figure 4. The main adenosine receptor antagonists divided into xanthine derivatives and non-xanthine derivatives.

4.1. Xanthine Derivates

Compounds belonging to this group result from modifications of the two main alkaloids, caffeine and theophylline [132]. These derivates show a high affinity for all the adenosine receptors, but in the GBM context, receptor affinity must be directed towards A2AAR in order to bind it selectively and competitively, reducing adenylate cyclase activity [133]. The main A2AAR xanthine antagonists are 8-(3-chlorostyryl) caffeine (CSC,7), 1,3-dipropyl-7-methyl-8-(3,4,-dimethoxystyryl)xanthine (KF 17837), 3,7-dimethyl-1-propargylxanthine derivates (DMPX), and Istradefylline (KW-6002), which has a K_i of 2.2 nM, and is an extremely strong, selective, and orally active adenosine A2A receptor antagonist [134]. DMPX was the first selective A2AAR to be detected [135]. Many selective A2AAR antagonists have been obtained, some of which are being used in clinical trials for neurodegenerative diseases such as Parkinson's disease, given the interconnection between dopaminergic D2 receptors and adenosine [136,137].

4.2. Polyheterocyclic Nitrogen System

Another group of A2AAR antagonists is represented by the polyheterocyclic nitrogen system, including Preladenant (SCH-420814), Ciforadenant (CPI-444) [138], Taminadenant (NIR178) [139], Imaradenant (AZD4635) [131], SCH442416 [140], and ZM241385 [141], characterized by small molecules that selectively bind to the A2A receptor, competitively inhibiting adenosine binding and signaling [142]. In the GBM context, this compound presents troubles that prevent its use in clinical trials, as it has a high binding affinity for the A2B receptor subtype [138]. With a K_i of 0.048 for human A2AAR, the SCH442416 antagonist is considered a strong, selective, and brain-penetrant antagonist of A2AAR [143]. However, strong evidence has been shown by Ciforadenant being active in multiple preclinical tumor models, both as monotherapy and in combination with PDL1 targets, and it has over 66-fold selectivity over the adenosine A1 receptor [144] (Table 1). Clinical studies conducted on GBM patients under 1 and 4 months of treatment with Ciforadenant have shown that it possesses immunomodulatory effects [145]. Through in vitro studies, it was possible to characterize adenosine-related gene expression with the production of chemokines and cytokines, including CXCL5, CCl2, IL-8, and CXCL1, of monocytic, CD14+ origin, using the receptor agonist NECA [146], and how Ciforadenant is able to neutralize them [145]. Thus, these reports suggest that adenosine signaling not only directly reduces T lymphocyte immunity but also shifts the balance from T effector responses to both recruitment and myeloid suppressor functions [138].

Table 1. Summary of the binding selectivity of adenosine receptor antagonists.

Adenosine Receptor Antagonists	Summary of Adenosine Receptor Antagonists				
	A1	A2$_A$	A2$_B$	A3	References
Xanthine derivates					
Caffeine	+	+	+	+	[132]
Theophylline	+	+	+	+	[132]
DMPX	+	+++	++	+	[135]
Istradefylline	+	+++	+	+	[130]
Taminadenant	+	++	+	++	[139]
Non-Xanthine derivates					
Ciforadenant	+++	+++	++	+	[138]
Imaradenant	++	+++	+	+	[131]
SCH442416	+	+++	++	+	[140]
ZM241385	+	+++	++	++	[141]

+ Low selectivity for adenosine ++ Halfway selectivity for adenosine +++ High selectivity for adenosine.

4.3. Enhancement of Immunotherapy Induced by Adenosine Receptor Antagonists

Another therapeutic approach to enhance immunotherapy targets the immune cells in the TME [56]. As previously reported, the A2AAR is expressed on the surface of many cells of the immune system, the activation of which induced an immunosuppressive effect [56]. Consequently, a selective A2AAR antagonist reducing intracellular cAMP levels allows lymphocytes to effectively fight tumor cells. Since A2A and A2B adenosine receptors are coupled to the G proteins, and both increase intracellular cAMP levels [71], the use of A2BAR antagonists leads to a reduction in cAMP by restoring the anti-tumor functions of lymphocytes [145]. It is of interest to note the relationship between A2A and A2B adenosine receptors: A2A is involved in the expression of A2BAR [67]; furthermore, its activity is influenced by the expression of A2BAR, and both proteins can interact to form new functional units [147]. This evidence, therefore, suggests that blocking these receptors may be an effective means of combating cancer [147]. In this regard, clinical trials are already underway in patients with different tumor types where either the use of selective antagonists for individual receptors or dual antagonists is employed [56].

For the treatment of advanced malignant tumors, such as GBM, a trial has been updated for 2021, showing the combined treatment of the dual A2AAR/A2BAR antagonist with the AB122 antibody and standard chemotherapy [56].

5. Future Perspectives

Given the increasing mortality rate caused by GBM and despite the many strategies adopted to counteract the tumor's progression, current treatments do not appear to be effective in influencing tumor growth. It is clear that each tumor is unique and different from the others, and that is why the development of drugs capable of blocking its growth and at the same time reducing the impact of therapy on the body requires a better understanding of the mechanisms triggered by the tumor. Here, the knowledge about the adenosine pathway and its involvement in the TME has been established and would support research and the discovery of new strategies, including the development of adenosine receptor antagonists. Other approaches to boost immunotherapy would be the use of dual antagonists, both for the A2A and A2B adenosine receptors, given their functional interconnection as immunosuppressive agents.

6. Conclusions

Despite the positive results and the numerous clinical trials underway, there are limitations to the development of these new candidates due to the pharmacokinetic complexity. Therefore, considering the promising effect of adenosine receptor antagonists, they could represent alternative treatments for GBM by using them alone or in combination with chemotherapy to improve patients' quality of life.

Author Contributions: I.P., E.E. and S.C. contributed to the conception and design of the review; G.C. (Giovanna Casili), M.L., M.C., A.P.C., A.R. and L.C. contributed to the interpretation of studies included in the review; V.B. and A.F. drafted the text; V.B. and A.F. contributed to preparing the figures; G.M., C.C. and G.C. (Giulia Chisari) contributed to the revision of the review. All authors have read and agreed to the published version of the manuscript.

Funding: This research received no external funding.

Conflicts of Interest: The authors declare no conflict of interest.

References

1. Bondy, M.L.; Scheurer, M.E.; Malmer, B.; Barnholtz-Sloan, J.S.; Davis, F.G.; Il'yasova, D.; Kruchko, C.; McCarthy, B.J.; Rajaraman, P.; Schwartzbaum, J.A.; et al. Brain tumor epidemiology: Consensus from the Brain Tumor Epidemiology Consortium. *Cancer* **2008**, *113*, 1953–1968. [CrossRef] [PubMed]
2. Daneman, R.; Zhou, L.; Kebede, A.A.; Barres, B.A. Pericytes are required for blood-brain barrier integrity during embryogenesis. *Nature* **2010**, *468*, 562–566. [CrossRef] [PubMed]
3. Wu, K.L.; Chan, S.H.; Chan, J.Y. Neuroinflammation and oxidative stress in rostral ventrolateral medulla contribute to neurogenic hypertension induced by systemic inflammation. *J. Neuroinflamm.* **2012**, *9*, 212. [CrossRef]
4. McFaline-Figueroa, J.R.; Lee, E.Q. Brain Tumors. *Am. J. Med.* **2018**, *131*, 874–882. [CrossRef] [PubMed]
5. Ansell, P.; Johnston, T.; Simpson, J.; Crouch, S.; Roman, E.; Picton, S. Brain tumor signs and symptoms: Analysis of primary health care records from the UKCCS. *Pediatrics* **2010**, *125*, 112–119. [CrossRef]
6. Minniti, G.; Traish, D.; Ashley, S.; Gonsalves, A.; Brada, M. Risk of second brain tumor after conservative surgery and radiotherapy for pituitary adenoma: Update after an additional 10 years. *J. Clin. Endocrinol. Metab.* **2005**, *90*, 800–804. [CrossRef]
7. Wirsching, H.G.; Galanis, E.; Weller, M. Glioblastoma. *Handb. Clin. Neurol.* **2016**, *134*, 381–397. [CrossRef]
8. Kaplan, K.; Kaya, Y.; Kuncan, M.; Ertunc, H.M. Brain tumor classification using modified local binary patterns (LBP) feature extraction methods. *Med. Hypotheses* **2020**, *139*, 109696. [CrossRef]

9. Ardizzone, A.; Scuderi, S.A.; Giuffrida, D.; Colarossi, C.; Puglisi, C.; Campolo, M.; Cuzzocrea, S.; Esposito, E.; Paterniti, I. Role of Fibroblast Growth Factors Receptors (FGFRs) in Brain Tumors, Focus on Astrocytoma and Glioblastoma. *Cancers* **2020**, *12*, 3825. [CrossRef]
10. Jiang, Y.; Uhrbom, L. On the origin of glioma. *Upsala J. Med. Sci.* **2012**, *117*, 113–121. [CrossRef]
11. Watanabe, T.; Nobusawa, S.; Kleihues, P.; Ohgaki, H. IDH1 mutations are early events in the development of astrocytomas and oligodendrogliomas. *Am. J. Pathol.* **2009**, *174*, 1149–1153. [CrossRef] [PubMed]
12. Al-Ali, F.; Hendon, A.J.; Liepman, M.K.; Wisniewski, J.L.; Krinock, M.J.; Beckman, K. Oligodendroglioma metastatic to bone marrow. *AJNR Am. J. Neuroradiol.* **2005**, *26*, 2410–2414. [PubMed]
13. Neumann, J.E.; Spohn, M.; Obrecht, D.; Mynarek, M.; Thomas, C.; Hasselblatt, M.; Dorostkar, M.M.; Wefers, A.K.; Frank, S.; Monoranu, C.M.; et al. Molecular characterization of histopathological ependymoma variants. *Acta Neuropathol.* **2020**, *139*, 305–318. [CrossRef] [PubMed]
14. Kim, W.; Yoo, H.; Shin, S.H.; Gwak, H.S.; Lee, S.H. Extraneural Metastases of Glioblastoma without Simultaneous Central Nervous System Recurrence. *Brain Tumor Res. Treat.* **2014**, *2*, 124–127. [CrossRef]
15. Scuderi, S.A.; Casili, G.; Ardizzone, A.; Forte, S.; Colarossi, L.; Sava, S.; Paterniti, I.; Esposito, E.; Cuzzocrea, S.; Campolo, M. KYP-2047, an Inhibitor of Prolyl-Oligopeptidase, Reduces GlioBlastoma Proliferation through Angiogenesis and Apoptosis Modulation. *Cancers* **2021**, *13*, 3444. [CrossRef]
16. Ohgaki, H.; Kleihues, P. Genetic pathways to primary and secondary glioblastoma. *Am. J. Pathol.* **2007**, *170*, 1445–1453. [CrossRef]
17. Louis, D.N. Molecular pathology of malignant gliomas. *Annu. Rev. Pathol.* **2006**, *1*, 97–117. [CrossRef]
18. Colwell, N.; Larion, M.; Giles, A.J.; Seldomridge, A.N.; Sizdahkhani, S.; Gilbert, M.R.; Park, D.M. Hypoxia in the glioblastoma microenvironment: Shaping the phenotype of cancer stem-like cells. *Neuro Oncol.* **2017**, *19*, 887–896. [CrossRef]
19. Jovcevska, I. Genetic secrets of long-term glioblastoma survivors. *Bosn. J. Basic Med. Sci.* **2019**, *19*, 116–124. [CrossRef]
20. Kim, H.J.; Park, J.W.; Lee, J.H. Genetic Architectures and Cell-of-Origin in Glioblastoma. *Front. Oncol.* **2020**, *10*, 615400. [CrossRef]
21. Dirkse, A.; Golebiewska, A.; Buder, T.; Nazarov, P.V.; Muller, A.; Poovathingal, S.; Brons, N.H.C.; Leite, S.; Sauvageot, N.; Sarkisjan, D.; et al. Stem cell-associated heterogeneity in Glioblastoma results from intrinsic tumor plasticity shaped by the microenvironment. *Nat. Commun.* **2019**, *10*, 1787. [CrossRef] [PubMed]
22. Anderson, N.M.; Simon, M.C. The tumor microenvironment. *Curr. Biol.* **2020**, *30*, R921–R925. [CrossRef] [PubMed]
23. Heiland, D.H.; Ravi, V.M.; Behringer, S.P.; Frenking, J.H.; Wurm, J.; Joseph, K.; Garrelfs, N.W.C.; Strahle, J.; Heynckes, S.; Grauvogel, J.; et al. Tumor-associated reactive astrocytes aid the evolution of immunosuppressive environment in glioblastoma. *Nat. Commun.* **2019**, *10*, 2541. [CrossRef] [PubMed]
24. Zong, H.; Verhaak, R.G.; Canoll, P. The cellular origin for malignant glioma and prospects for clinical advancements. *Expert Rev. Mol. Diagn.* **2012**, *12*, 383–394. [CrossRef]
25. Ohta, A.; Sitkovsky, M. Role of G-protein-coupled adenosine receptors in downregulation of inflammation and protection from tissue damage. *Nature* **2001**, *414*, 916–920. [CrossRef]
26. Koritzinsky, M.; Seigneuric, R.; Magagnin, M.G.; van den Beucken, T.; Lambin, P.; Wouters, B.G. The hypoxic proteome is influenced by gene-specific changes in mRNA translation. *Radiother. Oncol.* **2005**, *76*, 177–186. [CrossRef]
27. Liebelt, B.D.; Shingu, T.; Zhou, X.; Ren, J.; Shin, S.A.; Hu, J. Glioma Stem Cells: Signaling, Microenvironment, and Therapy. *Stem. Cells Int.* **2016**, *2016*, 7849890. [CrossRef]
28. Kietzmann, T.; Mennerich, D.; Dimova, E.Y. Hypoxia-Inducible Factors (HIFs) and Phosphorylation: Impact on Stability, Localization, and Transactivity. *Front. Cell Dev. Biol.* **2016**, *4*, 11. [CrossRef]
29. Das, S.; Marsden, P.A. Angiogenesis in glioblastoma. *N. Engl. J. Med.* **2013**, *369*, 1561–1563. [CrossRef]
30. Gabler, L.; Jaunecker, C.N.; Katz, S.; van Schoonhoven, S.; Englinger, B.; Pirker, C.; Mohr, T.; Vician, P.; Stojanovic, M.; Woitzuck, V.; et al. Fibroblast growth factor receptor 4 promotes glioblastoma progression: A central role of integrin-mediated cell invasiveness. *Acta Neuropathol. Commun.* **2022**, *10*, 65. [CrossRef]
31. Westermark, B. Platelet-derived growth factor in glioblastoma-driver or biomarker? *Upsala J. Med. Sci.* **2014**, *119*, 298–305. [CrossRef] [PubMed]
32. Pearson, J.R.D.; Cuzzubbo, S.; McArthur, S.; Durrant, L.G.; Adhikaree, J.; Tinsley, C.J.; Pockley, A.G.; McArdle, S.E.B. Immune Escape in Glioblastoma Multiforme and the Adaptation of Immunotherapies for Treatment. *Front. Immunol.* **2020**, *11*, 582106. [CrossRef] [PubMed]
33. Chouaib, S.; El Hage, F.; Benlalam, H.; Mami-Chouaib, F. Immunotherapy of cancer: Promise and reality. *Med. Sci.* **2006**, *22*, 755–759. [CrossRef]
34. Nakamura, K.; Smyth, M.J. Myeloid immunosuppression and immune checkpoints in the tumor microenvironment. *Cell. Mol. Immunol.* **2020**, *17*, 1–12. [CrossRef] [PubMed]
35. Goswami, S.; Walle, T.; Cornish, A.E.; Basu, S.; Anandhan, S.; Fernandez, I.; Vence, L.; Blando, J.; Zhao, H.; Yadav, S.S.; et al. Immune profiling of human tumors identifies CD73 as a combinatorial target in glioblastoma. *Nat. Med.* **2020**, *26*, 39–46. [CrossRef] [PubMed]
36. Fishman, P.; Bar-Yehuda, S.; Synowitz, M.; Powell, J.D.; Klotz, K.N.; Gessi, S.; Borea, P.A. Adenosine receptors and cancer. *Handb. Exp. Pharmacol.* **2009**, *193*, 399–441. [CrossRef]
37. Borea, P.A.; Gessi, S.; Merighi, S.; Vincenzi, F.; Varani, K. Pharmacology of adenosine receptors: The state of the art. *Physiol. Rev.* **2018**, *98*, 1591–1625. [CrossRef]

38. O'Hayre, M.; Vazquez-Prado, J.; Kufareva, I.; Stawiski, E.W.; Handel, T.M.; Seshagiri, S.; Gutkind, J.S. The emerging mutational landscape of G proteins and G-protein-coupled receptors in cancer. *Nat. Rev. Cancer* **2013**, *13*, 412–424. [CrossRef]
39. Geraldo, L.H.M.; Garcia, C.; da Fonseca, A.C.C.; Dubois, L.G.F.; de Sampaio, E.S.T.C.L.; Matias, D.; de Camargo Magalhaes, E.S.; do Amaral, R.F.; da Rosa, B.G.; Grimaldi, I.; et al. Glioblastoma Therapy in the Age of Molecular Medicine. *Trends Cancer* **2019**, *5*, 46–65. [CrossRef]
40. Stupp, R.; Dietrich, P.Y.; Ostermann Kraljevic, S.; Pica, A.; Maillard, I.; Maeder, P.; Meuli, R.; Janzer, R.; Pizzolato, G.; Miralbell, R.; et al. Promising survival for patients with newly diagnosed glioblastoma multiforme treated with concomitant radiation plus temozolomide followed by adjuvant temozolomide. *J. Clin. Oncol.* **2002**, *20*, 1375–1382. [CrossRef]
41. Ghiaseddin, A.; Peters, K.B. Use of bevacizumab in recurrent glioblastoma. *CNS Oncol.* **2015**, *4*, 157–169. [CrossRef] [PubMed]
42. Lombardi, G.; Caccese, M.; Padovan, M.; Cerretti, G.; Pintacuda, G.; Manara, R.; Di Sarra, F.; Zagonel, V. Regorafenib in Recurrent Glioblastoma Patients: A Large and Monocentric Real-Life Study. *Cancers* **2021**, *13*, 4731. [CrossRef] [PubMed]
43. Green, A.L.; Mulcahy Levy, J.M.; Vibhakar, R.; Hemenway, M.; Madden, J.; Foreman, N.; Dorris, K. Tumor treating fields in pediatric high-grade glioma. *Childs Nerv. Syst.* **2017**, *33*, 1043–1045. [CrossRef] [PubMed]
44. Mehta, M.; Wen, P.; Nishikawa, R.; Reardon, D.; Peters, K. Critical review of the addition of tumor treating fields (TTFields) to the existing standard of care for newly diagnosed glioblastoma patients. *Crit. Rev. Oncol. Hematol.* **2017**, *111*, 60–65. [CrossRef] [PubMed]
45. Ram, Z.; Culver, K.W.; Oshiro, E.M.; Viola, J.J.; DeVroom, H.L.; Otto, E.; Long, Z.; Chiang, Y.; McGarrity, G.J.; Muul, L.M.; et al. Therapy of malignant brain tumors by intratumoral implantation of retroviral vector-producing cells. *Nat. Med.* **1997**, *3*, 1354–1361. [CrossRef]
46. Klatzmann, D.; Valery, C.A.; Bensimon, G.; Marro, B.; Boyer, O.; Mokhtari, K.; Diquet, B.; Salzmann, J.L.; Philippon, J. A phase I/II study of herpes simplex virus type 1 thymidine kinase "suicide" gene therapy for recurrent glioblastoma. Study Group on Gene Therapy for Glioblastoma. *Hum. Gene Ther.* **1998**, *9*, 2595–2604. [CrossRef]
47. Raffel, C.; Culver, K.; Kohn, D.; Nelson, M.; Siegel, S.; Gillis, F.; Link, C.J.; Villablanca, J.G.; Anderson, W.F. Gene therapy for the treatment of recurrent pediatric malignant astrocytomas with in vivo tumor transduction with the herpes simplex thymidine kinase gene/ganciclovir system. *Hum. Gene Ther.* **1994**, *5*, 863–890. [CrossRef]
48. Zhou, W.; Qing, H.; Tong, Y.; Song, W. BACE1 gene expression and protein degradation. *Ann. N. Y. Acad. Sci.* **2004**, *1035*, 49–67. [CrossRef]
49. Cloughesy, T.F.; Mochizuki, A.Y.; Orpilla, J.R.; Hugo, W.; Lee, A.H.; Davidson, T.B.; Wang, A.C.; Ellingson, B.M.; Rytlewski, J.A.; Sanders, C.M.; et al. Neoadjuvant anti-PD-1 immunotherapy promotes a survival benefit with intratumoral and systemic immune responses in recurrent glioblastoma. *Nat. Med.* **2019**, *25*, 477–486. [CrossRef]
50. Bagley, S.J.; Desai, A.S.; Linette, G.P.; June, C.H.; O'Rourke, D.M. CAR T-cell therapy for glioblastoma: Recent clinical advances and future challenges. *Neuro Oncol.* **2018**, *20*, 1429–1438. [CrossRef]
51. Decking, U.K.; Schlieper, G.; Kroll, K.; Schrader, J. Hypoxia-induced inhibition of adenosine kinase potentiates cardiac adenosine release. *Circ. Res.* **1997**, *81*, 154–164. [CrossRef] [PubMed]
52. Li, J.; Fenton, R.A.; Wheeler, H.B.; Powell, C.C.; Peyton, B.D.; Cutler, B.S.; Dobson, J.G., Jr. Adenosine A2a receptors increase arterial endothelial cell nitric oxide. *J. Surg. Res.* **1998**, *80*, 357–364. [CrossRef] [PubMed]
53. Bouma, M.G.; Stad, R.K.; van den Wildenberg, F.A.; Buurman, W.A. Differential regulatory effects of adenosine on cytokine release by activated human monocytes. *J. Immunol.* **1994**, *153*, 4159–4168. [PubMed]
54. Van der Graaf, P.H.; Van Schaick, E.A.; Visser, S.A.; De Greef, H.J.; Ijzerman, A.P.; Danhof, M. Mechanism-based pharmacokinetic-pharmacodynamic modeling of antilipolytic effects of adenosine A(1) receptor agonists in rats: Prediction of tissue-dependent efficacy in vivo. *J. Pharmacol. Exp. Ther.* **1999**, *290*, 702–709. [PubMed]
55. Williams-Karnesky, R.L.; Stenzel-Poore, M.P. Adenosine and stroke: Maximizing the therapeutic potential of adenosine as a prophylactic and acute neuroprotectant. *Curr. Neuropharmacol.* **2009**, *7*, 217–227. [CrossRef]
56. Franco, R.; Rivas-Santisteban, R.; Navarro, G.; Reyes-Resina, I. Adenosine Receptor Antagonists to Combat Cancer and to Boost Anti-Cancer Chemotherapy and Immunotherapy. *Cells* **2021**, *10*, 2831. [CrossRef]
57. Coney, A.M.; Marshall, J.M. Role of adenosine and its receptors in the vasodilatation induced in the cerebral cortex of the rat by systemic hypoxia. *J. Physiol.* **1998**, *509 Pt 2*, 507–518. [CrossRef]
58. Manjunath, S.; Sakhare, P.M. Adenosine and adenosine receptors: Newer therapeutic perspective. *Indian J. Pharmacol.* **2009**, *41*, 97–105. [CrossRef]
59. Marcelino, H.; Carvalho, T.M.A.; Tomas, J.; Teles, F.I.; Honorio, A.C.; Rosa, C.B.; Costa, A.R.; Costa, B.M.; Santos, C.R.A.; Sebastiao, A.M.; et al. Adenosine Inhibits Cell Proliferation Differently in Human Astrocytes and in Glioblastoma Cell Lines. *Neuroscience* **2021**, *467*, 122–133. [CrossRef]
60. Deussen, A.; Stappert, M.; Schafer, S.; Kelm, M. Quantification of extracellular and intracellular adenosine production: Understanding the transmembranous concentration gradient. *Circulation* **1999**, *99*, 2041–2047. [CrossRef]
61. Collins, J.F.; Ghishan, F.K. Molecular cloning, functional expression, tissue distribution, and in situ hybridization of the renal sodium phosphate (Na+/P(i)) transporter in the control and hypophosphatemic mouse. *FASEB J.* **1994**, *8*, 862–868. [CrossRef] [PubMed]
62. Chen, J.F.; Eltzschig, H.K.; Fredholm, B.B. Adenosine receptors as drug targets—What are the challenges? *Nat. Rev. Drug Discov.* **2013**, *12*, 265–286. [CrossRef] [PubMed]

63. Palmer, T.M.; Benovic, J.L.; Stiles, G.L. Molecular basis for subtype-specific desensitization of inhibitory adenosine receptors. Analysis of a chimeric A1-A3 adenosine receptor. *J. Biol. Chem.* **1996**, *271*, 15272–15278. [CrossRef]
64. Sidders, B.; Zhang, P.; Goodwin, K.; O'Connor, G.; Russell, D.L.; Borodovsky, A.; Armenia, J.; McEwen, R.; Linghu, B.; Bendell, J.C.; et al. Adenosine Signaling Is Prognostic for Cancer Outcome and Has Predictive Utility for Immunotherapeutic Response. *Clin. Cancer Res.* **2020**, *26*, 2176–2187. [CrossRef]
65. Luongo, L.; Guida, F.; Imperatore, R.; Napolitano, F.; Gatta, L.; Cristino, L.; Giordano, C.; Siniscalco, D.; Di Marzo, V.; Bellini, G.; et al. The A1 adenosine receptor as a new player in microglia physiology. *Glia* **2014**, *62*, 122–132. [CrossRef] [PubMed]
66. Synowitz, M.; Glass, R.; Farber, K.; Markovic, D.; Kronenberg, G.; Herrmann, K.; Schnermann, J.; Nolte, C.; van Rooijen, N.; Kiwit, J.; et al. A1 adenosine receptors in microglia control glioblastoma-host interaction. *Cancer Res.* **2006**, *66*, 8550–8557. [CrossRef]
67. Marti Navia, A.; Dal Ben, D.; Lambertucci, C.; Spinaci, A.; Volpini, R.; Marques-Morgado, I.; Coelho, J.E.; Lopes, L.V.; Marucci, G.; Buccioni, M. Adenosine Receptors as Neuroinflammation Modulators: Role of A1 Agonists and A2A Antagonists. *Cells* **2020**, *9*, 1739. [CrossRef]
68. Muroi, Y.; Ishii, T.; Teramoto, K.; Hori, M.; Nishimura, M. Calcineurin contributes to the enhancing effect of adenosine on nerve growth factor-induced neurite outgrowth via the decreased duration of p38 mitogen-activated protein kinase phosphorylation. *J. Pharmacol. Sci.* **2004**, *95*, 124–131. [CrossRef]
69. Barkan, K.; Lagarias, P.; Stampelou, M.; Stamatis, D.; Hoare, S.; Safitri, D.; Klotz, K.N.; Vrontaki, E.; Kolocouris, A.; Ladds, G. Pharmacological characterisation of novel adenosine A3 receptor antagonists. *Sci. Rep.* **2020**, *10*, 20781. [CrossRef]
70. Rocha, R.; Torres, A.; Ojeda, K.; Uribe, D.; Rocha, D.; Erices, J.; Niechi, I.; Ehrenfeld, P.; San Martin, R.; Quezada, C. The Adenosine A(3) Receptor Regulates Differentiation of Glioblastoma Stem-Like Cells to Endothelial Cells under Hypoxia. *Int. J. Mol. Sci.* **2018**, *19*, 1228. [CrossRef]
71. Weaver, D.R. A2a adenosine receptor gene expression in developing rat brain. *Brain Res. Mol. Brain Res.* **1993**, *20*, 313–327. [CrossRef]
72. Singh, B.L.; Chen, L.; Cai, H.; Shi, H.; Wang, Y.; Yu, C.; Chen, X.; Han, X.; Cai, X. Activation of adenosine A2a receptor accelerates and A2a receptor antagonist reduces intermittent hypoxia induced PC12 cell injury via PKC-KATP pathway. *Brain Res. Bull.* **2019**, *150*, 118–126. [CrossRef] [PubMed]
73. Luongo, L.; Guida, F.; Maione, S.; Jacobson, K.A.; Salvemini, D. Adenosine Metabotropic Receptors in Chronic Pain Management. *Front. Pharmacol.* **2021**, *12*, 651038. [CrossRef] [PubMed]
74. Cunha, R.A.; Almeida, T.; Ribeiro, J.A. Modification by arachidonic acid of extracellular adenosine metabolism and neuromodulatory action in the rat hippocampus. *J. Biol. Chem.* **2000**, *275*, 37572–37581. [CrossRef]
75. Rebola, N.; Rodrigues, R.J.; Oliveira, C.R.; Cunha, R.A. Different roles of adenosine A1, A2A and A3 receptors in controlling kainate-induced toxicity in cortical cultured neurons. *Neurochem. Int.* **2005**, *47*, 317–325. [CrossRef]
76. Li, X.X.; Nomura, T.; Aihara, H.; Nishizaki, T. Adenosine enhances glial glutamate efflux via A2a adenosine receptors. *Life Sci.* **2001**, *68*, 1343–1350. [CrossRef]
77. Melani, A.; Cipriani, S.; Vannucchi, M.G.; Nosi, D.; Donati, C.; Bruni, P.; Giovannini, M.G.; Pedata, F. Selective adenosine A2a receptor antagonism reduces JNK activation in oligodendrocytes after cerebral ischaemia. *Brain* **2009**, *132*, 1480–1495. [CrossRef]
78. Huang, S.; Apasov, S.; Koshiba, M.; Sitkovsky, M. Role of A2a extracellular adenosine receptor-mediated signaling in adenosine-mediated inhibition of T-cell activation and expansion. *Blood* **1997**, *90*, 1600–1610. [CrossRef]
79. Young, A.; Ngiow, S.F.; Gao, Y.; Patch, A.M.; Barkauskas, D.S.; Messaoudene, M.; Lin, G.; Coudert, J.D.; Stannard, K.A.; Zitvogel, L.; et al. A2AR Adenosine Signaling Suppresses Natural Killer Cell Maturation in the Tumor Microenvironment. *Cancer Res.* **2018**, *78*, 1003–1016. [CrossRef]
80. Ott, M.; Tomaszowski, K.H.; Marisetty, A.; Kong, L.Y.; Wei, J.; Duna, M.; Blumberg, K.; Ji, X.; Jacobs, C.; Fuller, G.N.; et al. Profiling of patients with glioma reveals the dominant immunosuppressive axis is refractory to immune function restoration. *JCI Insight* **2020**, *5*. [CrossRef]
81. Block, E.T.; Cronstein, B.N. Interferon-gamma inhibits adenosine A2A receptor function in hepatic stellate cells by STAT1-mediated repression of adenylyl cyclase. *Int. J. Interferon Cytok. Mediat. Res.* **2010**, *2010*, 113–126. [CrossRef] [PubMed]
82. Cohen, H.B.; Ward, A.; Hamidzadeh, K.; Ravid, K.; Mosser, D.M. IFN-gamma Prevents Adenosine Receptor (A2bR) Upregulation To Sustain the Macrophage Activation Response. *J. Immunol.* **2015**, *195*, 3828–3837. [CrossRef] [PubMed]
83. Arslan, G.; Kontny, E.; Fredholm, B.B. Down-regulation of adenosine A2A receptors upon NGF-induced differentiation of PC12 cells. *Neuropharmacology* **1997**, *36*, 1319–1326. [CrossRef]
84. Orr, A.G.; Orr, A.L.; Li, X.J.; Gross, R.E.; Traynelis, S.F. Adenosine A(2A) receptor mediates microglial process retraction. *Nat. Neurosci.* **2009**, *12*, 872–878. [CrossRef]
85. Simoes, A.P.; Duarte, J.A.; Agasse, F.; Canas, P.M.; Tome, A.R.; Agostinho, P.; Cunha, R.A. Blockade of adenosine A2A receptors prevents interleukin-1beta-induced exacerbation of neuronal toxicity through a p38 mitogen-activated protein kinase pathway. *J. Neuroinflammation* **2012**, *9*, 204. [CrossRef]
86. Real, J.I.; Simoes, A.P.; Cunha, R.A.; Ferreira, S.G.; Rial, D. Adenosine A2A receptors modulate the dopamine D2 receptor-mediated inhibition of synaptic transmission in the mouse prefrontal cortex. *Eur. J. Neurosci.* **2018**, *47*, 1127–1134. [CrossRef]
87. Ray, C.J.; Marshall, J.M. The cellular mechanisms by which adenosine evokes release of nitric oxide from rat aortic endothelium. *J. Physiol.* **2006**, *570*, 85–96. [CrossRef]

88. Peng, W.; Wu, Z.; Song, K.; Zhang, S.; Li, Y.; Xu, M. Regulation of sleep homeostasis mediator adenosine by basal forebrain glutamatergic neurons. *Science* **2020**, *369*, eabb0556. [CrossRef]
89. Antonioli, L.; Yegutkin, G.G.; Pacher, P.; Blandizzi, C.; Hasko, G. Anti-CD73 in cancer immunotherapy: Awakening new opportunities. *Trends Cancer* **2016**, *2*, 95–109. [CrossRef]
90. Li, X.Y.; Moesta, A.K.; Xiao, C.; Nakamura, K.; Casey, M.; Zhang, H.; Madore, J.; Lepletier, A.; Aguilera, A.R.; Sundarrajan, A.; et al. Targeting CD39 in Cancer Reveals an Extracellular ATP- and Inflammasome-Driven Tumor Immunity. *Cancer Discov.* **2019**, *9*, 1754–1773. [CrossRef]
91. Maj, T.; Wang, W.; Crespo, J.; Zhang, H.; Wang, W.; Wei, S.; Zhao, L.; Vatan, L.; Shao, I.; Szeliga, W.; et al. Oxidative stress controls regulatory T cell apoptosis and suppressor activity and PD-L1-blockade resistance in tumor. *Nat. Immunol.* **2017**, *18*, 1332–1341. [CrossRef] [PubMed]
92. Arab, S.; Hadjati, J. Adenosine Blockage in Tumor Microenvironment and Improvement of Cancer Immunotherapy. *Immune. Netw.* **2019**, *19*, e23. [CrossRef] [PubMed]
93. MacKenzie, W.M.; Hoskin, D.W.; Blay, J. Adenosine suppresses alpha(4)beta(7) integrin-mediated adhesion of T lymphocytes to colon adenocarcinoma cells. *Exp. Cell Res.* **2002**, *276*, 90–100. [CrossRef] [PubMed]
94. Seydyousefi, M.; Moghanlou, A.E.; Metz, G.A.S.; Gursoy, R.; Faghfoori, M.H.; Mirghani, S.J.; Faghfoori, Z. Exogenous adenosine facilitates neuroprotection and functional recovery following cerebral ischemia in rats. *Brain Res. Bull.* **2019**, *153*, 250–256. [CrossRef] [PubMed]
95. Yang, R.; Elsaadi, S.; Misund, K.; Abdollahi, P.; Vandsemb, E.N.; Moen, S.H.; Kusnierczyk, A.; Slupphaug, G.; Standal, T.; Waage, A.; et al. Conversion of ATP to adenosine by CD39 and CD73 in multiple myeloma can be successfully targeted together with adenosine receptor A2A blockade. *J. Immunother. Cancer* **2020**, *8*, e000610. [CrossRef]
96. Volmer, J.B.; Thompson, L.F.; Blackburn, M.R. Ecto-5′-nucleotidase (CD73)-mediated adenosine production is tissue protective in a model of bleomycin-induced lung injury. *J. Immunol.* **2006**, *176*, 4449–4458. [CrossRef]
97. Antonioli, L.; Fornai, M.; Pellegrini, C.; D'Antongiovanni, V.; Turiello, R.; Morello, S.; Hasko, G.; Blandizzi, C. Adenosine Signaling in the Tumor Microenvironment. *Adv. Exp. Med. Biol.* **2021**, *1270*, 145–167. [CrossRef]
98. Koussemou, M.; Lorenz, K.; Klotz, K.N. The A2B adenosine receptor in MDA-MB-231 breast cancer cells diminishes ERK1/2 phosphorylation by activation of MAPK-phosphatase-1. *PLoS ONE* **2018**, *13*, e0202914. [CrossRef]
99. Ohta, A.; Gorelik, E.; Prasad, S.J.; Ronchese, F.; Lukashev, D.; Wong, M.K.; Huang, X.; Caldwell, S.; Liu, K.; Smith, P.; et al. A2A adenosine receptor protects tumors from antitumor T cells. *Proc. Natl. Acad. Sci. USA* **2006**, *103*, 13132–13137. [CrossRef]
100. Overwijk, W.W.; Restifo, N.P. Creating therapeutic cancer vaccines: Notes from the battlefield. *Trends Immunol.* **2001**, *22*, 5–7. [CrossRef]
101. Ablamunits, V. The importance of APC. *J. Autoimmune Dis.* **2005**, *2*, 3. [CrossRef] [PubMed]
102. Gonzalez, H.; Hagerling, C.; Werb, Z. Roles of the immune system in cancer: From tumor initiation to metastatic progression. *Genes Dev.* **2018**, *32*, 1267–1284. [CrossRef]
103. Leone, R.D.; Lo, Y.C.; Powell, J.D. A2aR antagonists: Next generation checkpoint blockade for cancer immunotherapy. *Comput. Struct. Biotechnol. J.* **2015**, *13*, 265–272. [CrossRef] [PubMed]
104. Mapara, M.Y.; Sykes, M. Tolerance and cancer: Mechanisms of tumor evasion and strategies for breaking tolerance. *J. Clin. Oncol.* **2004**, *22*, 1136–1151. [CrossRef] [PubMed]
105. Sitkovsky, M.; Lukashev, D.; Deaglio, S.; Dwyer, K.; Robson, S.C.; Ohta, A. Adenosine A2A receptor antagonists: Blockade of adenosinergic effects and T regulatory cells. *Br. J. Pharmacol.* **2008**, *153* (Suppl. S1), S457–S464. [CrossRef]
106. Gabrilovich, D.I.; Chen, H.L.; Girgis, K.R.; Cunningham, H.T.; Meny, G.M.; Nadaf, S.; Kavanaugh, D.; Carbone, D.P. Production of vascular endothelial growth factor by human tumors inhibits the functional maturation of dendritic cells. *Nat. Med.* **1996**, *2*, 1096–1103. [CrossRef]
107. Antonioli, L.; Lucarini, E.; Lambertucci, C.; Fornai, M.; Pellegrini, C.; Benvenuti, L.; Di Cesare Mannelli, L.; Spinaci, A.; Marucci, G.; Blandizzi, C.; et al. The Anti-Inflammatory and Pain-Relieving Effects of AR170, an Adenosine A3 Receptor Agonist, in a Rat Model of Colitis. *Cells* **2020**, *9*, 1509. [CrossRef]
108. Litchfield, K.; Reading, J.L.; Puttick, C.; Thakkar, K.; Abbosh, C.; Bentham, R.; Watkins, T.B.K.; Rosenthal, R.; Biswas, D.; Rowan, A.; et al. Meta-analysis of tumor- and T cell-intrinsic mechanisms of sensitization to checkpoint inhibition. *Cell* **2021**, *184*, 596–614.e514. [CrossRef]
109. Boison, D. Adenosine kinase: Exploitation for therapeutic gain. *Pharmacol. Rev.* **2013**, *65*, 906–943. [CrossRef]
110. Reisser, D.; Martin, F. CD4+ T cells recovered from a mixed immune lymphocyte-tumor cell culture induce thymidine incorporation by naive rat lymphocytes in response to tumor cells. *Int. J. Cancer* **1994**, *57*, 254–258. [CrossRef]
111. Mediavilla-Varela, M.; Luddy, K.; Noyes, D.; Khalil, F.K.; Neuger, A.M.; Soliman, H.; Antonia, S.J. Antagonism of adenosine A2A receptor expressed by lung adenocarcinoma tumor cells and cancer associated fibroblasts inhibits their growth. *Cancer Biol. Ther.* **2013**, *14*, 860–868. [CrossRef] [PubMed]
112. Torres, A.; Erices, J.I.; Sanchez, F.; Ehrenfeld, P.; Turchi, L.; Virolle, T.; Uribe, D.; Niechi, I.; Spichiger, C.; Rocha, J.D.; et al. Extracellular adenosine promotes cell migration/invasion of Glioblastoma Stem-like Cells through A3 Adenosine Receptor activation under hypoxia. *Cancer Lett.* **2019**, *446*, 112–122. [CrossRef] [PubMed]
113. Waickman, A.T.; Alme, A.; Senaldi, L.; Zarek, P.E.; Horton, M.; Powell, J.D. Enhancement of tumor immunotherapy by deletion of the A2A adenosine receptor. *Cancer Immunol. Immunother.* **2012**, *61*, 917–926. [CrossRef] [PubMed]

114. Sun, Y.; Huang, P. Adenosine A2B Receptor: From Cell Biology to Human Diseases. *Front. Chem.* **2016**, *4*, 37. [CrossRef] [PubMed]
115. Vigano, S.; Alatzoglou, D.; Irving, M.; Menetrier-Caux, C.; Caux, C.; Romero, P.; Coukos, G. Targeting Adenosine in Cancer Immunotherapy to Enhance T-Cell Function. *Front. Immunol.* **2019**, *10*, 925. [CrossRef]
116. Vijayan, D.; Young, A.; Teng, M.W.L.; Smyth, M.J. Targeting immunosuppressive adenosine in cancer. *Nat. Rev. Cancer* **2017**, *17*, 709–724. [CrossRef]
117. Hatfield, S.M.; Kjaergaard, J.; Lukashev, D.; Belikoff, B.; Schreiber, T.H.; Sethumadhavan, S.; Abbott, R.; Philbrook, P.; Thayer, M.; Shujia, D.; et al. Systemic oxygenation weakens the hypoxia and hypoxia inducible factor 1alpha-dependent and extracellular adenosine-mediated tumor protection. *J. Mol. Med.* **2014**, *92*, 1283–1292. [CrossRef]
118. Yan, A.; Joachims, M.L.; Thompson, L.F.; Miller, A.D.; Canoll, P.D.; Bynoe, M.S. CD73 Promotes Glioblastoma Pathogenesis and Enhances Its Chemoresistance via A2B Adenosine Receptor Signaling. *J. Neurosci.* **2019**, *39*, 4387–4402. [CrossRef]
119. Daniele, S.; Zappelli, E.; Natali, L.; Martini, C.; Trincavelli, M.L. Modulation of A1 and A2B adenosine receptor activity: A new strategy to sensitise glioblastoma stem cells to chemotherapy. *Cell Death Dis.* **2014**, *5*, e1539. [CrossRef]
120. Wink, M.R.; Lenz, G.; Braganhol, E.; Tamajusuku, A.S.; Schwartsmann, G.; Sarkis, J.J.; Battastini, A.M. Altered extracellular ATP, ADP and AMP catabolism in glioma cell lines. *Cancer Lett.* **2003**, *198*, 211–218. [CrossRef]
121. Cascalheira, J.F.; Goncalves, M.; Barroso, M.; Castro, R.; Palmeira, M.; Serpa, A.; Dias-Cabral, A.C.; Domingues, F.C.; Almeida, S. Association of the transcobalamin II gene 776C → G polymorphism with Alzheimer's type dementia: Dependence on the 5, 10-methylenetetrahydrofolate reductase 1298A → C polymorphism genotype. *Ann. Clin. Biochem.* **2015**, *52*, 448–455. [CrossRef] [PubMed]
122. Semmler, A.; Simon, M.; Moskau, S.; Linnebank, M. The methionine synthase polymorphism c.2756A>G alters susceptibility to glioblastoma multiforme. *Cancer Epidemiol. Biomark. Prev.* **2006**, *15*, 2314–2316. [CrossRef] [PubMed]
123. Carmeliet, P.; Dor, Y.; Herbert, J.M.; Fukumura, D.; Brusselmans, K.; Dewerchin, M.; Neeman, M.; Bono, F.; Abramovitch, R.; Maxwell, P.; et al. Role of HIF-1alpha in hypoxia-mediated apoptosis, cell proliferation and tumour angiogenesis. *Nature* **1998**, *394*, 485–490. [CrossRef]
124. Kust, B.M.; Biber, K.; van Calker, D.; Gebicke-Haerter, P.J. Regulation of K+ channel mRNA expression by stimulation of adenosine A2a-receptors in cultured rat microglia. *Glia* **1999**, *25*, 120–130. [CrossRef]
125. Heese, K.; Fiebich, B.L.; Bauer, J.; Otten, U. Nerve growth factor (NGF) expression in rat microglia is induced by adenosine A2a-receptors. *Neurosci. Lett.* **1997**, *231*, 83–86. [CrossRef]
126. Fiebich, B.L.; Biber, K.; Lieb, K.; van Calker, D.; Berger, M.; Bauer, J.; Gebicke-Haerter, P.J. Cyclooxygenase-2 expression in rat microglia is induced by adenosine A2a-receptors. *Glia* **1996**, *18*, 152–160. [CrossRef]
127. Ma, S.R.; Deng, W.W.; Liu, J.F.; Mao, L.; Yu, G.T.; Bu, L.L.; Kulkarni, A.B.; Zhang, W.F.; Sun, Z.J. Blockade of adenosine A2A receptor enhances CD8(+) T cells response and decreases regulatory T cells in head and neck squamous cell carcinoma. *Mol. Cancer* **2017**, *16*, 99. [CrossRef] [PubMed]
128. Liu, T.Z.; Wang, X.; Bai, Y.F.; Liao, H.Z.; Qiu, S.C.; Yang, Y.Q.; Yan, X.H.; Chen, J.; Guo, H.B.; Zhang, S.Z. The HIF-2alpha dependent induction of PAP and adenosine synthesis regulates glioblastoma stem cell function through the A2B adenosine receptor. *Int. J. Biochem. Cell Biol.* **2014**, *49*, 8–16. [CrossRef]
129. Wrensch, M.; Jenkins, R.B.; Chang, J.S.; Yeh, R.F.; Xiao, Y.; Decker, P.A.; Ballman, K.V.; Berger, M.; Buckner, J.C.; Chang, S.; et al. Variants in the CDKN2B and RTEL1 regions are associated with high-grade glioma susceptibility. *Nat. Genet.* **2009**, *41*, 905–908. [CrossRef]
130. Jacobson, K.A.; Nikodijevic, O.; Padgett, W.L.; Gallo-Rodriguez, C.; Maillard, M.; Daly, J.W. 8-(3-Chlorostyryl)caffeine (CSC) is a selective A2-adenosine antagonist in vitro and in vivo. *FEBS Lett.* **1993**, *323*, 141–144. [CrossRef]
131. Borodovsky, A.; Barbon, C.M.; Wang, Y.; Ye, M.; Prickett, L.; Chandra, D.; Shaw, J.; Deng, N.; Sachsenmeier, K.; Clarke, J.D.; et al. Small molecule AZD4635 inhibitor of A2AR signaling rescues immune cell function including CD103(+) dendritic cells enhancing anti-tumor immunity. *J. Immunother. Cancer* **2020**, *8*, e000417. [CrossRef] [PubMed]
132. Harmse, R.; van der Walt, M.M.; Petzer, J.P.; Terre'Blanche, G. Discovery of 1,3-diethyl-7-methyl-8-(phenoxymethyl)-xanthine derivatives as novel adenosine A1 and A2A receptor antagonists. *Bioorg. Med. Chem. Lett.* **2016**, *26*, 5951–5955. [CrossRef] [PubMed]
133. Schwabe, U.; Ukena, D.; Lohse, M.J. Xanthine derivatives as antagonists at A1 and A2 adenosine receptors. *Naunyn Schmiedebergs Arch. Pharmacol.* **1985**, *330*, 212–221. [CrossRef] [PubMed]
134. Chen, J.F.; Xu, K.; Petzer, J.P.; Staal, R.; Xu, Y.H.; Beilstein, M.; Sonsalla, P.K.; Castagnoli, K.; Castagnoli, N., Jr.; Schwarzschild, M.A. Neuroprotection by caffeine and A(2A) adenosine receptor inactivation in a model of Parkinson's disease. *J. Neurosci.* **2001**, *21*, RC143. [CrossRef] [PubMed]
135. Szopa, A.; Bogatko, K.; Serefko, A.; Wyska, E.; Wosko, S.; Swiader, K.; Doboszewska, U.; Wlaz, A.; Wrobel, A.; Wlaz, P.; et al. Agomelatine and tianeptine antidepressant activity in mice behavioral despair tests is enhanced by DMPX, a selective adenosine A2A receptor antagonist, but not DPCPX, a selective adenosine A1 receptor antagonist. *Pharmacol. Rep.* **2019**, *71*, 676–681. [CrossRef] [PubMed]
136. Masjedi, A.; Ahmadi, A.; Ghani, S.; Malakotikhah, F.; Nabi Afjadi, M.; Irandoust, M.; Karoon Kiani, F.; Heydarzadeh Asl, S.; Atyabi, F.; Hassannia, H.; et al. Silencing adenosine A2a receptor enhances dendritic cell-based cancer immunotherapy. *Nanomedicine* **2020**, *29*, 102240. [CrossRef] [PubMed]

137. Pollack, A.E.; Fink, J.S. Adenosine antagonists potentiate D2 dopamine-dependent activation of Fos in the striatopallidal pathway. *Neuroscience* **1995**, *68*, 721–728. [CrossRef]
138. Fong, L.; Hotson, A.; Powderly, J.D.; Sznol, M.; Heist, R.S.; Choueiri, T.K.; George, S.; Hughes, B.G.M.; Hellmann, M.D.; Shepard, D.R.; et al. Adenosine 2A Receptor Blockade as an Immunotherapy for Treatment-Refractory Renal Cell Cancer. *Cancer Discov.* **2020**, *10*, 40–53. [CrossRef]
139. Chiappori, A.A.; Creelan, B.; Tanvetyanon, T.; Gray, J.E.; Haura, E.B.; Thapa, R.; Barlow, M.L.; Chen, Z.; Chen, D.T.; Beg, A.A.; et al. Phase I Study of Taminadenant (PBF509/NIR178), an Adenosine 2A Receptor Antagonist, with or without Spartalizumab (PDR001), in Patients with Advanced Non-Small Cell Lung Cancer. *Clin. Cancer Res.* **2022**, *28*, 2313–2320. [CrossRef]
140. Yu, J.; Zhong, Y.; Shen, X.; Cheng, Y.; Qi, J.; Wang, J. In vitro effect of adenosine A2A receptor antagonist SCH 442416 on the expression of glutamine synthetase and glutamate aspartate transporter in rat retinal Muller cells at elevated hydrostatic pressure. *Oncol. Rep.* **2012**, *27*, 748–752. [CrossRef]
141. Poucher, S.M.; Keddie, J.R.; Brooks, R.; Shaw, G.R.; McKillop, D. Pharmacodynamics of ZM 241385, a potent A2a adenosine receptor antagonist, after enteric administration in rat, cat and dog. *J. Pharm. Pharmacol.* **1996**, *48*, 601–606. [CrossRef] [PubMed]
142. Poucher, S.M.; Keddie, J.R.; Singh, P.; Stoggall, S.M.; Caulkett, P.W.; Jones, G.; Coll, M.G. The in vitro pharmacology of ZM 241385, a potent, non-xanthine A2a selective adenosine receptor antagonist. *Br. J. Pharmacol.* **1995**, *115*, 1096–1102. [CrossRef] [PubMed]
143. Todde, S.; Moresco, R.M.; Simonelli, P.; Baraldi, P.G.; Cacciari, B.; Spalluto, G.; Varani, K.; Monopoli, A.; Matarrese, M.; Carpinelli, A.; et al. Design, radiosynthesis, and biodistribution of a new potent and selective ligand for in vivo imaging of the adenosine A(2A) receptor system using positron emission tomography. *J. Med. Chem.* **2000**, *43*, 4359–4362. [CrossRef]
144. Gillespie, R.J.; Cliffe, I.A.; Dawson, C.E.; Dourish, C.T.; Gaur, S.; Jordan, A.M.; Knight, A.R.; Lerpiniere, J.; Misra, A.; Pratt, R.M.; et al. Antagonists of the human adenosine A2A receptor. Part 3: Design and synthesis of pyrazolo[3,4-d]pyrimidines, pyrrolo[2,3-d]pyrimidines and 6-arylpurines. *Bioorg. Med. Chem. Lett.* **2008**, *18*, 2924–2929. [CrossRef]
145. Willingham, S.B.; Hotson, A.N.; Miller, R.A. Targeting the A2AR in cancer; early lessons from the clinic. *Curr. Opin. Pharmacol.* **2020**, *53*, 126–133. [CrossRef] [PubMed]
146. Gnad, T.; Navarro, G.; Lahesmaa, M.; Reverte-Salisa, L.; Copperi, F.; Cordomi, A.; Naumann, J.; Hochhauser, A.; Haufs-Brusberg, S.; Wenzel, D.; et al. Adenosine/A2B Receptor Signaling Ameliorates the Effects of Aging and Counteracts Obesity. *Cell Metab.* **2020**, *32*, 56–70.e57. [CrossRef] [PubMed]
147. Hinz, S.; Navarro, G.; Borroto-Escuela, D.; Seibt, B.F.; Ammon, Y.C.; de Filippo, E.; Danish, A.; Lacher, S.K.; Cervinkova, B.; Rafehi, M.; et al. Adenosine A2A receptor ligand recognition and signaling is blocked by A2B receptors. *Oncotarget* **2018**, *9*, 13593–13611. [CrossRef] [PubMed]

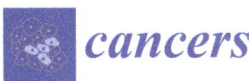

Article

Comprehensive Metabolic Profiling of MYC-Amplified Medulloblastoma Tumors Reveals Key Dependencies on Amino Acid, Tricarboxylic Acid and Hexosamine Pathways

Khoa Pham [1], Allison R. Hanaford [1], Brad A. Poore [1], Micah J. Maxwell [2,3], Heather Sweeney [2], Akhila Parthasarathy [2], Jesse Alt [4], Rana Rais [4,5], Barbara S. Slusher [4,5], Charles G. Eberhart [1,3] and Eric H. Raabe [2,3,*]

[1] Division of Neuropathology, Department of Pathology, School of Medicine, Johns Hopkins University, Baltimore, MD 21205, USA; kpham8@jhmi.edu (K.P.); allison.hanaford@seattlechildrens.org (A.R.H.); brad.a.poore@gmail.com (B.A.P.); ceberha@jhmi.edu (C.G.E.)
[2] Division of Pediatric Oncology, Department of Oncology, School of Medicine, Johns Hopkins University, Baltimore, MD 21287, USA; mmaxwel1@jhmi.edu (M.J.M.); hsweene1@jh.edu (H.S.); apartha1@jhu.edu (A.P.)
[3] Sidney Kimmel Comprehensive Cancer Center, School of Medicine, Johns Hopkins University, Baltimore, MD 21287, USA
[4] Johns Hopkins Drug Discovery, Baltimore, MD 21205, USA; jalt1@jhmi.edu (J.A.); rrais2@jhmi.edu (R.R.); bslusher@jhmi.edu (B.S.S.)
[5] Department of Neurology, School of Medicine, Johns Hopkins University, Baltimore, MD 21205, USA
* Correspondence: eraabe2@jhmi.edu

Simple Summary: The oncogene *MYC* alters cellular metabolism. Medulloblastoma is the most common malignant pediatric brain tumor. *MYC*-amplified medulloblastoma has a poor prognosis, and the metabolism of *MYC*-amplified medulloblastoma is poorly understood. We performed comprehensive metabolic profiling of *MYC*-amplified medulloblastoma and found increased reliance on potentially targetable pathways. We also found that the metabolism of *MYC*-amplified cell lines differed from orthotopic brain tumors in vitro and in flank tumors, suggesting that analyses conducted in vitro or in flank tumors may miss key vulnerabilities.

Abstract: Reprograming of cellular metabolism is a hallmark of cancer. Altering metabolism allows cancer cells to overcome unfavorable microenvironment conditions and to proliferate and invade. Medulloblastoma is the most common malignant brain tumor of children. Genomic amplification of *MYC* defines a subset of poor-prognosis medulloblastoma. We performed comprehensive metabolic studies of human *MYC*-amplified medulloblastoma by comparing the metabolic profiles of tumor cells in three different conditions—in vitro, in flank xenografts and in orthotopic xenografts in the cerebellum. Principal component analysis showed that the metabolic profiles of brain and flank high-MYC medulloblastoma tumors clustered closely together and separated away from normal brain and in vitro MYC-amplified cells. Compared to normal brain, *MYC*-amplified medulloblastoma orthotopic xenograft tumors showed upregulation of the TCA cycle as well as the synthesis of nucleotides, hexosamines, amino acids and glutathione. There was significantly higher glucose uptake and usage in orthotopic xenograft tumors compared to flank xenograft tumors and cells in culture. In orthotopic tumors, glucose was the main carbon source for the *de novo* synthesis of glutamate, glutamine and glutathione through the TCA cycle. In vivo, the glutaminase II pathway was the main pathway utilizing glutamine. Glutathione was the most abundant upregulated metabolite in orthotopic tumors compared to normal brain. Glutamine-derived glutathione was synthesized through the glutamine transaminase K (GTK) enzyme in vivo. In conclusion, high *MYC* medulloblastoma cells have different metabolic profiles in vitro compared to in vivo, and key vulnerabilities may be missed by not performing in vivo metabolic analyses.

Keywords: Warburg effect; mass spectrometry; isotope labeling; cancer metabolism; pediatric brain tumor

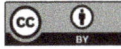

1. Introduction

Malignant transformation is a process that drives normal cells to become cancerous through the accumulation of alterations in proto-oncogenes and tumor suppressors [1–4]. Among different types of tumors, genetic alterations in PI3/mTOR, RAS/BRAF, MYC and TP53 reprogram metabolic pathways, allowing cancer cells to overcome unfavorable conditions and enabling them to proliferate at a pathologic rate and metastasize [5–11]. Identifying and interrupting the abnormal metabolic pathways that benefit cancer cells could yield a therapeutic index in which cancer cells are targeted while normal cells are not harmed [12–14].

In vitro metabolic studies and flux analysis using stable isotopes can provide a picture of the intracellular metabolite levels and how those metabolites change in response to therapy. However, in vitro models miss the influence from the native microenvironment, such as physiologic or hypoxic oxygen tension and pH and limited availability of nutrients as well as interaction with stromal cells and tumor-associated macrophages, all of which could have a significant impact on the intracellular metabolites of cancer cells [15–18]. These differences could potentially confound the applicability of cell culture metabolic and therapeutic findings to in vivo tumors, as shown in some type of cancers [19–22]. We therefore sought to assess how different types of in vitro and in vivo microenvironments affected the metabolic profiles of medulloblastoma.

Medulloblastoma is the most common malignant brain tumor in children. Survival depends on the molecular genetics and epigenetics of the patient's tumor [23]. *MYC*-amplified medulloblastoma has a worse outcome compared to non-*MYC* amplified medulloblastoma [24]. The poor prognosis for "Group 3", *MYC*-amplified medulloblastoma patients [25,26] and the severe complications faced by survivors due to the intensity of the therapy they receive indicate an urgent need for more effective and less toxic therapies.

We performed comprehensive metabolic studies—employing liquid chromatography/mass spectrometry (LC/MS) and uniformly labeled glucose and glutamine—of human *MYC*-amplified medulloblastoma by comparing the metabolic profiles of tumor cells in three different environments—in vitro, in flank xenografts and in orthotopic xenografts. Our goals were to: (1) identify changes in the metabolic pathways in the orthotopic tumors compared to normal brain; and (2) test if glucose and glutamine had the same metabolic fates in different tumor cell environments. We hypothesized that due to alterations in oxygen tension, nutrient availability and the microenvironment there would be significant discrepancies between the metabolic profile of the same *MYC*-amplified medulloblastoma cells in vitro, in flank tumors and in orthotopic tumors.

2. Materials and Methods

2.1. Cell Lines and Culture Conditions

2.1.1. Cell Culture

The patient-derived medulloblastoma cell line D425MED, first established at Duke University, Durham, NC, USA, was grown in MEM media (Gibco, Waltham, MA, USA) supplemented with 5% FBS (Gibco, Waltham, MA, USA) and 1% NEAA (Gibco, Waltham, MA, USA) [27–31]. The MED211 patient-derived xenograft was obtained from the Brain Tumor Resource Lab, Seattle, WA, USA and has been previously described [27–30]. We developed a cell line from the MED211 PDX model by removing tumor tissue from the tumor as described [28]. MED211 cells were grown in EGF/FGF (Peprotech, Rocky Hill, NJ, USA) neurobasal media.

In vitro metabolic flux experiments involved the media in confluent cells being changed just prior to the experiment. Three biological replicate samples of each cell line were pulsed with 10 µM U-glucose (13C6 99% purity) label from Cambridge Isotope (No. CLM-1396-1) or 4 µM U-glutamine (13C5, 15N2, 99% purity) label from Cambridge Isotope (No. CNLM-1275-H-0.5) for 2 h. Following the pulse, cells were spun down and washed with PBS. 1 mL of 80% UPLC-grade ice cold methanol was added to each pellet. Pellets were vortexed for 1 min and incubated at −80 °C to extract metabolites. Analysis of metabolites is described below.

2.1.2. Animal Studies

Orthotopic xenografting D425MED and MED211 involved the following process. After induction of general anesthesia with ketamine/xylazine in Nu/Nu mice, a burr hole was made in the skull of female Nu/Nu mice Charles River (Wilmington, MA, USA) 1 mm to the right of and 2 mm posterior to the lambdoid suture with an 18 gauge needle. The needle of a Hamilton syringe was inserted to a depth of 2.5 mm into the cerebellum using a needle guard, and 100,000 D425MED cells or MED211 cells in 3 µL of media were injected. MED211 tumors were established by serial transplantation of the patient-derived xenograft and not from cells in culture. All animals were monitored daily until they became symptomatic, exhibiting weight loss, hunching and ataxia. Mice were sacrificed to harvest tumor and uninvolved cerebellum and cortex in the same mouse for histology and metabolic studies.

Prior to tumor implantation, flank xenografting of D425MED and MED211 involved, animals being anesthetized with a mixture of 10% ketamine and 5% xylazine. One million cells of D425MED or MED211 suspended in 200 µL of a 50:50 mix of Matrigel (Corning) and media were injected for each flank tumor. Cells were injected using an 18 gauge needle. One tumor was implanted behind each flank, so each mouse carried four flank tumors [32].

2.2. In Vivo Stable Isotope Labeling and Metabolite Extraction and Analyses

Uniformly labeled glutamine was prepared at a 100 µM concentration in PBS and uniformly labeled glucose was prepared as a 20% solution in PBS. Three animals per group were given three 100 µL IP injections of isotope spaced 15 min apart. Euthanasia occurred two hours after the second isotope injection. Tumors were visually identified in the right cerebellar hemisphere due to their more grey/white appearance compared to the normal cerebellum and were dissected and immediately removed and flash frozen in liquid nitrogen. All uniformly labeled isotopes were obtained from Cambridge Isotope Labs, Tewksbury, MA, USA.

Frozen tumors were manually homogenized in liquid nitrogen using a mortar and pestle chilled by dry ice and liquid nitrogen. As the flank tumors were very large, an aliquot of tumor powder was weighed and incubated at −80 °C with 5 volumes of 80% ice-cold HPLC grade methanol to extract metabolites.

2.3. Mass Spectrometry Analysis

Samples (both in vivo and in vitro) were centrifuged at $14,000\times g$ rpm for 10 min at 4 °C, and the supernatants were transferred to glass insert liquid chromatography vials. Analyses occurred on an Agilent 1290 liquid chromatography system coupled to an Agilent 6520 quadrupole time of flight mass spectrometer. Samples (5 µL) were injected and separated on a Waters Acquity UPLC BEH (bridged ethyl hybrid) Amide 1.7 µm 2.1 × 100 mm HILIC (hydrophilic interaction liquid chromatography) column with a flow rate of 0.3 mL/minute. Mobile phases consisted of A (water + 0.1% formic acid) and B (acetonitrile + 0.1% formic acid). The column was equilibrated at 2.5/97.5 (A/B) and maintained for 1 min post injection. Mobile-phase A increased in a linear gradient from 2.5% to 65% from 1 to 9 min post injection then stepped to 97.5% A from 9 to 11 min to wash the column. Column was equilibrated in starting condition for 3 min before the next injection. The mass spectrometer, equipped with a dual electrospray ionization source, was run in negative ion and then in positive ion mode. The scan range was 50–1600 m/z. The source settings consisted of drying gas flow rate: 11 L/min; nebulizer: 40 pounds per square inch gauge; gas temp: 350 °C; capillary voltage: 3000 V (neg), 2500 V (pos).

2.3.1. Metabolite Analysis

Liquid chromatography–mass spectrometry data were analyzed using Agilent Qualitative Analysis B.07.00 and Elucidata Metabolomic Analysis and Visualization ENgine

(El-MAVEN) [33]. Metabolite identification was determined using standards and fragmentation database.

2.3.2. Sample Normalization and Statistical Analysis

Sample normalization and statistical analysis was performed with MetaboAnalyst 5.0 version. Resulting non-labeled and labeled data for each sample were normalized using the total ion count and then logarithmically transformed (base = 10). For each metabolite, transformed values greater than six standard deviations from mean across sample groups were set to missing data. Processing of the raw data yielded 72 identified metabolites. Statistical analysis as well as pathway analysis were performed by the submission of normalized data to a web-based service for metabolic data analysis: MetaboAnalyst (http://www.metaboanalyst.ca/MetaboAnalyst/, accessed in 2021). MetaboAnalyst is a web-based tool that combines results from pathway enrichment analysis with pathway topology analysis, which allowed the identification of the most relevant pathways involved in the conditions under study [34]. Data for identified metabolites detected in all samples were submitted into MetaboAnalyst with annotation based on common chemical names. Verification of accepted metabolites was conducted manually using HMDB, KEGG, and PubChem DBs.

GraphPad Prism was used to represent data graphically and measure statistical significance by Student's t-test.

2.4. Human RNAseq Data

RNAseq data were accessed through cBioPortal for Cancer Genomics, with specific queries to the publicly available Pediatric Brain Tumor Atlas, a collaborative effort by Children's Brain Tumor Tissue Consortium and Pacific Pediatric Neuro-Oncology Consortium with patients and their families. A manuscript describing this dataset is currently in preparation (https://alexslemonade.github.io/OpenPBTA-manuscript/, accessed in January 2022). Raw data were loaded into GraphPad Prism and analyzed by one-way ANOVA with Dunnet's multiple comparison tests.

2.5. Antibodies and Reagents

Western Blots

Proteins from cultured cell pellets or snap frozen in vivo samples were homogenized and extracted using RIPA buffer (Millipore Sigma, Burlington, MA, USA) and quantified using a Bradford Assay. We used antibodies against GLUT1 (Novus biologicals (NB110-39113)), glutamine synthetase (Abcam (ab73593)); glutathione synthetase (abcam (ab91591); GTK (KAT1) (Santa Cruz Biotechnologies (sc-374531)), Nit2 (Origene (TA501138)) and beta actin (Santa Cruz (sc-47778)). The following dilutions were used for all primary antibodies (1:1000), beta actin (1:1000). Peroxidase-labeled secondary antibodies were from Cell Signaling Technologies (Danvers, MA, USA) and used at a 1:3500 dilution. Bands were quantified using ImageJ, verson 1.5. Uncropped western blots are included in supplementary material (Figure S5).

3. Results

3.1. Orthotopic D425MED and MED211 Xenografts Showed Upregulation of Nucleotide Metabolism, Amino Acid, and Glutathione Synthesis

Microscopic examination of hematoxylin and eosin (HE) stained sections confirmed the presence of cellular xenografts, with representative images shown in (Figure S1A,B). Tumors demonstrated a "large cell" histology, commonly associated with MYC amplification. Tumor cells invaded into and disrupted the surrounding cerebellar architecture. These HE stained sections demonstrate that the orthotopic xenograft tumors used in our study grew in the native microenvironment, with histology similar to that of human primary *MYC*-amplified medulloblastoma.

Metabolic analysis found 3000–4000 analytes in normal brain (normal cortex and contralateral and uninvolved cerebellum) and orthotopic *MYC*-amplified D425MED and MED211 medulloblastoma tumors. Principal component analysis of metabolomes found distinct metabolic profiles in normal brain (cortex and normal contralateral cerebellum) compared to *MYC*-amplified medulloblastoma D425MED and MED211 orthotopic tumors (Figure 1A). In one of the orthotopic MED211 tumors, we found that the tumor and normal brain metabolomes data were distinct from the other samples in the PCA, likely due to technical issues. However, the PCA demonstrated that even with this heterogeneity, the normal samples clustered together with clear separation from the MED211 tumor samples. We also found that the D425MED and MED211 orthotopic tumor samples clustered together and were distinct from all of the normal brain samples. Analysis of the known or targeted metabolites further showed clear separation between normal brain and the orthotopic tumors. There were 72 metabolites confirmed with fragmentation data based in both normal brain and tumors (52 upregulated and 20 downregulated metabolites compared to normal brain). A heat map of the top 20 statistically significantly different metabolites showed upregulation of glutathione, ornithine, citrulline, histidine, proline, glycine and asparagine in orthotopic tumors compared to normal cortex and cerebellum (Figure 1B). Interestingly, orthotopic medulloblastoma tumors had lower glutamine levels compared to normal brain.

The enrichment and pathway impact analysis of the 52 upregulated metabolites revealed that the activity of the TCA cycle as well as the synthesis of nucleotides, glutathione and amino acids were upregulated in tumors compared to normal brain (Figure 1C,D). Of novel therapeutic interest, we also identified multiple metabolites of the urea cycle as being upregulated in medulloblastoma orthotopic tumors compared to normal brain, and this manifested as showing alteration in arginine metabolism in C and D. Glutamate, glutamine and glutathione were the most abundant metabolites detected in both tumors and normal brain. However, glutamate and glutamine were lower in tumors when compared to normal brain whereas glutathione was the most abundant upregulated metabolite found in tumors (Figure 1E,F).

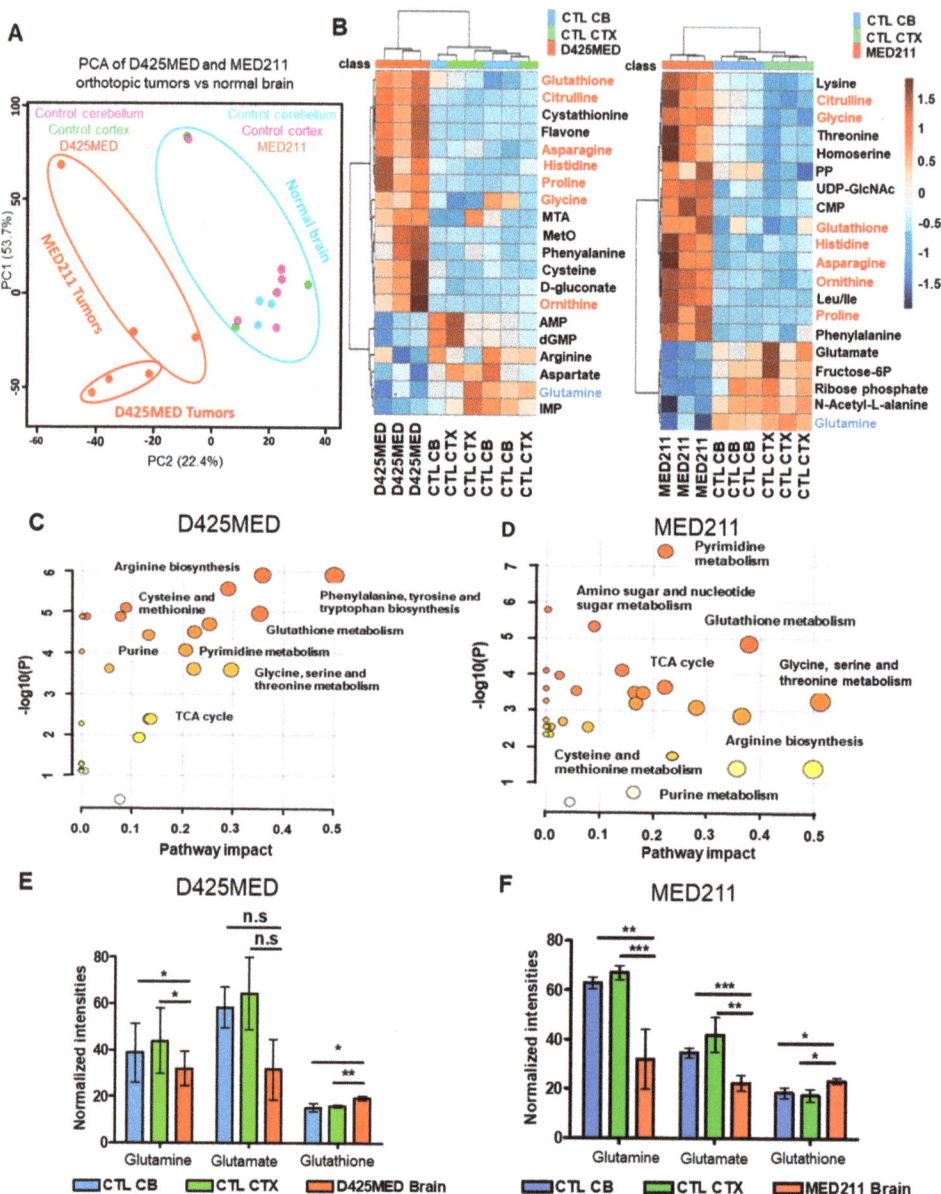

Figure 1. Orthotopic high *MYC*-amplified medulloblastoma tumors show upregulation of TCA cycle activities, nucleotides, amino acids and glutathione synthesis compared to normal brain (**A**). Principal component analysis shows distinct metabolic profiles of high MYC amplified D425MED and MED211 medulloblastoma tumors versus normal brain. D425MED and MED211 tumors segregate from both normal cerebellum and normal cortex. (**B**). Heat map of 20 metabolites that were statistically significantly different in D425MED and MED211 orthotopic tumors compared to normal cortex (CTL CTX) and cerebellum (CTL CB). Commonly increased metabolites in *MYC*-amplified medulloblastoma compared to normal brain included amino acids, glutathione and polyamines such as ornithine. Metabolites upregulated in both D425MED and MED211 compared to normal brain are highlighted

in red. Glutamine was decreased in orthotopic tumors compared to normal brain (highlighted in blue). Abbreviations: MTA = S-methyl-5′-thiaoadenosine, MetO = methionine sulfoxide, AMP = adenosine monophosphate, dGMP = deoxyguanine monophosphate, IMP = inosine monophosphate, CMP = cytidine monophosphate, PP = pyrophosphate, UDP-GlcNAc = uridine diphosphate N-acetylglucosamine. (**C,D**) Enrichment and pathways analysis using MetaboAnalyst 5.0 showed upregulation of the TCA cycle, glutathione synthesis and the metabolism of arginine, nucleotides and amino acids in both D425MED and MED211 orthotopic tumors. The y-axis is the log10 p value and the x-axis represents the pathway impact value computed from pathway topological analysis. The color and the size of the circles are based on the p-value and the number of hits. Larger circles indicate more metabolites are upregulated in that pathway and more red color indicates increasing statistical significance. (**E,F**) The three most abundant metabolites found in orthotopic D425MED (**E**) and MED211 (**F**) tumors compared to normal brain were glutamine, glutamate and glutathione. Glutamine and glutamate were observed at lower levels compared to normal brain, but the ratio of glutamate/glutamine was significantly higher in tumor compared to normal brain, suggesting higher glutamine usage in tumors. Glutathione (GSH) was also upregulated in tumors compared to normal brain. Abbreviations: normal (control) cerebellum = CTL CB; normal (control) cortex = CTL CTX; D425MED orthotopic tumor = D425MED; MED211 orthotopic tumor = MED211. The bar graphs show the mean intensities with the SD as error bar. Each group has three biological replicate samples. * $p < 0.05$, ** $p < 0.01$, *** $p < 0.001$, Student's t-test, n.s. = not significant.

3.2. The Metabolic Profile of MYC-Amplified Medulloblastoma In Vitro Models Was Distinct from In Vivo Flank and Orthotopic Xenograft Tumor Models

A major aim of our study was to learn how cancer cells alter their metabolic pathways to adapt to different growth environments, and the degree to which in vitro models recapitulated in vivo conditions. We therefore performed PCA comparing known metabolites of D425MED and MED211 MYC—amplified medulloblastoma in three different environments: in vitro, flank xenograft and orthotopic xenograft tumors growing in the cerebellum. The analysis showed that the metabolic profiles of in vivo settings (orthotopic and flank xenograft tumors) clustered closely together, but separated away from normal brain and the profile of the in vitro models (Figure 2A,B). We applied stable isotope uniformly labeled glucose (13C6) and glutamine (13C515N2) metabolomics to further understand how cancer cells utilize these substrates in different tumor environments.

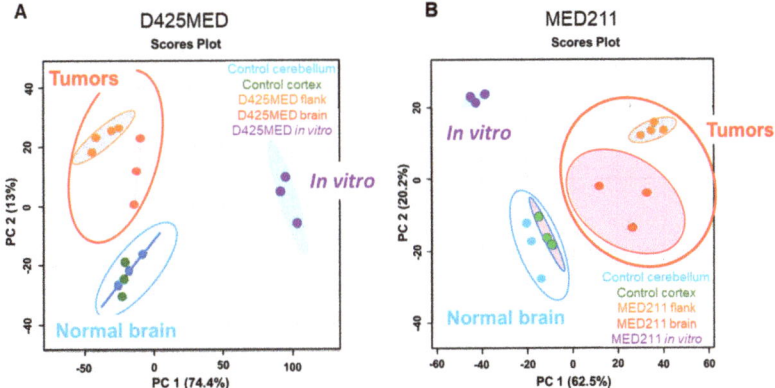

Figure 2. (**A,B**). Principal component analysis shows the metabolomes of orthotopic and flank xenograft tumors of D425MED (**A**) and MED211 (**B**) cluster closely together and are separated from normal brain and the metabolome of D425MED and MED211 cells grown in an in vitro environment. Abbreviations: normal (control) cerebellum = CTL CB; normal (control) cortex = CTL CTX; D425MED orthotopic tumor = D425MED brain; D425MED flank xenograft tumor = D425MED flank; MED211 orthotopic tumor = MED211 brain; MED211 flank xenograft tumor = MED211 flank.

3.3. Glucose Is the Main Carbon Source Fueling the TCA Cycle in Normal Brain and Orthotopic D425MED High MYC Medulloblastoma

Glucose is the main energy source in the normal brain. After entering cells, glucose is converted to glucose-6-phosphate, which is used in different metabolic pathways, such as the pentose phosphate pathway (PPP), the hexosamine biosynthetic pathway (HBP), amino acid synthesis, glycolysis and oxidative phosphorylation (Figure 3A). In normal brain, glucose is one of the critical energy sources, and normal brain expresses high levels of the glucose transporter GLUT1 (encoded by *SLC2A1*). We detected increased levels of GLUT1 in normal brain and in orthotopic medulloblastoma tumor compared to flank tumors (Figure 3B).

While glucose is a key energy source in normal brain, the normal brain also produces lactate at high levels. Lactate is one of the products of glycolysis that is highly present in normal brain and is transported from glia to neurons to provide an additional energy source through the astrocyte–neuron lactate shuttle [35]. We detected much higher lactate in normal brain and in orthotopic medulloblastoma tumor than in flank tumors or cells in culture (Figure 3C).

We then applied uniformly labeled glucose to study the contribution of glucose carbons into different downstream metabolic pathways. Isotope tracing using uniformly labeled glucose (13C6, m + 6) showed that glucose carbons contributed significantly to glutamate synthesis (which had the highest intensities of labeled 13C among other downstream glucose derived metabolites) in orthotopic xenograft tumor and normal brain (Figure 3D). The glucose-derived pyruvate m + 2 (derived through the pentose phosphate pathway) and m + 3 (generated by glycolysis) lose one carbon to yield Acetyl-coA m + 1 and m + 2 when entering the TCA cycle. As a result, cells yield m + 1 and m + 2 glucose-derived glutamate, as the product of the first completed TCA cycle turn. There were also glucose-derived glutamate m + 3, m + 4 and m + 5 (which are derived from citrate m + 3, m + 4, m + 5 as the products of m + 1, m + 2, m + 3 OAA combining with Acetyl-coA m + 1, m + 2) in normal brain and MYC-amplified medulloblastoma tumors, that represented the products of the TCA after the second turn and third turns. These data demonstrate that glucose is incorporated into the TCA cycle in high MYC medulloblastoma orthotopic tumors. There was even higher glucose incorporation into the TCA cycle in orthotopic tumors compared to normal brain, and this was confirmed upon analysis of the TCA cycle intermediate metabolites found in tumor and normal brain (Figure S2A). These findings confirmed that tumor cells simultaneously use glycolysis and oxidative phosphorylation.

We found the highest intensities of glucose-derived glutamate in orthotopic xenograft tumors, indicating that these tumors robustly synthesize glutamate through the TCA cycle. By comparing the intensities of glutamate isotopologues and other intermediate metabolites found in the TCA cycle in our three different settings, we found there was significantly higher glucose anaplerosis in orthotopic tumors compared to flank xenograft tumors and in vitro culture (Figure 3E, Figure S2B). These findings show that orthotopic D425MED *MYC*-amplified medulloblastoma and the control normal brain had higher uptake and use of glucose compared to D425MED flank xenograft tumors or D425MED cells in culture.

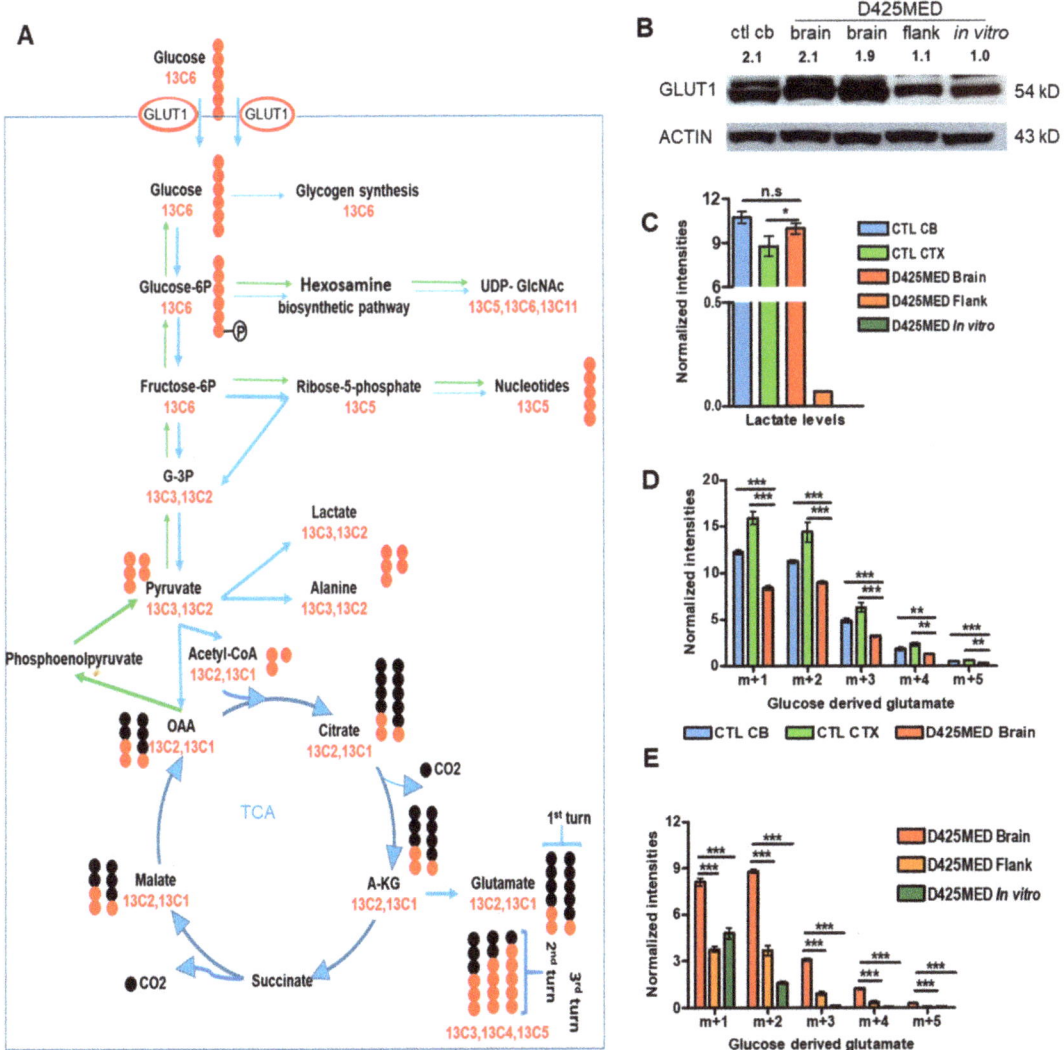

Figure 3. Glucose is the main carbon source for the TCA cycle in MYC-amplified medulloblastoma in vivo and xenograft tumors actively synthesize glutamate from glucose. (**A**) Cartoon illustrating the tracing method of uniformly labeled 13C6 glucose after being transported into cells by the glucose transporter GLUT1 and its contribution to different metabolic pathways. Red dots represent stable isotope labeled carbon C13 with one extra mass on the regular carbon 12C. Black dots represent for unlabeled carbon, or 12C. By tracing down the number of labeled carbon 13C (from uniformly labeled glucose 13C6) appearing in the downstream glucose-derived metabolites, we are able to tell how much glucose carbon contributes to the TCA cycle, glutamate synthesis, and other metabolites through different metabolic pathways. (**B**) Western blot showing higher expression of the glucose transporter GLUT1 (encoded by SLC2A1) in normal brain (ctl cb) and orthotopic tumor (D425MED brain) versus flank tumor (D425MED flank) and in vitro D425MED cells. Numbers above the blot indicate the densitometry normalized to ACTIN and compared to the in vitro condition. Uncropped

western blots are included in supplementary materials. (**C**) Bar graph showing increased lactate intensities in normal brain (NCB and CTX) and D425MED orthotopic tumors compared to flank tumors and D425MED cells in culture (in vitro). (**D**) Bar graph showing glucose-derived glutamate levels in normal brain (NCB and CTX) and lower levels in D425MED Brain (orthotopic tumor). Glutamate was the most abundant glucose-derived metabolite found in tumor and normal brain. (**E**) Bar graph showing increased glucose-derived glutamate levels in orthotopic tumor (D425MED Brain) compared to flank tumor and D425MED cells in culture. The highest intensities of glucose derived glutamate were found in orthotopic xenograft tumors (m + 1, m + 2, m + 3) compared to flank tumors and D425MED cells in culture. Abbreviations: normal (control) cerebellum = CTL CB; normal (control) cortex = CTL CTX; D425MED orthotopic tumor = D425MED brain; D425MED flank xenograft tumor = D425MED flank; D425MED cells in culture = D425MED in vitro. TCA = tricarboxylic acid. The bar graph shows the mean intensities with the SD as error bar. Each group has three biological replicate samples. * $p < 0.05$, ** $p < 0.01$, *** $p < 0.001$, Student's *t*-test.

3.4. Glucose-Derived Glutamate Was Used Differently in the In Vitro vs. In Vivo Setting

Glutamate is a major excitatory neurotransmitter in the brain [36]. Glutamate can also be converted to glutamine by glutamine synthetase (GS) [37–39] or incorporated into glutathione synthesis [40]. We detected significantly higher glucose-derived glutathione in tumors compared to normal brain, indicating that *MYC*-amplified medulloblastoma was using carbons from glucose to synthesize glutamate, which was then being incorporated into glutathione and glutamine (Figure 4A,B). Interestingly, we observed decreased m + 1, m + 2, and m + 3 glucose-derived glutamate and glutamine in orthotopic tumor compared to normal brain, but increased m + 1, m + 2, and m + 3 glutathione. One explanation for this would be that the tumor cells have increased glutathione needs and so are preferentially shunting the glucose carbons into glutathione, rather than allowing them to accumulate in glutamate and glutamine.

We also found significantly higher glutamine synthesis in orthotopic tumors compared to flank tumors and cells in culture. We found increased glucose-derived glutamine isotopologue intensities as well as increased glutamine synthetase (GS) protein expression by Western blot in orthotopic brain tumor compared to flank or cells in culture (Figure 4C,D). Although orthotopic tumors used glucose carbons to synthesize glutathione to a greater degree than normal brain, in comparing orthotopic, flank and in vitro D425MED, we found that in vitro tumor cells incorporated glucose carbons to the greatest extent into glutathione (Figure 4E). We confirmed that in vitro D425MED had the highest glutathione levels with non-labeled glutathione intensities (Figure 4F). Western blot showed increased expression of glutathione synthetase in cells in culture compared to orthotopic or flank D425MED tumor and normal cerebellum (Figure 4G), which was consistent with an increased glutathione production in cells in culture compared to orthotopic or flank tumors.

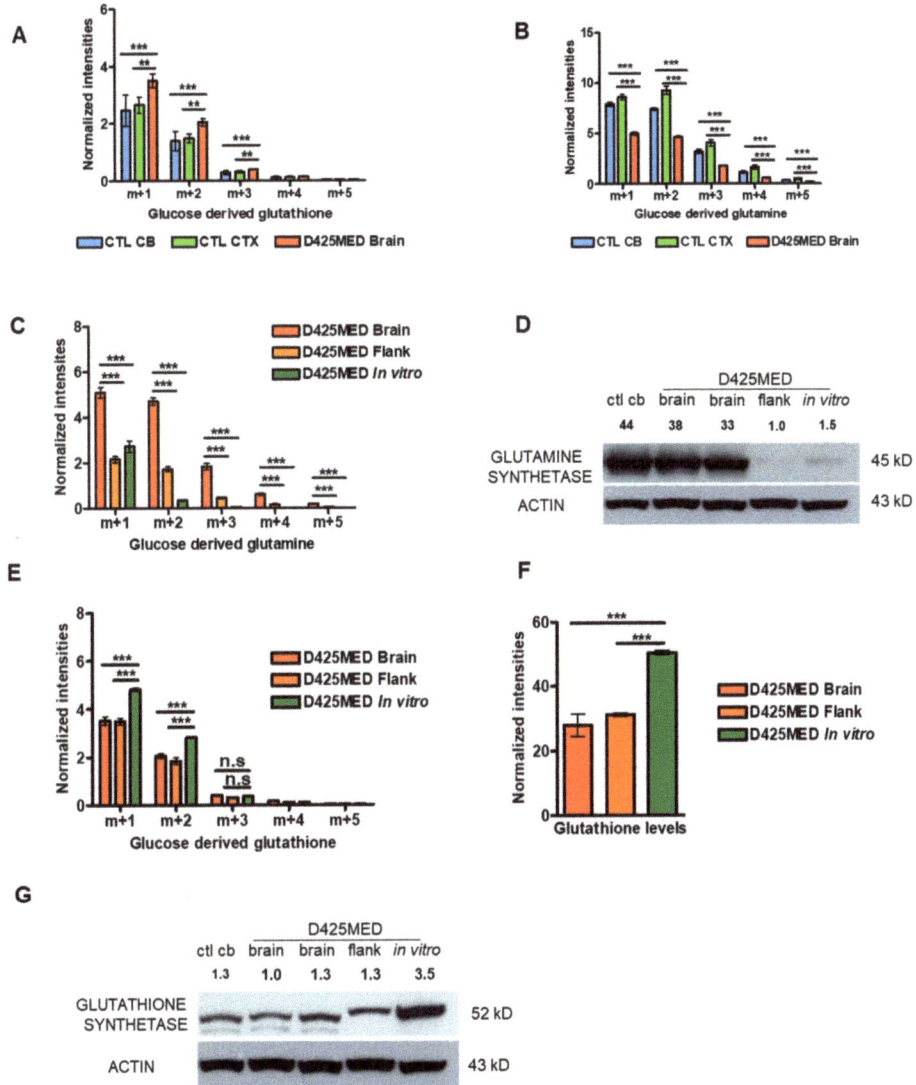

Figure 4. Glucose is the main carbon source for the TCA cycle in *MYC*-amplified medulloblastoma in vivo and xenograft tumors actively synthesize glutamine and glutathione. (**A**) Bar graph showing increased glucose-derived glutathione in orthotopic tumor compared to normal brain. (**B**) Bar graph showing lower intensities of glucose-derived glutamine found in orthotopic tumor compared to normal brain. (**C**) Bar graph showing increased m + 1, m + 2, m + 3 glucose-derived-glutamine in orthotopic D425MED tumors compared to flank tumors and cells in culture. (**D**) Western blot showing increased glutamine synthetase expression in normal cerebellum (ctl cb) and orthotopic tumor (D425MED brain) compared to flank tumor and D425MED cells in in vitro. Numbers above the graph indicate densitometry of the band normalized to ACTIN, compared to the "flank" condition. (**E**) Bar graph showing increased m + 1, m + 2, m + 3 glucose-derived glutathione in D425MED cells in vitro compared to orthotopic and flank tumors. (**F**) Bar graph showing unlabeled glutathione levels are highest in D425MED cells in culture compared to flank and orthotopic tumors. (**G**) Western

blot showing increased glutathione synthetase in D425MED cells in culture compared to flank and orthotopic tumors and normal brain (ctl cb). Numbers above the blot indicate densitometry normalized to ACTIN and compared to the lowest expression in normal brain. Uncropped western blots are included in supplementary materials. Abbreviations: normal (control) cerebellum = CTL CB; normal (control) cortex = CTL CTX; D425MED orthotopic tumor = D425MED brain; D425MED flank xenograft tumor = D425MED flank. The bar graph shows the mean intensities with the SD as error bar. Each group has three biological replicate samples. n.s. not significant, ** $p < 0.01$, *** $p < 0.001$, Student's t-test.

3.5. Gluconeogenesis Contributed to the Hexosamine Biosynthetic Pathway and Was Upregulated in Orthotopic D425MED High-MYC Medulloblastoma Tumor Compared to Normal Brain

Orthotopic *MYC*-amplified medulloblastoma D425MED tumors had increased levels of glucosamine-6-phosphate compared to normal brain, suggesting increased reliance on the hexosamine biosynthetic pathway, which is the main pathway used for glycosylation of proteins [41] (Figure 5A). Consistent with increased activity of the hexosamine pathway, we detected increased incorporation of glucose carbons in uridine diphosphate n-acetylglucosamine (UDP-GlcNAc) in our in vivo orthotopic xenografts compared to normal brain (Figure 5A). These metabolites were generated through the gluconeogenesis pathway because m + 1 was the most abundant intensity found among the isotopologues. The HBP is more active in vivo compared to in vitro, with significantly increased total Glucosamine-6P and m + 1 UDP-GlcNAc in flank and orthotopic xenografts compared to cells in culture (Figure 5B).

Interrogation of the Children's Brain Tumor Network/KidsFirst Pediatric Brain Tumor Atlas RNAseq data showed increased expression of mRNAs encoding key enzymes of the hexosamine biosynthetic pathway in medulloblastoma compared to other pediatric brain tumors (Figure 5C). Specifically, compared to pediatric low-grade glioma, we detected in medulloblastoma increased *GFPT1*, which encodes for the enzyme GFAT that converts fructose-6P to glucosamine-6P, the rate-limiting step in hexosamine synthesis [41]. We also found upregulated *GNA1*, which encodes enzyme that converts glucosamine-6P to N-acetylglucosamine 6P (GlcNac-6P). We found increased RNA levels of *AGX1*, which encodes the enzyme that converts GlcNac-1P to UDP-GlcNAc, as well as *OGT*, an enzyme that transfers N-acetyl-glucosamine (GlcNAc) to proteins. Figure 5D shows a cartoon overview of the pathway highlighting the metabolites we identified as upregulated and the corresponding upregulated enzymes.

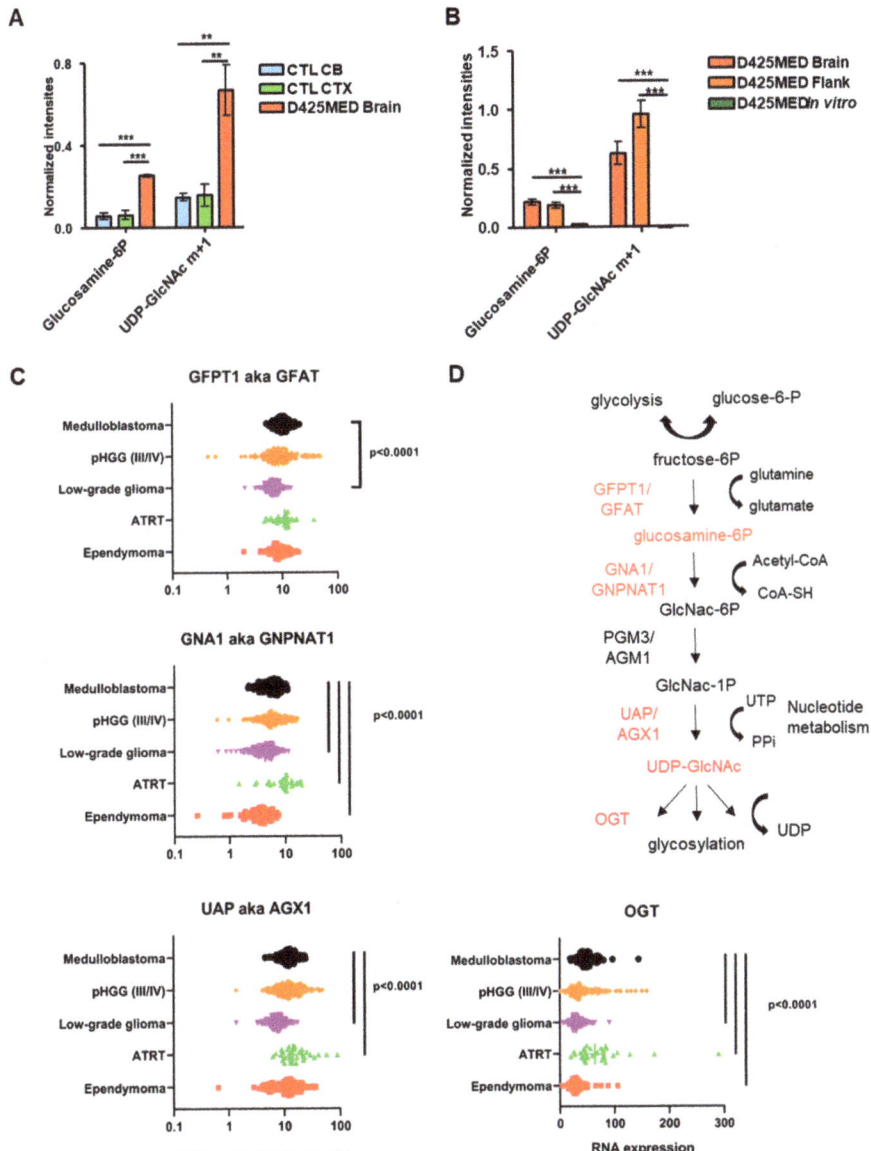

Figure 5. Upregulation of hexosamine biosynthetic pathway in the D425MED orthotopic tumor. (**A**) Bar graph showing that intermediate metabolites found in the hexosamine pathway were significantly higher in tumor compared to normal brain. Total levels of glucosamine-6-phosphate were increased in the D425MED tumor compared to normal brain. We also detected increased levels of Uridine diphosphate-N-acetyl Glucosamine (UDP-GlcNAc) in our studies of incorporation of uniformly labeled glucose. Metabolites were found mostly as m + 1 isotopes, suggesting they were generated through gluconeogenesis. (**B**) Bar graph showing increased hexosamine pathway metabolites in flank and orthotopic D425MED compared to cells in culture. We found increased Glucoseamine-6P and m + 1 UDP-GlcNAc in orthotopic and flank tumors compared to D425MED in culture. The bar graph

shows the mean intensities with the SD as error bar. Each group has three biological replicate samples. ** $p < 0.01$, *** $p < 0.001$, Student's t-test. (**C**) Interrogation of the Children's Brain Tumor Network Pediatric Brain Tumor Atlas RNAseq dataset showed that primary medulloblastoma tumors have increased expression of enzymes in the hexosamine biosynthetic pathway, including *GFAT, GNA1, UAP* and *OGT*, compared to other pediatric brain tumors, particularly low-grade glioma. Bars indicate statistical significance by one-way ANOVA with Dunnet multiple comparisons correction. ATRT tumors had increased average expression of *GNA1, UAP,* and *OGT* compared to medulloblastoma. (**D**) Cartoon showing the hexosamine biosynthetic pathway, with metabolites and their corresponding enzymes that are upregulated in medulloblastoma tumors highlighted in red. The bi-directional arrow at top indicates that glycolysis is reversible and gluconeogenesis may also occur. Abbreviations: Normal (control) cerebellum = CTL CB; Normal (control) cortex = CTL CTX; D425MED orthotopic tumor = D425MED brain; D425MED flank xenograft tumor = D425MED flank. ATRT = atypical teratoid/rhabdoid tumor; pHGG = pediatric high-grade glioma.

3.6. The Glutaminase II Pathway Was the Main Pathway Metabolizing Glutamine In Vivo

Glutamine is another major nutrient source for cells. Glutamine is used to synthesize amino acids, nucleotides and glutathione [42]. After conversion to alpha-ketoglutarate, glutamine can replenish the TCA cycle. We used uniformly labeled glutamine (13C5, 15N2) to understand how high MYC medulloblastoma in different environments metabolized glutamine.

The glutaminase 1 pathway is the most known pathway of glutamine metabolism. In this pathway, the glutaminase 1 (GLS1) enzyme converts glutamine to glutamate [43,44]. However, there is another series of enzymatic reactions (starting with glutamine transaminase K (GTK also known as KYAT1) followed by NIT2 called the "glutaminase II pathway" that is the main pathway to utilize glutamine in the brain [32,45–47]. In Figure 6A, we show how uniformly labeled glutamine (m + 7) is utilized under both pathways to generate glutamate isotopologues.

We found glutamine-derived glutamate was metabolized through both glutaminase 1 (yielding m + 6) and glutaminase ii pathways (yielding m + 1, m + 5) in cultured D425MED cells (Figure 6B). However, D425MED flank xenograft tumors showed a different pattern of glutamate isotopologues (Figure 6C) in which glutamate m + 1 was the most abundant. In the orthotopic D425MED tumor, this pattern became even more biased toward the glutaminase II pathway, in that almost all of the glutamine-derived glutamate was m + 1 and m + 5, and there was virtually undetectable amounts of glutamate m + 6. The glutaminase II pathway was also predominant in normal cortex and cerebellum (Figure 6D,E). The changing pattern among glutamine-derived glutamate isotopologues showed that most glutamine-derived glutamate was generated through the glutaminase II pathways (GTK) in vivo. We found similar changes in MED211 high MYC amplified medulloblastoma in flank xenograft tumors compared to MED211 cells in culture (Supplemental Figure S3A,B).

In the brain and orthotopic MYC-driven medulloblastoma tumor in addition to m + 1, we also detected at a much lower level in the orthotopic tumor, m + 2, m + 3 and m + 5 glutamate. These other species may represent glutamine carbons that were incorporated into the TCA cycle through alpha-ketoglutarate and then cycled back out after several turns to resynthesize glutamine. Alternatively, the m + 2 and m + 3 isotopologues may represent glutamine carbons that were incorporated in another organ in the mouse into glucose through gluconeogenesis. The resulting circulating glucose then contributed to glutamate and glutamine in tumor and brain via glycolysis and the TCA cycle. However, other glutamine-derived TCA metabolites were virtually undetectable in vivo.

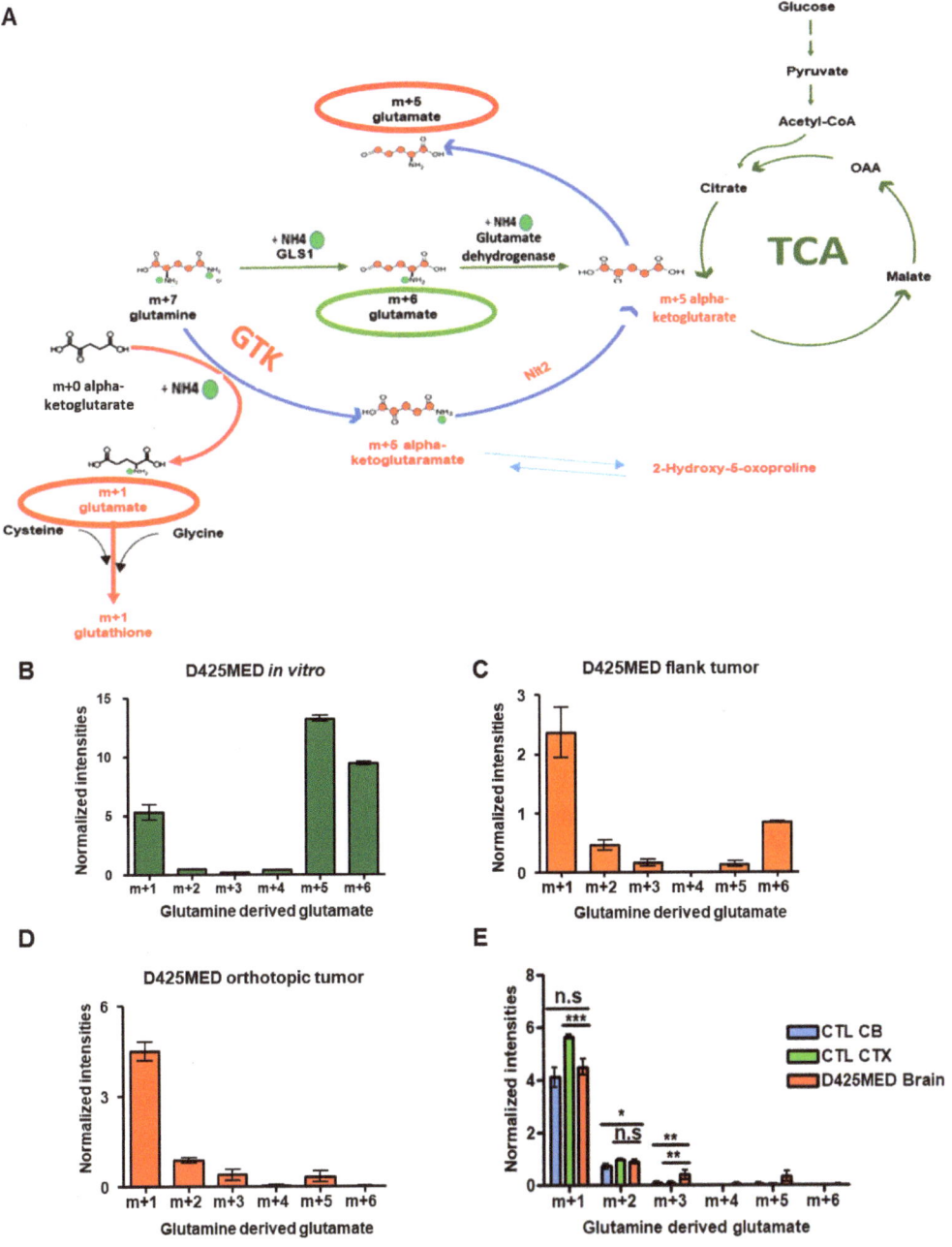

Figure 6. D425MED orthotopic tumors preferentially use the glutaminase II (GTK) pathway over the glutaminase 1 (GLS1) pathway. (**A**) Cartoon illustrating how glutamine is metabolized through GLS1 to yield glutamate m + 6 isotope (green arrows). The glutaminase II pathway (blue arrows) uses glutamine transaminase K (GTK) to generate glutamate m + 1 by adding the amino group from labeled glutamine to alpha-KG. The Nit2 enzyme converts m + 6 alpha-ketoglutaramate (KGM) to m + 5 alpha-KG. This can in turn be converted to m + 5 glutamate by glutamate dehydrogenasae. (**B**) Bar graph showing glutamine-derived glutamate in D425MED cells in vitro, with predominance

of m + 6. (**C**) Bar graph showing glutamine-derived glutamate in D425MED cells in flank tumors, showing increasing prominence of m + 1. (**D**) Bar graph showing glutamine-derived glutamate in D425MED cells in orthotopic tumors, showing predominance of m + 1 and near-absence of m + 6. (**E**) Bar graph comparing glutamine-derived glutamate in D425MED cells in orthotopic tumors and normal brain, showing predominance of m + 1 isotopologue. Abbreviations: normal (control) cerebellum = CTL CB; normal (control) cortex = CTL CTX; D425MED orthotopic tumor = D425MED brain; D425MED flank xenograft tumor = D425MED flank. The bar graph shows the mean intensities with the SD as error bar. Each group has three biological replicate samples. n.s. not significant, * $p < 0.05$, ** $p < 0.01$, *** $p < 0.001$, Student's *t*-test.

3.7. Glutamine Derived Glutathione Synthesis Was Mainly through GTK, and It Was Upregulated in Orthotopic D425MED High MYC Xenograft Tumors Compared to Normal Brain

For in vitro and in vivo D425MED, the most abundant labeled glutathione isotopologue was m + 1 (Figure 7A–C). Glutamate m + 1 derived glutathione was synthesized mainly through the glutaminase II pathway. The glutamine transaminase K (GTK or KYAT1) enzyme used endogenous alpha ketoglutarate (alpha-keto acid of glutamate) to incorporate the amino group from uniformly labeled glutamine to form glutamate m + 1. This m + 1 glutamate, together with cysteine and glycine, formed glutathione m + 1 (as demonstrated in the cartoon in Figure 6A). We found similar changes in MED211 in cell culture and flank xenograft tumors (Figure S3C,D).

Orthotopic tumors had significantly higher m + 1 glutamine-derived glutathione compared to normal brain (Figure 7D). Increased activity of GTK in orthotopic tumors was also confirmed with the ratio of m + 1 glutamate to total glutamine in D425MED tumor compared to normal cerebellum (Figure 7E). Western blot of GLS1, GTK, and NIT2 showed increased expression of GTK in orthotopic D452MED tumors compared to normal brain. (Figure 7F).

To extend our findings to additional medulloblastoma tumors, we interrogated the Children's Brain Tumor Network/KidsFirst Pediatric Brain Tumor Atlas RNAseq dataset (PedscBioportal). We found that medulloblastoma expresses significantly higher mRNA for *KYAT*, the gene that encodes GTK compared to other pediatric brain tumors, including ependymoma, low-grade glioma and atypical teratoid/rhabdoid tumor (ATRT). Expression of *KYAT* was not statistically significant compared to pediatric high-grade glioma (Figure S4).

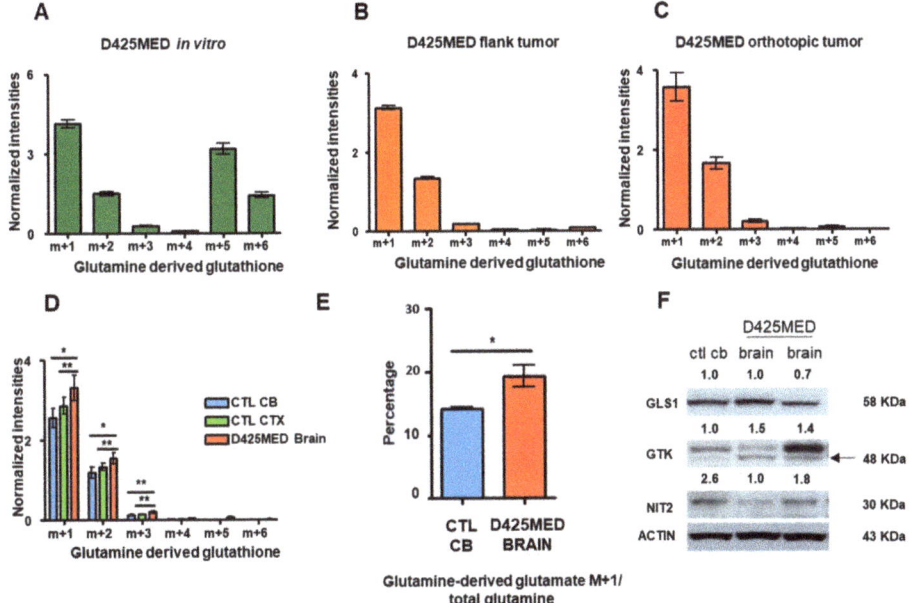

Figure 7. GTK is the main enzyme responsible for glutathione synthesis in vivo. (**A–C**). Bar graphs showing the contribution of glutamine-derived carbons and nitrogens to glutathione in D425MED in different environments. The majority of glutathione was synthesized through GTK because the highest glutamine-derived glutathione was the m + 1 isotopologue, in all models. The predominance is most stark in orthotopic tumors, where the m + 6 isotopologue is virtually undetectable. (**D**) Bar graph showing increased glutamine-derived glutathione in orthotopic tumor compared to normal brain. (**E**) Bar graph showing m + 1 glutamate to glutamine ratio in D425MED cells in orthotopic tumors. (**F**) Western blot of glutaminase II pathway enzymes showing increased GTK (arrow) in D425MED orthotopic tumors (D425MED brain) compared to uninvolved cerebellum (CTL CB). The upper band is likely non-specific. ACTIN shows equal loading in all lanes. In contrast to GTK, we did not detect increased NIT2 or GLS1 protein expression MED tumor compared to normal cerebellum. Numbers above each blot show densitometry normalized to ACTIN. Abbreviations: normal (control) cerebellum = CTL CB; normal (control) cortex = CTL CTX; D425MED orthotopic tumor = D425MED brain; D425MED flank xenograft tumor = D425MED flank. The bar graphs show the mean intensities with the SD as error bar. Each group has three biological replicate samples. * $p < 0.05$, ** $p < 0.01$, Student's *t*-test.

3.8. Overall Model of the Metabolomics of Orthotopic MYC-Amplified Medulloblastoma Reveals Key Dependencies That May Be Therapeutically Targetable

Our metabolic analysis of MYC-amplified medulloblastoma revealed upregulation in the metabolism of nucleotides, glutathione, the hexosamine biosynthetic pathway, the urea cycle and amino acids compared to normal brain. We also found increases in TCA cycle components malate, succinate and fumarate. Figure 8A shows a cartoon of the relationship between the TCA and urea cycles, with metabolites found to be upregulated in orthotopic MYC-amplified tumors highlighted in red. Outside of the liver, the urea cycle is not complete, in that there is no expression of the enzyme ornithine transcarbamylase (OTC1) that converts ornithine to citrulline and scavenges ammonia [48–50]. The urea cycle is a critical synthetic pathway to produce polyamines by production of ornithine. The urea cycle also produces the signaling molecule nitric oxide (NO) from arginine [48], generating citrulline. Citrulline is combined with aspartate by arginosuccinate synthetase (ASS1) to produce arginoosuccinate. The TCA cycle and urea cycle are linked by fumarate, which shuttles between the pathways in a reversible fashion catalyzed by the enzyme arginosuccinate lyase (ASL) [51]. ASL combines arginosuccinate and fumarate to make arginine.

While we did not detect increased arginine itself, we did identify increased citrulline and ornithine in MYC-amplified orthotopic tumors compared to normal brain. Ornithine is produced by arginase (ARG) or separately in several enzymatic steps from proline. ARG2 is the arginase enzyme most highly expressed in brain tissue [52]. Proline was also increased in MYC-amplified medulloblastoma compared to normal brain. Ornithine is subsequently incorporated into the polyamine biosynthetic pathway by ornithine decarboxylase (ODC1). Polyamines are post-translational protein modifications that promote invasion and growth of cancer cells [53].

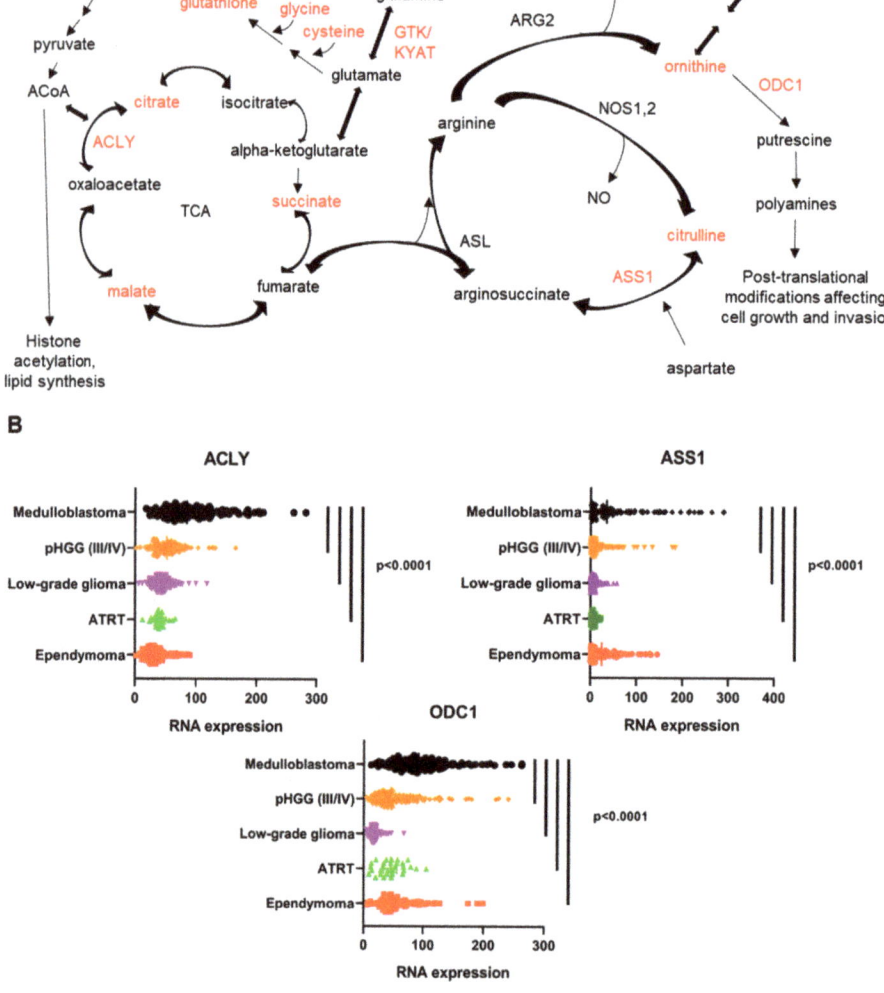

Figure 8. A Cartoon overview of some of the metabolic vulnerabilities identified in our study. Metabolites that we identified as being upregulated in orthotopic MYC-amplified medulloblastoma

compared to normal brain are highlighted in red. We identified upregulation of the hexosamine biosynthetic pathway, which is key for the glycosylation of proteins. We also found increased glutathione and elevated levels of the amino acids glycine and cysteine that are combined with glutamate to produce glutathione. We identified upregulation of TCA cycle intermediates succinate and malate and detected glucose-derived carbons in these metabolites, indicating that oxidative phosphorylation was likely occurring in orthotopic tumors. The glutaminase II pathway, featuring glutamine transaminase K (GTK) (encoded by the gene *KYAT*) is the predominate glutaminase pathway in the brain and in orthotopic MYC-amplified tumors. The enzyme ATP citrate lyase (ACLY) converts citate to oxaloacetate and acetyl-CoA, fueling fatty acid biosynthesis and also facilitating the reversal of the TCA cycle. The cartoon highlights the interaction between the tricarboxylic acid (TCA) cycle and urea cycle, in which fumarate shuttles between the two metabolic pathways through the reversible activity of arginosuccinate lyase (ASL). We identified upregulation of the urea cycle intermediates citrulline and ornithine. Citrulline is generated by the degradation of arginine during nitric oxide (NO) production. The enzyme arginosuccinate synthetase 1 (ASS1) combines citrulline with aspartate to generate arginosuccinate. Arginase 2 (ARG2) converts arginine to ornithine, releasing urea. Ornithine can also be synthesized in several steps from proline, which was also increased in *MYC*-amplified medulloblastoma compared to normal brain. Ornithine is a precursor of polyamines, which are intermediates for post-translational protein modification. Ornithine decarboxylase (ODC1) converts ornithine to putrescine, the first step in polyamine synthesis. Outside of the liver, the urea cycle does not generate citrulline from ornithine due to the low expression of ornithine transcarbamylase. Analysis of the Children's Brain Tumor Network Pediatric Brain Tumor Atlas RNAseq dataset shows increased expression of the mRNA encoding ATP citrate lyase (ACLY), arginosuccinate synthetase 1 (ASS1), and ornithine decarboxylase (ODC1) in medulloblastoma compared to other pediatric brain tumor subtypes. (**B**). *p* values indicated at the right represent results of one-way ANOVA with Dunnet multiple comparisons correction. Each dot represents RNA from a single tumor sample. The vertical bar in each tumor type shows the mean intensity of normalized RNA expression. Metabolic enzymes that we identified as being upregulated in 8B or in other figures in this paper are highlighted in red in (**A**).

To determine if some of the metabolic pathways we identified might be active in human patients with medulloblastoma, we queried the Children's Brain Tumor Network/KidsFirst Pediatric Brain Tumor Atlas RNAseq dataset (PedscBioportal). We identified increased mRNA levels of *ACLY*, *ASS1* and *ODC1* in medulloblastoma primary tumors compared to other pediatric brain tumors, suggesting an increased reliance in medulloblastoma on polyamines, arginine biosynthesis and the TCA cycle/production of acetyl-CoA (Figure 8B). Of note, we did not detect increased expression in medulloblastoma compared to other pediatric brain tumors of mRNA for pyruvate carboxylase (which would allow direct incorporation of pyruvate carbons to oxaloacetate) or any of the other TCA cycle or urea cycle enzymes).

4. Discussion

We identified significant differences in glucose and glutamine metabolism in high MYC medulloblastoma comparing in vitro, flank xenografts and orthotopic xenograft medulloblastoma models. *MYC*-amplified D425MED and MED211 medulloblastoma orthotopic xenograft brain tumors upregulated nucleotide, hexosamine, amino acid and glutathione synthesis compared to normal brain. Glutathione was the most abundant upregulated metabolite found in tumors compared to normal brain. Our findings were consistent with recently reported proteomics data in *MYC*-amplified medulloblastoma, showing upregulation of the glutathione biosynthetic pathway compared to non-MYC-amplified medulloblastoma and normal brain [54].

We found significantly higher glucose uptake and usage in normal brain and orthotopic xenografts compared to flank xenografts and in cells in culture. Glycolysis and incorporation of glucose into the TCA cycle were concurrently found in all settings. Similar findings showing incorporation of glucose carbons into the TCA cycle were reported in metabolic profiling of orthotopic glioblastomas [55].

Medulloblastoma tumors in our studies had higher activity of glucose anaplerosis compared to normal brain. D425MED orthotopic xenografts exhibited the strongest oxidative phosphorylation activities, even at presumably the lowest oxygen tension (3–5% in the brain compared to 21% for cells in culture) [56]. Glucose was the main carbon source for glutamate synthesis through the TCA cycle in high MYC amplified medulloblastoma. This finding confirms robust metabolism of glucose through glycolysis and into the TCA cycle in cancer cells in orthotopic xenografts. The incorporation of glucose into the TCA cycle contradicts a key claim of the "Warburg effect", namely that cancer cells are reliant on glycolysis for ATP generation and that glucose carbons would not be significantly incorporated into the TCA cycle [57,58].

Rather than being reliant on glutamine from the microenvironment, we found that MYC-amplified medulloblastoma tumor cells synthesized glutamine. Keeping with this theme of glutamine synthesis, the majority of glutamate in vivo became the precursor for glutamine via the activity of glutamine synthetase. This phenomenon may be considered as an anaplerotic reaction to replenish the neurotransmitter pool and for macromolecular synthesis through the TCA cycle in the brain [59]. The differences in metabolic profile between the orthotopic, flank and in vitro settings reflect the plasticity of D425-MED and MED211 MYC amplified medulloblastoma. There are as-yet unknown factors driving de novo glutamine synthesis in orthotopic tumors compared to the emphasis on glutathione production in vitro.

The differences in metabolic data found in D425MED and MED211 among settings reflect that metabolic reprograming is not only the consequence of genetic mutations but also the crosstalk of cancer cells to the microenvironment. Genetics define metabolic pathways to an extent, but the differences in nutrient availability, oxygen levels, pH and interactions with stromal cells in the different environments also regulate metabolic gene expression [52,60].

Metabolic analysis of orthotopic MYC-amplified tumors was key for identification of de novo biosynthesis of glutamine, since this was not noted in cells in culture, where glutamine is abundant in the culture media. Based on the abundance of m + 1 glutamate and the absence of m + 6 glutamate in orthotopic tumors, we conclude that the glutaminase II pathway is the main pathway utilizing glutamine in MYC-amplified medulloblastoma. Supporting this conclusion, we identified increased expression of GTK in tumor compared to normal brain. GTK functions to salvage alpha-keto acids, transfer alpha-keto acid/amino acid carbons between cellular and intracellular compartments, and in the methionine salvage pathway [61]. Uniformly labeled glutamine metabolic analyses demonstrated that the two most abundant glutamine-derived metabolites were glutamate and glutathione in vivo and these were synthesized through the glutamine transaminase K (GTK) enzyme. The glutaminase II pathway is important in normal brain metabolism [61]. However, we believe our report here is the first to describe the glutaminase II pathway as being predominant in MYC-amplified medulloblastoma. While we cannot fully exclude the activity of GLS1 in generating an m + 1 amino group that could be incorporated into m + 1 glutamate, the lack of m + 6 glutamate suggests that GLS is not as active in the brain compared to cells in culture and flank tumors and that GTK is the predominant glutaminase enzyme.

The accumulation of glutamine carbons in glutamate rather than in TCA cycle intermediates emphasizes the importance of glutamine and glutamate as key amino acids for MYC-driven medulloblastoma and is concordant with our finding that these tumor cells use glucose carbons via the TCA cycle to synthesize glutamate and glutamine (Figures 3E and 4C). Our data suggest there is very little glutamine carbon that contributes to the TCA cycle in MYC-amplified medulloblastoma in vivo.

The work presented here also identifies some key metabolic differences between normal cerebellum and cortex and MYC-amplified medulloblastoma tumors. Specifically, we identified upregulation of multiple amino acids, such as proline, glycine, histidine and asparagine in medulloblastoma compared to normal brain. We also found upregulation of urea cycle components citrulline and ornithine. The prominence of arginine biosynthesis in the pathway impact analysis (Figure 1C,D) highlights the upregulation of the citrulline–arginine cycle, in both *MYC*-driven medulloblastoma orthotopic xenograft models compared to normal brain. Arginine is used for the synthesis of polyamines, nitric oxide and urea [48,49,62,63]. Polyamines promote oncogenesis by supporting production of nucleic acids and proteins and regulating chromatin and transcription [53,64]. This work also confirmed and extended our prior finding that glutathione was upregulated in *MYC*-amplified medulloblastoma compared to normal brain [40]. Validating our metabolic data, we found that enzymes regulating the TCA and urea cycle are upregulated in medulloblastoma compared to other pediatric brain tumors in the Children's Brain Tumor Network/KidsFirst Pediatric Brain Tumor Atlas RNAseq dataset. Specifically, we found increased *KYAT*, the mRNA encoding GTK the key step in the glutaminase II pathway. We also found increased arginosuccinate synthetase 1 (ASS1), which reversibly catalyzes the production of arginosuccinate from citrulline and aspartate [65]. This finding is consistent with an independent analysis of a separate dataset that showed high level expression of mRNA for *ASS1*, *ASL* and *ARG2* and low expression of *OTC1* in primary medulloblastoma tumors [49]. We also found increased ornithine decarboxylase 1 (ODC1), which catalyzes the conversion of ornithine to putrescine, the first step in polyamine production. Lastly, we found increased ATP-citrate lyase (ACLY), which cleaves citrate to release acetyl-CoA and produce oxaloacetate [66]. Increased activity of ACLY allows the TCA cycle to run in reverse to potentially produce fumarate to fuel the urea cycle, as shown in Figure 8A.

Targeting these novel vulnerabilities may lead to improved outcomes in *MYC*-amplified medulloblastoma. We previously demonstrated that disrupting glutathione metabolism extended survival of mice bearing *MYC*-driven medulloblastoma orthotopic xenografts, further validating our metabolic findings and showing the value of our metabolic profiling approach [40]. The drug difluromethylornithine (DFMO) blocks ODC1 and has had success in high-risk neuroblastoma clinical trials [67–69]. There are encouraging preclinical data combining DFMO and the polyamine transporter inhibitor in diffuse intrinsic pontine glioma [70], and this pathway is upregulated in Hedgehog-driven medulloblastoma as well [71].

Multiple drugs are in development in other tumors that target the urea cycle through inhibition of aspartate or ASS1 [72,73], and some of these agents could be applied to medulloblastoma tumors with vulnerable metabolic profiles. Recent publications suggest that clinical metabolic profiling can be performed on pediatric primary tumor samples, suggesting that targeting metabolic profiles could be a new frontier in pediatric cancer and in brain tumors in general [74].

Limitations of our study include a lack of primary human tumor samples for metabolic profiling. We also use only two human cell models of MYC-amplified medulloblastoma. Uniformly labeled metabolomic experiments in MED211 were performed in vitro and in flank tumors. The high degree of concordance between MED211 and D425MED in all analyses suggests reliance on common metabolic pathways in MYC-amplified medulloblastoma. In addition, these limitations are addressed in part by the corroborating data from our laboratory and other groups, showing increased expression of mRNA and proteins related to the synthesis of key metabolic targets in medulloblastoma patient tumors compared to other pediatric brain tumors [49,54,71]. Our laboratory has already validated the increased reliance on glutathione as a vulnerability by demonstrating the in vivo combinatorial efficacy of treatments that decrease glutathione and chemotherapy, such as carboplatin, that are detoxified by glutathione [40].

5. Conclusions

The metabolism of MYC-amplified medulloblastoma cancer cells is different in vitro compared to in vivo. Our study revealed the limitations of metabolic profiling conducted in non-native tumor environments (in cell culture and flank xenografts). We identified multiple metabolites that are altered in orthotopic MYC-amplified medulloblastoma xenografts compared to normal brain and showed in a large clinical dataset that the mRNAs for key enzymes in these pathways are upregulated. Targeting these pathways may represent novel therapeutic approaches for medulloblastoma patients.

Supplementary Materials: The following are available online at https://www.mdpi.com/article/10.3390/cancers14051311/s1, Figure S1: Histology of high MYC amplified medulloblastoma orthotopic D425MED, Figure S2: Orthotopic MYC-amplified medulloblastoma has upregulated TCA intermediates compared to normal brain. Figure S3: In vivo preponderance of glutaminase II pathway in generating glutamine-derived glutamate and glutamine-derived glutathione. Figure S4: Increased expression of KYAT1, the gene encoding GTK, in primary pediatric medulloblastoma compared to other pediatric brain tumor samples, Figure S5: Uncropped Western blots used in this manuscript.

Author Contributions: Conceptualization, K.P., B.A.P., A.R.H. and E.H.R.; methodology, K.P., H.S. and B.A.P.; software, K.P. and H.S.; validation, K.P.; formal analysis, K.P., J.A. and B.A.P.; investigation, K.P., A.R.H., A.P. and B.A.P.; resources, R.R., B.S.S., E.H.R. and C.G.E.; data curation, B.A.P. and K.P.; writing—original draft preparation, K.P.; writing—review and editing, E.H.R., M.J.M., C.G.E., A.R.H. and B.A.P.; visualization, K.P.; supervision, R.R., B.S.S. and E.H.R.; project administration, E.H.R. and B.S.S.; funding acquisition, E.H.R. and B.S.S. All authors have read and agreed to the published version of the manuscript.

Funding: NINDS 1R01NS103927 (BSS and EHR); The Spencer Grace Foundation (EHR), The Ace for a Cure Foundation (EHR); Hyundai Hope on Wheels (MJM), Giant Food Pediatric Cancer Research Fund; National Cancer Institute Core Grant to the Johns Hopkins Sidney Kimmel Comprehensive Cancer Center (P30CA006973).

Institutional Review Board Statement: "Principles of laboratory animal care" (NIH publication No. 8623, revised 1985) was followed, using a protocol approved by the Johns Hopkins Animal Care and Use Committee, in compliance with the United States Animal Welfare Act regulations and Public Health Service Policy.

Informed Consent Statement: Not applicable.

Data Availability Statement: The metabolomics data from this study will be uploaded to the NIH Common Fund's National Metabolomics Data Repository (NMDR) and will be available from the corresponding author on request.

Conflicts of Interest: Slusher and Rais are founders of and hold equity in Dracen Pharmaceuticals, Inc. This arrangement has been reviewed and approved by the Johns Hopkins University in accordance with its conflict of interest policies. The other authors declare no competing interest.

Abbreviations

α-KG = alpha-ketoglutamate, HE = hematoxylin and eosin, HBP = hexosamine biosynthetic pathway, PCA = principal component analysis, PPP = pentose phosphate pathway, TCA = tricarboxylic acid, GTK = glutamine transaminase K, KGM = alpha-ketoglutaramate.

References

1. Fearon, E.R.; Vogelstein, B. A genetic model for colorectal tumorigenesis. *Cell* **1990**, *61*, 759–767. [CrossRef]
2. Land, H.; Parada, L.F.; Weinberg, R.A. Tumorigenic conversion of primary embryo fibroblasts requires at least two cooperating oncogenes. *Nature* **1983**, *304*, 596–602. [CrossRef]
3. Kim, N.W.; Piatyszek, M.A.; Prowse, K.R.; Harley, C.B.; West, M.D.; Ho, P.D.L.; Coviello, G.M.; Wright, W.E.; Weinrich, S.L.; Shay, J.W. Specific association of human telomerase activity with immortal cells and cancer. *Science* **1994**, *266*, 2011–2015. [CrossRef] [PubMed]
4. Vogelstein, B.; Fearon, E.R.; Hamilton, S.R.; Kern, S.E.; Preisinger, A.C.; Leppert, M.; Smits, A.M.; Bos, J.L. Genetic Alterations during Colorectal-Tumor Development. *N. Engl. J. Med.* **1988**, *319*, 525–532. [CrossRef] [PubMed]
5. Yuan, T.L.; Cantley, L.C. PI3K pathway alterations in cancer: Variations on a theme. *Oncogene* **2008**, *27*, 5497–5510. [CrossRef] [PubMed]

6. Hobbs, A.; Der, C.J.; Rossman, K.L. RAS isoforms and mutations in cancer at a glance. *J. Cell Sci.* **2016**, *129*, 1287–1292. [CrossRef] [PubMed]
7. Stine, Z.E.; Walton, Z.E.; Altman, B.; Hsieh, A.L.; Dang, C.V. MYC, Metabolism, and Cancer. *Cancer Discov.* **2015**, *5*, 1024–1039. [CrossRef] [PubMed]
8. Kruiswijk, F.; Labuschagne, C.F.; Vousden, K.H. p53 in survival, death and metabolic health: A lifeguard with a licence to kill. *Nat. Rev. Mol. Cell Biol.* **2015**, *16*, 393–405. [CrossRef]
9. Jiang, L.; Kon, N.; Li, T.; Wang, S.-J.; Su, T.; Hibshoosh, H.; Baer, R.; Gu, W. Ferroptosis as a p53-mediated activity during tumour suppression. *Nature* **2015**, *520*, 57–62. [CrossRef]
10. Li, T.; Kon, N.; Jiang, L.; Tan, M.; Ludwig, T.; Zhao, Y.; Baer, R.; Gu, W. Tumor Suppression in the Absence of p53-Mediated Cell-Cycle Arrest, Apoptosis, and Senescence. *Cell* **2012**, *149*, 1269–1283. [CrossRef]
11. Cantor, J.R.; Sabatini, D.M. Cancer Cell Metabolism: One Hallmark, Many Faces. *Cancer Discov.* **2012**, *2*, 881–898. [CrossRef]
12. Patra, K.C.; Wang, Q.; Bhaskar, P.T.; Miller, L.; Wang, Z.; Wheaton, W.; Chandel, N.; Laakso, M.; Muller, W.J.; Allen, E.L.; et al. Hexokinase 2 Is Required for Tumor Initiation and Maintenance and Its Systemic Deletion Is Therapeutic in Mouse Models of Cancer. *Cancer Cell* **2013**, *24*, 213–228. [CrossRef] [PubMed]
13. Shroff, E.H.; Eberlin, L.S.; Dang, V.M.; Gouw, A.M.; Gabay, M.; Adam, S.J.; Bellovin, D.I.; Tran, P.T.; Philbrick, W.M.; Garcia-Ocana, A.; et al. MYC oncogene overexpression drives renal cell carcinoma in a mouse model through glutamine metabolism. *Proc. Natl. Acad. Sci. USA* **2015**, *112*, 6539–6544. [CrossRef] [PubMed]
14. Clavell, L.A.; Gelber, R.D.; Cohen, H.J.; Hitchcock-Bryan, S.; Cassady, J.R.; Tarbell, N.J.; Blattner, S.R.; Tantravahi, R.; Leavitt, P.; Sallan, S.E. Four-Agent Induction and Intensive Asparaginase Therapy for Treatment of Childhood Acute Lymphoblastic Leukemia. *N. Engl. J. Med.* **1986**, *315*, 657–663. [CrossRef] [PubMed]
15. Dibble, C.C.; Manning, B.D. Signal integration by mTORC1 coordinates nutrient input with biosynthetic output. *Nat. Cell Biol.* **2013**, *15*, 555–564. [CrossRef]
16. Ochocki, J.D.; Simon, M.C. Nutrient-sensing pathways and metabolic regulation in stem cells. *J. Cell Biol.* **2013**, *203*, 23–33. [CrossRef]
17. Yuan, H.-X.; Xiong, Y.; Guan, K.-L. Nutrient Sensing, Metabolism, and Cell Growth Control. *Mol. Cell* **2013**, *49*, 379–387. [CrossRef]
18. Metallo, C.M.; Heiden, M.G.V. Understanding Metabolic Regulation and Its Influence on Cell Physiology. *Mol. Cell* **2013**, *49*, 388–398. [CrossRef]
19. Huang, D.; Ding, Y.; Zhou, M.; Rini, B.I.; Petillo, D.; Qian, C.-N.; Kahnoski, R.; Futreal, P.A.; Furge, K.A.; Teh, B.T. Interleukin-8 Mediates Resistance to Antiangiogenic Agent Sunitinib in Renal Cell Carcinoma. *Cancer Res.* **2010**, *70*, 1063–1071. [CrossRef]
20. Rini, B.I.; Atkins, M.B. Resistance to targeted therapy in renal-cell carcinoma. *Lancet Oncol.* **2009**, *10*, 992–1000. [CrossRef]
21. Smit, E.F.; de Vries, E.G.E.; Timmer-Bosscha, H.; de Leij, L.F.H.M.; Oosterhuis, J.W.; Scheper, R.J.; Weening, J.J.; Postmus, P.E.; Mulder, N.H. In vitro response of human small-cell lung-cancer cell lines to chemotherapeutic drugs; no correlation with clinical data. *Int. J. Cancer* **1992**, *51*, 72–78. [CrossRef] [PubMed]
22. Gaglio, D.; Valtorta, S.; Ripamonti, M.; Bonanomi, M.; Damiani, C.; Todde, S.; Negri, A.S.; Sanvito, F.; Mastroianni, F.; Di Campli, A.; et al. Divergent in vitro/in vivo responses to drug treatments of highly aggressive NIH-Ras cancer cells: A PET imaging and metabolomics-mass-spectrometry study. *Oncotarget* **2016**, *7*, 52017–52031. [CrossRef] [PubMed]
23. Weil, A.G.; Wang, A.C.; Westwick, H.J.; Ibrahim, G.M.; Ariani, R.T.; Crevier, L.; Perreault, S.; Davidson, T.; Tseng, C.-H.; Fallah, A. Survival in pediatric medulloblastoma: A population-based observational study to improve prognostication. *J. Neuro-Oncology* **2016**, *132*, 99–107. [CrossRef] [PubMed]
24. Eberhart, C.G.; Kratz, J.; Wang, Y.; Summers, K.; Stearns, D.; Cohen, K.; Dang, C.V.; Burger, P.C. Histopathological and Molecular Prognostic Markers in Medulloblastoma. *J. Neuropathol. Exp. Neurol.* **2004**, *63*, 441–449. [CrossRef] [PubMed]
25. Cho, Y.-J.; Tsherniak, A.; Tamayo, P.; Santagata, S.; Ligon, A.; Greulich, H.; Berhoukim, R.; Amani, V.; Goumnerova, L.; Eberhart, C.G.; et al. Integrative Genomic Analysis of Medulloblastoma Identifies a Molecular Subgroup That Drives Poor Clinical Outcome. *J. Clin. Oncol.* **2011**, *29*, 1424–1430. [CrossRef]
26. Taylor, M.D.; Northcott, P.A.; Korshunov, A.; Remke, M.; Cho, Y.-J.; Clifford, S.C.; Eberhart, C.G.; Parsons, D.W.; Rutkowski, S.; Gajjar, A.; et al. Molecular subgroups of medulloblastoma: The current consensus. *Acta Neuropathol.* **2011**, *123*, 465–472. [CrossRef]
27. He, X.M.; Wikstrand, C.J.; Friedman, H.S.; Bigner, S.H.; Pleasure, S.; Trojanowski, J.Q.; Bigner, D.D. Differentiation characteristics of newly established medulloblastoma cell lines (D384 Med, D425 Med, and D458 Med) and their transplantable xenografts. *Lab. Investig.* **1991**, *64*, 833–843.
28. Hanaford, A.R.; Alt, J.; Rais, R.; Wang, S.Z.; Kaur, H.; Thorek, D.L.; Eberhart, C.G.; Slusher, B.S.; Martin, A.M.; Raabe, E.H. Orally bioavailable glutamine antagonist prodrug JHU-083 penetrates mouse brain and suppresses the growth of MYC-driven medulloblastoma. *Transl. Oncol.* **2019**, *12*, 1314–1322. [CrossRef]
29. Nedelcovych, M.T.; Tenora, L.; Kim, B.-H.; Kelschenbach, J.; Chao, W.; Hadas, E.; Jančařík, A.; Prchalová, E.; Zimmermann, S.C.; Dash, R.P.; et al. N-(Pivaloyloxy)alkoxy-carbonyl Prodrugs of the Glutamine Antagonist 6-Diazo-5-oxo-l-norleucine (DON) as a Potential Treatment for HIV Associated Neurocognitive Disorders. *J. Med. Chem.* **2017**, *60*, 7186–7198. [CrossRef]
30. Brabetz, S.; Leary, S.E.S.; Gröbner, S.N.; Nakamoto, M.W.; Şeker-Cin, H.; Girard, E.; Cole, B.; Strand, A.D.; Bloom, K.L.; Hovestadt, V.; et al. A biobank of patient-derived pediatric brain tumor models. *Nat. Med.* **2018**, *24*, 1752–1761. [CrossRef]

31. Stearns, D.; Chaudhry, A.; Abel, T.W.; Burger, P.C.; Dang, C.V.; Eberhart, C.G. c-myc overexpression causes anaplasia in medul-loblastoma. *Cancer Res.* **2006**, *66*, 673–681. [CrossRef] [PubMed]
32. Meister, A.; Tice, S.V. Transamination from glutamine to α-keto acids. *J. Biol. Chem.* **1950**, *187*, 173–187. [CrossRef]
33. Agrawal, S.; Kumar, S.; Sehgal, R.; George, S.; Gupta, R.; Poddar, S.; Jha, A.; Pathak, S. El-MAVEN: A Fast, Robust, and User-Friendly Mass Spectrometry Data Processing Engine for Metabolomics. In *Methods in Pharmacology and Toxicology*; Springer Science and Business Media LLC: Berlin/Heidelberg, Germany, 2019; Volume 1978, pp. 301–321.
34. Chong, J.; Wishart, D.S.; Xia, J. Using MetaboAnalyst 4.0 for Comprehensive and Integrative Metabolomics Data Analysis. *Curr. Protoc. Bioinform.* **2019**, *68*, e86. [CrossRef] [PubMed]
35. Mason, S. Lactate Shuttles in Neuroenergetics—Homeostasis, Allostasis and Beyond. *Front. Neurosci.* **2017**, *11*, 43. [CrossRef] [PubMed]
36. Meldrum, B.S. Glutamate as a Neurotransmitter in the Brain: Review of Physiology and Pathology. *J. Nutr.* **2000**, *130*, 1007S–1015S. [CrossRef]
37. Yelamanchi, S.D.; Jayaram, S.; Thomas, J.K.; Gundimeda, S.; Khan, A.A.; Singhal, A.; Prasad, T.S.K.; Pandey, A.; Somani, B.L.; Gowda, H. A pathway map of glutamate metabolism. *J. Cell Commun. Signal.* **2016**, *10*, 69–75. [CrossRef] [PubMed]
38. Walker, M.; van der Donk, W.A. The many roles of glutamate in metabolism. *J. Ind. Microbiol. Biotechnol.* **2016**, *43*, 419–430. [CrossRef]
39. Cooper, A.J.L.; Jeitner, T.M. Central Role of Glutamate Metabolism in the Maintenance of Nitrogen Homeostasis in Normal and Hyperammonemic Brain. *Biomol.* **2016**, *6*, 16. [CrossRef]
40. Maynard, R.E.; Poore, B.; Hanaford, A.R.; Pham, K.; James, M.; Alt, J.; Park, Y.; Slusher, B.S.; Tamayo, P.; Mesirov, J.; et al. TORC1/2 kinase inhibition depletes glutathione and synergizes with carboplatin to suppress the growth of MYC-driven medulloblastoma. *Cancer Lett.* **2021**, *504*, 137–145. [CrossRef]
41. Akella, N.M.; Ciraku, L.; Reginato, M.J. Fueling the fire: Emerging role of the hexosamine biosynthetic pathway in cancer. *BMC Biol.* **2019**, *17*, 1–14. [CrossRef]
42. Yoo, H.C.; Yu, Y.C.; Sung, Y.; Han, J.M. Glutamine reliance in cell metabolism. *Exp. Mol. Med.* **2020**, *52*, 1496–1516. [CrossRef] [PubMed]
43. Gao, P.; Tchernyshyov, I.; Chang, T.-C.; Lee, Y.-S.; Kita, K.; Ochi, T.; Zeller, K.I.; De Marzo, A.M.; Van Eyk, J.E.; Mendell, J.T.; et al. c-Myc suppression of miR-23a/b enhances mitochondrial glutaminase expression and glutamine metabolism. *Nat.* **2009**, *458*, 762–765. [CrossRef]
44. Errera, M.; Greenstein, J.P. Phosphate-activated glutaminase in kidney and other tissues. *J. Biol. Chem.* **1949**, *178*, 495–502. [CrossRef]
45. Meister, A.; Sober, H.A.; Tice, S.V.; Fraser, P.E. Transamination and associated deamidation of asparagine and glutamine. *J. Biol. Chem.* **1952**, *197*, 319–330. [CrossRef]
46. Copper, A.J.L.; Meister, A. Isolation and properties of highly purified glutamine transaminase. *Biochemistry* **1972**, *11*, 661–671. [CrossRef]
47. Cooper, A.J.; Meister, A. Isolation and Properties of a New Glutamine Transaminase from Rat Kidney. *J. Biol. Chem.* **1974**, *249*, 2554–2561. [CrossRef]
48. Caldwell, R.W.; Rodriguez, P.C.; Toque, H.A.; Narayanan, S.P. Arginase: A Multifaceted Enzyme Important in Health and Disease. *Physiol. Rev.* **2018**, *98*, 641–665. [CrossRef]
49. Vardon, A.; Dandapani, M.; Cheng, D.; Cheng, P.; De Santo, C.; Mussai, F. Arginine auxotrophic gene signature in paediatric sarcomas and brain tumours provides a viable target for arginine depletion therapies. *Oncotarget* **2017**, *8*, 63506–63517. [CrossRef] [PubMed]
50. Albaugh, V.L.; Mukherjee, K.; Barbul, A. Proline Precursors and Collagen Synthesis: Biochemical Challenges of Nutrient Supplementation and Wound Healing. *J. Nutr.* **2017**, *147*, 2011–2017. [CrossRef] [PubMed]
51. Zheng, L.; MacKenzie, E.D.; Karim, S.A.; Hedley, A.; Blyth, K.; Kalna, G.; Watson, D.G.; Szlosarek, P.; Frezza, C.; Gottlieb, E. Reversed argininosuccinate lyase activity in fumarate hydratase-deficient cancer cells. *Cancer Metab.* **2013**, *1*, 12. [CrossRef]
52. Towle, H.C. Metabolic Regulation of Gene Transcription in Mammals. *J. Biol. Chem.* **1995**, *270*, 23235–23238. [CrossRef] [PubMed]
53. Li, J.; Meng, Y.; Wu, X.; Sun, Y. Polyamines and related signaling pathways in cancer. *Cancer Cell Int.* **2020**, *20*, 1–16. [CrossRef]
54. Kp, M.; Kumar, A.; Biswas, D.; Moiyadi, A.; Shetty, P.; Gupta, T.; Epari, S.; Shirsat, N.; Srivastava, S. The proteomic analysis shows enrichment of RNA surveillance pathways in adult SHH and extensive metabolic reprogramming in Group 3 medulloblastomas. *Brain Tumor Pathol.* **2021**, *38*, 96–108. [CrossRef] [PubMed]
55. Marin-Valencia, I.; Yang, C.; Mashimo, T.; Cho, S.; Baek, H.; Yang, X.-L.; Rajagopalan, K.N.; Maddie, M.; Vemireddy, V.; Zhao, Z.; et al. Analysis of Tumor Metabolism Reveals Mitochondrial Glucose Oxidation in Genetically Diverse Human Glioblastomas in the Mouse Brain In Vivo. *Cell Metab.* **2012**, *15*, 827–837. [CrossRef] [PubMed]
56. Ast, T.; Mootha, V.K. Oxygen and mammalian cell culture: Are we repeating the experiment of Dr. Ox? *Nat. Metab.* **2019**, *1*, 858–860. [CrossRef] [PubMed]
57. Warburg, O. On the Origin of Cancer Cells. *Science* **1956**, *123*, 309–314. [CrossRef] [PubMed]
58. Warburg, O. On Respiratory Impairment in Cancer Cells. *Sci.* **1956**, *124*, 269–270. [CrossRef]
59. Owen, O.E.; Kalhan, S.; Hanson, R.W. The Key Role of Anaplerosis and Cataplerosis for Citric Acid Cycle Function. *J. Biol. Chem.* **2002**, *277*, 30409–30412. [CrossRef]

60. Boukouris, A.E.; Zervopoulos, S.; Michelakis, E.D. Metabolic Enzymes Moonlighting in the Nucleus: Metabolic Regulation of Gene Transcription. *Trends Biochem. Sci.* **2016**, *41*, 712–730. [CrossRef]
61. Dorai, T.; Pinto, J.T.; Denton, T.T.; Krasnikov, B.F.; Cooper, A.J. The metabolic importance of the glutaminase II pathway in normal and cancerous cells. *Anal. Biochem.* **2020**, 114083. [CrossRef]
62. Fagerberg, L.; Hallström, B.M.; Oksvold, P.; Kampf, C.; Djureinovic, D.; Odeberg, J.; Habuka, M.; Tahmasebpoor, S.; Danielsson, A.; Edlund, K.; et al. Analysis of the Human Tissue-specific Expression by Genome-wide Integration of Transcriptomics and Antibody-based Proteomics. *Mol. Cell. Proteom.* **2014**, *13*, 397–406. [CrossRef] [PubMed]
63. Nagamani, S.C.; Erez, A. A metabolic link between the urea cycle and cancer cell proliferation. *Mol. Cell. Oncol.* **2016**, *3*, e1127314. [CrossRef] [PubMed]
64. Paz, E.A.; LaFleur, B.; Gerner, E.W. Polyamines are oncometabolites that regulate the LIN28/let-7 pathway in colorectal cancer cells. *Mol. Carcinog.* **2014**, *53*, E96–E106. [CrossRef] [PubMed]
65. Chiu, M.; Taurino, G.; Bianchi, M.G.; Kilberg, M.S.; Bussolati, O. Asparagine Synthetase in Cancer: Beyond Acute Lymphoblastic Leukemia. *Front. Oncol.* **2019**, *9*, 1480. [CrossRef]
66. Dominguez, M.; Brüne, B.; Namgaladze, D. Exploring the Role of ATP-Citrate Lyase in the Immune System. *Front. Immunol.* **2021**, *12*, 632526. [CrossRef]
67. Gamble, L.D.; Purgato, S.; Murray, J.; Xiao, L.; Yu, D.M.T.; Hanssen, K.M.; Giorgi, F.M.; Carter, D.R.; Gifford, A.J.; Valli, E.; et al. Inhibition of polyamine synthesis and uptake reduces tumor progression and prolongs survival in mouse models of neuroblastoma. *Sci. Transl. Med.* **2019**, *11*, eaau1099. [CrossRef]
68. Evageliou, N.F.; Haber, M.; Vu, A.; Laetsch, T.W.; Murray, J.; Gamble, L.; Cheng, N.C.; Liu, K.; Reese, M.; Corrigan, K.A.; et al. Polyamine Antagonist Therapies Inhibit Neuroblastoma Initiation and Progression. *Clin. Cancer Res.* **2016**, *22*, 4391–4404. [CrossRef] [PubMed]
69. Hogarty, M.D.; Norris, M.D.; Davis, K.; Liu, X.; Evageliou, N.F.; Hayes, C.S.; Pawel, B.; Guo, R.; Zhao, H.; Sekyere, E.; et al. ODC1 Is a Critical Determinant of MYCN Oncogenesis and a Therapeutic Target in Neuroblastoma. *Cancer Res.* **2008**, *68*, 9735–9745. [CrossRef]
70. Khan, A.; Gamble, L.D.; Upton, D.H.; Ung, C.; Yu, D.M.T.; Ehteda, A.; Pandher, R.; Mayoh, C.; Hébert, S.; Jabado, N.; et al. Dual targeting of polyamine synthesis and uptake in diffuse intrinsic pontine gliomas. *Nat. Commun.* **2021**, *12*, 1–13. [CrossRef]
71. D'Amico, D.; Antonucci, L.; Di Magno, L.; Coni, S.; Sdruscia, G.; Macone, A.; Miele, E.; Infante, P.; Di Marcotullio, L.; De Smaele, E.; et al. Non-canonical Hedgehog/AMPK-Mediated Control of Polyamine Metabolism Supports Neuronal and Medulloblastoma Cell Growth. *Dev. Cell* **2015**, *35*, 21–35. [CrossRef]
72. Delage, B.; Fennell, D.A.; Nicholson, L.; McNeish, I.; Lemoine, N.R.; Crook, T.; Szlosarek, P.W. Arginine deprivation and argininosuccinate synthetase expression in the treatment of cancer. *Int. J. Cancer* **2010**, *126*, 2762–2772. [CrossRef] [PubMed]
73. Helenius, I.T.; Madala, H.R.; Yeh, J.-R.J. An Asp to Strike Out Cancer? Therapeutic Possibilities Arising from Aspartate's Emerging Roles in Cell Proliferation and Survival. *Biomolecules* **2021**, *11*, 1666. [CrossRef] [PubMed]
74. Johnston, K.; Pachnis, P.; Tasdogan, A.; Faubert, B.; Zacharias, L.G.; Vu, H.S.; Rodgers-Augustyniak, L.; Johnson, A.; Huang, F.; Ricciardio, S.; et al. Isotope tracing reveals glycolysis and oxidative metabolism in childhood tumors of multiple histologies. *Med* **2021**, *2*, 395–410.e4. [CrossRef] [PubMed]

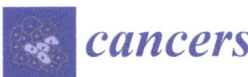

Review

Updates on Molecular Targeted Therapies for Intraparenchymal CNS Metastases

Akanksha Sharma [1,*], Lauren Singer [2] and Priya Kumthekar [2]

1. Department of Translational Neurosciences, Pacific Neuroscience Institute, Saint John Cancer Institute, Santa Monica, CA 90404, USA
2. Malnati Brain Tumor Institute at the Robert H. Lurie Comprehensive Cancer Center, Department of Neurology at the Feinberg School of Medicine, Northwestern University, Chicago, IL 60611, USA; lauren.singer@nm.org (L.S.); priya.kumthekar@nm.org (P.K.)
* Correspondence: asharma@pacificneuro.org; Tel.: +1-310-829-8265

Simple Summary: Metastatic disease to the central nervous system is an advanced-stage complication with historically devastating consequences and high mortality. Significant progress has been made in treatment in the last two decades, especially with the identification and targeting of specific mutations in the cancer pathway. In this review, we provide an updated overview of specific targets and highlight the numerous drugs that have demonstrated penetration and efficacy within the central nervous system.

Abstract: Central nervous system (CNS) metastases can occur in a high percentage of systemic cancer patients and is a major cause of morbidity and mortality in these patients. Almost any histology can find its way to the brain, but lung, breast, and melanoma are the most common pathologies seen in the CNS from metastatic disease. Identification of many key targets in the tumorigenesis pathway has been crucial to the development of a number of drugs that have demonstrated successful penetration of the blood–brain, blood–cerebrospinal fluid, and blood–tumor barriers. Targeted therapy and immunotherapy have dramatically revolutionized the field with treatment options that can provide successful and durable control of even CNS disease. In this review, we discuss major targets with successful treatment options as demonstrated in clinical trials. These include tyrosine kinase inhibitors, monoclonal antibodies, and antibody–drug conjugates. We also provide an update on the state of the field and highlight key upcoming trials. Patient-specific molecular information combined with novel therapeutic approaches and new agents has demonstrated and continues to promise significant progress in the management of patients with CNS metastases.

Keywords: intraparenchymal metastases; CNS disease; metastatic disease; targeted therapy; immunotherapy; tyrosine kinase inhibitors; monoclonal antibodies

Citation: Sharma, A.; Singer, L.; Kumthekar, P. Updates on Molecular Targeted Therapies for Intraparenchymal CNS Metastases. *Cancers* 2022, 14, 17. https://doi.org/10.3390/cancers14010017

Academic Editors: Edward Pan and Jose Manuel Lopes

Received: 7 November 2021
Accepted: 13 December 2021
Published: 21 December 2021

Publisher's Note: MDPI stays neutral with regard to jurisdictional claims in published maps and institutional affiliations.

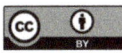

Copyright: © 2021 by the authors. Licensee MDPI, Basel, Switzerland. This article is an open access article distributed under the terms and conditions of the Creative Commons Attribution (CC BY) license (https://creativecommons.org/licenses/by/4.0/).

1. Introduction

Metastatic cancer can often find its way to the brain, where deposits may form either in the brain parenchyma itself resulting in intracranial or intraparenchymal metastases (IPM) or colonize the cerebrospinal fluid (CSF) surrounding the brain and spinal cord, resulting in leptomeningeal disease (LMD). Central nervous system (CNS) spread of systemic cancer as IPM or LMD is estimated to occur in 5–40% of patients with metastatic cancer; however, the actual prevalence may be even higher given CNS spread is not always identified before death and not routinely reported to state cancer registries [1,2]. Lung, breast, and melanoma are the most common sources of CNS metastases, though any cancer may metastasize to the parenchyma or CSF. IPM result in significant morbidity and negatively impact median overall survival (OS); indeed, patients with IPM are considered to have late or advanced stage cancer with a survival typically estimated to be less than six months [3]. Radiation therapy (RT), either via stereotactic radiosurgery (SRS) or whole brain radiation therapy

(WBRT), remain the primary modalities of treatment. However, there has been a notable increase in systemic therapy options for patients with IPM over the last decade, which has dramatically improved the landscape in terms of both progression-free survival (PFS) and OS for patients with several of these cancers.

Systemic options that have been more successful in controlling intracranial and extracranial disease are those that specifically target genomic alterations in the tumor. Several actionable genetic alterations have been identified in a range of primary cancers. In this review, we aim to discuss the most common and significant mutations and their respective targeted therapies. Figure 1 provides a visual overview of these targets and highlights the key drugs currently available that can target these mutations to inhibit downstream signaling pathways and also have been noted to have some degree of penetration and efficacy in the CNS. It is important to note, however, that IPM may not always share the same alterations as the extracranial disease. Genetic makeup of the primary cancer is not necessarily always a surrogate for the alterations that may be seen within CNS disease through a phenomenon called "branched evolution," suggesting the need for sampling directly from the CNS when feasible [4,5].

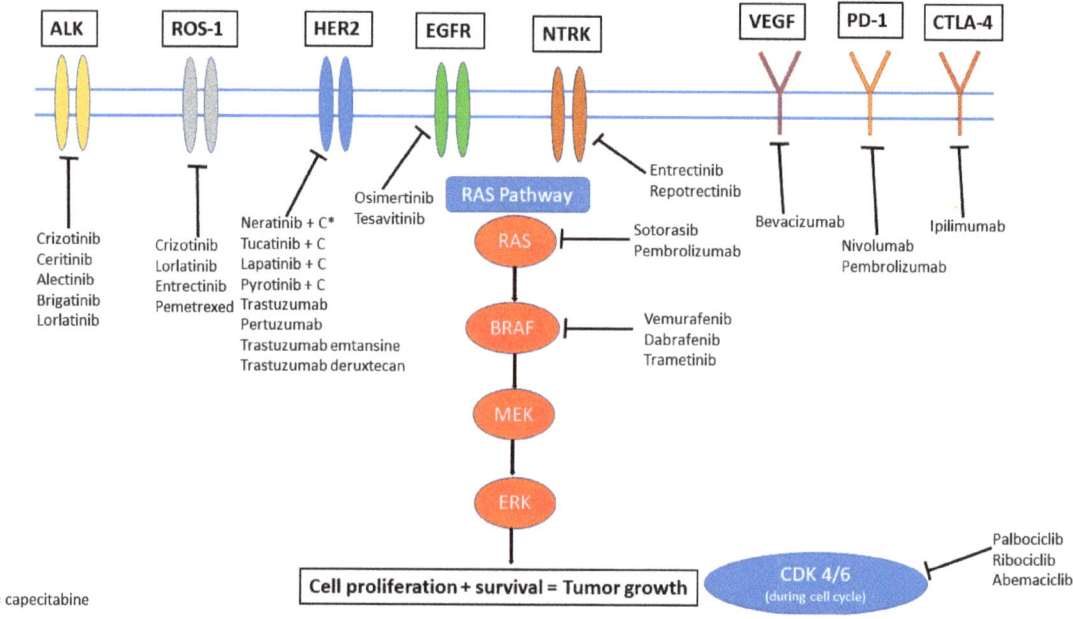

Figure 1. Therapeutic options illustrated by molecular target.

2. ALK-Targeted Therapies

The anaplastic lymphoma kinase (ALK) gene translocation is noted in 4–7% of non-small cell lung cancer (NSCLC) cases and results in a fusion between ALK and a second gene (most commonly EML4). ALK is a key regulator of tumor cell growth and survival, and this translocation results in increased activation of the signaling pathway, promoting oncogenic cell proliferation and survival. The tyrosine kinase domain of ALK can be targeted by a number of tyrosine kinase inhibitors (TKIs) (Figure 1). Crizotinib was the first of this class of drugs but demonstrated only marginally improved intracranial activity compared to chemotherapy. The newer generations of ALK inhibitors including ceritinib, alectinib, brigatinib, lorlatinib all demonstrated greater blood–brain barrier (BBB) penetration and CNS activity. Phase III trials in NSCLC with ceritinib have demonstrated an improved PFS when compared to chemotherapy (5.4 ms vs. 1.6 ms) [6]. In a phase II trial with pre-treated NSCLC patients, median PFS was 16.6 months and median overall survival

(OS) was 51.3 months [7]. Intracranial disease control rate (DCR) was as high as 80% with a median duration of response (DOR) of 24 months [7]. A trial with leptomeningeal disease (LMD) from NSCLC also demonstrated an overall response rate (ORR) of 16.7% with OS of 7.2 months in the LMD group [8].

Alectinib similarly demonstrates CNS activity and PFS benefit in patients regardless of IPM status. When compared to crizotinib, alectinib demonstrates a significantly high PFS (not reached vs. 10.2 months) [9]. In addition, alectinib has been shown to be protective against CNS disease progression based on results from a Phase III study in which only 12% in the alectinib arm had intracranial disease progression versus 45% in the crizotinib arm [10]. Alectinib generally was well tolerated, with primary side effects being anemia, myalgias, weight gain, and photosensitivity. Crizotinib, on the other hand, has a higher rate of nausea, diarrhea, and vomiting [10].

Brigatinib similarly demonstrates a better profile when compared to crizotinib and appears to be well tolerated. In a trial involving patients with NSCLC, median PFS was 29 months with brigatinib versus 9.2 months with crizotinib, with a confirmed rate of intracranial response rate of 78% vs. 29%, respectively [11]. Diarrhea is more common with brigatinib than alectinib, and other side effects included elevated creatine phosphokinase, cough, hypertension, and increased liver function tests [11].

Lorlatinib is a third generation TKI that has been designed to cross the BBB. In a phase III trial comparing lorlatinib to crizotinib that enrolled untreated patients with ALK rearrangements, intracranial response was 66% vs. 20%. As many as 71% of patients were noted to have complete response (CR) intracranially and at 12 months 72% still maintained response suggesting impressive durability to treatment. Similar to alectinib, lorlatinib tends to delay time to CNS progression, with the risk of CNS progression as low as 3% with lorlatinib versus 33% with crizotinib [12]. Lorlatinib is noted to have an added risk of memory impairment and cognitive issues.

Given the robust response data seen even in untreated patients with these later generation TKIs, the question arises if radiation therapy (RT) should be deferred or included for IPM from ALK rearranged NSCLC. No prospective data is available, and retrospective studies still suggest that there is benefit of added RT [13]. In specific clinical scenarios, including patients with small or asymptomatic IPM, IT may be reasonable to defer upfront RT for systemic therapy first.

ALK rearrangements are generally mutually exclusive to the other mutations discussed here with the exception of ROS1, which may co-exist with the ALK translocation and is discussed separately in this review. It is rare now in most countries where these drugs are available to use standard chemotherapy as first-line therapy and for patients with known IPM or relapsed/progressive disease with IPM, we recommend the use of lorlatinib or brigatinib to achieve disease control given the increased CNS penetration and excellent demonstrated efficacy as discussed above. Careful consideration of individual patient tolerance and risk of side effects should also be part of the decision-making process.

3. EGFR Targeted Therapies

The epidermal growth factor receptor (EGFR) is a member of the ErbB family of receptors. This transmembrane protein has important activity that can encourage growth factor signaling—over-expression or activation of the EGFR pathway results in increased cell proliferation and cell survival, via downstream activation of the phosphatidylinositol-3-kinase (PI3K/AKT) and Janus kinase (JAK/STAT) pathways. This mutation has been noted to occur in up to 35% of primary NSCLC patients, with a higher rate in those with an Asian ethnicity. The third-generation drug osimertinib is especially effective as a TKI for EGFR especially given it can also target the T790M mutation, an escape mutation on exon 20 that has been seen to confer resistance to TKI therapy. Osimertinib has demonstrated efficacy in treating EGFR-mutant NSCLC with CNS extension when compared to chemotherapy (platinum/pemetrexed) and to previous generation TKIs (gefitinib or erlotinib), a situation which prior to this would have had few therapeutic options. In the AURA 3 trial, osimertinib was compared to the previous standard chemotherapy (a combination of platinum/pemetrexed), and the CNS overall response rate was 70% vs. 31%. Median CNS response duration was noted to be 8.9 months [14]. When osimertinib was compared to gefitinib or erlotinib in the FLAURA trial, osimertinib demonstrated a CNS objective response rate of 91% and a median PFS that was not reached vs. 13.9 months in the control arm [15]. New CNS lesions only occurred in 12% of the osimertinib arm vs. 30% of the control arm, also suggesting a protective effect, with an overall median OS of 39 months vs. 32 months [15,16]. For LMD, a phase II prospective study found an impressive intracranial response rate of 55% and a median OS of 16.9 months for NSCLC with LMD. Osimertinib is generally well tolerated, with the most common side effects being diarrhea, dry skin, rash, and mucositis.

Osimertinib monotherapy is therefore becoming the standard first line therapy for EGFR mutated lung cancer. Inclusion of RT, specifically SRS, is also being questioned. While SRS may help with drug penetration or sensitize existing IPM, there is no clear randomized data to support this currently. Previous retrospective studies looked at this question with previous generation TKIs and found that addition of SRS did appear to improve survival [17]. Osimertinib is notably superior to these previous generations, however, in terms of IC response rate, and retrospective data demonstrates that RT may not add much benefit [18]. An ongoing prospective trial evaluating osimertinib versus osimertinib with SRS aims to better answer this question (NCT03769103, Table 1).

On the horizon is tesevatinib, a novel TKI with selectivity towards both EGFR and vascular endothelial growth factor (VEGF) that has demonstrated promising CNS penetration [19]. A phase II clinical trial in NSCLC brain metastases is evaluating this drug (NCT02616393, Table 1).

EGFR mutations are noted in other solid cancers such as colon cancer, esophageal cancer, glioblastoma, etc. However, at this time, studies utilizing EGFR TKIs in these other pathologies have not demonstrated the same level of efficacy or success in arresting tumor growth (especially when it comes to the CNS) as what has been seen in NSCLC. In our practice, the development of osimertinib has truly changed the landscape for patients with EGFR-mutant NSCLC, allowing for a prolonged period of disease remission even with CNS IPM, with relatively tolerable side effects. Osimertinib may also be used in the setting of small and asymptomatic brain metastases where RT is being deferred.

Table 1. Ongoing trials targeting IPM with targetable mutations.

Targeted Mutations	Trial	Phase	Population	Investigational Drug(s)	Total n	Primary Outcome	Comments
ALK, ROS1	NCT02927340	II	NSCLC	Lorlatinib	30	Intracranial disease control rate	
ALK, ROS1	NCT01970865	I/II	NSCLC	PF-0646392 vs. Crizotinib monotherapy	334	Participants with DLT, percentage of participants with overall and intracranial ORR	PF-0643922—ALK/ROS1 inhibitor
ALK, ROS1, or NTRK1-3	NCT03093116	I/II	Any IPM	Repotrectinib	450	DLT, recommended Phase II dose, ORR	Multiple arms comparing prior TKI and/or chemotherapy and treatment naive
ALK, ROS1, NTRK1-3	NCT05004116	I/II	Any IPM	Repotrectinib + Irinotecan + Temozolomide	50	Incidence of DLT, MTD	
EGFR	NCT03769103	II	NSCLC	SRS + Osimertinib vs. Osimertinib monotherapy	76	Intracranial PFS	Treatment naive brain mets included
ROS1	NCT04621188	II	NSCLC	Lorlatinib	84	ORR	Recurrence after failure of first-line TKI
ROS1	NCT03612154	II	NSCLC	Lorlatinib	35	ORR	
ROS1	NCT04919811	II	NSCLC or other IPM	Taletrectinib (DS-6051b)	119	ORR	
ROS1, NTRK	NCT02675491	I	Any IPM	DS-6051b	15	Number and severity of adverse events	
CDK, PI3K, NTRK/ROS1	NCT03994796	II	Any IPM	Abemaciclib or Paxalisib or Entrectinib	150	ORR	CDK population—Ademaciclib, PI3K—Paxalisib, NTRK/ROS1—Entrectinib
KRAS, EGFR	NCT01859026	I/IB	NSCLC	Erlotinib + MEK162	43	MTD	CDK4/6 inhibitor + MEK inhibitor
KRAS	NCT03299088	I	NSCLC	Pembrolizumab + Trametinib	15	Incidence of DLT	
KRAS	NCT03170206	I/II	NSCLC	Palbociclib or Binimetinib monotherapy vs. combination therapy	72	MTD, safety and tolerability, PFS	
KRAS	NCT03808558	II	NSCLC	TVB-2640	12	Disease control rate and response rate	
KRAS	NCT04111458	I	Any IPM	BI-1701963 monotherapy vs. co-administration with Trametinib	80	MTD based on DLI, number of patients with DLI, ORR	
KRAS G12C	NCT03785249	I/II	Any IPM	MRTX849 (Adagrasib) monotherapy vs. combination therapy with Pembrolizumab, Cetuximab, or Afatinib	565	Safety, pharmacokinetics, and clinical activity/efficacy of MRTX849	
CDK	NCT02896335	II	Any IPM	Palbociclib	30	Clinical benefit rate (intracranial)	
HER-2 negative	NCT04647916	II	Breast cancer	Sacituzumab Govitecan	44	ORR	
BRAFV600	NCT03911869	II	Melanoma	Encorafenib + Binimetinib vs. high dose	13	Incidence of DLT, incidence and severity of AE, incidence of dose modifications and discontinuations due to AE, brain metastasis response rate	
Checkpoint inhibition	NCT03340129	II	Melanoma	Ipilimumab + nivolumab w/ RT vs. Ipilimumab + Nivolumab alone	218	Neurological specific cause of death	

AE: adverse effects, DLT: dose-limiting toxicity, IPM: intraparenchymal metastases, MTD: maximum tolerated dose, NSLC: non-small cell lung cancer, ORR: overall response rate, PFS: progression free survival, TKI: tyrosine kinase inhibitor.

4. ROS-1 Alterations

A rare alteration, seen in only 1–2% of NSCLC, ROS1 is a receptor tyrosine kinase that is downstream of the c-ros oncogene. This rearrangement is similar to that of ALK and is seen also in glioblastoma, cholangiocarcinoma, ovarian carcinoma, angiosarcomas, etc. Aberrant ROS1 can activate multiple oncogenic pathways downstream, thus leading to tumor proliferation and survival.

It is noted that in NSCLC, a ROS1 fusion mutation predicts better response to pemetrexed based therapy, an agent which has been known to have CNS penetration [20,21]. Amidst the TKIs, crizotinib has been evaluated in the NSCLC population and trials have included IPM [22]. Median PFS for those with IPM was 10.2 months, and 13.8 months for those without IPM [23]. Lorlatinib has a higher potency against ROS1 and as discussed previously has excellent BBB penetration. An early phase study has demonstrated response intracranially in three patients with ROS1 mutated IPM but additional studies are ongoing (see Table 1) [22]. Entrectinib, discussed in the next section, may also be used to treat ROS1 fusion NSCLC. Anecdotal evidence and case reports suggest that other pathologies may also respond to these drugs or other ROS1-specific targeted TKIs, but additional data is needed and trials are ongoing at this time.

5. NTRK

Neurotrophic tyrosine receptor kinase or NTRK gene fusions can be seen in colorectal cancer, NSCLC, cholangiocarcinoma, glioblastoma, sarcoma, and thyroid cancers, amidst others. They involve NTRK1, 2 OR 3, which encode for the respective neurotrophin receptors (TRKA, TRKB, TRKC) and in turn this activation leads to oncogenesis. Entrectinib and repotrectinib are TKIs with affinity for these tyrosine receptor kinases (TRKs) and CNS penetration [24,25]. A pooled analysis of entrectinib in patients with NSCLC who had NTRK1 and ROS1 mutations demonstrated that 11 of 20 patients (55%) with baseline CNS metastases had a response, with median DOR of 12.9 months. Median intracranial PFS was 7.7 months [26,27]. A recent updated analysis of NCT02576431 and NCT021122913 presented this year demonstrated that heavily treated patients with advanced lung cancer and known IPM demonstrated an overall response rate to larotrectinib of 63%. Twelve-month PFS was 65% and median OS was 40 months, which is quite encouraging [28]. The drug was tolerable, with the most common side effects being fatigue, dysgeusia, paresthesias, nausea, and myalgias [27,28]. Additional larger trials are being conducted in other solid cancers that may carry this mutation, including glioblastoma. For NTRK and ROS mutated lung cancer, consideration of this class of drugs is highly advised in clinical practice both in the post RT setting as well as in the small and asymptomatic brain metastases setting where deferring RT may be preferred.

6. KRAS

The Kirsten rat sarcoma viral oncogene homolog or KRAS gene is aberrant in NSCLC (up to 25% of cases), colorectal cancers, and pancreatic ductal adenocarcinomas. An activating mutation in the KRAS gene results in increased formation of the K-Ras protein, a notable part of the RAS/MAPK pathway (Figure 1). This protein provides signals for cells to grow and proliferate, thus contributing to tumorigenesis. Until recently, the KRAS mutation was noted to be a poor prognostic indicator due to the lack of targeted options available and the fact that it appears to drive resistance to EGFR inhibition [29]. In recent years, however, more exciting options have emerged that suggest that KRAS inhibition is possible. Sotorasib was examined in advanced solid tumors that included NSCLC and colorectal cancers that had failed multiple lines of treatment. There was an objective complete response of 32% noted. This trial included patients with IPM though that subset has not been separately reported yet, but this holds promise for the future [30]. Other drugs being investigated in solid tumors include combinations with selumetinib or binimetinib, drugs that do have CNS penetration. This will be an area that will hold continued interest in the coming years, both for NSCLC and for other solid tumors that might also have the KRAS mutation.

Of note, immunotherapy with pembrolizumab demonstrates response in NSCLC regardless of KRAS status. When compared to chemotherapy, patients on pembrolizumab had a response rate of 57% (vs. 18%) in the KRAS subgroup of a larger trial [31]. This drug does have CNS penetration and activity against IPM as discussed in another section.

7. CDK4/6

The activation of cyclin-dependent kinases CDK4 and CDK6 in several cancers leads to increased, unregulated cell proliferation. Inhibiting these kinases can lead to cell cycle arrest and apoptosis of tumor cells. Currently, there are three FDA-approved CDK4/6 inhibitors—palbociclib (inhibits both CKD4 and CDK6), ribociclib (similar to palbociclib in structure but more potent against CDK4), and abemaciclib (different in structure and more potent against CDK4 also) [32]. These drugs have demonstrated efficacy and survival benefit in hormone positive breast cancer but intracranial response and benefit remains unclear and yet to be explored. Abemaciclib has better CNS penetration and early efficacy for IPM has been demonstrated with a phase II study demonstrating an intracranial benefit rate of 24% specifically for patients with HR+, HER2 negative, previously treated IPM [33]. Importantly, in this study, abemaciclib achieved therapeutic concentrations in the tissues of IPM, beyond what is required for CDK4 and CDK6 inhibition. The drug appears safe and is well-tolerated with mainly gastrointestinal side effects. Currently, additional evidence is being gathered in IPM specific clinical trials, but at this time it is clinically used for breast cancer with CNS spread (NCT03994796, Table 1).

8. Her2+ Targeted Therapies

The HER2 membrane tyrosine kinase is a member of the epidermal growth factor receptor family. Overexpression and gene amplification is an aberrancy noted in several solid cancers including breast, esophageal, ovarian, colorectal, etc. The upregulated expression of HER2 leads to downstream signaling pathway activation, thus leading to cell growth and proliferation, and preventing cell death. HER2 is noted to be upregulated in IPM when compared to the systemic disease, which explains the increased risk of HER2 tumors of colonizing the CNS. Small molecular TKIs including lapatinib, neratinib, and tucatinib have shown to have intracranial benefit in IPM from breast cancer, but only when used as combination therapy with capecitabine, with or without trastuzumab. Lapatinib combined with capecitabine demonstrates relatively low toxicity as well as an intracranial response rate of 38% with a PFS of 5.5 months in metastatic breast cancer to the brain [34]. Neratinib plus capecitabine has been compared to lapatinib plus capecitabine and the former demonstrated a higher PFS of 7.8 months with a combined intracranial response rate of 35% in the same population [35]. Tucatinib, when combined with both capecitabine and trastuzumab, has demonstrated the highest efficacy in reducing intracranial progression, with an intracranial response rate as high as 50% in metastatic breast cancer patients already previously treated with pertuzumab/trastuzumab [36,37]. Phase I studies have also demonstrated that even without capecitabine, tucatinib and trastuzumab combined results in a successful intracranial response and a clinical benefit (in patients with breast cancer previously treated with trastuzumab and ado-trastuzumab emtansine) [38,39]. This combination may also benefit patients with LMD, and this is being further explored in clinical trial (NCT03501979, Table 1).

Pyrotinib is a newer TKI that has been evaluated in patients with IPM with promising results. In a small cohort of 39 patients with IPM from breast cancer, median PFS was 8.7 ms and OS was 14 ms, with a response rate of 24% [40]. A similar response rate was seen in a prospective analysis from China, where intracranial response rate was 28% in previously treated breast cancer patients [41]. A similar response rate of 25% has been noted in patients with the more rare group of patients with HER2+ NSCLC treated with pyrotinib monotherapy [42]. Radiotherapy-naïve breast cancer patients with IPM were evaluated in a phase II trial where CNS response rates with pyrotinib in combination with capecitabine were noted to be as high as 75% and median PFS was 12.2 months, higher than the group that had been treated with RT [43]. Patients included in this study were required to be TKI naïve, and therefore while there is likely a role for pyrotinib in IPM, the appropriate sequencing with regards to other TKIs needs further clarification.

HER2 can also be targeted by monoclonal antibodies that have traditionally been considered to be unable to traverse the BBB. However, preclinical studies have demonstrated that at higher doses, trastuzumab does have BBB penetration [44,45]. This work provided the foundation of the PATRICIA study, evaluating high dose pertuzumab and trastuzumab together in patients with IPM from breast cancer [44]. This therapy was generally well tolerated and while the primary endpoint was not met due to a modest overall response rate (11%), the clinical benefit rate for these predominantly pretreated patients was 68% at 4 months and 51% at 6 months [44]. With all of this data in mind, at this time, our clinical practice recommendation is to consider the use of a TKI (most commonly tucatinib) with pertuzumab or trastuzumab, and capecitabine, in patients presenting with IPM to the brain from breast cancer. RT still has a critical role in IPM from breast cancer, and these patients may also receive combination SRS and/or WBRT in most cases for intracranial disease, at least until additional data shows non-inferiority of these treatment regimens.

HER2 targeted monoclonal antibodies may be conjugated to drugs (antibody—drug conjugates, or ADCs) to increase CNS penetration and efficacy. Trastuzumab conjugated to emtansine (T-DM1) is one such agent that was evaluated in the KAMILLA single arm phase IIIb trial. Patients with previously treated metastatic breast cancer were enrolled and in the IPM subgroup the median PFS was 5.5 months with an OS of 18.9 months, and an intracranial response rate of 21% [46]. T-Dxd or trastuzumab deruxtecan is an ADC that combines a topoisomerase I inhibitor to trastuzumab and is FDA-approved for patients with HER2+ advanced breast cancer after ≥ 2 lines of systemic therapy, based on data from the DESTINY-Breast01 phase 2 trial. Although patients with active, symptomatic IPM were excluded, those with asymptomatic IPM demonstrated a response rate of 41% and median PFS of 18 months, showing activity in the brain [47].

Trastuzumab may also be utilized intrathecally for patients with HER2 positive LMD. Doses ranging from 30 to 150 mg have been explored in phase I and II studies with no dose limiting toxicities and improvement in survival and clinical response as compared to historical controls [48–50]. A phase II study is ongoing (NCT01373710). Intrathecally delivered trastuzumab is not thought to have the same impact on parenchymal brain metastases and therefore its use is currently limited to the LMD setting BRAF inhibitors.

The most common BRAF mutations include the V600E substitution (valine substituted for glutamic acid) or the V600K mutation (valine substituted for lysine). As a consequence of these mutations, the MAPK pathway is upregulated, and cell cycle proliferation is encouraged. This mutation is most common in melanoma, where 50% of IPM might harbor a BRAF mutation. BRAF inhibitors include vemurafenib, dabrafenib, and encorafenib. Vemurafenib can have CNS efficacy as monotherapy, with a phase II study demonstrating response rates of 20% for treated and untreated IPM [51]. Dabrafenib monotherapy in the BREAK-MB trial demonstrated an intracranial response rate of 39% in BRAFV600E mutated IPM from melanoma; V600K mutated tumors had a lower response rate [52,53]. Combining MEK inhibition aides in overcoming drug resistance and improves the efficacy of BRAF inhibition, and thus the COMBI-MB trial combined dabrafenib with trametinib in patients with BRAFV600 mutant IPM. Intracranial responses as high as 58% were seen in these patients, which included cohorts of previously treated (with RT) and untreated patients [54]. At this point, BRAF therapy is a routine part of metastatic melanoma care and has dramatically changed the landscape in terms of PFS and OS for these patients, including for those with IPM. Combinations with concurrent immunotherapy, as well as the benefit of RT in this population, are questions still undergoing investigation. BRAF therapy may be utilized both in the post brain RT setting as well as can be a very reasonable treatment option for small and asymptomatic brain metastases without RT.

9. PD-1/PD-L1 Inhibition

Monoclonal antibodies targeting the programmed cell death protein 1 (PD-1) receptor, or its ligand (PD-L1), have increasingly emerged as a highly efficacious treatment for several cancers, including lung and melanoma. A tumor cell that overexpresses PD-L1 is able to attract PD-1 and thus protect itself from the body's own cytotoxic T-cell mediated immune mechanism which would kill aberrant and proliferating cells. Antibodies that inhibit this process by targeting either the protein or the ligand can boost the immune response against these tumor cells. A number of these checkpoint inhibitors have been approved in recent years and many others are being investigated. Nivolumab and pembrolizumab are the two most utilized PD-1 inhibitors, while atezolizumab, avelumab, and durvalumab are gaining prominence as PD-L1 inhibitors. Nivolumab has been combined with an antibody against the cytotoxic T-lymphocyte-associated protein 4 (CTLA-4) receptor, ipilimumab, to increase the immune response generated against cancer cells.

The phase II Checkmate 204 study combining nivolumab and ipilimumab recently released five-year follow up data. This trial included asymptomatic melanoma IPM and at 36 months OS had not yet been reached for 72% of patients, which demonstrated both the efficacy and durability of this response. An intracranial response rate of 55% was noted [55,56]. Of note, neurologically symptomatic patients and those already on steroids did not appear to glean significant benefit from this treatment combination. The ABC study from Australia was also a phase II trial that included cohorts with and without prior brain therapy. Again, intracranial response rate was high at 59%. Patients who had IPM that were previously treated, and those with LMD, responded less than those with untreated IPM [52].

BRAF inhibition may be combined with these monoclonal antibodies in patients with melanoma who have both PD-1 positivity and BRAF mutations, but trial data for this combination treatment is still pending at this time. There also remains question on the benefit of RT in these patients—radiation may provide increased durability to response and retrospective data suggests better survival and lower rate of CNS progression, but this has not yet been demonstrated prospectively [57–59] There also may be a higher rate of radiation necrosis and unnecessary toxicity in these patients that can be compounded by the use of immunotherapy, the rate of this complication is variable but may be as high as 15–20% [59,60].

Pembrolizumab, another PD-1 inhibitor, when combined with chemotherapy for NSCLC patients with IPM provides a notably higher clinical benefit, with a response rate of 39% (vs. 19.7% for chemo alone) and a durable response with a median OS of 18 months vs. 7.6 months [61]. These monoclonal antibodies have been overall very instrumental in transforming the landscape for patients with melanoma and lung cancer, completely changing survival even with advanced stage cancer with IPM. Their utility is not limited to these cancers alone—in fact, immunotherapy is rapidly integrating into regimens for a number of solid cancers including gastric, bladder, head and neck, esophageal, squamous cell, etc., resulting in higher rates of survival and improved outcomes for a large percentage of cancer patients. Immunotherapy is not without toxicity, of course, and patients are at risk for immune-mediated complications such as skin rashes, pneumonitis, colitis, hepatitis, and may have life-threatening or heavily disabling neurological complications. The data supports immunotherapy to be used for specific primary histologies (i.e., NSCLC, melanoma) even in the absence of RT particularly for small and asymptomatic brain metastases.

10. Other Agents

Another ADC composed of an antibody targeting the trophoblast cell-surface antigen 2 (Trop 2) coupled with a topoisomerase I inhibitor govitecan led to the development of sacitizumab govitecan (not included in Figure 1). Recently, results from a randomized phase 3 trial comparing sacituzumab govitecan to single agent chemotherapy in relapsed and refractory triple negative breast cancer were reported, demonstrating promising response with a median OS of 12.1 months compared to 6.7 months [62]. This trial, however, excluded IPM. A separate study, ASCENT 3, did allow for stable asymptomatic IPM and intracranial response rate for the sacituzumab govitecan group was 3% vs. 0% with chemotherapy [63]. Additional clinical trials evaluating sacituzumab govitecan in brain metastases are ongoing (NCT04647916).

BRCA1 and 2 can be targeted by PARP inhibitors such as olaparib and talazoparib, but intracranial response rate in active IPM is still to be explored and reported. The phase III EMBRACA trial with talazoparib did include a subgroup of treated and stable IPM patients who appeared to still benefit in terms of PFS [64]. An ongoing trial with veliparib is aiming to further answer this question (NCT02595905). At this time, additional data is awaited to make additional assessments on the utility of these therapies for patients with known IPM.

Medical therapy is often pursued after patients progress after standard of care radiation therapy and if there are no other targeted or immunotherapy options available. In a Phase II study enrolling solid tumor IPM patients who progressed following WBRT, patients were treated with bevacizumab at a dose of 10 mg/kg IV every two weeks until CNS disease progression. Response rate was 25% and the 6-month PFS: 46% (95% CI: 25–67%) and median PFS was 5.3 months. Median OS was 9.5 months (95% confidence interval 6.3 m–15.0 m) and QOL was maintained through treatment and there was no noted central nervous system bleeding. Of the 24 evaluable patients, 81% (22/24) experienced clinical benefit defined as stable disease or better [65]. Bevacizumab also may have a notable role in treating radiation necrosis from SRS in patients with IPM who cannot tolerate steroids due to side effects or where the necrosis and edema is proving to be steroid-refractory [66,67].

11. Conclusions/Future Directions

Systemic advancements over the past decade in oncologic care have led to improved outcomes for solid tumor cancer patients. Despite these advancements, the incidence of IPM continues to increase as patients live longer and as many of the currently utilized therapeutics do not cross the blood—brain barrier. The development of novel compounds including targeted therapies, ADCs, and immunotherapy amongst other advancements including more sophisticated imaging techniques have brought CNS metastases to the center stage. While there have been improvements in patient outcomes with these advents, there is still much more to understand and explore, and many unanswered question. This is in-part due to the lack of inclusion of patients with active IPM in the key clinical trials which have led to regulatory approval of many of these agents as well as inspired the design of additional studies. Given the only increasing incidence of IPM, it is crucial that these patients be included in clinical trials as they reflect the true populations seen in oncology clinics across the world. While trial design is challenging in this population, the incidence of IPM is 10-fold that of primary brain tumors, and as such should be given appropriate spotlight. This focus will ideally lead to better outcomes for our IPM patients across all primary tumor histologies.

Author Contributions: Conceptualization and data curation A.S. and P.K.; writing—original draft preparation, A.S.; writing—review and editing, P.K., supervision, P.K., figure, A.S., table, L.S. All authors have read and agreed to the published version of the manuscript.

Funding: This research received no external funding.

Conflicts of Interest: A.S and L.S have no conflicts of interest. P.K has research and grant support from Genentech, Novocure, DNAtrix and Orbus Therapeutics. P.K. has served on medical advisory boards for Biocept, Sintetica, Novocure, Janssen, Affinia, Celularity, and SDP Oncology. P.K. has provided consulting to Bliss Bio, Biocept, Enclear Therapies, Angiochem, Affinia Therapeutics.

References

1. Kromer, C.; Xu, J.; Ostrom, Q.; Gittleman, H.; Kruchko, C.; Sawaya, R.; Barnholtz-Sloan, J.S. Estimating the annual frequency of synchronous brain metastasis in the United States 2010–2013: A population-based study. *J. Neuro-Oncol.* **2017**, *134*, 55–64. [CrossRef] [PubMed]
2. Schouten, L.J.; Rutten, J.; Huveneers, H.A.M.; Twijnstra, A. Incidence of brain metastases in a cohort of patients with carcinoma of the breast, colon, kidney, and lung and melanoma. *Cancer* **2002**, *94*, 2698–2705. [CrossRef] [PubMed]
3. Villano, J.L.; Durbin, E.B.; Normandeau, C.; Thakkar, J.P.; Moirangthem, V.; Davis, F.G. Incidence of brain metastasis at initial presentation of lung cancer. *Neuro Oncol.* **2014**, *17*, 122–128. [CrossRef] [PubMed]
4. Brastianos, P.K.; Carter, S.L.; Santagata, S.; Cahill, D.; Taylor-Weiner, A.; Jones, R.T.; Van Allen, E.M.; Lawrence, M.S.; Horowitz, P.; Cibulskis, K.; et al. Genomic Characterization of Brain Metastases Reveals Branched Evolution and Potential Therapeutic Targets. *Cancer Discov.* **2015**, *5*, 1164–1177. [CrossRef]
5. Wang, H.; Ou, Q.; Li, D.; Qin, T.; Bao, H.; Hou, X.; Wang, K.; Wang, F.; Deng, Q.; Liang, J.; et al. Genes associated with increased brain metastasis risk in non–small cell lung cancer: Comprehensive genomic profiling of 61 resected brain metastases versus primary non–small cell lung cancer (Guangdong Association Study of Thoracic Oncology 1036). *Cancer* **2019**, *125*, 3535–3544. [CrossRef]
6. Shaw, A.T.; Kim, T.M.; Crinò, L.; Gridelli, C.; Kiura, K.; Liu, G.; Novello, S.; Bearz, A.; Gautschi, O.; Mok, T.; et al. Ceritinib versus chemotherapy in patients with ALK-rearranged non-small-cell lung cancer previously given chemotherapy and crizotinib (ASCEND-5): a randomised, controlled, open-label, phase 3 trial. *Lancet Oncol.* **2017**, *18*, 874–886. [CrossRef]
7. Nishio, M.; Felip, E.; Orlov, S.; Park, K.; Yu, C.-J.; Tsai, C.-M.; Cobo, M.; McKeage, M.; Su, W.-C.; Mok, T.; et al. Final Overall Survival and Other Efficacy and Safety Results From ASCEND-3: Phase II Study of Ceritinib in ALKi-Naive Patients With ALK-Rearranged NSCLC. *J. Thorac. Oncol.* **2019**, *15*, 609–617. [CrossRef]
8. Chow, L.; Barlesi, F.; Bertino, E.; Bent, M.V.D.; Wakelee, H.; Wen, P.; Chiu, C.-H.; Orlov, S.; Majem, M.; Chiari, R.; et al. Results of the ASCEND-7 phase II study evaluating ALK inhibitor (ALKi) ceritinib in patients (pts) with ALK+ non-small cell lung cancer (NSCLC) metastatic to the brain. *Ann. Oncol.* **2019**, *30*, v602–v603. [CrossRef]
9. Hida, T.; Nokihara, H.; Kondo, M.; Kim, Y.H.; Azuma, K.; Seto, T.; Takiguchi, Y.; Nishio, M.; Yoshioka, H.; Imamura, F.; et al. Alectinib versus crizotinib in patients with ALK -positive non-small-cell lung cancer (J-ALEX): An open-label, randomised phase 3 trial. *Lancet* **2017**, *390*, 29–39. [CrossRef]
10. Peters, S.; Camidge, D.R.; Shaw, A.T.; Gadgeel, S.; Ahn, J.S.; Kim, D.W.; Ou, S.-H.I.; Pérol, M.; Dziadziuszko, R.; Rosell, R.; et al. Alectinib versus Crizotinib in Untreated ALK-Positive Non–Small-Cell Lung Cancer. *N. Engl. J. Med.* **2017**, *377*, 829–838. [CrossRef]
11. Camidge, D.R.; Kim, H.R.; Ahn, M.-J.; Yang, J.C.H.; Han, J.-Y.; Hochmair, M.J.; Lee, K.H.; Delmonte, A.; Campelo, M.R.G.; Kim, D.-W.; et al. Brigatinib Versus Crizotinib in Advanced ALK Inhibitor–Naive ALK-Positive Non-Small Cell Lung Cancer: Second Interim Analysis of the Phase III ALTA-1L Trial. *J. Clin. Oncol.* **2020**, *38*. [CrossRef]
12. Shaw, A.T.; Bauer, T.M.; De Marinis, F.; Felip, E.; Goto, Y.; Liu, G.; Mazieres, J.; Kim, D.-W.; Mok, T.; Polli, A.; et al. First-Line Lorlatinib or Crizotinib in Advanced ALK-Positive Lung Cancer. *N. Engl. J. Med.* **2020**, *383*, 2018–2029. [CrossRef]
13. Johung, K.L.; Yeh, N.; Desai, N.B.; Williams, T.M.; Lautenschlaeger, T.; Arvold, N.D.; Ning, M.S.; Attia, A.; Lovly, C.; Goldberg, S.; et al. Extended Survival and Prognostic Factors for Patients With ALK-Rearranged Non–Small-Cell Lung Cancer and Brain Metastasis. *J. Clin. Oncol.* **2016**, *34*, 123–129. [CrossRef]
14. Wu, Y.-L.; Ahn, M.-J.; Garassino, M.C.; Han, J.-Y.; Katakami, N.; Kim, H.R.; Hodge, R.; Kaur, P.; Brown, A.P.; Ghiorghiu, D.; et al. CNS Efficacy of Osimertinib in Patients With T790M-Positive Advanced Non–Small-Cell Lung Cancer: Data From a Randomized Phase III Trial (AURA3). *J. Clin. Oncol.* **2018**, *36*, 2702–2709. [CrossRef]
15. Reungwetwattana, T.; Nakagawa, K.; Cho, B.C.; Cobo, M.; Cho, E.K.; Bertolini, A.; Bohnet, S.; Zhou, C.; Lee, K.H.; Nogami, N.; et al. CNS Response to Osimertinib Versus Standard Epidermal Growth Factor Receptor Tyrosine Kinase Inhibitors in Patients With Untreated EGFR-Mutated Advanced Non–Small-Cell Lung Cancer. *J. Clin. Oncol.* **2018**, *36*, 3290–3297. [CrossRef]
16. Ramalingam, S.S.; Vansteenkiste, J.; Planchard, D.; Cho, B.C.; Gray, J.E.; Ohe, Y.; Zhou, C.; Reungwetwattana, T.; Cheng, Y.; Chewaskulyong, B.; et al. Overall Survival with Osimertinib in Untreated, EGFR-Mutated Advanced NSCLC. *N. Engl. J. Med.* **2020**, *382*, 41–50. [CrossRef]
17. Magnuson, W.J.; Lester-Coll, N.; Wu, A.J.; Yang, T.J.; Lockney, N.; Gerber, N.K.; Beal, K.; Amini, A.; Patil, T.; Kavanagh, B.D.; et al. Management of Brain Metastases in Tyrosine Kinase Inhibitor–Naïve Epidermal Growth Factor Receptor–Mutant Non-Small-Cell Lung Cancer: A Retrospective Multi-Institutional Analysis. *J. Clin. Oncol.* **2017**, *35*, 1070–1077. [CrossRef]
18. Xie, L.; Nagpal, S.; Wakelee, H.A.; Li, G.; Soltys, S.G.; Neal, J.W. Osimertinib for EGFR-Mutant Lung Cancer with Brain Metastases: Results from a Single-Center Retrospective Study. *Oncologist* **2018**, *24*, 836–843. [CrossRef]
19. Lin, N.U.; Freedman, R.A.; Miller, K.; Jhaveri, K.L.; Eiznhamer, D.A.; Berger, M.S.; Hamilton, E.P. Determination of the maximum tolerated dose (MTD) of the CNS penetrant tyrosine kinase inhibitor (TKI) tesevatinib administered in combination with trastuzumab in HER2+ patients with metastatic breast cancer (BC). *J. Clin. Oncol.* **2016**, *34*, 514. [CrossRef]
20. Chen, Y.-F.; Hsieh, M.-S.; Wu, S.-G.; Chang, Y.-L.; Yu, C.-J.; Yang, J.C.-H.; Yang, P.-C.; Shih, J.-Y. Efficacy of Pemetrexed-Based Chemotherapy in Patients with ROS1 Fusion–Positive Lung Adenocarcinoma Compared with in Patients Harboring Other Driver Mutations in East Asian Populations. *J. Thorac. Oncol.* **2016**, *11*, 1140–1152. [CrossRef]

21. Kumthekar, P.; Grimm, S.A.; Avram, M.J.; Kaklamani, V.; Helenowski, I.; Rademaker, A.; Cianfrocca, M.; Gradishar, W.; Patel, J.; Mulcahy, M.; et al. Pharmacokinetics and efficacy of pemetrexed in patients with brain or leptomeningeal metastases. *J. Neuro-Oncology* **2013**, *112*, 247–255. [CrossRef]
22. Shaw, A.T.; Felip, E.; Bauer, T.M.; Besse, B.; Navarro, A.; Postel-Vinay, S.; Gainor, J.F.; Johnson, M.; Dietrich, J.; James, L.P.; et al. Lorlatinib in non-small-cell lung cancer with ALK or ROS1 rearrangement: an international, multicentre, open-label, single-arm first-in-man phase 1 trial. *Lancet Oncol.* **2017**, *18*, 1590–1599. [CrossRef]
23. Wu, Y.L.; Yang, J.C.; Kim, D.W.; Lu, S.; Zhou, J.; Seto, T.; Yang, J.J.; Yamamoto, N.; Ahn, M.J.; Takahashi, T.; et al. Phase II Study of Crizotinib in East Asian Patients With ROS1-Positive Advanced Non-Small-Cell Lung Cancer. *J. Clin. Oncol. Off. J. Am. Soc. Clin. Oncol.* **2018**, *36*, 1405–1411. [CrossRef]
24. Drilon, A.E.; Ou, S.-H.I.; Cho, B.C.; Kim, D.-W.; Lee, J.; Lin, J.J.; Zhu, V.W.; Kim, H.; Kim, T.M.; Ahn, M.-J.; et al. A phase 1 study of the next-generation ALK/ROS1/TRK inhibitor ropotrectinib (TPX-0005) in patients with advanced ALK/ROS1/NTRK+ cancers (TRIDENT-1). *J. Clin. Oncol.* **2018**, *36*, 2513. [CrossRef]
25. Yun, M.R.; Kim, D.H.; Kim, S.-Y.; Joo, H.-S.; Lee, Y.W.; Choi, H.M.; Park, C.W.; Heo, S.G.; Kang, H.N.; Lee, S.S.; et al. Repotrectinib Exhibits Potent Antitumor Activity in Treatment-Naïve and Solvent-Front–Mutant ROS1-Rearranged Non–Small Cell Lung Cancer. *Clin. Cancer Res.* **2020**. [CrossRef]
26. Drilon, A.; Siena, S.; Dziadziuszko, R.; Barlesi, F.; Krebs, M.G.; Shaw, A.T.; de Braud, F.; Rolfo, C.; Ahn, M.-J.; Wolf, J.; et al. Entrectinib in ROS1 fusion-positive non-small-cell lung cancer: Integrated analysis of three phase 1–2 trials. *Lancet Oncol.* **2019**, *21*, 261–270. [CrossRef]
27. Drilon, A.; Siena, S.; Ou, S.-H.I.; Patel, M.; Ahn, M.J.; Lee, J.; Bauer, T.M.; Farago, A.F.; Wheler, J.J.; Liu, S.V.; et al. Safety and Antitumor Activity of the Multitargeted Pan-TRK, ROS1, and ALK Inhibitor Entrectinib: Combined Results from Two Phase I Trials (ALKA-372-001 and STARTRK-1). *Cancer Discov.* **2017**, *7*, 400–409. [CrossRef]
28. Lin, J.J.; Kummar, S.; Tan, D.S.-W.; Lassen, U.N.; Leyvraz, S.; Liu, Y.; Moreno, V.; Patel, J.D.; Rosen, L.S.; Solomon, B.M.; et al. Long-term efficacy and safety of larotrectinib in patients with TRK fusion-positive lung cancer. *J. Clin. Oncol.* **2021**, *39*, 9109. [CrossRef]
29. Marabese, M.; Ganzinelli, M.; Garassino, M.C.; Shepherd, F.A.; Piva, S.; Caiola, E.; Macerelli, M.; Bettini, A.; Lauricella, C.; Floriani, I.; et al. KRAS mutations affect prognosis of non-small-cell lung cancer patients treated with first-line platinum containing chemotherapy. *Oncotarget* **2015**, *6*, 34014–34022. [CrossRef]
30. Hong, D.S.; Fakih, M.G.; Strickler, J.H.; Desai, J.; Durm, G.A.; Shapiro, G.I.; Falchook, G.S.; Price, T.J.; Sacher, A.; Denlinger, C.S.; et al. KRASG12C Inhibition with Sotorasib in Advanced Solid Tumors. *N. Engl. J. Med.* **2020**, *383*, 1207–1217. [CrossRef]
31. Herbst, R.; Lopes, G.; Kowalski, D.; Kasahara, K.; Wu, Y.-L.; De Castro, G.; Cho, B.; Turna, H.; Cristescu, R.; Aurora-Garg, D.; et al. LBA4 Association of KRAS mutational status with response to pembrolizumab monotherapy given as first-line therapy for PD-L1-positive advanced non-squamous NSCLC in Keynote-042. *Ann. Oncol.* **2019**, *30*, xi63–xi64. [CrossRef]
32. Zhang, M.; Zhang, L.; Hei, R.; Li, X.; Cai, H.; Wu, X.; Zheng, Q.; Cai, C. CDK inhibitors in cancer therapy, an overview of recent development. *Am. J. Cancer Res.* **2021**, *11*, 1913–1935. [PubMed]
33. Tolaney, S.M.; Sahebjam, S.; Le Rhun, E.; Bachelot, T.; Kabos, P.; Awada, A.; Yardley, D.; Chan, A.; Conte, P.; Diéras, V.; et al. A Phase II Study of Abemaciclib in Patients with Brain Metastases Secondary to Hormone Receptor–Positive Breast Cancer. *Clin. Cancer Res.* **2020**, *26*, 5310–5319. [CrossRef] [PubMed]
34. Lin, N.U.; Eierman, W.; Greil, R.; Campone, M.; Kaufman, B.; Steplewski, K.; Lane, S.R.; Zembryki, D.; Rubin, S.D.; Winer, E.P. Randomized phase II study of lapatinib plus capecitabine or lapatinib plus topotecan for patients with HER2-positive breast cancer brain metastases. *J. Neuro-Oncol.* **2011**, *105*, 613–620. [CrossRef]
35. Hurvitz, S.A.; Saura, C.; Oliveira, M.; Trudeau, M.E.; Moy, B.; Delaloge, S.; Gradishar, W.; Kim, S.; Haley, B.; Ryvo, L.; et al. Efficacy of Neratinib Plus Capecitabine in the Subgroup of Patients with Central Nervous System Involvement from the NALA Trial. *Oncologist* **2021**, *26*, e1327–e1338. [CrossRef]
36. Lin, N.U.; Borges, V.; Anders, C.; Murthy, R.K.; Paplomata, E.; Hamilton, E.; Hurvitz, S.; Loi, S.; Okines, A.; Abramson, V.; et al. Intracranial Efficacy and Survival With Tucatinib Plus Trastuzumab and Capecitabine for Previously Treated HER2-Positive Breast Cancer With Brain Metastases in the HER2CLIMB Trial. *J. Clin. Oncol.* **2020**, *38*, 2610–2619. [CrossRef]
37. Murthy, R.K.; Loi, S.; Okines, A.; Paplomata, E.; Hamilton, E.; Hurvitz, S.A.; Lin, N.U.; Borges, V.; Abramson, V.; Anders, C.; et al. Tucatinib, Trastuzumab, and Capecitabine for HER2-Positive Metastatic Breast Cancer. *N. Engl. J. Med.* **2020**, *382*, 597–609, Erratum in **2020**, *382*, 586. [CrossRef]
38. Borges, V.F.; Ferrario, C.; Aucoin, N.; Falkson, C.; Khan, Q.; Krop, I.; Welch, S.; Conlin, A.; Chaves, J.; Bedard, P.L.; et al. Tucatinib Combined With Ado-Trastuzumab Emtansine in Advanced ERBB2/HER2-Positive Metastatic Breast Cancer: A Phase 1b Clinical Trial. *JAMA Oncol.* **2018**, *4*, 1214–1220. [CrossRef]
39. Metzger Filho, O.; Leone, J.P.; Li, T.; Tan-Wasielewski, Z.; Trippa, L.; Barry, W.T.; Younger, J.; Lawler, E.; Walker, L.; Freedman, R.A.; et al. Phase I dose-escalation trial of tucatinib in combination with trastuzumab in patients with HER2-positive breast cancer brain metastases. *Ann. Oncol.* **2020**, *31*, 1231–1239. [CrossRef]
40. Anwar, M.; Chen, Q.; Ouyang, D.; Wang, S.; Xie, N.; Ouyang, Q.; Fan, P.; Qian, L.; Chen, G.; Zhou, E.; et al. Pyrotinib Treatment in Patients With HER2-positive Metastatic Breast Cancer and Brain Metastasis: Exploratory Final Analysis of Real-World, Multicenter Data. *Clin. Cancer Res.* **2021**, *27*, 4634–4641. [CrossRef]

41. Lin, Y.; Lin, M.; Zhang, J.; Wang, B.; Tao, Z.; Du, Y.; Zhang, S.; Cao, J.; Wang, L.; Hu, X. Real-World Data of Pyrotinib-Based Therapy in Metastatic HER2-Positive Breast Cancer: Promising Efficacy in Lapatinib-Treated Patients and in Brain Metastasis. *Cancer Res. Treat.* **2020**, *52*, 1059–1066. [CrossRef]
42. Zhou, C.; Li, X.; Wang, Q.; Gao, G.; Zhang, Y.; Chen, J.; Shu, Y.; Hu, Y.; Fan, Y.; Fang, J.; et al. Pyrotinib in HER2-Mutant Advanced Lung Adenocarcinoma After Platinum-Based Chemotherapy: A Multicenter, Open-Label, Single-Arm, Phase II Study. *J. Clin. Oncol.* **2020**, *38*, 2753–2761. [CrossRef]
43. Yan, M.; Ouyang, Q.; Sun, T.; Niu, L.; Yang, J.; Li, L.; Song, Y.; Hao, C.; Chen, Z. Pyrotinib plus capecitabine for HER2-positive metastatic breast cancer patients with brain metastases (PERMEATE): A multicenter, single-arm phase II study. *J. Clin. Oncol.* **2021**, *39*, 1037. [CrossRef]
44. Lin, N.U.; Pegram, M.; Sahebjam, S.; Ibrahim, N.; Fung, A.; Cheng, A.; Nicholas, A.; Kirschbrown, W.; Kumthekar, P. Pertuzumab Plus High-Dose Trastuzumab in Patients With Progressive Brain Metastases and HER2-Positive Metastatic Breast Cancer: Primary Analysis of a Phase II Study. *J. Clin. Oncol.* **2021**, *39*, 2667–2675. [CrossRef]
45. Terrell-Hall, T.B.; Nounou, M.I.; El-Amrawy, F.; Griffith, J.; Lockman, P.R. Trastuzumab distribution in an in-vivo and in-vitro model of brain metastases of breast cancer. *Oncotarget* **2017**, *8*, 83734–83744. [CrossRef]
46. Montemurro, F.; Delaloge, S.; Barrios, C.; Wuerstlein, R.; Anton, A.; Brain, E.; Hatschek, T.; Kelly, C.M.; Peña-Murillo, C.; Yilmaz, M.; et al. Trastuzumab emtansine (T-DM1) in patients with HER2-positive metastatic breast cancer and brain metastases: Exploratory final analysis of cohort 1 from KAMILLA, a single-arm phase IIIb clinical trial☆. *Ann. Oncol.* **2020**, *31*, 1350–1358. [CrossRef]
47. Jerusalem, G.H.M.; Park, Y.H.; Yamashita, T.; Hurvitz, S.A.; Modi, S.; Andre, F.; Krop, I.E.; Gonzalez, X.; Hall, P.S.; You, B.; et al. Trastuzumab deruxtecan (T-DXd) in patients with HER2+ metastatic breast cancer with brain metastases: A subgroup analysis of the DESTINY-Breast01 trial. *J. Clin. Oncol.* **2021**, *39*, 526. [CrossRef]
48. Bonneau, C.; Paintaud, G.; Tredan, O.; Dubot, C.; Desvignes, C.; Dieras, V.; Taillibert, S.; Tresca, P.; Turbiez, I.; Li, J.; et al. Phase I feasibility study for intrathecal administration of trastuzumab in patients with HER2 positive breast carcinomatous meningitis. *Eur. J. Cancer* **2018**, *95*, 75–84. [CrossRef]
49. Figura, N.B.; Rizk, V.T.; Mohammadi, H.; Evernden, B.; Mokhtari, S.; Yu, H.M.; Robinson, T.J.; Etame, A.B.; Tran, N.D.; Liu, J.; et al. Clinical outcomes of breast leptomeningeal disease treated with intrathecal trastuzumab, intrathecal chemotherapy, or whole brain radiation therapy. *Breast Cancer Res. Treat.* **2019**, *175*, 781–788. [CrossRef]
50. Kumthekar, P.; Lassman, A.B.; Lin, N.; Grimm, S.; Gradishar, W.; Pentsova, E.; Jeyapalan, S.; Groves, M.; Melisko, M.; Raizer, J. LPTO-02. INTRATHECAL (IT) TRASTUZUMAB (T) FOR THE TREATMENT OF LEPTOMENINGEAL DISEASE (LM) IN PATIENTS (PTS) WITH HUMAN EPIDERMAL RECEPTOR-2 POSITIVE (HER2+) CANCER: A MULTICENTER PHASE 1/2 STUDY. *Neuro-Oncol. Adv.* **2019**, *1*, i6. [CrossRef]
51. McArthur, G.A.; Maio, M.; Arance, A.; Nathan, P.; Blank, C.; Avril, M.-F.; Garbe, C.; Hauschild, A.; Schadendorf, D.; Hamid, O.; et al. Vemurafenib in metastatic melanoma patients with brain metastases: an open-label, single-arm, phase 2, multicentre study. *Ann. Oncol.* **2016**, *28*, 634–641. [CrossRef]
52. Long, G.V.; Atkinson, V.; Lo, S.; Guminski, A.D.; Sandhu, S.K.; Brown, M.P.; Gonzalez, M.; Scolyer, R.A.; Emmett, L.; McArthur, G.A.; et al. Five-year overall survival from the anti-PD1 brain collaboration (ABC Study): Randomized phase 2 study of nivolumab (nivo) or nivo+ipilimumab (ipi) in patients (pts) with melanoma brain metastases (mets). *J. Clin. Oncol.* **2021**, *39*, 9508. [CrossRef]
53. Long, G.V.; Atkinson, V.; Lo, S.; Sandhu, S.; Guminski, A.D.; Brown, M.P.; Wilmott, J.S.; Edwards, J.; Gonzalez, M.; Scolyer, R.A.; et al. Combination nivolumab and ipilimumab or nivolumab alone in melanoma brain metastases: a multicentre randomised phase 2 study. *Lancet Oncol.* **2018**, *19*, 672–681. [CrossRef]
54. A Davies, M.; Saiag, P.; Robert, C.; Grob, J.-J.; Flaherty, K.T.; Arance, A.; Sileni, V.C.; Thomas, L.; Lesimple, T.; Mortier, L.; et al. Dabrafenib plus trametinib in patients with BRAFV600-mutant melanoma brain metastases (COMBI-MB): A multicentre, multicohort, open-label, phase 2 trial. *Lancet Oncol.* **2017**, *18*, 863–873. [CrossRef]
55. Tawbi, H.A.-H.; Forsyth, P.A.J.; Hodi, F.S.; Lao, C.D.; Moschos, S.J.; Hamid, O.; Atkins, M.B.; Lewis, K.D.; Thomas, R.P.; Glaspy, J.A.; et al. Efficacy and safety of the combination of nivolumab (NIVO) plus ipilimumab (IPI) in patients with symptomatic melanoma brain metastases (CheckMate 204). *J. Clin. Oncol.* **2019**, *37*, 9501. [CrossRef]
56. A Tawbi, H.; A Forsyth, P.; Hodi, F.S.; Lao, C.D.; Moschos, S.J.; Hamid, O.; Atkins, M.B.; Lewis, K.; Thomas, R.P.; A Glaspy, J.; et al. Safety and efficacy of the combination of nivolumab plus ipilimumab in patients with melanoma and asymptomatic or symptomatic brain metastases (CheckMate 204). *Neuro-Oncol.* **2021**, *23*, 1961–1973. [CrossRef]
57. Khan, M.; Lin, J.; Liao, G.; Tian, Y.; Liang, Y.; Li, R.; Liu, M.; Yuan, Y. SRS in Combination With Ipilimumab: A Promising New Dimension for Treating Melanoma Brain Metastases. *Technol. Cancer Res. Treat.* **2018**, *17*. [CrossRef]
58. Kiess, A.P.; Wolchok, J.D.; Barker, C.; Postow, M.A.; Tabar, V.; Huse, J.T.; Chan, T.A.; Yamada, Y.; Beal, K. Stereotactic Radiosurgery for Melanoma Brain Metastases in Patients Receiving Ipilimumab: Safety Profile and Efficacy of Combined Treatment. *Int. J. Radiat. Oncol.* **2015**, *92*, 368–375. [CrossRef]
59. Skrepnik, T.; Sundararajan, S.; Cui, H.; Stea, B. Improved time to disease progression in the brain in patients with melanoma brain metastases treated with concurrent delivery of radiosurgery and ipilimumab. *OncoImmunology* **2017**, *6*, e1283461. [CrossRef]

60. Minniti, G.; Anzellini, D.; Reverberi, C.; Cappellini, G.C.A.; Marchetti, L.; Bianciardi, F.; Bozzao, A.; Osti, M.; Gentile, P.C.; Esposito, V. Stereotactic radiosurgery combined with nivolumab or Ipilimumab for patients with melanoma brain metastases: Evaluation of brain control and toxicity. *J. Immunother. Cancer* **2019**, *7*, 102. [CrossRef]
61. Powell, S.F.; Rodríguez-Abreu, D.; Langer, C.J.; Tafreshi, A.; Paz-Ares, L.; Kopp, H.-G.; Rodríguez-Cid, J.; Kowalski, D.M.; Cheng, Y.; Kurata, T.; et al. Outcomes With Pembrolizumab Plus Platinum-Based Chemotherapy for Patients With NSCLC and Stable Brain Metastases: Pooled Analysis of KEYNOTE-021, -189, and -407. *J. Thorac. Oncol.* **2021**, *16*, 1883–1892. [CrossRef] [PubMed]
62. Bardia, A.; Hurvitz, S.A.; Tolaney, S.M.; Loirat, D.; Punie, K.; Oliveira, M.; Brufsky, A.; Sardesai, S.D.; Kalinsky, K.; Zelnak, A.B.; et al. Sacituzumab Govitecan in Metastatic Triple-Negative Breast Cancer. *N. Engl. J. Med.* **2021**, *384*, 1529–1541. [CrossRef] [PubMed]
63. Diéras, V.; Weaver, R.; Tolaney, S.M.; Bardia, A.; Punie, K.; Brufsky, A.; Rugo, H.S.; Kalinsky, K.; Traina, T.; Klein, L.; et al. Abstract PD13-07: Subgroup analysis of patients with brain metastases from the phase 3 ASCENT study of sacituzumab govitecan versus chemotherapy in metastatic triple-negative breast cancer. *Cancer Res.* **2021**, *81*, PD13-07. [CrossRef]
64. Litton, J.K.; Scoggins, M.E.; Hess, K.R.; Adrada, B.E.; Murthy, R.K.; Damodaran, S.; DeSnyder, S.M.; Brewster, A.M.; Barcenas, C.H.; Valero, V.; et al. Neoadjuvant Talazoparib for Patients With Operable Breast Cancer With a Germline BRCA Pathogenic Variant. *J. Clin. Oncol.* **2020**, *38*, 388–394. [CrossRef]
65. Kumthekar, P.; Dixit, K.; Grimm, S.A.; Lukas, R.V.; Schwartz, M.A.; Rademaker, A.; Sharp, L.; Nelson, V.; Raizer, J.J. A phase II trial of bevacizumab in patients with recurrent solid tumor brain metastases who have failed whole brain radiation therapy (WBRT). *J. Clin. Oncol.* **2019**, *37*, 2070. [CrossRef]
66. Delishaj, D.; Ursino, S.; Pasqualetti, F.; Cristaudo, A.; Cosottini, M.; Fabrini, M.G.; Paiar, F. Bevacizumab for the Treatment of Radiation-Induced Cerebral Necrosis: A Systematic Review of the Literature. *J. Clin. Med. Res.* **2017**, *9*, 273–280. [CrossRef]
67. Levin, V.A.; Bidaut, L.; Hou, P.; Kumar, A.J.; Wefel, J.S.; Bekele, B.N.; Prabhu, S.; Loghin, M.; Gilbert, M.R.; Jackson, E. Randomized Double-Blind Placebo-Controlled Trial of Bevacizumab Therapy for Radiation Necrosis of the Central Nervous System. *Int. J. Radiat. Oncol.* **2011**, *79*, 1487–1495. [CrossRef]

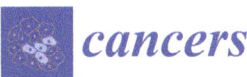

Article

Tumor Mutation Burden, Expressed Neoantigens and the Immune Microenvironment in Diffuse Gliomas

Guangyang Yu [1,†], Ying Pang [1,†], Mythili Merchant [1], Chimene Kesserwan [2], Vineela Gangalapudi [2], Abdalla Abdelmaksoud [2], Alice Ranjan [1], Olga Kim [1], Jun S. Wei [2], Hsien-Chao Chou [2], Xinyu Wen [2], Sivasish Sindiri [2], Young K. Song [2], Liqiang Xi [3], Rosandra N. Kaplan [4], Terri S. Armstrong [1], Mark R. Gilbert [1], Kenneth Aldape [3], Javed Khan [2,*] and Jing Wu [1,*]

1. Neuro-Oncology Branch, Center for Cancer Research, National Cancer Institute, National Institutes of Health, Bethesda, MD 20892, USA; guangyangyu11@fudan.edu.cn (G.Y.); ying.pang@nih.gov (Y.P.); mythili.merchant@nih.gov (M.M.); alice.ranjan@nih.gov (A.R.); olga.kim@nih.gov (O.K.); terri.armstrong@nih.gov (T.S.A.); mark.gilbert@nih.gov (M.R.G.)
2. Genetics Branch, Center for Cancer Research, National Cancer Institute, National Institutes of Health, Bethesda, MD 20892, USA; chimene.kesserwan@nih.gov (C.K.); vineela.gangalapudi@nih.gov (V.G.); abdalla.abdelmaksoud@nih.gov (A.A.); weij@mail.nih.gov (J.S.W.); hsien-chao.chou@nih.gov (H.-C.C.); wenxi@mail.nih.gov (X.W.); sivasish.sindiri@nih.gov (S.S.); songyo@mail.nih.gov (Y.K.S.)
3. Laboratory of Pathology, Center for Cancer Research, National Cancer Institute, National Institutes of Health, Bethesda, MD 20892, USA; xil2@mail.nih.gov (L.X.); kenneth.aldape@nih.gov (K.A.)
4. Pediatric Oncology Branch, Center for Cancer Research, National Cancer Institute, National Institutes of Health, Bethesda, MD 20892, USA; rosie.kaplan@nih.gov
* Correspondence: khanjav@mail.nih.gov (J.K.); jing.wu3@nih.gov (J.W.); Tel.: +1-240-760-6135 (J.K.); +1-240-760-6036 (J.W.)
† These authors contributed equally to this work.

Simple Summary: Tumor mutation burden (TMB) has shown promise as a biomarker for immune checkpoint blockade therapy in some cancers, but not consistently in gliomas. The goal of our study was to systematically investigate the association between TMB, expressed neoantigens, and the tumor immune microenvironment in IDH-mutant and IDH-wildtype gliomas, which are two types of biologically distinct gliomas. We demonstrated that TMB positively correlated with expressed neoantigens, but inversely correlated with immune score in IDH-wildtype tumors but showed no correlation in IDH-mutant tumors. The antigen processing and presenting (APP) score may have potential as a clinical biomarker to predict immune therapy response in gliomas. Lastly, 19% of patients had pathogenic or likely pathogenic germline mutations, primarily in DNA damage repair genes.

Abstract: Background: A consistent correlation between tumor mutation burden (TMB) and tumor immune microenvironment has not been observed in gliomas as in other cancers. Methods: Driver germline and somatic mutations, TMB, neoantigen, and immune cell signatures were analyzed using whole exome sequencing (WES) and transcriptome sequencing of tumor and WES of matched germline DNA in a cohort of 66 glioma samples (44 IDH-mutant and 22 IDH-wildtype). Results: Fourteen samples revealed a hypermutator phenotype (HMP). Eight pathogenic (P) or likely pathogenic (LP) germline variants were detected in 9 (19%) patients. Six of these 8 genes were DNA damage repair genes. P/LP germline variants were found in 22% of IDH-mutant gliomas and 12.5% of IDH-wildtype gliomas ($p = 0.7$). TMB was correlated with expressed neoantigen but showed an inverse correlation with immune score ($R = -0.46$, $p = 0.03$) in IDH-wildtype tumors and no correlation in IDH-mutant tumors. The Antigen Processing and Presentation (APP) score correlated with immune score and was surprisingly higher in NHMP versus HMP samples in IDH-wildtype gliomas, but higher in HMP versus NHMP in IDH-mutant gliomas. Conclusion: TMB was inversely correlated with immune score in IDH-wildtype gliomas and showed no correlation in IDH-mutant tumors. APP was correlated with immune score and may be further investigated as a biomarker for response to immunotherapy in gliomas. Studies of germline variants in a larger glioma cohort are warranted.

Keywords: glioma; tumor mutation burden; neoantigen; immune score; germline mutation; antigen processing and presentation; immunotherapy

1. Introduction

Gliomas are the most common primary malignant brain tumor and remain a fatal disease [1]. They are challenging to treat, largely due to the high level of intra- and intertumoral heterogeneity and a genomic landscape that constantly evolves due to selective pressure in response to therapies [2]. In addition, the immunosuppressive tumor microenvironment (TME) counteracts the efficacy of therapies, particularly immunotherapies [2].

In the past decade, immunotherapy such as immune checkpoint blockade has emerged as an effective therapeutic approach for several types of cancers, such as melanoma and lung cancer [3]. However, response to immunotherapy varies in patients with the same type of cancer, demonstrating the importance of identifying predictive biomarkers [3]. Tumor mutation burden (TMB), which is often proportional to the neoantigen burden, has emerged as a promising predictive biomarker of immune response in melanoma and lung cancer [4]. These efforts are highlighted in the KEYNOTE-158 study, which led to the recent US Food and Drug Administration (FDA) approval of using pembrolizumab, an anti-PD1 immune checkpoint inhibitor, in solid tumors with a TMB above 10 mutations per mega base (Mb) (defined as having a hypermutator phenotype (HMP)) [5]. However, this correlation between TMB and response to immunotherapy has not been consistently observed in gliomas [6,7].

A recently published seminal study by Touat et al. comprehensively analyzed the molecular determinants of TMB in over 10,000 glioma samples [6]. Two major pathways to hypermutation were elucidated: a de novo pathway associated with constitutional defects in mismatch repair (MMR) genes, and an acquired resistance driven by MMR deficiency following temozolomide (TMZ) treatment. While MMR deficient tumors are more likely to accumulate TMB, they were found to have a lack of T cell infiltrates and a low rate of response to anti-PD1 therapy. This study provided evidence that TMZ can drive the accumulation of mutations without promoting a response to immunotherapy. While detailed characterization of the phenotypic and molecular features of hypermutated gliomas has been performed, a systematic analysis of the associations between TMB, expressed neoantigens, and tumor microenvironment has not been previously performed and may provide a better understanding of the discordance between a high TMB and poor response to immunotherapy in gliomas.

In addition, the mechanisms underlying this discordance may not be the same in biologically distinct subsets of gliomas. Isocitrate dehydrogenase (IDH)-mutant gliomas have a distinct tumor biology compared to IDH-wildtype gliomas at genetic and epigenetic levels [8]. Moreover, *IDH* mutation status has been considered a favorable predictive biomarker for clinical outcomes [9]. The discovery of mutations in *IDH* genes has led to a better understanding of glioma biology as well as a major change in diagnostic criteria and standards of care.

In this study, we performed a comprehensive genomic analysis including whole exome sequencing (WES) and transcriptomic analysis of primary and recurrent tumor samples in both IDH-mutant and IDH-wildtype gliomas. Furthermore, we examined germline cancer predisposition genes (CPGs) by conducting WES of matched blood samples. The focus of our study was to analyze the correlations between TMB, expressed neoantigens, immune score of the tumor microenvironment, and antigen processing and presentation (APP) function in IDH-wildtype and -mutant gliomas separately. Our data shows promise for further investigating APP score as a clinical biomarker for determining immune response in glioma patients.

2. Results

2.1. Sample Characteristics

A total of 66 tumor samples and matched blood samples collected from 48 glioma patients from January 2016 to March 2020 were analyzed. As summarized in Table 1 and further expanded on in Table S1, the sample cohort included both IDH-mutant (n = 44) and IDH-wildtype (n = 22) tumors, as well as samples collected from primary (n = 13) and recurrent disease stages (n = 53), ranging from the 1st to more than 5th recurrence, which represent different stages of the disease (Table 1, Table S1). The samples used in this study also exhibited different histology and tumor World Health Organization (WHO) grades.

Table 1. Sample Characteristics by IDH mutation status.

	All Samples n = 66	IDH Mutant n = 44	IDH Wildtype n = 22
Tumor histological type			
Astrocytoma	54	32	22
Oligodendroglioma	12	12	0
WHO grade			
II	4	4	0
III	28	23	5
IV	34	17	17
Disease status			
Primary disease	13	7	6
Recurrent disease	53	37	16
No. recurrence			
0	13	7	6
1–2	33	19	14
3–5	18	16	2
>5	2	2	0
Tumor mutation burden *			
NHMP	51	32	19
HMP	14	11	3
Prior brain tumor therapies **			
TMZ/TMZ+RT	43	31	12
XRT	4	1	3
Others ***	19	12	7

Note: * Tumor mutation burden is available in 65 sample that has tumor DNA available. ** Treatments received by the patient prior to sample collection. *** Other therapies include surgical resection in newly diagnosed tumors, clinical trial therapies, and Tumor Treating Field. Abbreviations: IDH, isocitrate dehydrogenase; TMZ, temozolomide; RT, radiation therapy; HMP: hypermutator phenotype defined by more than 10 mutations per Mb.

2.2. Pathogenic Germline Mutations

Among 48 patients, nine (19%) were found to carry heterozygous pathogenic (P) or likely pathogenic (LP) germline alterations in eight cancer predisposition genes (CPGs): *TP53, MUTYH, BLM, RET, ERCC6, MITF, BRIP1,* and *MSH2* (Table 2). Importantly, six of them, except for *RET* and *MITF*, are involved in the DNA damage repair (DDR) pathway, indicating the importance of genomic instability in glioma genesis. Among these nine patients, seven had IDH-mutant gliomas and two had IDH-wildtype gliomas. No correlation was found between P/LP variants and the *IDH* somatic mutation status (P/LP germline variants in 21.9% of patients with IDH-mutant gliomas versus 12.5% of patients with IDH-wildtype gliomas, two-tailed Fisher's exact test, $p = 0.7$). Analysis of the TMB revealed HMP in two patients with IDH-mutant gliomas at the time of disease recurrence, each carrying P/LP germline variants in *MUTYH* and *ERCC6*, respectively and in one patient with de novo IDH-wildtype tumor (NCI0392) carrying a pathogenic variant in *MSH2*. Therefore, three of 11 (27.3%) patients with HMP tumors and three of 37 (7.9%) patients with NHMP tumors had P/LP germline mutations in DDR genes. However, we found no association between the hypermutation phenotype and the presence of P/LP germline variants in the DDR pathway (two-tailed Fisher's exact, $p = 0.12$). Taken together, mutations in DDR-related genes are common among P/LP germline variants. However, the association of DDR germline variants with HMP development needs to be further studied in a larger cohort.

Table 2. Pathogenic or likely pathogenic germline mutations detected in 9 patients.

Patient	Diagnosis *	Gene	Mutation	Associated Mendelian Disease	Mendelian Inheritance	ACMG-Based Classification [10]	HMP
OM161	Astrocytoma, IDH-mutant, WHO grade 4	TP53	p.R209Q	Li-Fraumeni syndrome	Autosomal Dominant	Likely pathogenic	No
CL0095	Astrocytoma, IDH-mutant, WHO grade 4	MUTYH	p.G396D	MUTYH associated polyposis	Autosomal Dominant	Likely pathogenic	No
CL0101	Astrocytoma, IDH-mutant, grade 4	BLM	p.Q548X	Bloom Syndrome	Autosomal Dominant	Pathogenic	No
CL0248	Astrocytoma, IDH-mutant, WHO grade 3	RET	p.K666N	Medullary thyroid carcinoma	Autosomal Dominant	Pathogenic/Likely pathogenic	No
CL0301	Astrocytoma, IDH-mutant, WHO grade 4	ERCC6	p.R670W	Cockayne syndrome	Autosomal Dominant	Likely pathogenic	Yes
CL0326	Astrocytoma, IDH-mutant, WHO grade 3	MITF	p.E419K	Susceptibility to cutaneous melanomaWaardenburg syndrome	Risk factorAutosomal Dominant	Risk factor/Likely pathogenic for cutaneous melanoma	No
CL0332	Astrocytoma, IDH-mutant, WHO grade 4	MUTYH	p.G396D	MUTYH associated polyposis	Autosomal Dominant	Likely pathogenic	Yes
NCI0391	Gliosarcoma, IDH-wildtype, WHO grade 4	BRIP1	p.T997fs	Fanconi Anemia	Autosomal Dominant	Pathogenic	No
NCI0392	Glioblastoma, IDH-wildtype, WHO grade 4	MSH2	c.1386+1G>A	Lynch syndrome	Autosomal Dominant	Pathogenic	Yes

Notes: * Diagnosis is based on "The Consortium to Inform Molecular and Practical Approaches to CNS Tumor Taxonomy" (cIMPCT-NOW update 6). Patients had multiple recurrence, the diagnosis in the table reflects the highest World Health Organization (WHO) grade. Abbreviations: WHO: World Health Organization; ACMG: American College of Medical Genetics; HMP: hypermutator phenotype defined by more than 10 mutations per Mb.

2.3. Mutational Landscape

Among the 66 samples, tumor DNA was available for 65 samples. A total of 28,630 high confidence somatic mutations were detected by WES analysis. Using our in-house tiering system, 353 pathogenic or hotspot mutations (tier 1) were detected [11]. The top somatic mutations in the tier 1 list are summarized in Figure 1A. The common genetic alterations include *IDH1* (58%), *TP53* (58%), *ATRX* (47%), *IDH2* (11%), CIC (13%), *SETD2* (13%), *PIK3CA* (11%), *PIK3R1*(11%), *PTEN* (8%), and *RB1*(8%), which are consistent with previously reported genomic alterations in gliomas [12]. To further understand the potential of these high confidence somatic mutations to generate tumor antigens, we examined the percentage of mutant genes that are expressed. We looked for the exact variant reads from RNAseq of the corresponding tumor using a set of filters (VAF ≥ 0.1, total RNA coverage ≥ 10, variant coverage ≥ 2) to identify the expressed somatic mutations from all high confidence somatic mutations. Tier 1 mutations were more likely to be expressed compared to all high confidence somatic mutations (52.4% vs. 30.1%, $p < 0.0001$; Fisher's exact test, two-tailed) (Figure 1B).

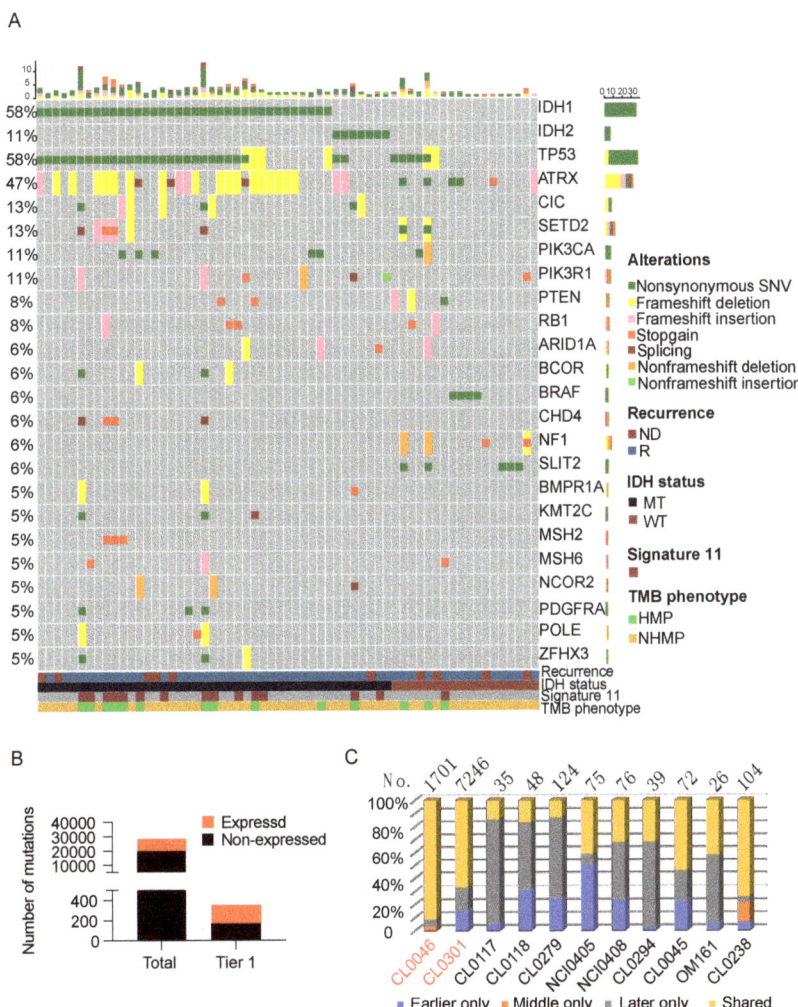

Figure 1. Somatic mutations detected in the sample cohort. (**A**) An integrated analysis of the sample cohort (66 samples) depicts the top tier 1 mutations. The samples are grouped by recurrence status, *IDH* mutation status, presence of mutational signature 11, and TMB phenotype. Complete information of all genetic alterations can be found in the database (https://clinomics.ccr.cancer.gov/clinomics/public/login accessed date: 20 November 2021) (**B**) High confidence somatic variants count analysis shows that tier 1 high confident somatic mutations contain a higher percentage of expressed mutations than the total high confident somatic mutations. (**C**) Matched recurrent glioma samples share expressed somatic mutations. Total number of expressed somatic mutations is labeled for each patient. Patients labeled in red carry HMP tumors, and patients labeled in black carry NHMP tumors. NHMP, TMB less than 10 mutations per Mb. HMP, TMB more than 10 mutations per Mb. ND, newly diagnosed tumor. R, recurrent tumor.

A comparison of the genetic alterations in recurrent IDH-mutant gliomas with those in the matched newly diagnosed tumors demonstrated a significant number of acquired mutations that are specific to the recurrent tumors [13]. To examine the genetic alterations that evolve through disease progression, we analyzed the high confidence somatic mutations in the samples collected at early recurrences to their matched samples collected at later recurrences. Patients CL0046 and CL0301, who developed HMP, had the highest number of shared mutations in the matched samples (Figure 1C). This suggests that recurrent HMP gliomas harbor mutations that persist, indicating the existence of a resistant clone. Patient CL0238, previously reported by our group to harbor a pathogenic fusion gene *BCR-ABL* [14], was diagnosed with a NHMP glioma that also had a high percentage of shared mutations, indicating that the fusion event of *BCR-ABL* occurred early and that it is an oncogenic driver leading to rapid progression of disease without significant clonal divergence.

To better understand the mutational profiles of gliomas, we calculated the TMB in our sample cohort using WES data of tumor samples and their matched blood samples. The TMB in all 65 samples ranged from 0.6 to 254 mutations per Mb. We then compared TMB in newly diagnosed (ND) and recurrent tumors in both IDH-wildtype and IDH-mutant gliomas. TMB values of recurrent samples were significantly higher than that of ND samples for IDH-mutant tumors (median: 1.17 versus 2.63, $p = 0.007$). However, no statistically significant difference in TMB values was found between recurrent and ND samples for IDH-wildtype tumors (Figure 2A). Using 10 mutations per Mb as the cutoff, 14 tumor samples were defined as HMP and 51 samples were NHMP. Among the 14 HMP samples, 11 samples were IDH-mutant and three were IDH-wildtype, and among the 51 NHMP samples, 32 were IDH-mutant and 19 were IDH-wildtype (Table S2). There was no difference in hypermutation phenotype incidence between IDH-mutant and IDH-wildtype gliomas (26% and 13.6%, respectively, two-tailed Fisher's exact test, $p = 0.35$).

The TMZ-induced mutational signature (G:C > A:T), defined as signature 11, is often observed in post-TMZ recurrent gliomas and relevant to clinical management of glioma patient [6]. Touat et al. demonstrated that over 98% of post-treatment HMP gliomas showed signature 11 and that exposing MMR-deficient cells to TMZ induces HMP with signature 11, suggesting that HMP and signature 11 represent MMR deficiency and TMZ resistance [6]. In order to examine the prevalence of signature 11 in all tumors exposed to TMZ, we analyzed the 52 samples that were collected at disease recurrence in our cohort. Among all recurrent samples, 43 were from tumors that had prior exposure to TMZ or TMZ + radiotherapy (Table 1), and 42 of them had DNA samples. Among all samples, 15 of them demonstrated signature 11. Interestingly, 35.7% (15 of 42) samples exposed to TMZ developed signature 11, and 93.3% (14 of 15) were IDH-mutant gliomas. Of the other 27 samples without signature 11, 16 were IDH-mutant and 11 were IDH-wildtype. With the exposure to TMZ, 45.2% (14 out of 30) IDH-mutant tumors and 8.3% (1 out of 12) IDH-wildtype tumors developed signature 11, suggesting that the IDH-mutant tumors were more likely to harbor signature 11 following TMZ exposure (two-tailed Fisher's exact test, $p = 0.02$).

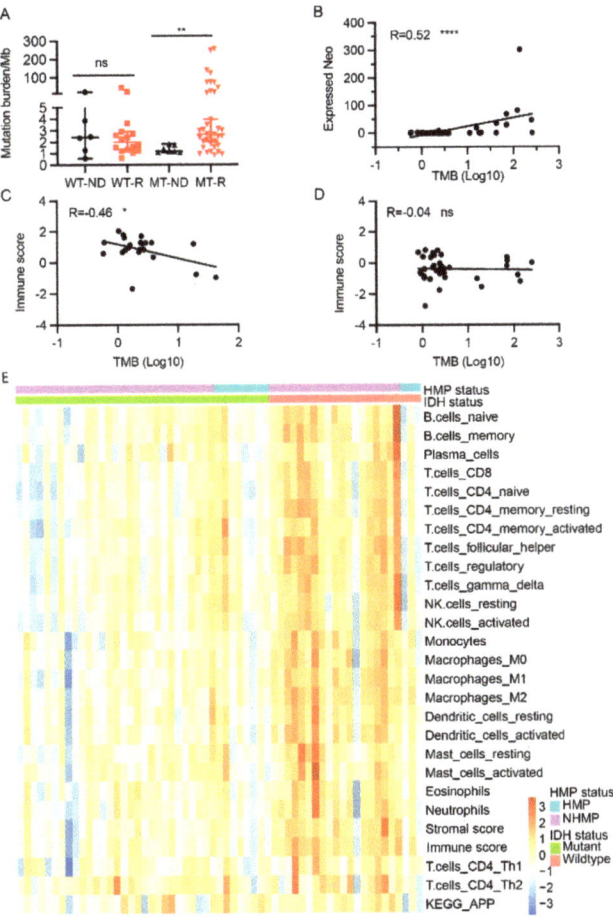

Figure 2. Neoantigen profile and immune signatures (n = 60). (**A**) Tumor mutation burden at initial diagnosis and recurrence in IDH-mutant (MT) and IDH-wildtype (WT) gliomas. (**B**) A significant correlation between expressed neoantigens and tumor mutation burden in all samples (R = 0.52, $p < 0.0001$). (**C**) An inverse correlation between TMB and immune score in IDH-wildtype glioma samples (R = −0.46, $p < 0.05$). (**D**) No correlation between TMB and immune score in IDH-mutant samples (R = 0.04, $p > 0.05$). (**E**) Heatmap of immune signatures in gliomas. Samples are grouped by their IDH mutation status and HMP status. Expressed neo, expressed neoantigen. ns: not statistically significant; *, $p < 0.05$; **, $p < 0.01$; ****, $p < 0.0001$. WT-ND, IDH-wildtype, newly diagnosed tumor. WT-R, IDH-wildtype, recurrent tumor. MT-ND, IDH-mutant, newly diagnosed tumor. MT-R, IDH-mutant, recurrent tumor. Wilcoxon rank sum test, ns: not statistically significant; *, $p < 0.05$.

2.4. TMB, Neoantigens, and Immune Signatures

Tumor neoantigens play a vital role in anti-tumor immunity. To better understand the immune landscape of gliomas, neoantigens from tumor samples in our cohort were predicted from mutations detected by WES of tumor DNA. In total, we found 1963 neoantigens (derived from 1325, 4.6% of all high confidence somatic variants) predicted to have a high binding affinity to human leukocyte antigen I (HLA-I) ($IC_{50} < 500$ nanomolar (nM)) and a lower HLA-I binding affinity ($IC_{50} > 500$ nM) to the corresponding wildtype peptides. Since immune cells must recognize neoantigens that are expressed and presented by HLA molecules on the tumor cell surface, we filtered out 619 expressed neoantigens from the predicted neoantigens by using a cut off total RNA read coverage ≥ 10, matched variant

RNA read coverage ≥ 2 and VAF ≥ 0.1 (Table S3) (31.5%, 619/1963). As fusion genes are also a source of neoantigens, fusion gene-derived neoantigens were also included in the neoantigen calculation. In our samples, 20 high-confidence fusion gene-derived neoantigens were detected (IC_{50} < 500 nM). While the predicted neoantigens are directly derived from somatic mutations and are expected to correlate with TMB, we confirmed that the expressed neoantigens also have a statistically significant correlation with TMB in all samples (Pearson R = 0.52, p < 0.0001) (Figure 2B).

Although a correlation between TMB and the tumor immune response has been reported in other cancers, there is a discordance in gliomas [15]. Given the overall strong correlation between TMB and the expressed neoantigens, we next examined the correlation between TMB and tumor immune scores. In our cohort, TMB showed an inverse correlation with immune score in IDH-wildtype samples (R = −0.46, p = 0.03) (Figure 2C), and no correlation in IDH-mutant gliomas (Figure 2D), suggesting that the *IDH* mutation has an impact on the correlation of TMB and immune score.

To characterize the tumor immune microenvironment of HMP and NHMP in IDH-mutant and IDH-wildtype tumors, we performed ssGSEA using the transcriptomic data that was available for 60 samples in our sample cohort. Immune cell specific gene sets were used to calculate enrichment scores for infiltrating immune cell types and describe overall "immune signature score" in each sample [16]. Most of the immune cell infiltration scores for CD8 T cells, CD4 T cells, subtypes of dendritic cells, and macrophages were higher in IDH-wildtype samples compared to IDH-mutant samples (Figure 2E and Figure S1), which is similar to previous findings in primary gliomas from The Cancer Genome Atlas (TCGA) dataset [17]. It was also notable that several subsets of T cells and NK cells had a higher score in NHMP compared to HMP in IDH-wildtype tumors. However, no significant difference was observed between HMP and NHMP in IDH-mutant tumors (Figure S1). Overall, the immune signature clustered better by *IDH* mutation status, IDH-wildtype versus IDH-mutant, than by TMB, HMP versus NHMP (Figure 2E).

In order to better understand the immune signatures of the tumor microenvironment, we examined the infiltrating immune cell subtypes inferred by CIBERSORT scores [16]. As shown in Figure S2, regardless of *IDH* status or TMB, all glioma groups showed similarly high percentage of immune cells classified as M2 macrophages, but no significant difference between groups (one-way ANOVA test, p = 0.78) (Figure S3A). Monocytes and activated mast cells also had relatively high percentages (total average 13.9% and 12.7%, respectively) of infiltration compared to other immune cells such as CD8 T cells (total average 3.5%). Furthermore, there was no significant difference in CD8 T cell infiltration between HMP and NHMP samples, irrespective of *IDH* mutation status (One-way ANOVA test, p = 0.28) (Figure S3B). These data are consistent with previous findings that M2 macrophages are the dominant immune cell in the glioma microenvironment, whereas CD8 T cells are a minority [15]. In addition, the similar proportions of these immune cells across all groups are unlikely to explain the different correlations of TMB and immune scores in IDH-mutant and IDH-wildtype gliomas.

2.5. Antigen Processing and Presentation

Effective immune responses against tumors largely depend on immune cells recognizing antigens presented on the tumor surface. HLA-I loss and defects in the antigen processing machinery were reported to be common in various cancers, including gliomas [18–21]. To assess the ability of antigen presentation in gliomas, we first explored the expression of the major histocompatibility complex class I. As shown in Figure 3A, no significant difference in the expression levels of HLA-A, B, or C was found between HMP and NHMP samples in either IDH-mutant or IDH-wildtype tumors. These results suggest that HLA expression is unlikely to be the cause of the different correlation of TMB and immune scores in IDH-mutant and IDH-wildtype gliomas.

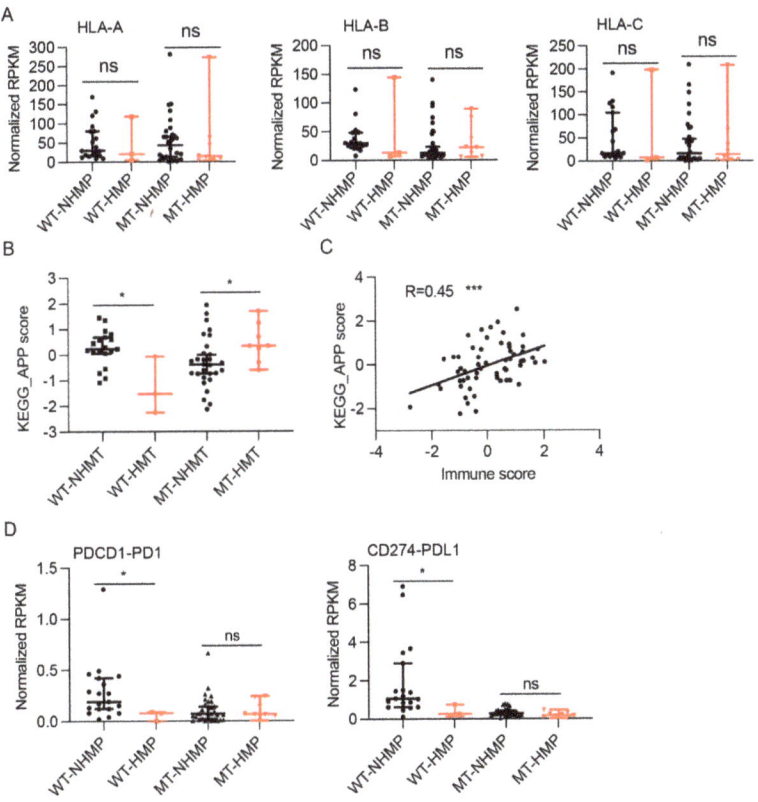

Figure 3. Antigen processing and presentation (APP) and immunosuppressive gene expression in HMP and NHMP glioma samples. (**A**) No difference in expression of type I HLAs between HMP and NHMP samples is detected in either IDH-wildtype or IDH-mutant tumors. (**B**) APP score is higher in NHMP than HMP for IDH-wildtype glioma samples ($p < 0.05$), but higher in HMP than NHMP for IDH-mutant glioma samples ($p < 0.05$). (**C**) KEGG_APP score correlates with immune score ($R = 0.45$, $p < 0.0001$). (**D**) RNA expression level of PDCD1 and CD274 in HMP and NHMP in both IDH-mutant and wildtype gliomas. APP, antigen -processing and -presentation. RPKM, reads per kilobase of transcript per million reads mapped. Wilcoxon rank sum test, ns: not statistically significant. *, $p < 0.05$. ***, $p < 0.001$.

To further understand the discordance between neoantigen burden and immune infiltrate function in the tumor microenvironment, the KEGG Antigen Processing and Presentation (APP) score between HMP and NHMP samples was compared in both IDH-mutant and -wildtype gliomas. As shown in Figure 3B, the KEGG APP score was significantly higher in NHMP samples compared to HMP samples in IDH-wildtype tumor (median 0.2385 versus −1.518, $p = 0.014$). In contrast, a significantly higher KEGG APP score was found in HMP samples versus NHMP samples in IDH-mutant gliomas (median 0.35 versus −0.39, $p = 0.03$). To better understand the effect of APP score on the tumor microenvironment, the correlation between APP score and immune score was analyzed. As shown in Figure 3C, the APP score had a statistically significant correlation with immune score in gliomas ($R = 0.45$, $p = 0.0003$). These data indicate that APP function is different between HMP and NHMP samples with different *IDH* mutation status but correlates with immune score in our sample cohort.

2.6. Immunosuppressive Gene Expression in Gliomas

To understand the role of immunosuppressive factors in the tumor microenvironment of HMP and NHMP gliomas, we analyzed the expression of well-known immunosuppressive genes. The expression levels of most examined immunosuppressive genes did not show significant differences between HMP and NHMP samples in IDH-mutant gliomas, except for *TGFB1*, which had a trend of higher expression in NHMP IDH-mutant samples (median 4.34 versus 2.9, $p = 0.054$) (Figure S4). In IDH-wildtype gliomas, the immunosuppressive genes that showed a statistically significant difference in expression between NHMP and HMP samples were *PD1* and *PDL1* (median *PD1*: 0.19 versus 0.08, $p = 0.04$; *PDL1*: 1.06 versus 0.27, $p = 0.04$) (Figure 3D). These data suggest a potential therapeutic role of targeting *TGFB1* and *PD1/PDL1* in IDH-mutant and IDH-wildtype gliomas, respectively.

3. Discussion

TMB has been used as a predictive biomarker of response to immune checkpoint blockade therapy in several cancers, including melanoma and lung cancer [4]. However, a correlation between TMB and response to immunotherapy has not been observed in gliomas consistently [6]. In this study, we focused on a systematic assessment of the TMB, expressed neoantigens, and the tumor immune microenvironment in both IDH-wildtype and IDH-mutant gliomas, which have distinct tumor biology. Compared to IDH-wildtype glioma, IDH-mutant gliomas were more likely to accumulate mutation burden during their disease progression and more likely to harbor signature 11 following the exposure to TMZ. Most importantly, while TMB had a positive correlation with expressed neoantigens, it showed an inverse correlation with immune scores in IDH-wildtype gliomas and no correlation in IDH-mutant gliomas. In addition, we found a significantly higher APP score in NHMP compared to HMP samples in IDH-wildtype gliomas, but a higher APP score in HMP compared to NHMP in IDH-mutant gliomas. Together with the strong correlation between APP score and immune score, the data suggests that APP score could be further investigated as a biomarker for predicting response to immunotherapy, and that the impact of TMB on the immune signature depends on the *IDH* mutation status. Finally, we also analyzed germline alterations of CPGs, particularly P/LP genes, and explored the correlation with other tumor driver genes, such as *IDH* and *TP53*. Our results provide evidence for further evaluating P/LP germline variants in a larger glioma cohort and a potential value in screening patients prior to receiving treatment.

3.1. Germline Variants of P/LP CPGs in Gliomas

Despite the fact that we only analyzed a small cohort of glioma patients, 19% of them carried a germline monoallelic P/LP variant in CPG. The prevalence in our cohort is higher than what is reported in the literature in both pediatric and adult cancer patients [22,23]. To understand the spectrum of CPGs, particularly the P/LP mutations of CPGs in IDH-mutant and IDH-wildtype gliomas, we collected and analyzed germline genomic information in all cases. Although there was no statistically significant association between *IDH* mutation status and the occurrence of P/LP mutations, interesting observations between CPGs and somatic variants in the tumors were made. First, a germline *TP53* mutation (p.R209Q) was detected in a patient with grade 3 astrocytoma (OM161). In addition to *TP53* mutation and loss of heterozygosity (LOH), a frame-shift deletion of *ATRX* and somatic *IDH1* mutation, which is considered a tumor driver gene in gliomas, were also detected in the tumor. *IDH* mutation was also detected in two patients with grade 4 astrocytoma (CL0095 and CL0332) who carried a monoallelic germline mutation of *MUTYH* (p.G396D), which is a common mutation in MUTYH-associated polyposis (MAP) with an autosomal recessive inheritance [24]. Another IDH-mutant grade 4 astrocytoma patient (CL0101) was found to have a monoallelic pathogenic nonsense *BLM* mutation (p.Q548X). Biallelic *BLM* mutation usually occurs in Bloom syndrome, which features abnormal DNA repair and high levels of chromosome breaks and rearrangements [25]. Evidently, *IDH* mutations frequently occurred in patients carrying P/LP germline mutations in our patient cohort. These observations raise a question about the role of another cancer driver gene such as *IDH* mutation in the presence of germline drivers such as *TP53* mutation. Thus, it would be interesting to review the P/LP germline mutations of CPGs in a large cohort of IDH-mutant tumors. However, based on our available data, it may not be possible to determine with certainty which P/LP variants are incidental and therefore, less likely to contribute to the primary tumor diagnosis. For instance, while the *TP53* variant reported in patient OM161 is likely causal of the patient's astrocytoma, it would be less likely for a monoallelic *MUTYH* in patients CL0095 or CL00332 to contribute to their respective tumor diagnoses.

3.2. TMB, Immune Signatures, and IDH Mutation Status

There has been increasing evidence that TMB does not consistently correlate with immune response in gliomas [6,15] Our analysis revealed that TMB and immune scores are correlated differently in IDH-mutant and -wildtype gliomas. As summarized in Figure 4, in IDH-wildtype tumors, NHMP tumors have better APP function and immune scores than HMP tumors. In contrast, HMP tumors have higher APP function than NHMP, but not a better immune score, in IDH-mutant gliomas. Furthermore, APP score strongly correlates with immune score in all gliomas. While one would expect a higher TMB to result in a higher number of expressed neoantigens, in turn increasing the immune response, our findings revealed the opposite in the case of IDH-wildtype gliomas. A similar finding was described by Gromeier et al., who reported that IDH-wildtype samples with a lower TMB had higher immune inflammation, which was explained by the mechanism of neoantigen depletion/immunoediting [26]. Of note, we also found that the CD8 T cells showed a non-significant trend of being suppressed alongside APP suppression in the IDH-wildtype HMP gliomas (Figure S1), potentially dampening the immune response. Interestingly, while APP scores were elevated in the HMP subgroup in IDH-mutant gliomas, no significant correlation between the immune signature and TMB in this subset of patients was revealed. Therefore, it is possible that despite the high APP score in IDH-mutant HMP gliomas, 2-hydroxygluarate (2-HG) induces T cell suppression in some capacity. The production of this oncometabolite is a unique feature of IDH-mutant gliomas and has been previously shown to impair T cell activation and reduce T cell migration to the tumor site. Importantly, our ssGSEA data supported this because comparison of the CD8 T cell score in IDH-wildtype and -mutant gliomas revealed a significant suppression of these immune cells in the latter (Figure S5), consistent with findings from other studies [27].

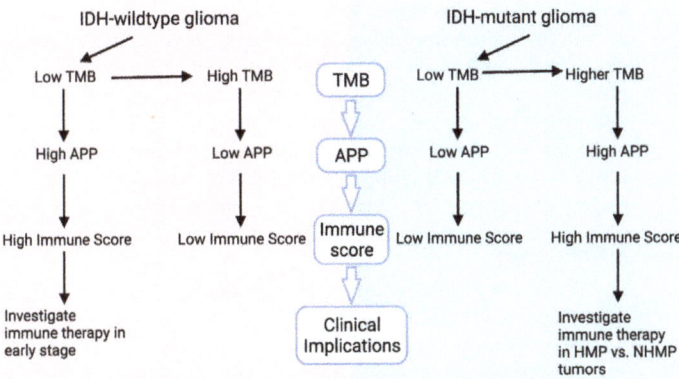

Figure 4. Graphic summary of study findings. In IDH-wildtype tumors, NHMP tumors have higher APP and immune scores than HMP, suggesting a need to investigate potential benefit for immunotherapy in early stage of the disease. However, in IDH-mutant gliomas, HMP tumors have higher APP scores than NHMP. Despite a lack of correlation between TMB and immune scores, investigation of immune therapy in HMP versus HNMP glioma is warranted and ongoing.

3.3. Clinical Implications, Prospectives and Limitations

While conferring tumorigenesis, P/LP germline mutations may also provide important applications to aid patient management. For example, previous studies have shown that patients who are *MSH6* mutation carriers should avoid treatment with alkylating agents such as TMZ [28]. In our patient cohort, we detected a *MSH2* germline mutation in an IDH-wildtype glioblastoma patient (NCI0392), who was diagnosed with Lynch syndrome and had a *de novo* HMP brain tumor. In this case, alkylating agents such as TMZ should have been avoided if more treatment options were available to the patient. A patient with an IDH-mutant grade 4 astrocytoma (CL0301) was found to have a germline mutation in *ERCC6*, an important gene in the DNA double-stranded breaks (DSBs) repair pathway. This patient received more than 24 cycles of TMZ after the initial diagnosis of a lower grade astrocytoma, and both tumors from later recurrences were found to be HMP, harboring 2200 high confidence somatic mutations, which indicated a likely pathogenic function of this mutation and a potential role in HMP development when treated with TMZ. Although the association between the hypermutation phenotype and the presence of P/LP germline variants in the DDR pathway was not found to be statistically significant, investigation in a larger patient cohort is needed. Screening of those germline mutations of CPGs may provide insights to assist the clinical management of cancer patients.

In addition, further studying potential clinical biomarkers is vital for selecting patients who will benefit from immunotherapy. For an expressed neoantigen to elicit an immune response, a high APP score and HLA expression level are necessary. Currently, we do not completely understand why IDH-wildtype HMP gliomas show a decreased APP score. It is possible that critical genes are mutated at the time of development of HMP in IDH-WT tumors that disrupts APP and thus cause resistance to immunotherapy. This potential resistance mechanism can be further explored in a longitudinal study where matched tumor samples are collected and analyzed. Our findings of the correlation between APP function and immune score support testing the use of immunotherapy at an early stage of the disease for IDH-wildtype glioma patients when the TMB is low and APP function is high in a larger cohort study. The anti-PD1/PDL1 therapies may be valuable because of the increased expression level of PD1/PDL1 when TMB is relatively lower in the IDH-wildtype tumors. Interestingly, in the case of IDH-mutant gliomas, an opposite trend is seen, wherein a high APP score is seen in HMP gliomas, suggesting a potential value in considering IDH-mutant HMP gliomas for immunotherapy rather than their NHMP counterparts (Figure 4). While the findings of our study expand the knowledge of TMB, expressed neoantigens, and the tumor immune microenvironment and provided insights for clinical investigations, certain limitations are present. The conclusions are drawn from bioinformatic analyses of a sample cohort from a single institution. Further validation using in vitro and in vivo glioma models as well as larger cohort studies are thus warranted. Due to the retrospective nature of the study, the percentage of IDH-mutant glioma may not be representative of the incidence in the entire malignant glioma population. Nevertheless, our ongoing clinical trial (NCT 03718767) will provide prospectively collected data to further elucidate the correlation between TMB, expressed neoantigens, and tumor immune signatures.

4. Conclusions

TMB was inversely correlated with immune score in IDH-wildtype and showed no correlation in IDH-mutant gliomas. APP was correlated with immune score and may be further investigated as a biomarker for response to immunotherapy in gliomas. Studies of germline variants in a larger glioma cohort are warranted.

5. Materials and Methods

5.1. Patients and Samples

Adult patients with primary malignant brain tumors, who were evaluated at the Neuro-Oncology Branch, Center for Cancer Research, National Cancer Institute (NCI), were enrolled in NCI 16-C-0151 (NCT02851706), NCI 19-C-0006 (NCT03718767), and NCI

10-C-0086 (NCT01109394). The protocols were approved by the Institutional Review Board of the National Institutes of Health. Written consents were obtained from all patients. Both matched whole blood and brain tumor samples were collected and analyzed using the ClinOmics platform, a clinical next-generation sequencing program at NCI [29]. Tumor samples were only collected for sequencing if sufficient tissue for clinical diagnosis was available. The schema of overall experimental approach for this study is summarized in Figure S6.

5.2. mRNA Sequencing (RNAseq)

Tumor RNA was extracted from Formalin Fixed Paraffin-Embedded (FFPE) tumor sections by the Rneasy FFPE kit (Qiagen, Germantown, MD, USA). RNA libraries were prepared by using Illumina TruSeq RNA Access Library Preparation Kit according to the manufacturer's protocol (TruSeq RNA Exome kits; Illumina, San Diego, CA, USA). The sequencing was performed on Illumina NextSeq500 (Illumina) according to the manufacturer's protocols. Samples were sequenced at a depth of 40 million reads per sample. All the RNAseq data was processed by using an RNAseq data analysis pipeline, where reads were mapped to the ENSEMBL human genome GRCh37 build 71 using STAR. Single-sample Gene Set Enrichment Analysis (ssGSEA) was used for the generation of immune cell infiltration scores, immune scores, and antigen processing and presentation scores based on the previously published gene sets [16,30]. CIBERSORT was used to analyze the proportions of immune cells [29].

5.3. Whole Exome Sequencing

Tumor DNA was extracted from FFPE samples. Genomic DNA, which was used as germline exome sequencing, was extracted from the peripheral blood cells of individual patients. The exome was enriched by using SureSelect Clinical Research Exome Kits according to the manufacturer's instructions (Agilent, Santa Clara, CA, USA). The prepared samples were sequenced on Illumina NextSeq500 (Illumina). Reportable germline mutations, which is defined as actionable genomic alterations to be targeted by the FDA approved drugs or clinical trials, were filtered out by in-house criteria [29]. TMB was defined as the number of somatic mutations in the coding region per Mb, which contain single nucleotide variants (SNVs), small insertions and deletions (INDELs) (usually less than 20 bases). TMB was calculated as indicated in the previous report [31].

5.4. Identification of Somatic Mutation

The bcl files of exome sequencing were converted to FASTQ files by using the bcl2fastq tool in CASAVA (Illumina). The sequences were then mapped to the human reference genome GRCH37 by using a customized NCI ClinOmics Bioinformatic Pipeline v3.2. MuTect and Strelka were used for somatic single nucleotide variant (SNV) and small indel calling respectively. The Genome Analysis Toolkit (GATK) and HaplotypeCaller (HAPLOC) for germline SNV and indel callings as previously described. High confidence somatic mutations were called by using the cutoffs: (1) tumor total coverage $\geq 20\times$, (2) normal total coverage $\geq 20\times$ and (3) variant allele frequency (VAF) ≥ 0.10. Using these parameters, our assay has a high sensitivity of 100% and a positive predictive value (PPV) of 90% for the exome sequencing.

5.5. Neoantigen Prediction from Mutations and Fusions, and Expressed Neoantigen Computation

The high confidence of somatic mutations was used for the neoantigen prediction according to the previous report [32]. The amino acid change and the transcript peptide sequence were annotated by seq2HLA v2.2, HLAminer_v1.3.1, in-house developed script consensusHLA.pl, consencusSomaticsVCF, pl, VEP v.86, pvacseqtools 1.3.5. NeoFuse v1.1.1 was used for the prediction of fusion neoantigens. NeoFuse internally runs OptiType for genotyping of class-1 HLA and Arriba for predicting of fusion peptides and MHC flurry for binding affinity prediction. The neoantigen candidates with a mutant HLA type I binding score (IC$_{50}$) lower than 500 nM, and a corresponding wild type binding IC$_{50}$ of greater than 500 nM were selected as predicted neoantigens. The expressed high confidence neoantigens from somatic mutations were called based on the high confidence neoantigens from somatic mutations by further using the cutoffs: (1) total RNA read coverage $\geq$ 10, (2) matched variant RNA read coverage $\geq$ 2, (3) VAF $\geq$ 0.1. The total expressed neoantigen load was calculated by adding the high confidence expressed neoantigen mutation and high confidence neoantigen from fusion.

5.6. Statistical Analysis

Wilcoxon rank sum test was used for differential analyses between two subgroups. One-way ANOVA test was used in the comparison of more than two groups. Categorical variables were compared using Fisher's exact test. All statistical analyses were performed by using GraphPad Prism software (Version 8, GraphPad Software, Inc., San Diego, CA, USA). p value < 0.05 was considered significant (*, $p < 0.05$; **, $p < 0.01$; ***, $p < 0.001$).

5.7. Data Availability

All Data has been deposited in dbGaP and RNAseq and Somatic Data is available on an online database (https://clinomics.ccr.cancer.gov/clinomics/public/login, accessed date: 20 November 2021).

Supplementary Materials: The following are available online at https://www.mdpi.com/article/10.3390/cancers13236092/s1, Figure S1. ssGSEA scores of immune cells, stromal score and immune score between HMP and NHMP samples with IDH status. MT, IDH-mutant, WT, IDH-wildtype. Figure S2. Different immune cell proportions are analyzed in HMP and NHMP samples by CIBERSORT. Figure S3. Comparison of percentages of M2 macrophages and CD8 T cells in HMP and NHMP samples. Figure S4. Immunosuppressive gene expressions are analyzed between HMP and NHMP samples. Figure S5. CD8 T cell scores in IDH-wildtype are higher than in IDH-mutant glioma. Figure S6. Schema of the experimental approach. Table S1. Sample cohort information. Table S2. HMP tumors. Table S3. High confidence expressed neoantigens from mutations.

Author Contributions: Conceptualization, G.Y., Y.P., J.K. and J.W.; Methodology, G.Y., Y.P., C.K., J.K. and J.W.; Software, V.G., A.A., H.-C.C., X.W. and S.S.; Formal Analysis, G.Y., Y.P., C.K., V.G., A.A., H.-C.C., J.K. and J.W.; Investigation, all authors; Resources, R.N.K., T.S.A., M.R.G., K.A., J.K. and J.W.; Data Curation, G.Y., Y.P., M.M., C.K., V.G., A.A., A.R., J.S.W., H.-C.C., X.W., S.S. and L.X.; Writing—Original Draft Preparation, G.Y., Y.P., M.M. and J.W.; Writing—Review & Editing, M.M., C.K., J.S.W., A.R., O.K. and J.K.; Supervision, J.K. and J.W.; Funding Acquisition, J.K. and J.W. All authors have read and agreed to the published version of the manuscript.

Funding: Supported by the NIH Lasker Clinical Research Scholars Program and NCI Intramural Research Program (1ZIABC011841 and 1ZIABC011840).

Institutional Review Board Statement: The study protocols for sample collection were reviewed and approved by the NCI Institutional Review Board. (Protocol code and date of approval, NCT02851706 2 August 2016, NCT03718767 24 October 2018, and NCT01109394 23 April 2010).

Informed Consent Statement: Informed consent was waived for data analysis report, due to all samples used in this analysis are deidentified.

Data Availability Statement: All Data has been deposited in dbGaP and RNAseq and Somatic Data is available on an online database (https://clinomics.ccr.cancer.gov/clinomics/public/login, accessed date: 20 November 2021).

Acknowledgments: This research was supported by the NIH Intramural Research Program and Lasker Clinical Research Scholar Program. We thank all the patients for participating in and supporting the clinical studies, which ultimately help other patients with brain tumors.

Conflicts of Interest: The authors declare no conflict of interest.

References

1. Lapointe, S.; Perry, A.; Butowski, N.A. Primary brain tumours in adults. *Lancet* **2018**, *392*, 432–446. [CrossRef]
2. Nicholson, J.G.; Fine, H.A. Diffuse Glioma Heterogeneity and Its Therapeutic Implications. *Cancer Discov.* **2021**, *11*, 575–590. [CrossRef] [PubMed]
3. Seidel, J.A.; Otsuka, A.; Kabashima, K. Anti-PD-1 and Anti-CTLA-4 Therapies in Cancer: Mechanisms of Action, Efficacy, and Limitations. *Front. Oncol.* **2018**, *8*, 86. [CrossRef]
4. Jardim, D.L.; Goodman, A.; de Melo Gagliato, D.; Kurzrock, R. The Challenges of Tumor Mutational Burden as an Immunotherapy Biomarker. *Cancer Cell* **2021**, *39*, 154–173. [CrossRef]
5. Prasad, V.; Addeo, A. The FDA approval of pembrolizumab for patients with TMB >10 mut/Mb: Was it a wise decision? No. *Ann. Oncol.* **2020**, *31*, 1112–1114. [CrossRef] [PubMed]
6. Touat, M.; Li, Y.Y.; Boynton, A.N.; Spurr, L.F.; Iorgulescu, J.B.; Bohrson, C.L.; Cortes-Ciriano, I.; Birzu, C.; Geduldig, J.E.; Pelton, K.J.N. Mechanisms and therapeutic implications of hypermutation in gliomas. *Nature* **2020**, *580*, 517–523. [CrossRef] [PubMed]
7. Merchant, M.; Ranjan, A.; Pang, Y.; Yu, G.; Kim, O.; Khan, J.; Wu, J. Tumor mutational burden and immunotherapy in gliomas. *Trends Cancer* **2021**, *7*, 1054–1058. [CrossRef] [PubMed]
8. Turkalp, Z.; Karamchandani, J.; Das, S. IDH mutation in glioma: New insights and promises for the future. *JAMA Neurol.* **2014**, *71*, 1319–1325. [CrossRef]
9. Cancer Genome Atlas Research Network; Brat, D.J.; Verhaak, R.G.; Aldape, K.D.; Yung, W.K.; Salama, S.R.; Cooper, L.A.; Rheinbay, E.; Miller, C.R.; Vitucci, M.; et al. Comprehensive, Integrative Genomic Analysis of Diffuse Lower-Grade Gliomas. *N. Engl. J. Med.* **2015**, *372*, 2481–2498.
10. Richards, S.; Aziz, N.; Bale, S.; Bick, D.; Das, S.; Gastier-Foster, J.; Grody, W.W.; Hegde, M.; Lyon, E.; Spector, E.; et al. Standards and guidelines for the interpretation of sequence variants: A joint consensus recommendation of the American College of Medical Genetics and Genomics and the Association for Molecular Pathology. *Genet. Med.* **2015**, *17*, 405–424. [CrossRef]
11. Roper, N.; Brown, A.L.; Wei, J.S.; Pack, S.; Trindade, C.; Kim, C.; Restifo, O.; Gao, S.; Sindiri, S.; Mehrabadi, F.; et al. Clonal Evolution and Heterogeneity of Osimertinib Acquired Resistance Mechanisms in EGFR Mutant Lung Cancer. *Cell Rep. Med.* **2020**, *1*, 100007. [CrossRef]
12. Ceccarelli, M.; Barthel, F.P.; Malta, T.M.; Sabedot, T.S.; Salama, S.R.; Murray, B.A.; Morozova, O.; Newton, Y.; Radenbaugh, A.; Pagnotta, S.M.; et al. Molecular Profiling Reveals Biologically Discrete Subsets and Pathways of Progression in Diffuse Glioma. *Cell* **2016**, *164*, 550–563. [CrossRef]
13. Bai, H.; Harmanci, A.S.; Erson-Omay, E.Z.; Li, J.; Coskun, S.; Simon, M.; Krischek, B.; Ozduman, K.; Omay, S.B.; Sorensen, E.A.; et al. Integrated genomic characterization of IDH1-mutant glioma malignant progression. *Nat. Genet.* **2016**, *48*, 59–66. [CrossRef] [PubMed]
14. Pang, Y.; Yu, G.; Butler, M.; Sindiri, S.; Song, Y.K.; Wei, J.S.; Wen, X.; Chou, H.C.; Quezado, M.; Pack, S.; et al. Report of Canonical BCR-ABL1 Fusion in Glioblastoma. *JCO Precis. Oncol.* **2021**, *5*, PO.20.00519. [CrossRef]
15. Thorsson, V.; Gibbs, D.L.; Brown, S.D.; Wolf, D.; Bortone, D.S.; Ou Yang, T.H.; Porta-Pardo, E.; Gao, G.F.; Plaisier, C.L.; Eddy, J.A.; et al. The Immune Landscape of Cancer. *Immunity* **2018**, *48*, 812–830.e14. [CrossRef]
16. Newman, A.M.; Liu, C.L.; Green, M.R.; Gentles, A.J.; Feng, W.; Xu, Y.; Hoang, C.D.; Diehn, M.; Alizadeh, A.A. Robust enumeration of cell subsets from tissue expression profiles. *Nat. Methods* **2015**, *12*, 453–457. [CrossRef] [PubMed]
17. Su, J.; Long, W.; Ma, Q.; Xiao, K.; Li, Y.; Xiao, Q.; Peng, G.; Yuan, J.; Liu, Q. Identification of a Tumor Microenvironment-Related Eight-Gene Signature for Predicting Prognosis in Lower-Grade Gliomas. *Front. Genet.* **2019**, *10*, 1143. [CrossRef] [PubMed]
18. Garrido, F.; Aptsiauri, N.; Doorduijn, E.M.; Garcia Lora, A.M.; van Hall, T. The urgent need to recover MHC class I in cancers for effective immunotherapy. *Curr. Opin. Immunol.* **2016**, *39*, 44–51. [CrossRef] [PubMed]
19. Mehling, M.; Simon, P.; Mittelbronn, M.; Meyermann, R.; Ferrone, S.; Weller, M.; Wiendl, H. WHO grade associated downregulation of MHC class I antigen-processing machinery components in human astrocytomas: Does it reflect a potential immune escape mechanism? *Acta Neuropathol.* **2007**, *114*, 111–119. [CrossRef]
20. Facoetti, A.; Nano, R.; Zelini, P.; Morbini, P.; Benericetti, E.; Ceroni, M.; Campoli, M.; Ferrone, S. Human leukocyte antigen and antigen processing machinery component defects in astrocytic tumors. *Clin. Cancer Res.* **2005**, *11*, 8304–8311. [CrossRef]
21. Yeung, J.T.; Hamilton, R.L.; Ohnishi, K.; Ikeura, M.; Potter, D.M.; Nikiforova, M.N.; Ferrone, S.; Jakacki, R.I.; Pollack, I.F.; Okada, H. LOH in the HLA class I region at 6p21 is associated with shorter survival in newly diagnosed adult glioblastoma. *Clin. Cancer Res.* **2013**, *19*, 1816–1826. [CrossRef]
22. Newman, S.; Nakitandwe, J.; Kesserwan, C.A.; Azzato, E.M.; Wheeler, D.A.; Rusch, M.; Shurtleff, S.; Hedges, D.J.; Hamilton, K.V.; Foy, S.G.; et al. Genomes for Kids: The scope of pathogenic mutations in pediatric cancer revealed by comprehensive DNA and RNA sequencing. *Cancer Discov.* **2021**, *11*, 1–20. [CrossRef]
23. Schrader, K.A.; Cheng, D.T.; Joseph, V.; Prasad, M.; Walsh, M.; Zehir, A.; Ni, A.; Thomas, T.; Benayed, R.; Ashraf, A.; et al. Germline Variants in Targeted Tumor Sequencing Using Matched Normal DNA. *JAMA Oncol.* **2016**, *2*, 104–111. [CrossRef] [PubMed]
24. Pitroski, C.E.; Cossio, S.L.; Koehler-Santos, P.; Graudenz, M.; Prolla, J.C.; Ashton-Prolla, P. Frequency of the common germline MUTYH mutations p.G396D and p.Y179C in patients diagnosed with colorectal cancer in Southern Brazil. *Int. J. Colorectal Dis.* **2011**, *26*, 841–846. [CrossRef]

25. Cunniff, C.; Bassetti, J.A.; Ellis, N.A. Bloom's Syndrome: Clinical Spectrum, Molecular Pathogenesis, and Cancer Predisposition. *Mol. Syndromol.* **2017**, *8*, 4–23. [CrossRef]
26. Gromeier, M.; Brown, M.C.; Zhang, G.; Lin, X.; Chen, Y.; Wei, Z.; Beaubier, N.; Yan, H.; He, Y.; Desjardins, A.; et al. Very low mutation burden is a feature of inflamed recurrent glioblastomas responsive to cancer immunotherapy. *Nat. Commun.* **2021**, *12*, 352. [CrossRef] [PubMed]
27. Amankulor, N.M.; Kim, Y.; Arora, S.; Kargl, J.; Szulzewsky, F.; Hanke, M.; Margineantu, D.H.; Rao, A.; Bolouri, H.; Delrow, J.; et al. Mutant IDH1 regulates the tumor-associated immune system in gliomas. *Genes Dev.* **2017**, *31*, 774–786. [CrossRef]
28. Scott, R.H.; Mansour, S.; Pritchard-Jones, K.; Kumar, D.; MacSweeney, F.; Rahman, N. Medulloblastoma, acute myelocytic leukemia and colonic carcinomas in a child with biallelic MSH6 mutations. *Nat. Clin. Pract. Oncol.* **2007**, *4*, 130–134. [CrossRef]
29. Chang, W.; Brohl, A.S.; Patidar, R.; Sindiri, S.; Shern, J.F.; Wei, J.S.; Song, Y.K.; Yohe, M.E.; Gryder, B.; Zhang, S.; et al. Multidimensional ClinOmics for Precision Therapy of Children and Adolescent Young Adults with Relapsed and Refractory Cancer: A Report from the Center for Cancer Research. *Clin. Cancer Res.* **2016**, *22*, 3810–3820. [CrossRef]
30. Yoshihara, K.; Shahmoradgoli, M.; Martinez, E.; Vegesna, R.; Kim, H.; Torres-Garcia, W.; Trevino, V.; Shen, H.; Laird, P.W.; Levine, D.A.; et al. Inferring tumour purity and stromal and immune cell admixture from expression data. *Nat. Commun.* **2013**, *4*, 2612. [CrossRef] [PubMed]
31. Zehir, A.; Benayed, R.; Shah, R.H.; Syed, A.; Middha, S.; Kim, H.R.; Srinivasan, P.; Gao, J.; Chakravarty, D.; Devlin, S.M.; et al. Mutational landscape of metastatic cancer revealed from prospective clinical sequencing of 10,000 patients. *Nat. Med.* **2017**, *23*, 703–713. [CrossRef] [PubMed]
32. McLaren, W.; Gil, L.; Hunt, S.E.; Riat, H.S.; Ritchie, G.R.; Thormann, A.; Flicek, P.; Cunningham, F. The Ensembl Variant Effect Predictor. *Genome Biol.* **2016**, *17*, 122. [CrossRef] [PubMed]

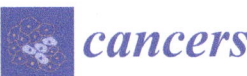

Review

Molecular Classification and Therapeutic Targets in Ependymoma

Thomas Larrew [1,†], Brian Fabian Saway [1,†], Stephen R. Lowe [2,‡] and Adriana Olar [3,*,‡]

1. Department of Neurosurgery, Medical University of South Carolina, Charleston, SC 29425, USA
2. Neurosurgical Associates, Knoxville, TN 37920, USA
3. NOMIX Laboratories, Denver, CO 80218, USA
* Correspondence: adriana_olar@yahoo.com or aolar@nomixlaboratories.com
† These authors contributed equally to this work.
‡ Equal senior contribution.

Simple Summary: Molecular characterization of ependymoma has revolutionized its categorization. This new molecular classification has implications particularly in targeted therapeutics. Amongst the ten subgroups of ependymoma currently described, three are found in the spinal compartment, and three in the infratentorial and supratentorial compartments respectively; the subependymoma subgroup is found in all these anatomic compartments. Each subgroup carries unique molecular features that lead to oncogenesis and to disparities in prognosis. Here, the molecular classification, key clinical features, current understanding of tumorigenesis, and potential molecular targets for cranial and spinal ependymoma are discussed.

Abstract: Ependymoma is a biologically diverse tumor wherein molecular classification has superseded traditional histological grading based on its superior ability to characterize behavior, prognosis, and possible targeted therapies. The current, updated molecular classification of ependymoma consists of ten distinct subgroups spread evenly among the spinal, infratentorial, and supratentorial compartments, each with its own distinct clinical and molecular characteristics. In this review, the history, histopathology, standard of care, prognosis, oncogenic drivers, and hypothesized molecular targets for all subgroups of ependymoma are explored. This review emphasizes that despite the varied behavior of the ependymoma subgroups, it remains clear that research must be performed to further elucidate molecular targets for these tumors. Although not all ependymoma subgroups are oncologically aggressive, development of targeted therapies is essential, particularly for cases where surgical resection is not an option without causing significant morbidity. The development of molecular therapies must rely on building upon our current understanding of ependymoma oncogenesis, as well as cultivating transfer of knowledge based on malignancies with similar genomic alterations.

Keywords: ependymoma; subependymoma; RELA; YAP1; ZFTA; PFA; PFB; MYCN; Group A; Group B; myxopapillary; targeted therapy

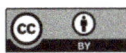

1. Introduction

Ependymomas are primary central nervous system (CNS) tumors derived from the ependymal lining of the ventricular system [1,2]. These tumors are found in both the pediatric and adult population and are found throughout the CNS, including the supratentorial (ST) space, the infratentorial (IT) space and the spinal (SP) compartment. They are most commonly found in the ventricular system, but also in the parenchyma.

Based on the Central Brain Tumor Registry of the United States, ependymal tumors represent approximately 1.6% of all primary CNS tumors. Incidence of ependymal tumors ranges from 0.29 to 0.6 per 100,000 person-years and is lowest in the first two decades of life and highest in the 65–74 years old age group [3]. Tumor location is largely dependent on the patient age, with nearly 90% of pediatric ependymal tumors occurring intracranially, and approximately 65% of adult tumors occurring in the spine [4]. Amongst patients with intracranial ependymomas, there is significant morbidity and mortality. In a multicenter study of 282 adult patients, the 5-year overall survival (OS) rate was 62% for ST tumors and 85% for IT tumors [5]. Patients with SP ependymomas fare better with a 5-year OS of 97%.

Management of adult patients with ependymoma involves surgical resection for its cytoreductive effects and, in many cases, to restore normal cerebrospinal fluid (CSF) dynamics [6–8]. Postoperative radiotherapy is usually employed, particularly in cases of World Health Organization (WHO) grade II intracranial ependymoma after subtotal resection (STR) and WHO grade III intracranial and spinal anaplastic ependymoma regardless of the extent of resection [5,8–11]. The use of radiotherapy remains controversial for WHO grade II intracranial ependymoma and spinal ependymoma after gross total resection (GTR) [12]. Chemotherapy is typically reserved for cases of advanced or recurrent ependymoma that cannot be further resected or irradiated [11]. There is very little description of efficacious use of chemotherapies for ependymoma in general. In a study of adult recurrent low-grade and anaplastic SP, ST, and IT ependymoma, a regimen of temozolomide and lapatinib was used with modest results and a median progression-free survival (PFS) of 8 months [13]. Among the small number of studies looking at the use of chemotherapy for ependymoma, there is a lack of any standard regimens with durable results, though use of platinum compounds or temozolomide has been suggested due their favorable safety profiles [11,13–18]. There has been limited use of immunotherapy for adult ependymoma, though there are a few documented cases of its use in pediatric recurrent ependymoma [19].

The management of pediatric patients with ependymoma follows a similar paradigm except for several key differences. Pediatric ependymoma management centers around GTR and radiotherapy. Based on National Cancer Institute recommendations, all intracranial pediatric ependymoma cases require surgery and postoperative radiotherapy unless the patient is under 1 year of age [20]. The European Association of Neuro-Oncology (EANO) has similar recommendations except it is recommended that postoperative radiotherapy should be used in children older than 18 months, or in children between 12 and 18 months with significant neurological deficits [11]. Traditionally, chemotherapy regimens were utilized in children younger than 3 years of age with newly diagnosed ependymoma to defer radiation. However, there is mounting evidence that earlier radiation may lead to improved outcomes [21–23] In comparing the trials POG-9233 trial and ACNS0121, which had similar protocols except for the use of radiotherapy, there was a 50–60% improvement in survival for patients under 3 years old who were treated with radiation therapy [24,25]. It is recommended that second-look surgery be performed when GTR is achievable, as it leads to better disease control [26]. In STR cases, the benefit of pre-radiation chemotherapy is still being investigated but may be used [27]. Pediatric patients with disease recurrence should undergo resection with postoperative radiotherapy [28]. Chemotherapy has been used in recurrent cases but the response generally lacks durability [29,30]. Chemotherapy regimens should be based on prior exposures, though clinical trials should be explored [11].

The management strategy of adult patients that suffer from relapse is currently evolving as our understanding of the molecular drivers of this disease are being further investigated [31]. Moreover, the most effective management of disseminated versus local recurrence is also not well delineated. Although there is a dearth of randomized clinical data, there is a consensus that recurrent lesions that are non-operable should receive radiotherapy in both the adult and pediatric populations. The utility of chemotherapy and immunotherapy for disease recurrence is also actively being explored. EANO recommends platinum or temozolomide based on their favorable toxicity profiles, though clinical trials should be considered [11,17]. Ongoing research on this topic includes locoregional delivery of chimeric antigen receptor T (CAR T) cells targeting various surface antigens expressed on recurrent ependymomas, which has been shown to be highly efficacious in a mouse model [32]. As our treatment modalities improve for this pathology, and longevity of this patient population subsequentially increases, optimization of treatment regimens for recurrence using a combination of surgery, radiation, and chemo-/immuno-therapies will need to be further investigated.

2. History

Ependymomas have classically been diagnosed based on the WHO histological classification strategy, which was designed to integrate histopathological characteristics to facilitate tumor diagnosis, guide treatment strategy, allow for prognostication, and aid research by allowing for interlaboratory comparisons. In 2016, the WHO classification for CNS tumors incorporated not only light microscopy, immunohistochemical lineage-associated proteins, and ultrastructural characteristics, but also a few molecular markers, namely *RELA*-fusion ependymoma, to enhance the diagnostic and prognostic utility of this classification strategy [1]. Despite this, controversy in the field remains regarding the use of primarily histology to guide tumor grading. This controversy stems from the notable histopathologic variations seen between and within specimens, the large inter-observer grading discrepancies among neuropathologists, and the lack of consistent prognostication based on WHO grading [33–36]. There was a clear paucity amongst scientists and clinicians on how to effectively categorize this diverse CNS pathology to better identify, analyze, and prognosticate in order to provide patients with accurate information regarding their diagnosis. Similar to other CNS malignancies, investigators began to focus on molecular signatures as a means to fill this void.

The introduction of molecular markers in the 2016 WHO classification and the expansion in the 2021 WHO classification, was a function of several investigations elucidating the genetic uniqueness within the histologically defined subgroups of ependymomas. These findings began as a series of multi-omics studies that separated genomic groups of ependymomas with clinical and prognostic correlation. Early studies focused on gene expression and copy number profiles, while late studies focused on epigenomics [37–44].

In 2015, a landmark clinical and genomic study by Pajtler et al., utilized DNA methylation profiling of 500 ependymomas to identify nine subgroups [40]. This project solidified and supported previous research emphasizing that despite similar histopathological features among ependymoma tumors, their diverse biological behavior could be better defined and categorized based on genomic markers. The nine subgroups of ependymomas were divided evenly amongst the three major compartments of the CNS. The SP compartment contained the subgroups of SP subependymoma (SP-SE), SP myxopapillary ependymoma (MPE), and SP ependymoma (SPE), all of which have predilection for the adult population. The IT compartment contained the subgroups posterior fossa subependymoma (PF-SE), posterior fossa ependymoma Group A (PFA), and posterior fossa ependymoma Group B (PFB), of which, the PFA alone has a strong preponderance for the pediatric population. Lastly, the ST compartment contained the subgroups of ST subependymoma (ST-SE), ST ependymoma with *YAP1* fusion (ST-YAP1), and ST ependymoma with *RELA* fusion (ST-RELA). All nine subgroups were found to have distinct DNA methylation patterns that correlated with pertinent clinicopathological variables, such as age and sex. The study was also able to demonstrate that risk stratification by molecular subgrouping is superior to the histopathological grading used by the 2007 WHO grading system. However, it is important to note that in this and following studies, many classic histology ependymomas (grade II) were classified into the SE and MPE subgroups [37,40]. Nevertheless, this study served as the foundation for subsequent studies validating and expanding upon these new molecular subgroups of ependymomas.

In 2021, the WHO Classification of Tumors of the CNS will be again updated with its 5th edition attempting to capture all of the recent updates in genomic profiling and to address some of the aforementioned issues. This update introduced the *C11orf95/ZFTA*-fusion subgroup (same as the former 2016 *RELA*-fusion subgroup), *YAP1*-fusion subgroup, PFA subgroup, PFB subgroup, and the SP ependymoma with *MYCN* amplification subgroup. These were added as unique genomic markers, and transcriptional patterns were identified that could better differentiate ependymomas despite similar histological features [45–50]. While this offers additional molecular categories, data is lacking to assign grading based solely on molecular alterations, as is seen in diffuse gliomas [49,50].

The 2021 WHO classification, the Pajtler study, and the subsequent studies that examined these distinct subgroups in the population, their underlying oncogenic drivers, as well as proposed molecular targets, are the subject of this review. Besides, SE and MPE which remain their own histological categories, ependymomas are now primarily defined by anatomic location (SP, PF, ST), histology (grade 2 or 3), and molecular features [49,50]. In this review, we describe the three subgroups of ependymoma found in each of the three anatomic compartments, as well as the SE subgroups found at every location. These 10 subgroups and their characteristics are summarized in Figure 1.

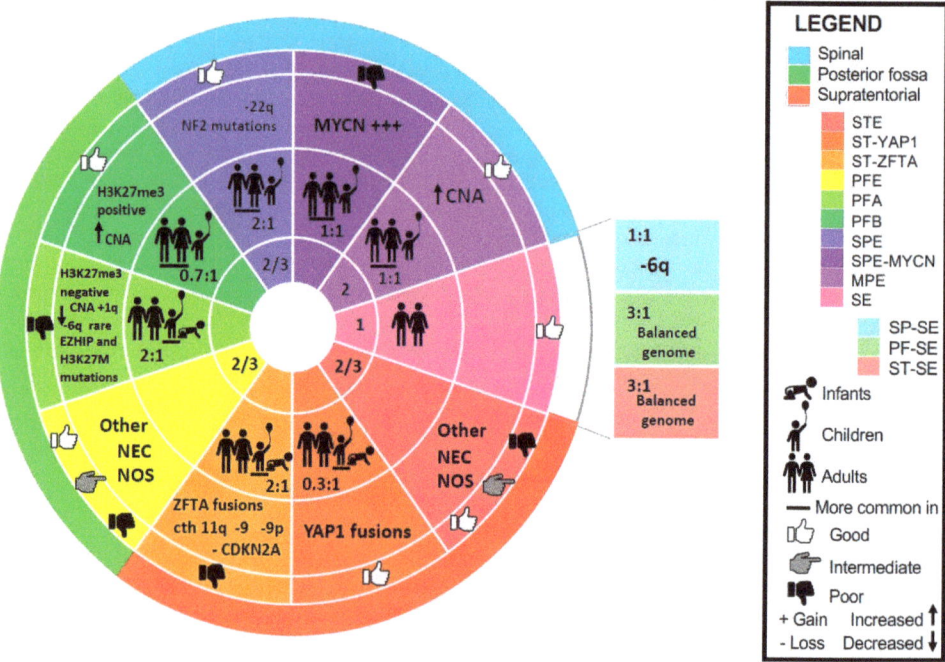

Figure 1. Ependymoma molecular classification per WHO 2021. Concentric discs represent (inner to outward): WHO grade, age and sex ratio (male to female), characteristic molecular features, outcome, location. Abbreviations: CNA—copy number alterations, cth—chromothripsis, MPE—myxopapillary ependymoma, NEC—not elsewhere classified (other molecular alteration, not described), NOS—not otherwise specified (molecular testing is not available), PFE—posterior fossa ependymoma, PFA—posterior fossa ependymoma Group A, PFB—posterior fossa ependymoma Group B, PF-SE—posterior fossa subependymoma, SE—subependymoma, SP-SE—spinal cord subependymoma, SPE—spinal cord ependymoma, SPE-MYCN—spinal cord ependymoma with *MYCN* amplification, STE—supratentorial ependymoma, ST-SE—supratentorial subependymoma, ST-YAP1—supratentorial ependymoma with *YAP1* fusion, ST-ZFTA—supratentorial ependymoma with *ZFTA* fusion.

3. Subependymoma (SE)

In the 2021 CNS WHO classification, subependymoma (SE) remains a separate entity (encompassing SP-SE, ST-SE and PF-SE–described below) identified by morphologic criteria (Figure 2A) as there is currently no clinical justification of SE molecular subgroups at each anatomic site [49,50]. Grossly, these tumors are tan-white-gray, nodular, and firm, bulging into the ventricles. The histopathology is defined as clusters of isomorphic nuclei embedded in a dense, fine, glial fibrillary background, mild nuclear pleomorphism, microcystic formations (especially in lateral ventricular tumors), with or without occasional hemorrhage, and/or calcification. SE express glial acidic fibrillary protein (GFAP) and ezrin-radixin-moesin binding protein 50 or Na+/H+ Exchanger Regulatory Factor (NHERF1/EBP50) microlumens, whereas epithelial membrane antigen (EMA) is rarely expressed [1,51,52]. They are considered slow growing WHO grade 1 tumors often presenting with symptoms related to CSF obstruction if intracranially located, given their predilection for the ventricular system. They can present with spinal cord/nerve root compression if located in the spine.

3.1. Spinal Subependymoma (SP-SE)

Spinal subependymomas (SP-SE) have a predilection for the cervical or cervicothoracic junction, and typically present with insidious myelopathy or radicular pain [53]. This subgroup commonly presents in the adult population with a mean age of presentation of 44 years old, and with an even sex distribution, based on the few case series that have been published [54,55].

Patients with SP-SE have an excellent prognosis when treated with the standard of care treatment strategy of microsurgical resection [55]. GTR with minimal disruption of adjacent vital structures via microsurgery is the gold standard treatment, and is often feasible with the advancement of microsurgical tools and intraoperative neuromonitoring. When GTR is not achievable given proximity to eloquent structures, STR is advised with serial follow-up imaging. A large systematic review assessing outcomes in 105 cases of SP-SE found that 65% of patients underwent GTR and that of these, 57% had worsened function after surgery, while only 41% of the patients that underwent STR or partial resection experienced worsened function [55]. No patients had tumors with malignant transformation; therefore, long-term survival for all patients was expected. This study emphasizes the significant morbidity associated with surgical intervention of this subtype of tumor given the eloquent adjacent structures despite the excellent mortality rates. The authors make the argument for the benefits of cure in this disease. However, when the demarcation margin is not very clear during surgical debulking, the benefits of cure via GTR may not outweigh the risks of causing significant neurological morbidity as disease progression is likely to be very slow. No adjuvant radiotherapy is needed as good clinical outcomes are seen following both gross and STR of SP-SE [56]. Altogether, while SP-SE have an excellent prognosis when treated with microsurgical resection, there is inherent risk taken when surgically removing these tumors from the eloquent spinal cord, which may limit therapeutic reach.

Research into the molecular drivers underlying oncogenesis of SP-SE has been sparse, and likely secondary to its benign clinical course. The two largest genetic analyses of this tumor subgroup both showed loss of 6q [37,40]. In addition, Witt et al. noted an almost 50% copy number reduction in 19p and 19q, while in the seven SP-SE patients in the Pajtler study no chromosome 19 copy number loss was noted. The one, uniformly defining characteristic of this subgroup is deletion of chromosome 6q [40]. Previously, the role of 6q deletion in all subsets of ependymoma has been controversial as studies have reported variable influence on patient prognosis. Specifically, 6q25.3 deletions were found to be markers of good prognosis and survival, as shown by the risk stratification scheme of intracranial ependymomas proposed by Korshunov et al. and confirmed in the pediatric population by Monoranu et al. [57,58]. Conversely, Rajaram et al. found 6q23 deletions to be a marker of disease progression in a mixed population of ependymoma subgroups [59]. While the role of 6q deletion in SE tumorigenesis and behavior requires further research, its involvement and targeting in other malignancies may provide avenues for future treatment strategies. Specifically, the c-myeloblastosis gene (c-MYB), a proto-oncogene encoding a transcription regulator that plays an essential role in regulation of hematopoiesis and located on chromosome 6q23.3, is being explored as a driver in the oncogenesis of this tumor [60]. Additionally, 6q cytogenetic abnormalities are commonly seen in T-cell lymphoblastic leukemia/lymphoma. Research in this field has recently identified EPHA7, a tumor suppressor gene found on 6q that encodes the protein Ephrin type-A receptor 7, a receptor tyrosine kinase that mediates developmental events in the nervous system [61]. EPHA7 may contribute in part to the onset of T-cell lymphomas.

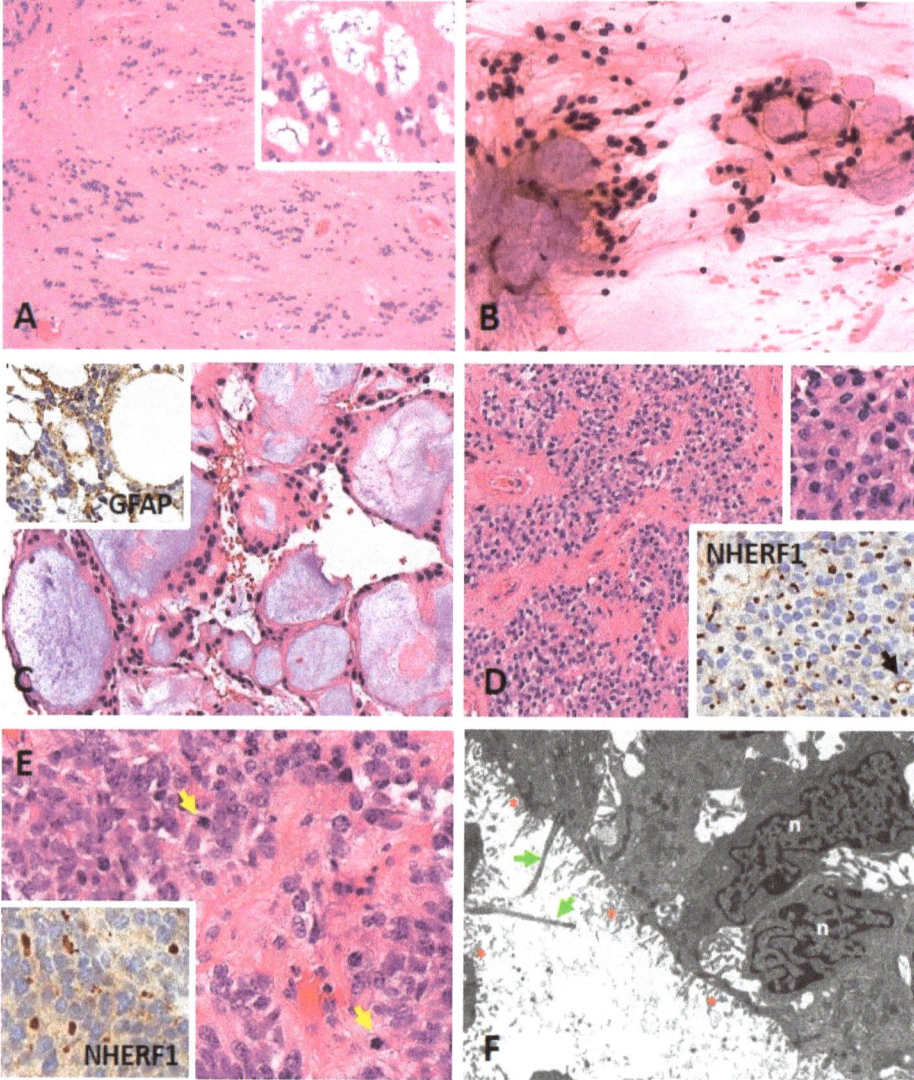

Figure 2. Morphology of subependymoma and ependymoma. (**A**) Subependymoma composed of clusters of isomorphic nuclei embedded in a fibrillary matrix of glial cell processes (HE, 100×). Cystic degeneration and nuclear pleomorphism (degeneration-related) can be present in larger tumors (inset) (HE, 200×). (**B**) Myxopapillary ependymoma showing ependymal cells with bland oval nuclei and fibrillary processes around aggregates of myxoid material (smear, HE, 200×). (**C**) Tissue section of myxopapillary ependymoma showing bland GFAP positive (inset, GFAP, 200×) ependymal cells around blood vessels with myxoid degeneration (HE, 200×). (**D**) Ependymoma composed of neoplastic glial cells arranged around blood vessels in pseudorosettes (HE, 100×). The tumor nuclei are round to oval, monomorphic with stippled chromatin (top inset) (HE, 200×). Anti-NHERF1/EBP50 immunohistochemistry showing numerous dot-like microlumens and a rare ring-like structure (arrow) (bottom inset) (200×). (**E**) Anaplastic ependymoma with enlarged pleomorphic nuclei and mitotic activity (arrows) (HE, 200×). Anti-NHERF1/EBP50 immunohistochemistry showing an area with microlumens (inset) (200×). (**F**) Electron micrograph showing the lumen of a true rosette lined by ependymal tumor cells with rare cilia (green arrows) and abundant microvilli (red asterisks) (18,000×). Abbreviations: HE—hematoxylin and eosin, n—nucleus Note: Photographs in D-F were kindly provided by Dr. Maria-Magdalena Georgescu, NeuroMarkers PLLC, Houston, TX, USA.

3.2. Posterior Fossa Subependymoma (PF-SE)

The histopathologic origin of SE in the IT compartment remains uncertain. Possible cell origins include ependymal-glial precursor cells, subependymal plate cells, and tanycytes [62,63]. Macroscopically, the tumors are firm, well-delineated, and lobulated masses bulging into the fourth ventricle (IVthV). The most common location for intracranial SE. PF-SE is typically found on the floor or the roof of the IVthV. Approximately 20% of these tumors are calcified. Unlike ST-SE, PF-SE is unlikely to be cystic. Dissimilar to most other ependymoma subgroups, PF-SE occurs in middle-aged to older patients, with the average age around 60 years old [40,62]. PF-SE is more common in the male population with almost a 3:1 ratio [62].

PF-SE carries low pathogenicity and, in fact, is often not discovered until postmortem examination [64,65]. GTR is generally thought to be curative, though recurrences can occur [62,66]. Radiotherapy may be used in cases of STR, but is typically reserved as salvage therapy if progression occurs. Chemotherapy and molecularly targeted therapy have not routinely been employed given the tumor's slow growth and low risk for recurrence or metastasis. The 5-year PFS and OS are generally high, at 86–90% and 91–100%, respectively [40,62,67].

Genomic analyses of PF-SE have had mixed results regarding copy number variations [37,40]. While the landmark paper by Pajtler et al. did not find any copy number loss or gain, there was over 50% copy number loss in chromosome 19p and 19q in the 24 PF-SE patients studied by Witt et al. Based on examination of the transcription profiles of PF-SE tumors, its tumorigenesis appears to be related to fatty acid metabolism, mast cell and leukocyte processes (KIT), signal transduction pathways (specifically STAT), as well as, chemotaxis [40]. In a study by Kong et al., an SE cell line was created and a tissue microarray analysis was performed demonstrating high tumor expression levels of topoisomerase II-β, HIF-1α, E3 ubiquitin-protein ligase Mdm2, and nucleolin on immunohistochemistry and Western blot analyses [68]. Topoisomerase II-β is encoded by *TOP2B* and is a key decatenating enzyme [69]. HIF-1α is encoded by *HIF1A* and functions as a master transcriptional regulator in the response to hypoxia. E3 ubiquitin-protein ligase Mdm2 is encoded by *MDM2* and functions to mediate ubiquitination of p53 leading to its degradation. Nucleolin is encoded by *NCL* and is a major nucleolar protein associated with intranucleolar chromatin and preribosomal particles that induces chromatin decondensation by binding to histone H1. Given the benign course of PF-SE, there are no chemotherapy regimens commonly used, nor are there any current targeted therapies for this disease. At the time of writing, there are no clinical trials for chemotherapies or molecularly targeted therapies for SE. *KIT* may be a viable target as it is only expressed at high levels in PF-SE tumors but not the other subgroups [40]. Multikinase inhibitors, such as imatinib, have been demonstrated to inhibit the autophosphorylation of c-KIT and could play a role in disease progression [70,71]. Topoisomerase inhibitors and p-STAT3/HIF-1α inhibitors appear to inhibit SE cell line growth suggesting a topoisomerase II inhibitor, such as FDA-approved etoposide and teniposide, could counteract PF-SE disease progression [68].

3.3. Supratentorial Subependymoma (ST-SE)

Supratentorial subependymoma (ST-SE) is often attached to the wall of the ventricular system. While the IVthV is a common intracranial location (40–60% of intracranial cases), SE is most commonly found supratentorially in the lateral ventricles (30–45% of intracranial cases), as subependymal glial cells are thought to play a large role in the origin of this neoplasm [72–74]. Similar to its IT counterpart, patients can present with symptoms related to CSF obstruction [67,75]. Presentation is common throughout adulthood but is most frequently seen in the third to sixth decades of life and in males rather than females [40,65,67,76,77].

The current gold standard treatment is maximal resection [67,76]. The use of adjuvant radiotherapy is generally not recommended as a good prognosis with surgery alone is seen if GTR is achieved [40,62,66,67]. Similar to its IT counterpart, there may be a role for radiotherapy if there is recurrence or symptomatic residual disease [67,76]. Unlike PF-SE, GTR may be more easily achievable given ST-SE is not in proximity to the brainstem. OS is excellent, at 96–100% for 1, 5, and 10-year [40,78].

Because of the uncommon nature of this subgroup, as well as the excellent prognosis following GTR, there has been little research regarding molecular targets for ST-SE. Similar to SP-SE and PF-SE, the two largest genomic studies have shown disputing results regarding copy number variations [37,40]. The Pajtler analysis of 21 ST-SE patients demonstrated a balanced genome, while the Witt analysis of 14 ST-SE patients demonstrated a 50% copy number loss in chromosome 19p and 19q. This discrepancy will have to be solved by future studies in all SEs. Regarding target development, the previously mentioned study by Kong et al. sought to identify and prioritize potential therapeutic targets for SE tumors through the use of tissue microarrays, ex vivo analysis, and in vitro cytotoxic assays [68]. This study derived the first-known human SE cell line from a resected SE and has laid the foundation for future research to identify potential molecular targets and develop therapeutic approaches. Of importance, this study demonstrated tumor expression of p53, MDM2, HIF-1α, topoisomerase II-b, p-STAT3 and nucleolin while also showing growth suppression of SE cells ex vivo utilizing a topoisomerase inhibitor (WP744) and the p-STAT3/HIF-1α inhibitors (WP1066 and WP1193). The targets highlighted in this molecular study may be applicable to SP-SE, IT-SE, and ST-SE; however, given the benign course of SE, development of targeted therapy may have a limited role in management in comparison to other ependymoma subgroups that may have malignant transformation. In rare instances of symptomatic residual or inability to resection, particularly in SP-SE cases, there may be a role for targeted therapies, but given the rarity of this, the authors encourage investigation into other ependymoma subgroups.

4. Myxopapillary Ependymoma (MPE)

Myxopapillary ependymoma (MPE) is a tumor originating almost exclusively in the spine (conus medullaris, cauda equina, and filum terminale). MPE was previously classified as WHO grade I in the 2016 WHO CNS classification, but because there is evidence that its outcomes are comparable to those of classic ependymoma, the new 2021 WHO CNS classification recommends assigning grade 2 to MPE [5,49,50]. MPE is defined by slow growth and favorable prognosis and accounts for 27% of all SP ependymoma [79]. Grossly, MPE are often encapsulated, lobulated, tan, and soft. They have a glistening cut surface with or without cyst formation and/or hemorrhage. Histopathologically, MPE is composed of well-differentiated cuboidal to elongated tumor cells radially oriented around hyalinized fibrovascular cores, commonly with degeneration-derived myxoid accumulation (Figure 2B,C) [1,80–82]. Patients frequently present with radicular pain and/or back pain [83]. While these tumors are found within all age groups, they are commonly found in the third and fourth decade of life, with a slight male predominance [84].

MPE is retained as a separate entity in WHO 2021 and defined by histological criteria. Methylation analysis by Pajtler et al., separated a MPE methylation subgroup from two SE and six classic ependymoma methylation subgroups [40]; however, that study, and an additional methylation analysis in a different study, grouped many classic histological ependymomas in the MPE and SE methylation subgroups, suggesting that methylation classification might not be reliable [37,40]. Moreover, such classification does not bring additional clinical significance to MPEs [49,50].

Similar to SP-SE, the gold standard treatment modality for MPE is maximal safe resection [85]. A systematic review of 28 articles demonstrated that overall recurrence rate after GTR (16%) was significantly lower than what was demonstrated following STR (33%) in the pooled cohort, with a mean follow-up of 75 months [84]. This review also demonstrated that adjuvant radiotherapy is not necessary as is not associated with a decrease in recurrence. There are reports, however, that radiotherapy may aid in disease control. An MD Anderson Cancer Center study showed that the addition of adjuvant radiotherapy to surgery was associated with significantly higher 10-year PFS rates (75%

for surgery and postoperative radiotherapy vs. 37% for surgery alone) and higher 10-year local tumor control rates (86% for surgery and postoperative radiotherapy vs. 46% for surgery alone) [86]. A 10-year OS of 75–100% has been demonstrated with STR followed by radiotherapy [87,88].

The current state of understanding of the oncogenic drivers that lead to MPE is still in its infancy as the excellent prognosis with surgery has not necessitated targeted therapies. While chromosomal instability is considered to be the defining genomic characteristic of this subgroup of ependymoma, as seen by the copy-number variation gains observed by Pajtler et al. in their DNA methylation array of 26 samples of MPE, there are three notable genes that are areas of current research and possible future molecular targets [40]. Overexpression of *homeobox B13* (*HOXB13*), a gene encoding a transcription factor that regulates skin development, has been shown by multiple studies [40,89]. The key involvement of this gene in developmental pathways has led researchers to hypothesize it plays a role in MPE tumorigenesis. Confounding this hypothesis is that the upregulated HOX genes commonly seen in MPE are *HOXB13*, *homeobox A13* (*HOXA13*), *homeobox C10* (*HOXC10*), and *homeobox D10* (*HOXD10*), all of which are genes overexpressed in the developing lumbar spine [90]. Immunohistochemistry analysis of adult filum terminale did not demonstrate HOXB13 expression, supporting the hypothesis that HOX groups 10–13 are expressed in early development and switched off once segmentation has completed, and its presence in adult MPE represents aberrant expression [89]. Oncogenesis amongst HOX genes is a growing area of research as aberrant HOX expression has been demonstrated in other malignancies including acute myeloid leukemia, breast, cervical, small-cell and non-small cell lung, prostate, skin, and thyroid cancers [89]. HOXB13 protein overexpression must be recognized and further assessed as a potential future therapeutic target [89,91]. Two other genes with overexpression seen in MPE are *neurofilament light chain* (*NEFL*), encoding a Class IV intermediate neurofilament expressed in neurons and located on chromosome 8p21.2 in close proximity to transcription factor binding sites of HOX genes, and *platelet derived growth factor receptor alpha* (*PDGFRA*), a gene which encodes a tyrosine kinase [89,92]. While the ubiquitous expression of these genes in various processes throughout the CNS has thus far precluded any significant progress in developing targeted therapies, as seen by the lack of clinical trials addressing these overexpressed genes, these are promising targets for future research. Lastly, a recent study assessing DNA methylation and gene expression profiles of pediatric SP ependymomas also identified overexpression of *HOXB13*, lending further evidence towards the importance of this gene [93]. This study also demonstrated significant overexpression of genes involved in the mitochondrial oxidative phosphorylation respiratory chain, such as *cyclooxygenase-2* (*COX2*), a gene that encodes for cyclooxygenase, which plays a vital role in inflammation and has been shown to be overexpressed in various cancers as it also plays a role in cell proliferation, neovascularization, and tumor metastasis [93–96]. While this was a small series in the pediatric population, it has provided more insight into the complex molecular amalgam that drives the tumorigenesis of MPE. As surgical resection remains the mainstay treatment of those afflicted by this tumor, further research will attempt to identify key genes that are uniquely expressed that may be future targets.

5. Spinal Ependymoma (SPE)

Spinal ependymoma (SPE) (WHO grade 2 or 3) is a tan, soft, well-circumscribed tumor composed of monomorphic glial cells with round to oval nuclei with speckled chromatin. They form perivascular pseudorosettes and/or true ependymal rosettes. When hypercellularity, cellular atypia, frequent mitoses, abundant endothelial proliferation and/or palisading necrosis are present, the tumor is deemed to be WHO grade 3. Histological patterns (clear cell, papillary, tanycytic) can be seen but do not have clinical significance [1,49,50,97]. Ependymomas express GFAP, S100 protein, EMA, and NHERF1/EBP50. The latter is a protein involved in epithelial morphogenesis and is superior to EMA for diagnosis of complex cases or ambiguous tumors (AO unpublished observations) [51]. Ultrastructurally, ependymomas are characterized by cilia, blepharoblasts, microvilli, and junctional complexes (Figure 2D–F) [1]. SPE is associated with *neurofibromatosis type 2* (*NF2*) mutations or deletions as seen in the molecular study by Pajtler et al., which found 90.5% of samples categorized into the SP ependymoma group demonstrated copy number variations of chromosome 22q where this gene is located [40].

Unlike MPE and SE, which are easily distinguishable entities, the 2016 WHO classification of ependymoma into grades II or III is less consistent [1,98]. Studies have found there to be significant intratumoral heterogeneity and, moreover, significant grade inter-rater variability among neuropathologists [33,99]. Although there are a number of studies demonstrating prognosis correlating with WHO grade, there is controversy regarding the prognostic utility of WHO grading of ependymoma, as there are also studies demonstrating no significant difference in survival between cases stratified per WHO grade [99–103]. It is for this, and the aforementioned reasons, that the field has moved towards molecular characterization of ependymoma. This tumor can be found anywhere in the spinal column but is often found in the cervical spine, which leads to the common presenting symptoms of radicular pain, myelopathy, and neck pain [97]. Men are found to be more affected than women. This subgroup is frequently diagnosed in patients 30–40 years old [37,40].

The standard treatment modality is microsurgical resection with the goal of GTR with minimal normal tissue disruption; however, the role of adjuvant radiotherapy is a topic of debate. One series of 104 (101 grade II and 3 grade III) SPEs that underwent surgical resection found the median PFS of those that underwent microsurgical resection to be 14.9 years for grade II and 3.7 years for grade III SPEs. Furthermore, they reported no significant change in PFS for patients that underwent adjuvant radiotherapy following STR [104]. Another large case series assessing long-term outcomes of 88 patients with SPE that underwent microsurgical resection, with and without adjuvant radiotherapy, found the surgical extent of resection to be an independent predictor of longer PFS, while postoperative radiotherapy after incomplete resection did not significantly correlate with longer times to recurrence [105]. A more recent study of 69 patients with SPE found for grade II lesions, STR and radiotherapy yielded better outcomes than STR alone, with a 10-year PFS of 77% and 68%, respectively [106]. Altogether, there is moderate evidence that adjuvant radiotherapy should be considered for patients that undergo STR.

Despite this excellent prognostic profile, the presence of *NF2* alterations in other CNS tumors has led to extensive research being performed to better understand the function and oncogenesis that occurs in tumors harboring this genomic variation. *NF2* is a tumor suppressor gene, located on chromosome 22q12.2 and codes for the protein Merlin. Deletions or loss-of-function mutations of this gene leads to neurofibromatosis type II, which is inherited in an autosomal dominant pattern [107]. Merlin is a scaffolding protein that links F-actin, transmembrane receptors, and intracellular effectors that modulate receptor mediated signaling pathways controlling cell proliferation and survival. The vast number of signaling pathways that are affected by Merlin emphasize its importance in integrating these pathways to influence cell morphology, motility, proliferation and survival. While Merlin's role in all of these pathways is still not completely understood, there are three molecular pathways that have been well defined and provide insight into how loss-of-function of Merlin can lead to oncogenesis. First, Merlin serves to inhibit various membrane receptors and the RhoGTPase family signaling cascade. Through binding to the CD44 cell membrane protein, Merlin negatively regulates this protein, which functions to increase cell proliferation. Additionally, through interaction with P21 Activated Kinase (PAK), Merlin inhibits Rac Family Small GTPase 1 (Rac1)/Cell Division Cycle 42 (Cdc42) signaling which leads to downstream inhibition of effectors including Rat sarcoma virus (RAS), Phosphoinositide 3-kinase (PI3K), and Ras-related C3 botulinum toxin (RAC). This ultimately leads to reduction in downstream Rapidly Accelerated Fibrosarcoma (RAF)/Myocyte Enhancer Factor (MEF)/Extracellular Signal-Regulated Kinase (ERK), Mammalian Target of Rapamycin Complex 1 (mTORC1), and Focal Adhesion Kinase (FAK) signaling [108]. Second, through binding PI 3-Kinase Enhance-L (PIKE-L), Merlin regulates and inhibits the PI3K/Protein Kinase B (AKT) pathway, which influences and promotes cellular survival and growth. Lastly, through the mammalian Hippo pathway, Merlin is involved with inhibition of Yes-associated Protein (YAP), a protein responsible for cell proliferation control and which has important regulatory functions in regeneration, organ development and stem cell self-renewal [109]. In this pathway, Merlin functions to promote translocation of Large Tumor Suppressor Kinase 1 and 2 (LATS1/2) to the nucleus while also inhibiting Cullin Ring Ubiquitin Ligase 4 (CRL4), both leading to reduced transcriptional output of YAP and other domain transcription factors [109].

As robust research has allowed for the meticulous understanding of the role of Merlin in oncogenesis, there have been several treatments under investigation targeting these molecular pathways. Small molecular MEK inhibitors are currently under investigation as they seek to target and inhibit the RAF/MEK/ERK pathway for *NF2*-associated tumors (NCT02639546, NCT03095248 on www.clinicaltrials.gov, (accessed on 9 November 2021)). A phase 2 clinical trial is also looking at *NF2* specific molecular targets via a FAK inhibitor on *NF2* mutant meningiomas (NCT02523014/A071401). Another *NF2* specific molecular pathway target is verteporfin a benzoporphyrin derivative that is currently used as a photosensitizer in macular degeneration, as it has been shown to disrupt YAP oncogenic activity [110,111]. Other research regarding bevacizumab, a vascular endothelial growth factor (VEGF) inhibitor, has shown promise for *NF2*-associated schwannomas, meningiomas, and ependymomas [108,112]. Lastly, further proposed targets include the PD-1/PD-L1 axis, the chemokine receptor C-X-C chemokine receptor type 4 (CXCR4), and Ephrin receptor B2 [61,108,113–115]. As the function of Merlin and its interactions with various signaling pathways are better understood, additional molecular targets will be discovered, while clinical trials will continue to move forward to understand the utility of drugs for established targets.

6. Spinal Ependymoma with *MYCN* Amplification (SPE-MYCN)

Spinal ependymoma with *MYCN* amplification (SPE-MYCN) has recently been added as a new molecular category of ependymoma based on the updated 2021 CNS WHO classification, which was based upon several studies that have identified the presence of this molecular signature in a subgroup of highly aggressive SPEs. In 2001, Scheil et al. was the first to report on the amplification of *Myelocytomatosis-N* (*MYCN*), a gene located on chromosome 2p24.3 encoding a proto-oncogene transcription factor located in the cell nucleus that is critical for normal CNS development. This finding was based on a comparative genomic hybridization study of 26 ependymomas in 22 patients. Two cases of SPE-MYCN were identified with histological characterizations leading to a diagnosis of SP ependymoma WHO Grade III, one of which had relapse and intracranial metastases [116]. Later, Ghasemi et al., using DNA methylation analyses, observed *MYCN* amplification in a cohort of 13 tumors, of which 10 were WHO Grade III and three were WHO Grade II [117]. This series identified a strikingly worse prognosis than any other SP ependymoma subgroup, with a PFS of 17 months and a median OS of 7.3 years. These tumors were also unique in their location, favoring the cervical and thoracic spine, being predominately intradural and extramedullary. The presence of diffuse leptomeningeal spread, and dissemination was observed in 100% of cases. Further supporting the importance of this molecular marker was the retention of *MYCN* amplification in all recurrent tumors assessed, as well as the presence of MYCN protein overexpression by immunohistochemistry, suggesting malignant progression being driven by increased *MYCN* gene expression. Using a similar DNA methylation assay, two other studies recorded similar results, leading to a total of 27 published cases of ependymoma with *MYCN* amplification, which has led to the categorization of this subset of SPE [118,119]. Altogether, these studies demonstrate a slight predilection for the female sex with a mean age of diagnosis in the third decade of life. While these retrospective studies without prospective confirmation represent only a small number of patients, disallowing any clear incidence or strong epidemiological data to be extrapolated, what has thus been reported has called for this molecular marker to be further studied and used as a prognosticator of poor outcomes. *MYCN*, a member of the family of MYC oncogenes, plays a large role in neurogenesis and has been implicated in the genesis of various CNS malignancies such as neuroblastoma, pediatric glioblastoma, and medulloblastoma, as well as malignancies outside of the CNS such as leukemia and prostate cancer [120–124]. There are no current clinical trials targeting MYCN; however, there are several reported investigations assessing strategies for MYCN inhibition. Among these promising reports include inhibitors targeting histone deacetylase (HDAC), poly(ADP-ribose) polymerase (PARP), Auro A-kinase (AURKA), and Bromodomain and extraterminal domain (BET) proteins, as well as immunotherapy targeting through DNA vaccination [125].

7. Posterior Fossa Ependymoma (PFE)

Posterior fossa ependymoma (PFE) has been studied and classified by many studies. Initially these studies used gene expression and copy number profiles, and defined two groups of tumors: Groups 1 and 2 by Wani et al., and Groups A and B by Witt et al. and by Hoffman et al. [42–44]. The groups identified correlate across studies with Group 1/A associated with younger age and a more aggressive course compared to Group 2/B. With the introduction of DNA methylation profiling technology, additional studies confirmed these findings and made uniform the terminology for posterior fossa ependymoma Group A (PFA) and posterior fossa ependymoma Group B (PFB). These two groups are now part of the WHO 2021 classification [37–40,49,50,126]. PFE that are not PFA/B can be qualified as "other", "not otherwise specified (NOS)", which includes those that are not able to be molecularly analyzed, or "not elsewhere classified (NEC)", which includes those with other molecular alterations. In an analysis of 35 PFE, 14 (40%) patients had PFA, 17 (48.6%) patients had PFB, and 4 (11.4%) patients were not classified into either, and thus should be presumed to be PFE, NOS/NEC [42]. Many studies characterize PFE based on their unique DNA methylation signatures [40,126,127]. As DNA methylation testing is not widely available, the use of an antibody against the trimethylated histone H3 at lysine 27 (H3K27me3) has been used to differentiate PFA from PFB [127–130]. There is a reduction or loss of H3K27me3 immunoexpression in PFA and persistent H3K27me3 immunoexpression in PFB [127–130].

Although the molecular characterization of PFEs has caused significant change in the categorization of these tumors, the DNA methylation results should be interpreted with care and in context with histology. There are many reasons why bioinformatics analyses (of any kind) should be interpreted with care, but this is beyond the scope of this article. Briefly, this starts with the quality of the tissue processed (time stored in formalin vs. fresh), the accuracy of tissue selected (tumor vs something else) and the algorithms used for data normalization. Similarly, the parameters, cut-off scores, and functions used for the analysis proper are of outmost importance. In the case of methylation there is no gold standard as of yet, and although the bioinformatic strategy used in the largest study published so far on brain tumors is now being commercialized, this algorithm was not sufficiently validated. Moreover, although this study included a large number of samples overall, when divided per rare entities the number of samples was small [131]. Therefore, methylation analysis, despite some opinions, is far from being "gold standard" for brain tumor diagnosis. For example, in an adult study, DNA methylation profiling of 38 IT tumors (seven WHO grade I SE, twenty-five WHO grade II ependymoma, and six WHO grade III anaplastic ependymoma) recategorized them as 24 PF-SE subgroup, 1 PFA subgroup, and 13 PFB subgroup; therefore this classification should be questioned as many ependymomas ($n = 17$ in this study) were classified as SE [37]. Similarly in another study, 11 IT ependymomas were classified by DNA methylation profiling as PF-SE [40].

PFEs are histologically grade 2 or 3, as described above in the SPE section (Figure 2D–F). As the molecular classification of PFE tumors is fairly novel, there are few studies describing specific subgroup location and radiographic characteristics. PFE is characterized as arising from the ependymal lining of the IVthV, often extruding out of the foramina of Luschka and Magendie [132,133]. PFE demonstrates heterogeneous enhancement, and approximately 50% demonstrate calcifications, with early evidence that calcifications primarily occur in PFA. Among patients with PFE, signs and symptoms related to CSF obstruction including headaches, nausea/vomiting, and lethargy are common, given their location in the IVthV [67,77].

8. Posterior Fossa Ependymoma Group A (PFA)

PFA is primarily a pediatric disease, with a median age of 3 years, and age ranging from 6 months to 58 years old across studies [37,40–42,127]. Adult cases make up a small percentage of the total cases. In studies with adult and pediatric PFA patients, 1–18.5% of patients are adults while the remainder are pediatric [40,41]. In a study of 134 adult PFE patients, 12% of the cases were H3K27me3-negative and presumed to be PFA [134]. PFA occurs more commonly in males, with a 65% to 35% male to female predominance. Aside from the aforementioned general PFE radiographic and clinical presentation, initial research on PFA demonstrates approximately two-thirds occur laterally and approximately one-third occurs medially [39,43].

In regard to ependymal tumors of the IT region, PFA has the poorest prognosis. Additionally, its prognosis is among the most dismal of all ependymoma subgroups. In comparing patients older than 10 years to those younger, the 5-year PFS and OS was 54% and 71%, which was not significantly different than patients younger than 10 years [39,40]. Although studies of purely adult PFA are uncommon, one such study had similar findings with H3K27me3-negative PFE patients having a 5-year PFS and OS of 44% and 80%, respectively [134]. This study showed that Ki-67 (MIB-1) index <10%, use of first-line radiotherapy, and GTR, were positive prognostic factors.

Overall, PFA tumors appear to have balanced genomes with the most frequent copy number variations being 1q gains (17.3–25%) and 6q losses (6.4–8.6%), both of which are negative prognostic indicators [40,135,136]. It is, rather, epigenetic changes such as the loss of H3K27me3 expression that lead to the PFA tumorigenesis [41,127,128]. There is increasing evidence that pathogenesis may be similar to that of diffuse midline gliomas (DMG) with *H3K27M* mutations and, in very rare instances (0.6–4.2% of cases), PFAs share this mutation [128–130,136–138]. In DMG, *H3K27M* mutations induce derepression of pro-oncogenic transcription factors through global reduction of histone 3 K27 trimethylation, H3K27me3. In addition to sharing this global DNA hypomethylation, PFA tumors have increased H3K27me3 enrichment at select genomic loci similar to that of *H3K27M*-mutant DMG [128].

An important oncogenic driver in PFA is Cxorf67, or EZH Inhibitory Protein (EZHIP), and its interaction with polycomb repressive complex 2 (PRC2), a histone methyltransferase that primarily methylates H3K27. Both Histone H3K27M and Cxorf67/EZHIP have short sequences that bind and inhibit PRC2 [139]. These sequences bind to the Su(var)3-9/enhancer-of-zeste/trithorax (SET) domain of EZH2, which is part of PRC2 and inhibits its methyltransferase activity, mimicking the function of mutated K27M oncohistones and resulting in loss of methylation at residue K27 of Histone H3 (Figure 3) [136,139–141]. PFA ependymomas show increased expression of Cxorf67/EZHIP and absence of H3K27me3 [129,136]. Although rare, Cxorf67/EZHIP missense mutations (<10%) have been reported in PFA [136]. It was shown that these mutations do not alter the protein function [139]. Jain et al. hypothesized that these mutations increase EZHIP expression by altering the *cis*-acting gene regulatory elements [139]. Importantly, increased Cxorf67/EZHIP expression correlates with loss of H3K27me3 in PFE, and is mutually exclusive with *H3K27M* mutations [129]. The lack of trimethylation and the decrease in H3K27me3 level cause derepression/upregulation of PRC2 target genes, including genes involved in neurodevelopment, and likely contribute to PFA tumorigenesis [139,140,142]. Rarely, ATRX protein loss by immunohistochemistry (4–25%) has been reported in PFA [129,130]. Alpha-thalassemia, mental retardation, X-linked/death domain–associated protein (ATRX/DAXX) complex is involved in incorporating histone H3.3 at pericentric heterochromatin and telomers. ATRX loss leads to increased DNA damage and genomic instability [143].

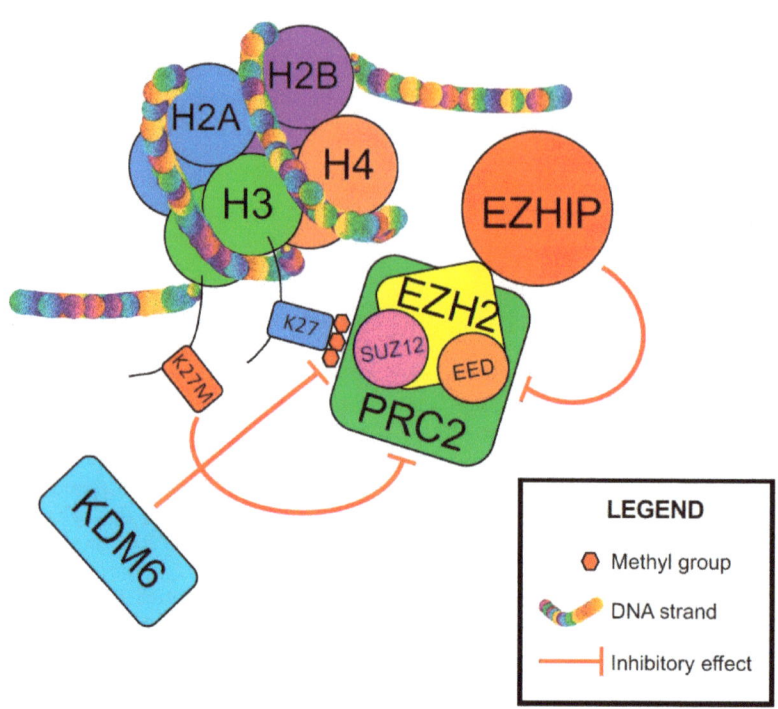

Figure 3. Mechanism of tumorigenesis in posterior fossa ependymoma Group A (PFA). EED—embryonic ectoderm development, EZH2—enhancer of zeste homolog 2, EZHIP—EZH inhibitory protein or Cxorf67, H2A—histone 2A, H2B—histone 2B, H3—histone 3, H4—histone 4, K27—lysine 27 on histone H3, K27M—methionine substitution for lysine on histone 3, KDM6—lysine-specific demethylase 6, PRC2—polycomb repressive complex 2, SUZ12—suppressor of zeste 12 homolog.

There is evidence that the microenvironment plays a strong role in PFA growth and propagation [144–146]. An inflammatory state driven by chronic IL-6 and STAT3 expression differentiates this subtype from PFB [145,146]. The master regulator of IL-6, NF-κB, and its pathway are enriched in PFA tumors. Leucine zipper downregulated in cancer 1 (LDOC1) is a transcriptional repressor of NF-κB and is a key regulator of this pathway. LDOC1 gene expression is decreased in PFA in comparison to other pediatric brain tumors. Moreover, ependymoma cells treated with 5AZA-DC, a DNA methylase transferase inhibitor, upregulate LDOC1 expression and decrease IL-6 secretion. PFA growth is also dependent on hypoxia, and even transient exposure of PFA cells to ambient oxygen causes irreversible cellular death [144]. Hypoxia induces restricted availability of S-adenosyl methionine (SAM), a substrate for methylation including H3K27 methyltransferase EZH2, which leads to the PFA-characteristic globally diminished histone methylation and increased demethylation and acetylation of H3K27. Gene ontology analysis of PFA has demonstrated overexpression of genes associated with wound healing, angiogenesis (VEGF and HIF-1α signaling), and migration and adhesion (integrin signaling and extracellular matrix assembly), a pattern similar to the mesenchymal signature in glioblastoma [43,44]. Telomerase activity has been found to be a significant player in PFA pathogenicity [147]. Epigenetic hypermethylation of *hTERT* promoter and chromosome 1q gain were both strongly associated with telomerase reactivation in PFA.

Currently, there are no established targeted therapies for PFA. As PFA tumorigenesis appears similar to *H3K27M*-mutant DMG, medications directed at this cancer may also have therapeutic value in PFA [148]. Quantitative high-throughput screening of 2706 approved and investigational drugs, followed by testing on patient-derived xenograft models of *H3K27M-mutant* DMG, revealed the combination multihistone deacetylase inhibitor panobinostat and the proteasome inhibitor marizomib to have the highest therapeutic value and thus may have applicability in the PFA setting [149]. Given the limited genomic foci of H3K27me3 hypermethylation, DNA methylation inhibitors may be suitable targeted therapies. A study by Michealraj et al. demonstrated this to be the case with inhibition of histone lysine methylation, leading to diminished survival of resected PFA cell lines [144]. In a pilot study, 5-Azacytidine, a DNA methylation inhibitor, was used in pediatric recurrent PFE, and although it was found to be safe, it was not found to limit progression of disease at the study dosage [150]. Lastly, as previously discussed, EZHIP appears to be crucial in the oncogenesis of PFA [136,140]. Interrupting the interaction between EZHIP and EZH2 may block the oncogenic upregulation of PRC2 downstream genes, similar to targeting the residual activity of PRC2 or "detoxification" of Histone H3K27M as attempted for diffuse midline glioma [139]. A recent study showed that tumor cells with increased EZHIP expression suppress DNA repair and respond to PARP inhibitors, especially when associated with radiotherapy [151].

9. Posterior Fossa Ependymoma Group B (PFB)

Posterior fossa ependymoma Group B (PFB) tumors occur in adolescent and adult populations, with a median age of approximately 30 years and an age range of 2 to 65 years across studies [37,40–42,127]. These same studies demonstrated a slight predilection of disease towards the female sex. Studies with adult and pediatric PFB patients have demonstrated 75–81% of patients are adult aged, while the remainder are pediatric [40,41]. In the largest study of adult PFE patients, 88% of the cases were H3K27me3-positive and presumably PFB, while the other cases were H3K27me3-negative (PFA) [134]. In addition to the previously described clinical and radiographic findings, over 90% of the PFB subgroup tumors are located medially within the posterior fossa [43]. In comparison to PFA, patients with PFB have a better prognosis [39,40]. These tumors are rarely invasive or metastatic, and are unlikely to recur. Five-year PFS and OS was 83% and 98% in patients older than 10. In a study of adult ependymoma, H3K27me3-positive PFE patients were found to have a 5-year PFS and OS of 87% and 99%, respectively [134]. Similarly to PFA, prognosis of PFB is not affected by age at diagnosis but does benefit from GTR and Ki-67 <10% [38,39,134]. In contrast to PFA, both 5-year PFS and OS in PFB patients do not appear to be affected by first-line radiotherapy.

In comparison to the balanced chromosomal composition of PFA, PFB is characterized by a high degree of chromosomal instability, with many copy number aberrations present [40]; most notably, over 50% copy number losses in 6p and 6q, and over 50% copy number gains in 15q, 18p, and 18q [37,40]. However, thus far, no recurrent mutation has been found in PFB tumors [38,126]. Genomic investigation of PFB has demonstrated this subgroup to be more differentiated with an ependymal-like trajectory [126,152]. It is also characterized by hyperactivity of gene sets involved in sonic hedgehog (Shh) signaling, oxidative metabolism, and ciliogenesis/microtubule assembly (including *FOXJ1*) [40,43,44,152]. *FOXJ1* encodes Forkhead box protein J1, which is an important regulator of motile ciliogenesis, has been associated with Shh signaling, and is highly expressed in ependyma and choroid plexus [153,154]. The expression of FOXJ1 has been associated with several tumors including ependymal and gastric cancers, though this has primarily been decreased expression [154,155]. However, there are several instances of FOXJ1 overexpression in tumors, such as clear cell renal cell carcinoma and colorectal cancer, that merit further investigation [156,157]. In a colorectal cancer study, the overexpression of FOXJ1 significantly promoted nuclear translocation of β-catenin, an important factor in the Wnt-β-catenin pathway and in intestinal tumorigenesis. An adaptor protein NHERF1/EBP50 has been found to suppress the Wnt-β-catenin pathway-driven intestinal neoplasia [158,159]. Interestingly, NHERF1/EBP50 is a strong diagnostic marker for ependymoma in general, is an organizer of polarity structures such as ependymal cilia, and as further discussed in the ST-YAP1 section, has a domain PDZ-2 that binds to both β-catenin and YAP1 [51]. There are several medications that indirectly affect the Wnt-β-catenin pathway, but the development of directed small molecule inhibitors is still in its infancy [160–162]. More recently, a first in class NHERF1 PDZ1-domain inhibitor has been developed that addresses the PDZ1-domain role of membrane recruitment/displacement [163]. Although these medications are being developed for other indications, the combination of NHERF1 PDZ1 inhibitors with β-catenin inhibitors may have a role in future care of ependymal tumors.

10. Supratentorial Ependymoma (STE)

The new 2021 WHO Classification of CNS tumors included two main subsets of ependymomas located in the ST space: those that have *YAP1-fusions* (ST-YAP1) and those that have *ZFTA-fusions* (ST-ZFTA) [49,50]. The non-YAP1/ZFTA STE are best classified as "other" or "NOS/NEC", and a histological grade can be offered. Further investigation will lead to other possible molecular subgroups. Additionally, as future studies begin to utilize these subcategories, further prognostic data will likely emerge. Earlier studies assessing prognosis of STE prior to molecular classification likely represent a heterogeneous population which include the now identified molecular subgroups, as well as tumors that would fall into the STE, NOS/NEC subgroup. Therefore, at the moment, no demographic or prognostic data are available for this subgroup, which remains, as of now, a subgroup of exclusion.

11. Supratentorial Ependymoma with *YAP1-Fusion* (ST-YAP1)

Supratentorial ependymoma with YAP1-fusion (ST-YAP1) is primarily a pediatric subgroup of ependymoma, with the median age of approximately 1 year and an age range from seven months to 51 years across studies [40,164,165]. Its occurrence in the adult population is extremely rare, though documented. Approximately 13–25% of ST-YAP1 cases occur in males [40,165]. Prognosis is significantly better than ST ependymoma with *ZFTA-fusion*, with most reports of 5-year OS at 100% [40,165]. The genomic origin of this tumor involves the fusion of chromosome 11 *YAP1* gene with chromosome X *MAMLD1* gene, though fusion with another gene, *FAM118B* [40,165]. YAP1 or yes-associated protein 1, the oncoprotein of *YAP1* gene, is a downstream effector in the Hippo signaling pathway [69]. YAP interacts with various transcription factors in the nucleus, including TEAD (transcriptional enhancer factor domain) transcription factors, which increases expression of genes involved in cell proliferation [166]. YAP works with another co-activator, TAZ, (also known as protein Tafazzin encoded by gene *TAZ*) in a similar but non-redundant fashion to complex with TEAD to act on gene targets [167]. Preventing the interaction of YAP with TEAD transcription factors resulted in lack of tumor formation in mice [166]. In another mouse study, ectopic expression of YAP1 led to generation of tumors with molecular and ultrastructural characteristics of human ependymoma [168]. This suggests their interaction is critical in formation of ST-YAP1 tumors, and may be a therapeutic target. YAP1 effects do not lie solely in the Hippo pathway; but have been linked to several pathways including the Wnt-β-catenin pathway and a mechanotransduction pathway [169,170]. YAP also interacts with adaptor molecule NHERF1/EBP50, an in vivo tumor repressor for intestinal adenoma development and an organizer of polarity structures such as ependymal cilia [51,158]. In a primarily adult study by Georgescu et al., NHERF1/EBP50 immunoexpression was shown to be diagnostic in a majority of ependymal tumors but not of other CNS tumors. YAP activity has also been implicated in drug resistance in a number of cancers, including esophageal cancer, oral squamous cell carcinoma, urothelial cell carcinoma, and radiation resistance in glioblastoma and medulloblastoma [171]. YAP has been demonstrated to assist in the immune escape of tumor cells by enhancing programmed death ligand-1 (*PD-L1*) gene expression, thus attenuating T-cell activation [171,172].

In the setting of breast cancer cell cultures that depend on YAP/TAZ, the use of on-market drugs dasatinib, fluvastatin, and pazopanib inhibit nuclear location of YAP/TAZ [173]. Dasatinib is a tyrosine kinase inhibitor used to treat chronic myeloid leukemia, fluvastatin is a statin class drug that has been used in cell lines with antitumor effects, and pazopanib is a multi-kinase inhibitor of VEFG receptor-1, -2, and -3, PDGFRA, and c-kit used sarcoma and renal cell carcinoma treatment [174–176]. Oku et al. demonstrated that all three drugs induce phosphorylation of YAP/TAZ, and pazopanib also induces proteasomal degradation of YAP/TAZ [173]. In addition, a combination of these compounds was shown to reduce cell proliferation in YAP/TAZ-dependent breast cancer cells. As previously discussed in the SPE, Verteporfin has been shown to have anti-oncogenic effects through inhibiting YAP1 activity [110]. In a study using a mouse model with patient gastric cancer xenografts, verteporfin treatment was shown to inhibit cancer growth in vivo [177]. Based on these studies, targeting YAP and/or its co-activators will likely be the mainstay of therapeutic candidates in ST-YAP1 and likely in other cancers as well.

12. Supratentorial Ependymoma with ZFTA-Fusion (ST-ZFTA)

ST-ZFTA is the second main subgroup of ependymoma in the ST compartment and harbors the worst outcome [1]. ST-ZFTA has a predilection for the lateral and third ventricle, with most occurring adjacent to the ventricular system, but it is not uncommon for this subset of ependymoma to be extraventricular and cortically based [178]. While the median age of patients with this tumor subgroup is 8 years, the range is 0 to 69 years, with 23% being adults and a peak incidence in the sixth decade of life for those diagnosed in adulthood [34,40]. There is a sex predilection towards males. Microsurgical resection with radiotherapy is considered the mainstay of treatment [2]. With resection and radiotherapy, this subgroup harbors a dismal prognosis with 10-year PFS of approximately 20% and OS of approximately 50% [40]. The role of chemotherapy for this subgroup is yet to be established; however, the recent introduction of this ependymoma subgroup into the WHO classification of CNS tumors will likely bolster research into the underpinnings of the oncogenesis of this tumor [2].

On immunohistochemistry, L1 Cell Adhesion Molecule (L1CAM)/(CD171) corresponds to the presence of *ZFTA fusion* but is neither sensitive nor specific, while p65/double immunostaining has a 92% positive predictive value and a 100% negative predictive value [179]. ST-ZFTA was originally classified as ST-RELA based on the presence of the gene *REL-associated protein* (RELA) fusing with the gene Zinc Finger Translocation Associated (ZFTA), also known as *C11orf95*, being thought to be the distinguishing molecular characteristic. The reason for this change in nosology is based on several studies showing that both *RELA* and *ZFTA* fuse with various genes secondary to chromothripsis. However, ST-ZFTA demonstrates a consistent histomolecular entity following *ZFTA* fusion with or without *RELA*, thus underscoring the molecular importance of the presence of *ZFTA* fusion, as opposed to *RELA* [50,180–184]. It is reported that about 2/3 of ST ependymomas in children harbor this *ZFTA* fusion, and Pajtler et al. observed the presence of this genomic fusion in 72% of ST ependymomas [40,181]. While the landscape is vast for the possible fusion partners with *ZFTA*, the main fusion partners that have been identified and shown to be sufficient for tumorigenesis are *Mastermind Like Transcription Coactivator 2* (MAML2), *Nuclear Receptor Coactivator 2* (NCOA2), and *Nuclear Receptor Coactivator 1* (NCOA1) [182–185].

The introduction of the *ZFTA-fusion* subgroup was, in large part, a result of the landmark study by Parker et al. that identified the fusion of *RELA* with *ZFTA* in two thirds of ST ependymoma [181]. These tumors were found to involve a chromothripsis event with chromosome 11q13.1, the location of *ZFTA*. While the fusion of *ZFTA* has been established as the molecular marker distinguishing this subgroup, the function and role of *ZFTA* is still not completely understood. However, the introduction of this molecular subgroup has bolstered investigation into the function of *ZFTA*, and a recent study by Kupp et al. utilized a combination of transcriptomics, chromatin immunoprecipitation sequencing, and proteomics to elucidate the mechanism behind this gene [186]. This work has provided evidence that ZFTA tethers fusion proteins across the genome, modifying chromatin to an active state and enabling its partner transcriptional coactivators to promote uninhibited expression of various genomic targets. The work demonstrating the shuttling and enabling function of ZFTA serves as the foundation for future studies to develop targeted therapies attacking this protein. While the role of ZFTA is only recently being unraveled, RELA, the principal effector of canonical Nuclear factor-κB (NF-κB), has been well studied, and its tumorigenesis mapped out. RELA is normally located in the cytoplasm via nuclear factor of kappa light polypeptide gene enhancer alpha (IkBα)-mediated sequestration; however, upon external pressures, RELA protein is translocated to the nucleus to influence the NF-κB pathway [187,188]. Parker et al. demonstrated in a mouse model that the ZFTA-RELA fusion protein spontaneously translocates to the nucleus of neural stem cells to activate NF-κB target genes, which lead to the transformation of these cells into ependymoma [181]. Therefore, as ZFTA-RELA preferentially localizes to the nucleus, persistent activation of the NF-κB pathway is the proposed mechanism of oncogenesis. The NF-κB transcriptional regulator protein family is closely linked to cellular inflammation, and while constitutive activation of these proteins are often seen in human tumors, the rarity of mutations in members of this pathway has obfuscated research attempts to understand and identify targetable areas [189,190]. Additionally, Arabzade et al. showed through a autochthonous mouse tumor model that in addition to direct activation of canonical NF-κB, that ZFTA-RELA fusion protein binds to thousands of PLAGL (PLAG1 Like Zinc Finger 1)-enriched sites across the genome [191]. Moreover, ZFTA-RELA fusion protein recruits various transcriptional coactivators such as bromodomain-containing protein 4 (Brd4), histone acetyltransferase p300 (Ep300), and CREB-binding protein (Cbp), all of which are possible areas for future pharmacologic inhibition. Another promising target is *Fibroblast Growth Factor Receptor 3* (*FGFR3*). *FGFR3*, a gene located on chromosome 4 and responsible for bone development, has been shown to be overexpressed in an in-vitro model of ST-ZFTA. This study also demonstrated the efficacy of a broad range of FGFR inhibitors in inducing maturation in their invitro model, a therapeutic concept currently considered of high potential in pediatric cancers [192]. Lastly, immune checkpoint molecules are another possible target currently being investigated. Wang et al. uncovered that expression of PD-L1 independently predicts outcomes in patients with ST, extraventricular ependymomas [193]. T-cell exhaustion induced by overexpression of PD-L1 is a mechanism by which tumors evade immune-mediated clearance [194]. This observed overexpression in high-grade STEs that independently predicts outcomes further emphasizes the importance of this molecular trait and underscores the need for further studies assessing the efficacy of PD-L1 inhibitors in treating ST-ZFTA. While this pathway of oncogenesis is the subject of ongoing research, and has been further elucidated, the driver of chromothripsis causing this fusion is still not understood. It is theorized that in the pediatric setting, the deletion of *cyclin-dependent kinase inhibitor 2A/B* (*CDKN2A/B*) may play a role, as it influences the TP53 pathway which has been linked to chromothripsis in other tumors [40,195]. Given the established mechanism of oncogenesis, it is vital that inhibitors of RELA pathways, i.e., NF-κB signaling pathways, be further researched as viable therapies [188].

13. Conclusions

The novel description of the molecular origin of ependymoma has led to further understanding of this genetically diverse tumor. When compared to histopathological classification, the molecular categorization of ependymal tumors into 10 distinct subgroups has led to a more refined characterization of clinical course and potential molecular targets.

Given the unique profile of each ependymoma subgroup, future research must rely on molecular characterization rather than classical histopathological categorization alone. Genomic profiling of ependymal tumors is essential in the further elucidation of molecular targets. While many of ependymoma subgroups are aggressive, even the benign subgroups urgently need targeted therapies, as many tumors are not amenable to surgical resection without causing substantial disability. Research must continue to build on studies that have elucidated ependymoma oncogenesis, as well as investigate novel targets based on malignancies with similar gene ontology. An up-to-date clinical trial list regarding targeted treatments for ependymoma is available on "clinicaltrials.gov" (accessed on 9 November 2021). As the molecular underpinnings of ependymomas are further unraveled through the groundbreaking work of investigators in the field, it is expected that this list will continue to grow.

Author Contributions: Concept and design A.O.; Supervision S.R.L., A.O.; literature review, data acquisition and interpretation, manuscript writing T.L., B.F.S.; critical review of manuscript T.L., B.F.S., S.R.L., A.O.; figure acquisition and design A.O. All authors have read and agreed to the published version of the manuscript.

Funding: This work was supported by funds from NOMIX Laboratories LLC, Denver, CO, USA.

Acknowledgments: This work is dedicated to all ependymoma patients out there. The authors kindly thank Maria-Magdalena Georgescu, NeuroMarkers PLLC, Houston, TX, USA for providing photographs for Figure 2D–F.

Conflicts of Interest: Authors declare no conflict of interest.

Abbreviations

Note of Nomenclature: As the new WHO classification of tumors of the CNS is currently being published and could be released at any moment, it is noteworthy to mention that in this paper we keep WHO 2016 grade terminology (aka roman numerals) when we refer (or cite) to previously published studies that used 2016 classification criteria.

IVthV	Fourth ventricle
5AZA-DC	DNA methylase transferase inhibitor 5-aza-2′-deoxycytidine
AKT	Protein kinase B
ATRX/DAXX	Alpha-thalassemia, mental retardation, X-linked/death domain–associated protein complex
AURKA	Auro A-kinase
BET	Bromodomain and extraterminal domain
Brd4	Bromodomain-containing protein 4
c-KIT	Proto-oncogene encoding tyrosine-protein kinase KIT, CD117, or stem cell growth factor receptor
c-MYB	c-myeloblastosis
CAR T	Chimeric antigen receptor T cell
Cbp	CREB-binding protein
Cdc42	Cell division cycle 42
COX2	Cyclooxygenase-2
CNS	Central nervous system
CRL4	Cullin Ring Ubiquitin Ligase 4
CSF	Cerebrospinal fluid
CXCR4	C-X-C chemokine receptor type 4
EANO	The European Association of Neuro-Oncology
EED	Embryonic ectoderm development
EMA	Epithelial membrane antigen
Ep300	Histone acetyltransferase p300
EPHA7	Ephrin type-A receptor 7
ERK	Extracellular Signal-Regulated Kinase
ERM	Ezrin, radixin, moesin binding protein
EZHIP	EZH Inhibitory Protein or CXorf67
EZH2	Enhancer of zeste homolog 2
FAK	Focal Adhesion Kinase
FAM 118B	Family with sequence similarity 118 member B
FGFR3	Fibroblast growth factor receptor 3
FOXJ1	Forkhead box protein J1
GFAP	Glial fibrillary acidic protein
GTR	Gross total resection
H3K27M	Histone H3 lysine 27 to methionine mutation
H3K27me3	Trimethylated histone H3 at lysine 27
HDAC	Histone deacetylase

HE	Hematoxylin and eosin
HIF-1a	Hypoxia inducible factor 1 alpha
HOXA13	Homeobox A13
HOXB13	Homeobox B13
HOXC10	Homeobox C10
HOXD10	Homeobox D10
hTERT	Human telomerase reverse transcriptase
IkBα	Nuclear factor of kappa light polypeptide gene enhancer in B cells alpha
IL-6	Interleukin-6
IT	Infratentorial
KDM6	Lysine-specific demethylase 6
KIT	Tyrosine protein kinase or stem cell growth factor receptor or CD117
L1CAM	L1 Cell Adhesion Molecule
LATS1/2	Large Tumor Suppressor Kinase 1 and 2
LDOC	Leucine zipper downregulated in cancer 1
MAML2	Mastermind like transcription coactivator 2
MAMLD1	Mastermind like domain containing 1
MDM2	Mouse double minute 2 homolog or E3 ubiquitin-protein ligase Mdm2
MEF	Myocyte enhancer factor
MPE	Spinal myxopapillary ependymoma
mTORC1	Mammalian Target of Rapamycin Complex 1
MYCN	Myelocytomatosis-N
NCOA1	Nuclear receptor coactivator 1
NCOA2	Nuclear receptor coactivator 2
NEFL	Neurofilament light chain
NEC	Not elsewhere classified
NF-κB	Nuclear factor-κB
NF2	Neurofibromatosis type 2
NHERF1/EBP50	Na+/H+ exchanger regulatory factor/ezrin-radixin-moesin binding protein 50
NOS	Not otherwise specified
OS	Overall survival
PAK	P21 activated kinase
PARP	Poly (ADP-ribose) polymerase
PDGFRA	Platelet derived growth factor alpha
PFA	Posterior fossa ependymoma Group A
PFB	Posterior fossa ependymoma Group B
PFE	Posterior fossa ependymoma
PF-SE	Posterior fossa subependymoma
PFS	Progression-free survival
PI3K	Phosphoinositide 3-kinase
PIKE-L	Phosphoinositide 3-Kinase Enhancer-brain specific isoform
PLAGL	PLAG1 like zinc finger 1
PRC2	Polycomb repressive complex 2
Rac1	Ras-related C3 botulinum toxin substrate 1
RAC	Ras-related C3 botulinum toxin
RAF	Rapidly accelerated fibrosarcoma
Ras	Rat sarcoma virus
RELA	REL-associated protein
SAM	S-adenosyl methionine
SE	Subependymoma
SET	Su(var)3-9/enhancer-of-zeste/trithorax
Shh	Sonic hedgehog
SP	Spinal
SPE	Spinal ependymoma
SPE-MYCN	Spinal ependymoma with MYCN amplification
SP-SE	Spinal subependymoma
ST	Supratentorial
ST-RELA	Supratentorial ependymoma with RELA fusion
ST-SE	Supratentorial subependymoma

ST-YAP1	Supratentorial ependymoma with YAP1 fusion
STAT	Signal transducer and activator of transcription
STE	Supratentorial ependymoma
STR	Subtotal resection
SUZ12	Suppressor of zeste 12 homolog
TEAD	Transcriptional enhancer factor domain
TAZ	Gene encoding protein Tafazzin
VEGF	Vascular endothelial growth factor
WHO	World Health Organization
WP744	4′-O-benzylated doxorubicin analog
WP1066	JAK2/STAT3 inhibitor
WP1193	JAK2/STAT3 inhibitor
YAP1	Yes1 associated transcriptional regulator or YAP or YAP65
ZFTA	Zinc finger translocation-associated

References

1. Louis, D.N.; Perry, A.; Reifenberger, G.; von Deimling, A.; Figarella-Branger, D.; Cavenee, W.K.; Ohgaki, H.; Wiestler, O.D.; Kleihues, P.; Ellison, D.W. The 2016 World Health Organization Classification of Tumors of the Central Nervous System: A summary. *Acta Neuropathol.* **2016**, *131*, 803–820. [CrossRef]
2. Wu, J.; Armstrong, T.S.; Gilbert, M.R. Biology and management of ependymomas. *Neuro-Oncology* **2016**, *18*, 902–913. [CrossRef] [PubMed]
3. Ostrom, Q.T.; Patil, N.; Cioffi, G.; Waite, K.; Kruchko, C.; Barnholtz-Sloan, J.S. CBTRUS statistical report: Primary brain and other central nervous system tumors diagnosed in the United States in 2013–2017. *Neuro-Oncology* **2020**, *22*, IV1–IV96. [CrossRef] [PubMed]
4. McGuire, C.S.; Sainani, K.L.; Fisher, P.G. Incidence patterns for ependymoma: A Surveillance, Epidemiology, and End Results study—Clinical article. *J. Neurosurg.* **2009**, *110*, 725–729. [CrossRef]
5. Vera-Bolanos, E.; Aldape, K.; Yuan, Y.; Wu, J.; Wani, K.; Necesito-Reyes, M.J.; Colman, H.; Dhall, G.; Lieberman, F.S.; Metellus, P.; et al. Clinical course and progression-free survival of adult intracranial and spinal ependymoma patients. *Neuro-Oncology* **2015**, *17*, 440–447. [CrossRef]
6. Pajtler, K.W.; Mack, S.C.; Ramaswamy, V.; Smith, C.A.; Witt, H.; Smith, A.; Hansford, J.R.; von Hoff, K.; Wright, K.D.; Hwang, E.; et al. The current consensus on the clinical management of intracranial ependymoma and its distinct molecular variants. *Acta Neuropathol.* **2017**, *133*, 5–12. [CrossRef] [PubMed]
7. Reni, M.; Gatta, G.; Mazza, E.; Vecht, C. Ependymoma. *Crit. Rev. Oncol. Hematol.* **2007**, *63*, 81–89. [CrossRef] [PubMed]
8. National Comprehensive Cancer Network. Central Nervous System Cancers. Available online: https://www.nccn.org/professionals/physician_gls/pdf/cns.pdf (accessed on 9 September 2021).
9. Metellus, P.; Guyotat, J.; Chinot, O.; Durand, A.; Barrie, M.; Giorgi, R.; Jouvet, A.; Figarella-Branger, D. Adult intracranial WHO grade II ependymomas: Long-term outcome and prognostic factor analysis in a series of 114 patients. *Neuro-Oncology* **2010**, *12*, 976–984. [CrossRef]
10. Rogers, L.; Pueschel, J.; Spetzler, R.; Shapiro, W.; Coons, S.; Thomas, T.; Speiser, B. Is gross-total resection sufficient treatment for posterior fossa ependymomas? *J. Neurosurg.* **2005**, *102*, 629–636. [CrossRef]
11. Rudà, R.; Reifenberger, G.; Frappaz, D.; Pfister, S.M.; Laprie, A.; Santarius, T.; Roth, P.; Tonn, J.C.; Soffietti, R.; Weller, M.; et al. EANO guidelines for the diagnosis and treatment of ependymal tumors. *Neuro-Oncology* **2018**, *20*, 445–456. [CrossRef]
12. Aizer, A.A.; Ancukiewicz, M.; Nguyen, P.L.; MacDonald, S.M.; Yock, T.I.; Tarbell, N.J.; Shih, H.A.; Loeffler, J.S.; Oh, K.S. Natural history and role of radiation in patients with supratentorial and infratentorial WHO grade II ependymomas: Results from a population-based study. *J. Neurooncol.* **2013**, *115*, 411–419. [CrossRef] [PubMed]
13. Gilbert, M.R.; Yuan, Y.; Wu, J.; Mendoza, T.; Vera, E.; Omuro, A.; Lieberman, F.; Robins, H.I.; Gerstner, E.R.; Wu, J.; et al. A phase II study of dose-dense temozolomide and lapatinib for recurrent low-grade and anaplastic supratentorial, infratentorial, and spinal cord ependymoma. *Neuro-Oncology* **2021**, *23*, 468–477. [CrossRef]
14. Brandes, A.A.; Cavallo, G.; Reni, M.; Tosoni, A.; Nicolardi, L.; Scopece, L.; Franceschi, E.; Sotti, G.; Talacchi, A.; Turazzi, S.; et al. A multicenter retrospective study of chemotherapy for recurrent intracranial ependymal tumors in adults by the Gruppo Italiano Cooperativo di Neuro-Oncologia. *Cancer* **2005**, *104*, 143–148. [CrossRef] [PubMed]
15. Chamberlain, M.C.; Johnston, S.K. Temozolomide for recurrent intracranial supratentorial platinum-refractory ependymoma. *Cancer* **2009**, *115*, 4775–4782. [CrossRef] [PubMed]
16. Green, R.M.; Cloughesy, T.F.; Stupp, R.; Deangelis, L.M.; Woyshner, E.A.; Ney, D.E.; Lassman, A.B. Bevacizumab for recurrent ependymoma. *Neurology* **2009**, *73*, 1677–1680. [CrossRef]
17. Rudà, R.; Bosa, C.; Magistrello, M.; Franchino, F.; Pellerino, A.; Fiano, V.; Trevisan, M.; Cassoni, P.; Soffietti, R. Temozolomide as salvage treatment for recurrent intracranial ependymomas of the adult: A retrospective study. *Neuro-Oncology* **2016**, *18*, 261–268. [CrossRef]

18. Gramatzki, D.; Roth, P.; Felsberg, J.; Hofer, S.; Rushing, E.J.; Hentschel, B.; Westphal, M.; Krex, D.; Simon, M.; Schnell, O.; et al. Chemotherapy for intracranial ependymoma in adults. *BMC Cancer* **2016**, *16*, 287. [CrossRef]
19. Kieran, M.W.; Goumnerova, L.; Manley, P.; Chi, S.N.; Marcus, K.J.; Manzanera, A.G.; Polanco, M.L.S.; Guzik, B.W.; Aguilar-Cordova, E.; Diaz-Montero, C.M.; et al. Phase I study of gene-mediated cytotoxic immunotherapy with AdV-tk as adjuvant to surgery and radiation for pediatric malignant glioma and recurrent ependymoma. *Neuro-Oncology* **2019**, *21*, 537–546. [CrossRef]
20. National Cancer Institute. Childhood Ependymoma Treatment (PDQ®)–Health Professional Version. Available online: https://www.cancer.gov/types/brain/hp/child-ependymoma-treatment-pdq (accessed on 30 November 2021).
21. Duffner, P.K.; Horowitz, M.E.; Krischer, J.P.; Friedman, H.S.; Burger, P.C.; Cohen, M.E.; Sanford, R.A.; Mulhern, R.K.; James, H.E.; Freeman, C.R.; et al. Postoperative Chemotherapy and Delayed Radiation in Children Less Than Three Years of Age with Malignant Brain Tumors. *N. Engl. J. Med.* **1993**, *328*, 1725–1731. [CrossRef]
22. Snider, C.A.; Yang, K.; Mack, S.C.; Suh, J.H.; Chao, S.T.; Merchant, T.E.; Murphy, E.S. Impact of radiation therapy and extent of resection for ependymoma in young children: A population-based study. *Pediatr. Blood Cancer* **2018**, *65*, e26880. [CrossRef]
23. Grundy, R.G.; Wilne, S.A.; Weston, C.L.; Robinson, K.; Lashford, L.S.; Ironside, J.; Cox, T.; Chong, W.K.; Campbell, R.H.; Bailey, C.C.; et al. Primary postoperative chemotherapy without radiotherapy for intracranial ependymoma in children: The UKCCSG/SIOP prospective study. *Lancet Oncol.* **2007**, *8*, 696–705. [CrossRef]
24. Strother, D.R.; Lafay-Cousin, L.; Boyett, J.M.; Burger, P.; Aronin, P.; Constine, L.; Duffner, P.; Kocak, M.; Kun, L.E.; Horowitz, M.E.; et al. Benefit from prolonged dose-intensive chemotherapy for infants with malignant brain tumors is restricted to patients with ependymoma: A report of the pediatric oncology group randomized controlled trial 9233/34. *Neuro-Oncology* **2014**, *16*, 457–465. [CrossRef]
25. Merchant, T.E.; Bendel, A.E.; Sabin, N.D.; Burger, P.C.; Shaw, D.W.; Chang, E.; Wu, S.; Zhou, T.; Eisenstat, D.D.; Foreman, N.K.; et al. Conformal radiation therapy for pediatric ependymoma, chemotherapy for incompletely resected ependymoma, and observation for completely resected, supratentorial ependymoma. *J. Clin. Oncol.* **2019**, *37*, 974–983. [CrossRef]
26. Massimino, M.; Solero, C.L.; Garrè, M.L.; Biassoni, V.; Cama, A.; Genitori, L.; Di Rocco, C.; Sardi, I.; Viscardi, E.; Modena, P.; et al. Second-look surgery for ependymoma: The Italian experience—Clinical article. *J. Neurosurg. Pediatr.* **2011**, *8*, 246–250. [CrossRef]
27. Garvin, J.H.; Selch, M.T.; Holmes, E.; Berger, M.S.; Finlay, J.L.; Flannery, A.; Goldwein, J.W.; Packer, R.J.; Rorke-Adams, L.B.; Shiminski-Maher, T.; et al. Phase II study of pre-irradiation chemotherapy for childhood intracranial ependymoma. Children's Cancer Group protocol 9942: A report from the Children's Oncology Group. *Pediatr. Blood Cancer* **2012**, *59*, 1183–1189. [CrossRef]
28. Zacharoulis, S.; Ashley, S.; Moreno, L.; Gentet, J.C.; Massimino, M.; Frappaz, D. Treatment and outcome of children with relapsed ependymoma: A multi-institutional retrospective analysis. *Childs Nerv. Syst.* **2010**, *26*, 905–911. [CrossRef]
29. Jakacki, R.I.; Foley, M.A.; Horan, J.; Wang, J.; Kieran, M.W.; Bowers, D.C.; Bouffet, E.; Zacharoulis, S.; Gill, S.C. Single-agent erlotinib versus oral etoposide in patients with recurrent or refractory pediatric ependymoma: A randomized open-label study. *J. Neurooncol.* **2016**, *129*, 131–138. [CrossRef]
30. Bouffet, E.; Capra, M.; Bartels, U. Salvage chemotherapy for metastatic and recurrent ependymoma of childhood. *Childs Nerv. Syst.* **2009**, *25*, 1293–1301. [CrossRef]
31. Iqbal, M.S.; Lewis, J. An overview of the management of adult ependymomas with emphasis on relapsed disease. *Clin. Oncol.* **2013**, *25*, 726–733. [CrossRef]
32. Donovan, L.K.; Delaidelli, A.; Joseph, S.K.; Bielamowicz, K.; Fousek, K.; Holgado, B.L.; Manno, A.; Srikanthan, D.; Gad, A.Z.; Van Ommeren, R.; et al. Locoregional delivery of CAR T cells to the cerebrospinal fluid for treatment of metastatic medulloblastoma and ependymoma. *Nat. Med.* **2020**, *26*, 720–731. [CrossRef]
33. Ellison, D.W.; Kocak, M.; Figarella-Branger, D.; Felice, G.; Catherine, G.; Pietsch, T.; Frappaz, D.; Massimino, M.; Grill, J.; Boyett, J.M.; et al. Histopathological grading of pediatric ependymoma: Reproducibility and clinical relevance in European trial cohorts. *J. Negat. Results Biomed.* **2011**, *10*, 7. [CrossRef]
34. Hübner, J.-M.; Kool, M.; Pfister, S.M.; Pajtler, K.W. Epidemiology, molecular classification and WHO grading of ependymoma. *J. Neurosurg. Sci.* **2018**, *62*, 46–50. [CrossRef]
35. Tihan, T.; Zhou, T.; Holmes, E.; Burger, P.C.; Ozuysal, S.; Rushing, E.J. The prognostic value of histological grading of posterior fossa ependymomas in children: A Children's Oncology Group study and a review of prognostic factors. *Mod. Pathol.* **2008**, *21*, 165–177. [CrossRef]
36. Xi, S.; Sai, K.; Hu, W.; Wang, F.; Chen, Y.; Wang, J.; Zeng, J.; Chen, Z. Clinical significance of the histological and molecular characteristics of ependymal tumors: A single institution case series from China. *BMC Cancer* **2019**, *19*, 717. [CrossRef]
37. Witt, H.; Gramatzki, D.; Hentschel, B.; Pajtler, K.W.; Felsberg, J.; Schackert, G.; Löffler, M.; Capper, D.; Sahm, F.; Sill, M.; et al. DNA methylation-based classification of ependymomas in adulthood: Implications for diagnosis and treatment. *Neuro-Oncology* **2018**, *20*, 1616–1624. [CrossRef]
38. Cavalli, F.M.G.; Hübner, J.M.; Sharma, T.; Luu, B.; Sill, M.; Zapotocky, M.; Mack, S.C.; Witt, H.; Lin, T.; Shih, D.J.H.; et al. Heterogeneity within the PF-EPN-B ependymoma subgroup. *Acta Neuropathol.* **2018**, *136*, 227–237. [CrossRef]
39. Ramaswamy, V.; Hielscher, T.; Mack, S.C.; Lassaletta, A.; Lin, T.; Pajtler, K.W.; Jones, D.T.W.; Luu, B.; Cavalli, F.M.G.; Aldape, K.; et al. Therapeutic impact of cytoreductive surgery and irradiation of posterior fossa ependymoma in the molecular era: A retrospective multicohort analysis. *J. Clin. Oncol.* **2016**, *34*, 2468–2477. [CrossRef]

40. Pajtler, K.W.; Witt, H.; Sill, M.; Jones, D.T.W.; Hovestadt, V.; Kratochwil, F.; Wani, K.; Tatevossian, R.; Punchihewa, C.; Johann, P.; et al. Molecular Classification of Ependymal Tumors across All CNS Compartments, Histopathological Grades, and Age Groups. *Cancer Cell* **2015**, *27*, 728–743. [CrossRef]
41. Mack, S.C.; Witt, H.; Piro, R.M.; Gu, L.; Zuyderduyn, S.; Stütz, A.M.; Wang, X.; Gallo, M.; Garzia, L.; Zayne, K.; et al. Epigenomic alterations define lethal CIMP-positive ependymomas of infancy. *Nature* **2014**, *506*, 445–450. [CrossRef] [PubMed]
42. Hoffman, L.M.; Donson, A.M.; Nakachi, I.; Griesinger, A.M.; Birks, D.K.; Amani, V.; Hemenway, M.S.; Liu, A.K.; Wang, M.; Hankinson, T.C.; et al. Molecular sub-group-specific immunophenotypic changes are associated with outcome in recurrent posterior fossa ependymoma. *Acta Neuropathol.* **2014**, *127*, 731–745. [CrossRef]
43. Witt, H.; Mack, S.C.; Ryzhova, M.; Bender, S.; Sill, M.; Isserlin, R.; Benner, A.; Hielscher, T.; Milde, T.; Remke, M.; et al. Delineation of two clinically and molecularly distinct subgroups of posterior fossa ependymoma. *Cancer Cell* **2011**, *20*, 143–157. [CrossRef]
44. Wani, K.; Armstrong, T.S.; Vera-Bolanos, E.; Raghunathan, A.; Ellison, D.; Gilbertson, R.; Vaillant, B.; Goldman, S.; Packer, R.J.; Fouladi, M.; et al. A prognostic gene expression signature in infratentorial ependymoma. *Acta Neuropathol.* **2012**, *123*, 727–738. [CrossRef]
45. Carter, M.; Nicholson, J.; Ross, F.; Crolla, J.; Allibone, R.; Balaji, V.; Perry, R.; Walker, D.; Gilbertson, R.; Ellison, D.W. Genetic abnormalities detected in ependymomas by comparative genomic hybridisation. *Br. J. Cancer* **2002**, *86*, 929–939. [CrossRef]
46. Puget, S.; Grill, J.; Valent, A.; Bieche, I.; Dantas-Barbosa, C.; Kauffmann, A.; Dessen, P.; Lacroix, L.; Geoerger, B.; Job, B.; et al. Candidate genes on chromosome 9q33-34 involved in the progression of childhood ependymomas. *J. Clin. Oncol.* **2009**, *27*, 1884–1892. [CrossRef]
47. Korshunov, A.; Hielscher, T.; Ryzhova, M. Molecular Staging of Intracranial Ependymoma in Children and Adults Structure and Mechanism of Key Nonsense-Mediated mRNA Decay Factor Complexes View project EURAT: Ethical and legal aspects of genome sequencing View project. *J. Clin. Oncol.* **2010**, *28*, 3182–3190. [CrossRef]
48. Modena, P.; Lualdi, E.; Facchinetti, F.; Veltman, J.; Reid, J.F.; Minardi, S.; Janssen, I.; Giangaspero, F.; Forni, M.; Finocchiaro, G.; et al. Identification of tumor-specific molecular signatures in intracranial ependymoma and association with clinical characteristics. *J. Clin. Oncol.* **2006**, *24*, 5223–5233. [CrossRef]
49. Louis, D.N.; Perry, A.; Wesseling, P.; Brat, D.J.; Cree, I.A.; Figarella-Branger, D.; Hawkins, C.; Ng, H.K.; Pfister, S.M.; Reifenberger, G.; et al. The 2021 WHO Classification of Tumors of the Central Nervous System: A summary. *Neuro-Oncology* **2021**, *23*, 1231–1251. [CrossRef]
50. Ellison, D.W.; Aldape, K.D.; Capper, D.; Fouladi, M.; Gilbert, M.R.; Gilbertson, R.J.; Hawkins, C.; Merchant, T.E.; Pajtler, K.; Venneti, S.; et al. cIMPACT-NOW update 7: Advancing the molecular classification of ependymal tumors. *Brain Pathol.* **2020**, *30*, 863–866. [CrossRef]
51. Georgescu, M.M.; Yell, P.; Mobley, B.C.; Shang, P.; Georgescu, T.; Wang, S.H.J.; Canoll, P.; Hatanpaa, K.J.; White, C.L.; Raisanen, J.M. NHERF1/EBP50 is an organizer of polarity structures and a diagnostic marker in ependymoma. *Acta Neuropathol. Commun.* **2015**, *3*, 11. [CrossRef]
52. D'Amico, R.S.; Praver, M.; Zanazzi, G.J.; Englander, Z.K.; Sims, J.S.; Samanamud, J.L.; Ogden, A.T.; McCormick, P.C.; Feldstein, N.A.; McKhann, G.M.; et al. Subependymomas Are Low-Grade Heterogeneous Glial Neoplasms Defined by Subventricular Zone Lineage Markers. *World Neurosurg.* **2017**, *107*, 451–463. [CrossRef] [PubMed]
53. Shimada, S.; Ishizawa, K.; Horiguchi, H.; Shimada, T.; Hirose, T. Subependymoma of the spinal cord and review of the literature. *Pathol. Int.* **2003**, *53*, 169–173. [CrossRef]
54. Krishnan, S.S.; Panigrahi, M.; Pendyala, S.; Rao, S.I.; Varma, D.R. Cervical Subependymoma: A rare case report with possible histogenesis. *J. Neurosci. Rural Pract.* **2012**, *3*, 366–369. [CrossRef]
55. Soleiman, H.A.; Ironside, J.; Kealey, S.; Demetriades, A.K. Spinal subependymoma surgery: Do no harm. Little may be more! *Neurosurg. Rev.* **2020**, *43*, 1047–1053. [CrossRef]
56. Wu, L.; Yang, T.; Deng, X.; Yang, C.; Zhao, L.; Fang, J.; Wang, G.; Yang, J.; Xu, Y. Surgical outcomes in spinal cord subependymomas: An institutional experience. *J. Neurooncol.* **2014**, *116*, 99–106. [CrossRef]
57. Korshunov, A.; Neben, K.; Wrobel, G.; Tews, B.; Benner, A.; Hahn, M.; Golanov, A.; Lichter, P. Gene Expression Patterns in Ependymomas Correlate with Tumor Location, Grade, and Patient Age. *Am. J. Pathol.* **2003**, *163*, 1721–1727. [CrossRef]
58. Monoranu, C.M.; Huang, B.; Zangen, I.L.; Rutkowski, S.; Vince, G.H.; Gerber, N.U.; Puppe, B.; Roggendorf, W. Correlation between 6q25.3 deletion status and survival in pediatric intracranial ependymomas. *Cancer Genet. Cytogenet.* **2008**, *182*, 18–26. [CrossRef]
59. Rajaram, V.; Gutmann, D.H.; Prasad, S.K.; Mansur, D.B.; Perry, A. Alterations of protein 4.1 family members in ependymomas: A study of 84 cases. *Mod. Pathol.* **2005**, *18*, 991–997. [CrossRef]
60. George, O.L.; Ness, S.A. Situational awareness: Regulation of the myb transcription factor in differentiation, the cell cycle and oncogenesis. *Cancers* **2014**, *6*, 2049–2071. [CrossRef]
61. López-Nieva, P.; Vaquero, C.; Fernández-Navarro, P.; González-Sánchez, L.; Villa-Morales, M.; Santos, J.; Esteller, M.; Fernández-Piqueras, J. EPHA7, a new target gene for 6q deletion in T-cell lymphoblastic lymphomas. *Carcinogenesis* **2012**, *33*, 452–458. [CrossRef] [PubMed]
62. Nguyen, H.S.; Doan, N.; Gelsomino, M.; Shabani, S. Intracranial Subependymoma: A SEER Analysis 2004–2013. *World Neurosurg.* **2017**, *101*, 599–605. [CrossRef] [PubMed]

63. Friede, R.L.; Pollak, A. The cytogenetic basis for classifying ependymomas. *J. Neuropathol. Exp. Neurol.* **1978**, *37*, 103–118. [CrossRef]
64. Ragel, B.T.; Osborn, A.G.; Whang, K.; Townsend, J.J.; Jensen, R.L.; Couldwell, W.T. Subependymomas: An analysis of clinical and imaging features. *Neurosurgery* **2006**, *58*, 881–889. [CrossRef]
65. Rushing, E.J.; Cooper, P.B.; Quezado, M.; Begnami, M.; Crespo, A.; Smirniotopoulos, J.G.; Ecklund, J.; Olsen, C.; Santi, M. Subependymoma revisited: Clinicopathological evaluation of 83 cases. *J. Neuro-Oncol.* **2007**, *85*, 297–305. [CrossRef]
66. Leeper, H.; Felicella, M.M.; Walbert, T. Recent Advances in the Classification and Treatment of Ependymomas. *Curr. Treat. Options Oncol.* **2017**, *18*, 55. [CrossRef]
67. Bi, Z.; Ren, X.; Zhang, J.; Jia, W. Clinical, radiological, and pathological features in 43 cases of intracranial subependymoma. *J. Neurosurg.* **2015**, *122*, 49–60. [CrossRef]
68. Kong, L.Y.; Wei, J.; Haider, A.S.; Liebelt, B.D.; Ling, X.; Conrad, C.A.; Fuller, G.N.; Levine, N.B.; Priebe, W.; Sawaya, R.; et al. Therapeutic targets in subependymoma. *J. Neuroimmunol.* **2014**, *277*, 168–175. [CrossRef]
69. Bateman, A.; Martin, M.J.; Orchard, S.; Magrane, M.; Agivetova, R.; Ahmad, S.; Alpi, E.; Bowler-Barnett, E.H.; Britto, R.; Bursteinas, B.; et al. UniProt: The universal protein knowledgebase in 2021. *Nucleic Acids Res.* **2021**, *49*, D480–D489. [CrossRef]
70. Capdeville, R.; Buchdunger, E.; Zimmermann, J.; Matter, A. Glivec (ST1571, imatinib), a rationally developed, targeted anticancer drug. *Nat. Rev. Drug Discov.* **2002**, *1*, 493–502. [CrossRef]
71. Donson, P.; Werner, E.; Amani, V.; Griesinger, A.; Witt, D.; Nellan, A.; Vibhakar, R.; Hankinson, T.; Handler, M.; Dorris, K.; et al. Tyrosine kinase inhibitors axitinib, imatinib and pazopanib are selectively potent in ependymoma. *Neuro-Oncology* **2017**, *19*, iv17. [CrossRef]
72. Newton, H.B.; Ray-Chaudhury, A. Overview of Brain Tumor Epidemiology and Histopathology. *Handb. Brain Tumor Chemother.* **2006**, 3–20. [CrossRef]
73. Kleihues, P.; Burger, P.C.; Scheithauer, B.W. *Histological Typing of Tumours of the Central Nervous System*; Springer: Berlin/Heidelberg, Germany, 1993. [CrossRef]
74. Kweh, B.T.S.; Rosenfeld, J.V.; Hunn, M.; Tee, J.W. Tumor characteristics and surgical outcomes of intracranial subependymomas: A systematic review and meta-analysis. *J. Neurosurg.* **2021**, *20*, 1–13. [CrossRef]
75. Jooma, R.; Torrens, M.J.; Bradshaw, J.; Brownell, B. Subependymomas of the fourth ventricle. Surgical treatment in 12 cases. *J. Neurosurg.* **1985**, *62*, 508–512. [CrossRef]
76. Varma, A.; Giraldi, D.; Mills, S.; Brodbelt, A.R.; Jenkinson, M.D. Surgical management and long-term outcome of intracranial subependymoma. *Acta Neurochir.* **2018**, *160*, 1793–1799. [CrossRef]
77. Scheithauer, B.W. Symptomatic subependymoma. Report of 21 cases with review of the literature. *J. Neurosurg.* **1978**, *49*, 689–696. [CrossRef]
78. Hou, Z.; Wu, Z.; Zhang, J.; Zhang, L.; Tian, R.; Liu, B.; Wang, Z. Lateral ventricular subependymomas: An analysis of the clinical features of 27 adult cases at a single institute. *Neurol. India* **2012**, *60*, 379. [CrossRef]
79. Limaiem, F.; Das, J.M. Myxopapillary Ependymoma. Available online: http://www.ncbi.nlm.nih.gov/pubmed/32644598 (accessed on 7 July 2021).
80. Sonneland, P.R.L.; Scheithauer, B.W.; Onofrio, B.M. Myxopapillary ependymoma. A clinicopathologic and immunocytochemical study of 77 cases. *Cancer* **1985**, *56*, 883–893. [CrossRef]
81. Mørk, S.J.; Løken, A.C. Ependymoma. A follow-up study of 101 cases. *Cancer* **1977**, *40*, 907–915. [CrossRef]
82. Kraetzig, T.; McLaughlin, L.; Bilsky, M.H.; Laufer, I. Metastases of spinal myxopapillary ependymoma: Unique characteristics and clinical management. *J. Neurosurg. Spine* **2018**, *28*, 201–208. [CrossRef]
83. Bagley, C.A.; Wilson, S.; Kothbauer, K.F.; Bookland, M.J.; Epstein, F.; Jallo, G.I. Long term outcomes following surgical resection of myxopapillary ependymomas. *Neurosurg. Rev.* **2009**, *32*, 321–334. [CrossRef]
84. Feldman, W.B.; Clark, A.J.; Safaee, M.; Ames, C.P.; Parsa, A.T. Tumor control after surgery for spinal myxopapillary ependymomas: Distinct outcomes in adults versus children. *J. Neurosurg. Spine* **2013**, *19*, 471–476. [CrossRef]
85. Liu, T.; Yang, C.; Deng, X.; Li, A.; Xin, Y.; Yang, J.; Xu, Y. Clinical characteristics and surgical outcomes of spinal myxopapillary ependymomas. *Neurosurg. Rev.* **2020**, *43*, 1351–1356. [CrossRef]
86. Akyurek, S.; Chang, E.L.; Yu, T.K.; Little, D.; Allen, P.K.; McCutcheon, I.; Mahajan, A.; Maor, M.H.; Woo, S.Y. Spinal myxopapillary ependymoma outcomes in patients treated with surgery and radiotherapy at M.D. Anderson Cancer Center. *J. Neurooncol.* **2006**, *80*, 177–183. [CrossRef]
87. Waldron, J.N.; Laperriere, N.J.; Jaakkimainen, L.; Simpson, W.J.; Payne, D.; Milosevic, M.; Wong, C.S. Spinal cord ependymomas: A retrospective analysis of 59 cases. *Int. J. Radiat. Oncol. Biol. Phys.* **1993**, *27*, 223–229. [CrossRef]
88. Whitaker, S.J.; Bessell, E.M.; Ashley, S.E.; Bloom, H.J.G.; Bell, B.A.; Brada, M. Postoperative radiotherapy in the management of spinal cord ependymoma. *J. Neurosurg.* **1991**, *74*, 720–728. [CrossRef] [PubMed]
89. Barton, V.N.; Donson, A.M.; Kleinschmidt-Demasters, B.K.; Birks, D.K.; Handler, M.H.; Foreman, N.K. Unique molecular characteristics of pediatric myxopapillary ependymoma. *Brain Pathol.* **2010**, *20*, 560–570. [CrossRef] [PubMed]
90. Wellik, D.M. Hox patterning of the vertebrate axial skeleton. *Dev. Dyn.* **2007**, *236*, 2454–2463. [CrossRef] [PubMed]
91. Alharbi, R.A.; Pandha, H.S.; Simpson, G.R.; Pettengell, R.; Poterlowicz, K.; Thompson, A.; Harrington, K.; El-Tanani, M.; Morgan, R. Inhibition of HOX/PBX dimer formation leads to necroptosis in acute myeloid leukemia cells. *Oncotarget* **2017**, *8*, 89566–89579. [CrossRef] [PubMed]

92. Takahashi, Y.; Hamada, J.I.; Murakawa, K.; Takada, M.; Tada, M.; Nogami, I.; Hayashi, N.; Nakamori, S.; Monden, M.; Miyamoto, M.; et al. Expression profiles of 39 HOX genes in normal human adult organs and anaplastic thyroid cancer cell lines by quantitative real-time RT-PCR system. *Exp. Cell Res.* **2004**, *293*, 144–153. [CrossRef] [PubMed]
93. Ahmad, O.; Chapman, R.; Storer, L.C.; Luo, L.; Heath, P.R.; Resar, L.; Cohen, K.J.; Grundy, R.G.; Lourdusamy, A. Integrative molecular characterization of pediatric spinal ependymoma: The UK Children's Cancer and Leukaemia Group study. *Neuro-Oncol. Adv.* **2021**, *3*, vdab043. [CrossRef]
94. Toomey, D.P.; Murphy, J.F.; Conlon, K.C. COX-2, VEGF and tumour angiogenesis. *Surgeon* **2009**, *7*, 174–180. [CrossRef]
95. Schonthal, A.H. Exploiting Cyclooxygenase-(in)Dependent Properties of COX-2 Inhibitors for Malignant Glioma Therapy. *Anticancer Agents Med. Chem.* **2012**, *10*, 450–461. [CrossRef]
96. Axelsson, H.; Lönnroth, C.; Wang, W.; Svanberg, E.; Lundholm, K. Cyclooxygenase inhibition in early onset of tumor growth and related angiogenesis evaluated in EP1 and EP3 knockout tumor-bearing mice. *Angiogenesis* **2006**, *8*, 339–348. [CrossRef]
97. Celano, E.; Salehani, A.; Malcolm, J.G.; Reinertsen, E.; Hadjipanayis, C.G. Spinal cord ependymoma: A review of the literature and case series of ten patients. *J. Neurooncol.* **2016**, *128*, 377–386. [CrossRef] [PubMed]
98. Gupta, K.; Salunke, P. Understanding Ependymoma Oncogenesis: An Update on Recent Molecular Advances and Current Perspectives. *Mol. Neurobiol.* **2017**, *54*, 15–21. [CrossRef] [PubMed]
99. Guyotat, J.; Metellus, P.; Giorgi, R.; Barrie, M.; Jouvet, A.; Fevre-Montange, M.; Chinot, O.; Durand, A.; Figarella-Branger, D. Infratentorial ependymomas: Prognostic factors and outcome analysis in a multi-center retrospective series of 106 adult patients. *Acta Neurochir.* **2009**, *151*, 947–960. [CrossRef] [PubMed]
100. Gerszten, P.C.; Pollack, I.F.; Martínez, A.J.; Lo, K.H.; Janosky, J.; Albright, A.L. Intracranial ependymomas of childhood lack of correlation of histopathology and clinical outcome. *Pathol. Res. Pract.* **1996**, *192*, 515–522. [CrossRef]
101. Schiffer, D.; Chiò, A.; Giordana, M.T.; Migheli, A.; Palma, L.; Pollo, B.; Soffietti, R.; Tribolo, A. Histologic prognostic factors in ependymoma. *Childs Nerv. Syst.* **1991**, *7*, 177–182. [CrossRef]
102. Korshunov, A.; Golanov, A.; Sycheva, R.; Timirgaz, V. The Histologic Grade Is a Main Prognostic Factor for Patients with Intracranial Ependymomas Treated in the Microneurosurgical Era: An Analysis of 258 Patients. *Cancer* **2004**, *100*, 1230–1237. [CrossRef] [PubMed]
103. Lopez-Rivera, V.; Dono, A.; Abdelkhaleq, R.; Sheth, S.A.; Chen, P.R.; Chandra, A.; Ballester, L.Y.; Esquenazi, Y. Treatment trends and overall survival in patients with grade II/III ependymoma: The role of tumor grade and location. *Clin. Neurol. Neurosurg.* **2020**, *199*, 106282. [CrossRef]
104. Tarapore, P.E.; Modera, P.; Naujokas, A.; Oh, M.C.; Amin, B.; Tihan, T.; Parsa, A.T.; Ames, C.P.; Chou, D.; Mummaneni, P.V.; et al. Pathology of spinal ependymomas: An institutional experience over 25 years in 134 patients. *Neurosurgery* **2013**, *73*, 247–255. [CrossRef] [PubMed]
105. Lee, S.H.; Chung, C.K.; Kim, C.H.; Yoon, S.H.; Hyun, S.J.; Kim, K.J.; Kim, E.S.; Eoh, W.; Kim, H.J. Long-term outcomes of surgical resection with or without adjuvant radiation therapy for treatment of spinal ependymoma: A retrospective multicenter study by the Korea Spinal Oncology Research Group. *Neuro-Oncology* **2013**, *15*, 921–929. [CrossRef]
106. Savoor, R.; Sita, T.L.; Dahdaleh, N.S.; Helenowski, I.; Kalapurakal, J.A.; Marymont, M.H.; Lukas, R.; Kruser, T.J.; Smith, Z.A.; Koski, T.; et al. Long-term outcomes of spinal ependymomas: An institutional experience of more than 60 cases. *J. Neuro-Oncol.* **2020**, *151*, 241–247. [CrossRef] [PubMed]
107. Petrilli, A.M.; Fernández-Valle, C. Role of Merlin/NF2 inactivation in tumor biology. *Oncogene* **2016**, *35*, 537–548. [CrossRef] [PubMed]
108. Coy, S.; Rashid, R.; Stemmer-Rachamimov, A.; Santagata, S. An update on the CNS manifestations of neurofibromatosis type 2. *Acta Neuropathol.* **2020**, *139*, 643–665. [CrossRef] [PubMed]
109. Abylkassov, R.; Xie, Y. Role of yes-associated protein in cancer: An update (Review). *Oncol. Lett.* **2016**, *12*, 2277–2282. [CrossRef]
110. Liu-Chittenden, Y.; Huang, B.; Shim, J.S.; Chen, Q.; Lee, S.J.; Anders, R.A.; Liu, J.O.; Pan, D. Genetic and pharmacological disruption of the TEAD-YAP complex suppresses the oncogenic activity of YAP. *Genes Dev.* **2012**, *26*, 1300–1305. [CrossRef] [PubMed]
111. Soria, J.C.; Gan, H.K.; Blagden, S.P.; Plummer, R.; Arkenau, H.T.; Ranson, M.; Evans, T.R.J.; Zalcman, G.; Bahleda, R.; Hollebecque, A.; et al. A phase I, pharmacokinetic and pharmacodynamic study of GSK2256098, a focal adhesion kinase inhibitor, in patients with advanced solid tumors. *Ann. Oncol.* **2016**, *27*, 2268–2274. [CrossRef]
112. Sato, T.; Sekido, Y. NF2/merlin inactivation and potential therapeutic targets in mesothelioma. *Int. J. Mol. Sci.* **2018**, *19*, 988. [CrossRef]
113. Chen, P.; Rossi, N.; Priddy, S.; Pierson, C.R.; Studebaker, A.W.; Johnson, R.A. EphB2 activation is required for ependymoma development as well as inhibits differentiation and promotes proliferation of the transformed cell. *Sci. Rep.* **2015**, *5*, 9248. [CrossRef] [PubMed]
114. Han, Y.; Liu, D.; Li, L. PD-1/PD-L1 pathway: Current researches in cancer. *Am. J. Cancer Res.* **2020**, *10*, 724–742.
115. Pavon, L.F.; Sibov, T.T.; de Toledo, S.R.C.; de Oliveira, D.M.; Cabral, F.R.; de Souza, J.G.; Boufleur, P.; Marti, L.C.; Malheiros, J.M.; da Cruz, E.F.; et al. Establishment of primary cell culture and an intracranial xenograft model of pediatric ependymoma: A prospect for therapy development and understanding of tumor biology. *Oncotarget* **2018**, *9*, 21731. [CrossRef]

116. Scheil, S.; Brüderlein, S.; Eicker, M.; Herms, J.; Herold-Mende, C.; Steiner, H.H.; Barth, T.F.E.; Möller, P. Low frequency of chromosomal imbalances in anaplastic ependymomas as detected by comparative genomic hybridization. *Brain Pathol.* **2001**, *11*, 133–143. [CrossRef] [PubMed]
117. Ghasemi, D.R.; Sill, M.; Okonechnikov, K.; Korshunov, A.; Yip, S.; Schutz, P.W.; Scheie, D.; Kruse, A.; Harter, P.N.; Kastelan, M.; et al. MYCN amplification drives an aggressive form of spinal ependymoma. *Acta Neuropathol.* **2019**, *138*, 1075–1089. [CrossRef]
118. Raffeld, M.; Abdullaev, Z.; Pack, S.D.; Xi, L.; Nagaraj, S.; Briceno, N.; Vera, E.; Pittaluga, S.; Lopes Abath Neto, O.; Quezado, M.; et al. High level MYCN amplification and distinct methylation signature define an aggressive subtype of spinal cord ependymoma. *Acta Neuropathol. Commun.* **2020**, *8*, 101. [CrossRef]
119. Swanson, A.A.; Raghunathan, A.; Jenkins, R.B.; Messing-Jünger, M.; Pietsch, T.; Clarke, M.J.; Kaufmann, T.J.; Giannini, C. Spinal cord ependymomas with MYCN amplification show aggressive clinical behavior. *J. Neuropathol. Exp. Neurol.* **2019**, *78*, 791–797. [CrossRef] [PubMed]
120. Astolfi, A.; Vendemini, F.; Urbini, M.; Melchionda, F.; Masetti, R.; Franzoni, M.; Libri, V.; Serravalle, S.; Togni, M.; Paone, G.; et al. MYCN is a novel oncogenic target in pediatric T-cell Acute Lymphoblastic Leukemia. *Oncotarget* **2014**, *5*, 120–130. [CrossRef]
121. Barone, G.; Anderson, J.; Pearson, A.D.J.; Petrie, K.; Chesler, L. New strategies in neuroblastoma: Therapeutic targeting of MYCN and ALK. *Clin. Cancer Res.* **2013**, *19*, 5814–5821. [CrossRef] [PubMed]
122. Korshunov, A.; Schrimpf, D.; Ryzhova, M.; Sturm, D.; Chavez, L.; Hovestadt, V.; Sharma, T.; Habel, A.; Burford, A.; Jones, C.; et al. H3-/IDH-wild type pediatric glioblastoma is comprised of molecularly and prognostically distinct subtypes with associated oncogenic drivers. *Acta Neuropathol.* **2017**, *134*, 507–516. [CrossRef] [PubMed]
123. Lee, J.K.; Phillips, J.W.; Smith, B.A.; Park, J.W.; Stoyanova, T.; McCaffrey, E.F.; Baertsch, R.; Sokolov, A.; Meyerowitz, J.G.; Mathis, C.; et al. N-Myc Drives Neuroendocrine Prostate Cancer Initiated from Human Prostate Epithelial Cells. *Cancer Cell* **2016**, *29*, 536–547. [CrossRef] [PubMed]
124. Ruiz-Pérez, M.V.; Henley, A.B.; Arsenian-Henriksson, M. The MYCN protein in health and disease. *Genes* **2017**, *8*, 113. [CrossRef]
125. Stermann, A.; Huebener, N.; Seidel, D.; Fest, S.; Eschenburg, G.; Stauder, M.; Schramm, A.; Eggert, A.; Lode, H.N. Targeting of MYCN by means of DNA vaccination is effective against neuroblastoma in mice. *Cancer Immunol. Immunother.* **2015**, *64*, 1215–1227. [CrossRef]
126. Mack, S.C.; Pajtler, K.W.; Chavez, L.; Okonechnikov, K.; Bertrand, K.C.; Wang, X.X.; Erkek, S.; Federation, A.; Song, A.; Lee, C.; et al. Therapeutic targeting of ependymoma as informed by oncogenic enhancer profiling. *Nature* **2018**, *553*, 101–105. [CrossRef]
127. Panwalkar, P.; Clark, J.; Ramaswamy, V.; Hawes, D.; Yang, F.; Dunham, C.; Yip, S.; Hukin, J.; Sun, Y.; Schipper, M.J.; et al. Immunohistochemical analysis of H3K27me3 demonstrates global reduction in group-A childhood posterior fossa ependymoma and is a powerful predictor of outcome. *Acta Neuropathol.* **2017**, *134*, 705–714. [CrossRef]
128. Bayliss, J.; Mukherjee, P.; Lu, C.; Jain, S.U.; Chung, C.; Martinez, D.; Sabari, B.; Margol, A.S.; Panwalkar, P.; Parolia, A.; et al. Lowered H3K27me3 and DNA hypomethylation define poorly prognostic pediatric posterior fossa ependymomas. *Sci. Transl. Med.* **2016**, *8*, 366ra161. [CrossRef]
129. Nambirajan, A.; Sharma, A.; Rajeshwari, M.; Boorgula, M.T.; Doddamani, R.; Garg, A.; Suri, V.; Sarkar, C.; Sharma, M.C. EZH2 inhibitory protein (EZHIP/Cxorf67) expression correlates strongly with H3K27me3 loss in posterior fossa ependymomas and is mutually exclusive with H3K27M mutations. *Brain Tumor Pathol.* **2021**, *38*, 30–40. [CrossRef]
130. Tanrıkulu, B.; Danyeli, A.E.; Özek, M.M. Is H3K27me3 status really a strong prognostic indicator for pediatric posterior fossa ependymomas? A single surgeon, single center experience. *Childs Nerv. Syst.* **2020**, *36*, 941–949. [CrossRef]
131. Capper, D.; Jones, D.T.W.; Sill, M.; Hovestadt, V.; Schrimpf, D.; Sturm, D.; Koelsche, C.; Sahm, F.; Chavez, L.; Reuss, D.E.; et al. DNA methylation-based classification of central nervous system tumours. *Nature* **2018**, *555*, 469–474. [CrossRef]
132. Yuh, E.L.; Barkovich, A.J.; Gupta, N. Imaging of ependymomas: MRI and CT. *Childs Nerv. Syst.* **2009**, *25*, 1203–1213. [CrossRef] [PubMed]
133. Yonezawa, U.; Karlowee, V.; Amatya, V.J.; Takayasu, T.; Takano, M.; Takeshima, Y.; Sugiyama, K.; Kurisu, K.; Yamasaki, F. Radiology Profile as a Potential Instrument to Differentiate Between Posterior Fossa Ependymoma (PF-EPN) Group A and B. *World Neurosurg.* **2020**, *140*, e320–e327. [CrossRef]
134. Zhao, F.; Wu, T.; Wang, L.M.; Zhang, J.; Zhang, H.; Li, S.W.; Zhang, S.; Li, P.; Wang, B.; Luo, L.; et al. Survival and Prognostic Factors of Adult Intracranial Ependymoma: A Single-institutional Analysis of 236 Patients. *Am. J. Surg. Pathol.* **2021**, *45*, 979–987. [CrossRef]
135. Baroni, L.V.; Sundaresan, L.; Heled, A.; Coltin, H.; Pajtler, K.W.; Lin, T.; Merchant, T.E.; McLendon, R.; Faria, C.; Buntine, M.; et al. Ultra high-risk PFA ependymoma is characterized by loss of chromosome 6q. *Neuro-Oncology* **2021**, *23*, 1360–1370. [CrossRef] [PubMed]
136. Pajtler, K.W.; Wen, J.; Sill, M.; Lin, T.; Orisme, W.; Tang, B.; Hübner, J.M.; Ramaswamy, V.; Jia, S.; Dalton, J.D.; et al. Molecular heterogeneity and CXorf67 alterations in posterior fossa group A (PFA) ependymomas. *Acta Neuropathol.* **2018**, *136*, 211–226. [CrossRef] [PubMed]
137. Ryall, S.; Guzman, M.; Elbabaa, S.K.; Luu, B.; Mack, S.C.; Zapotocky, M.; Taylor, M.D.; Hawkins, C.; Ramaswamy, V. H3 K27M mutations are extremely rare in posterior fossa group A ependymoma. *Childs Nerv. Syst.* **2017**, *33*, 1047–1051. [CrossRef]
138. De Sousa, G.R.; Lira, R.C.P.; de Almeida Magalhães, T.; da Silva, K.R.; Nagano, L.F.P.; Saggioro, F.P.; Baroni, M.; Marie, S.K.N.; Oba-Shinjo, S.M.; Brandelise, S.; et al. A coordinated approach for the assessment of molecular subgroups in pediatric ependymomas using low-cost methods. *J. Mol. Med.* **2021**, *99*, 1101–1113. [CrossRef]

139. Jain, S.U.; Do, T.J.; Lund, P.J.; Rashoff, A.Q.; Diehl, K.L.; Cieslik, M.; Bajic, A.; Juretic, N.; Deshmukh, S.; Venneti, S.; et al. PFA ependymoma-associated protein EZHIP inhibits PRC2 activity through a H3 K27M-like mechanism. *Nat. Commun.* **2019**, *10*, 2146. [CrossRef] [PubMed]
140. Hübner, J.M.; Müller, T.; Papageorgiou, D.N.; Mauermann, M.; Krijgsveld, J.; Russell, R.B.; Ellison, D.W.; Pfister, S.M.; Pajtler, K.W.; Kool, M. EZHIP/CXorf67 mimics K27M mutated oncohistones and functions as an intrinsic inhibitor of PRC2 function in aggressive posterior fossa ependymoma. *Neuro-Oncology* **2019**, *21*, 878–889. [CrossRef]
141. Krug, B.; Harutyunyan, A.S.; Deshmukh, S.; Jabado, N. Polycomb repressive complex 2 in the driver's seat of childhood and young adult brain tumours. *Trends Cell Biol.* **2021**, *31*, 814–828. [CrossRef]
142. Jain, S.U.; Rashoff, A.Q.; Krabbenhoft, S.D.; Hoelper, D.; Do, T.J.; Gibson, T.J.; Lundgren, S.M.; Bondra, E.R.; Deshmukh, S.; Harutyunyan, A.S.; et al. H3 K27M and EZHIP Impede H3K27-Methylation Spreading by Inhibiting Allosterically Stimulated PRC2. *Mol. Cell* **2020**, *80*, 726–735. [CrossRef]
143. Dyer, M.A.; Qadeer, Z.A.; Valle-Garcia, D.; Bernstein, E. ATRX and DAXX: Mechanisms and mutations. *Cold Spring Harb. Perspect. Med.* **2017**, *7*, a026567. [CrossRef]
144. Michealraj, K.A.; Kumar, S.A.; Kim, L.J.Y.; Cavalli, F.M.G.; Przelicki, D.; Wojcik, J.B.; Delaidelli, A.; Bajic, A.; Saulnier, O.; MacLeod, G.; et al. Metabolic Regulation of the Epigenome Drives Lethal Infantile Ependymoma. *Cell* **2020**, *181*, 1329–1345. [CrossRef]
145. Griesinger, A.M.; Witt, D.A.; Grob, S.T.; Georgio Westover, S.R.; Donson, A.M.; Sanford, B.; Mulcahy Levy, J.M.; Wong, R.; Moreira, D.C.; Desisto, J.A.; et al. NF-κB upregulation through epigenetic silencing of LDOC1 drives tumor biology and specific immunophenotype in Group A ependymoma. *Neuro-Oncology* **2017**, *19*, 1350–1360. [CrossRef]
146. Griesinger, A.M.; Josephson, R.J.; Donson, A.M.; Levy, J.M.M.; Amani, V.; Birks, D.K.; Hoffman, L.M.; Furtek, S.L.; Reigan, P.; Handler, M.H.; et al. Interleukin-6/STAT3 pathway signaling drives an inflammatory phenotype in group a ependymoma. *Cancer Immunol. Res.* **2015**, *3*, 1165–1174. [CrossRef]
147. Gojo, J.; Lötsch, D.; Spiegl-Kreinecker, S.; Pajtler, K.W.; Neumayer, K.; Korbel, P.; Araki, A.; Brandstetter, A.; Mohr, T.; Hovestadt, V.; et al. Telomerase activation in posterior fossa group A ependymomas is associated with dismal prognosis and chromosome 1q gain. *Neuro-Oncology* **2017**, *19*, 1183–1194. [CrossRef]
148. Meel, M.H.; Kaspers, G.J.L.; Hulleman, E. Preclinical therapeutic targets in diffuse midline glioma. *Drug Resist. Updates* **2019**, *44*, 15–25. [CrossRef]
149. Lin, G.L.; Wilson, K.M.; Ceribelli, M.; Stanton, B.Z.; Woo, P.J.; Kreimer, S.; Qin, E.Y.; Zhang, X.; Lennon, J.; Nagaraja, S.; et al. Therapeutic strategies for diffuse midline glioma from high-throughput combination drug screening. *Sci. Transl. Med.* **2019**, *11*. [CrossRef]
150. Sandberg, D.I.; Yu, B.; Patel, R.; Hagan, J.; Miesner, E.; Sabin, J.; Smith, S.; Fletcher, S.; Shah, M.N.; Sirianni, R.W.; et al. Infusion of 5-Azacytidine (5-AZA) into the fourth ventricle or resection cavity in children with recurrent posterior Fossa Ependymoma: A pilot clinical trial. *J. Neurooncol.* **2019**, *141*, 449–457. [CrossRef]
151. Han, J.; Yu, M.; Bai, Y.; Yu, J.; Jin, F.; Li, C.; Zeng, R.; Peng, J.; Li, A.; Song, X.; et al. Elevated CXorf67 Expression in PFA Ependymomas Suppresses DNA Repair and Sensitizes to PARP Inhibitors. *Cancer Cell* **2020**, *38*, 844–856. [CrossRef]
152. Gojo, J.; Englinger, B.; Jiang, L.; Hübner, J.M.; Shaw, M.L.; Hack, O.A.; Madlener, S.; Kirchhofer, D.; Liu, I.; Pyrdol, J.; et al. Single-Cell RNA-Seq Reveals Cellular Hierarchies and Impaired Developmental Trajectories in Pediatric Ependymoma. *Cancer Cell* **2020**, *38*, 44–59. [CrossRef]
153. Cruz, C.; Ribes, V.; Kutejova, E.; Cayuso, J.; Lawson, V.; Norris, D.; Stevens, J.; Davey, M.; Blight, K.; Bangs, F.; et al. Foxj1 regulates floor plate cilia architecture and modifies the response of cells to sonic hedgehog signalling. *Development* **2010**, *137*, 4271–4282. [CrossRef]
154. Abedalthagafi, M.S.; Wu, M.P.; Merrill, P.H.; Du, Z.; Woo, T.; Sheu, S.H.; Hurwitz, S.; Ligon, K.L.; Santagata, S. Decreased FOXJ1 expression and its ciliogenesis programme in aggressive ependymoma and choroid plexus tumours. *J. Pathol.* **2016**, *238*, 584–597. [CrossRef]
155. Wang, J.; Cai, X.; Xia, L.; Zhou, J.; Xin, J.; Liu, M.; Shang, X.; Liu, J.; Li, X.; Chen, Z.; et al. Decreased Expression of FOXJ1 is a Potential Prognostic Predictor for Progression and Poor Survival of Gastric Cancer. *Ann. Surg. Oncol.* **2015**, *22*, 685–692. [CrossRef]
156. Zhu, P.; Piao, Y.; Dong, X.; Jin, Z. Forkhead box J1 expression is upregulated and correlated with prognosis in patients with clear cell renal cell carcinoma. *Oncol. Lett.* **2015**, *10*, 1487–1494. [CrossRef]
157. Liu, K.; Fan, J.; Wu, J. Forkhead box protein J1 (FOXJ1) is overexpressed in colorectal cancer and promotes nuclear translocation of β-catenin in SW620 cells. *Med. Sci. Monit.* **2017**, *23*, 856–866. [CrossRef] [PubMed]
158. Georgescu, M.M.; Gagea, M.; Cote, G. NHERF1/EBP50 Suppresses Wnt-β-Catenin Pathway–Driven Intestinal Neoplasia. *Neoplasia* **2016**, *18*, 512–523. [CrossRef]
159. Kreimann, E.L.; Morales, F.C.; De Orbeta-Cruz, J.; Takahashi, Y.; Adams, H.; Liu, T.J.; McCrea, P.D.; Georgescu, M.M. Cortical stabilization of β-catenin contributes to NHERF1/EBP50 tumor suppressor function. *Oncogene* **2007**, *26*, 5290–5299. [CrossRef] [PubMed]
160. Dihlmann, S.; Von Knebel Doeberitz, M. Wnt/β-catenin-pathway as a molecular target for future anti-cancer therapeutics. *Int. J. Cancer* **2005**, *113*, 515–524. [CrossRef]

161. Jang, G.B.; Hong, I.S.; Kim, R.J.; Lee, S.Y.; Park, S.J.; Lee, E.S.; Park, J.H.; Yun, C.H.; Chung, J.U.; Lee, K.J.; et al. Wnt/β-catenin small-molecule inhibitor CWP232228 preferentially inhibits the growth of breast cancer stem-like cells. *Cancer Res.* **2015**, *75*, 1691–1702. [CrossRef]
162. Pak, S.; Park, S.; Kim, Y.; Park, J.H.; Park, C.H.; Lee, K.J.; Kim, C.S.; Ahn, H. The small molecule WNT/β-catenin inhibitor CWP232291 blocks the growth of castration-resistant prostate cancer by activating the endoplasmic reticulum stress pathway. *J. Exp. Clin. Cancer Res.* **2019**, *38*, 342. [CrossRef]
163. Coluccia, A.; La Regina, G.; Naccarato, V.; Nalli, M.; Orlando, V.; Biagioni, S.; De Angelis, M.L.; Baiocchi, M.; Gautier, C.; Gianni, S.; et al. Drug Design and Synthesis of First in Class PDZ1 Targeting NHERF1 Inhibitors as Anticancer Agents. *ACS Med. Chem. Lett.* **2019**, *10*, 499–503. [CrossRef]
164. Lester, A.; McDonald, K.L. Intracranial ependymomas: Molecular insights and translation to treatment. *Brain Pathol.* **2020**, *30*, 3–12. [CrossRef]
165. Andreiuolo, F.; Varlet, P.; Tauziède-Espariat, A.; Jünger, S.T.; Dörner, E.; Dreschmann, V.; Kuchelmeister, K.; Waha, A.; Haberler, C.; Slavc, I.; et al. Childhood supratentorial ependymomas with YAP1-MAMLD1 fusion: An entity with characteristic clinical, radiological, cytogenetic and histopathological features. *Brain Pathol.* **2019**, *29*, 205–216. [CrossRef] [PubMed]
166. Pajtler, K.W.; Wei, Y.; Okonechnikov, K.; Silva, P.B.G.; Vouri, M.; Zhang, L.; Brabetz, S.; Sieber, L.; Gulley, M.; Mauermann, M.; et al. YAP1 subgroup supratentorial ependymoma requires TEAD and nuclear factor I-mediated transcriptional programmes for tumorigenesis. *Nat. Commun.* **2019**, *10*, 3914. [CrossRef] [PubMed]
167. Kristal Kaan, H.Y.; Chan, S.W.; Tan, S.K.J.; Guo, F.; Lim, C.J.; Hong, W.; Song, H. Crystal structure of TAZ-TEAD complex reveals a distinct interaction mode from that of YAP-TEAD complex. *Sci. Rep.* **2017**, *7*, 2035. [CrossRef]
168. Eder, N.; Roncaroli, F.; Dolmart, M.C.; Horswell, S.; Andreiuolo, F.; Flynn, H.R.; Lopes, A.T.; Claxton, S.; Kilday, J.P.; Collinson, L.; et al. YAP1/TAZ drives ependymoma-like tumour formation in mice. *Nat. Commun.* **2020**, *11*, 2380. [CrossRef]
169. Rosenbluh, J.; Nijhawan, D.; Cox, A.G.; Li, X.; Neal, J.T.; Schafer, E.J.; Zack, T.I.; Wang, X.; Tsherniak, A.; Schinzel, A.C.; et al. β-catenin driven cancers require a YAP1 transcriptional complex for survival and tumorigenesis. *Cell* **2012**, *151*. [CrossRef]
170. Dupont, S.; Morsut, L.; Aragona, M.; Enzo, E.; Giulitti, S.; Cordenonsi, M.; Zanconato, F.; Le Digabel, J.; Forcato, M.; Bicciato, S.; et al. Role of YAP/TAZ in mechanotransduction. *Nature* **2011**, *474*, 179–184. [CrossRef] [PubMed]
171. Szulzewsky, F.; Holland, E.C.; Vasioukhin, V. YAP1 and its fusion proteins in cancer initiation, progression and therapeutic resistance. *Dev. Biol.* **2021**, *475*, 205–221. [CrossRef]
172. Pan, Z.; Tian, Y.; Cao, C.; Niu, G. The emerging role of YAP/TAZ in tumor immunity. *Mol. Cancer Res.* **2019**, *17*, 1777–1786. [CrossRef]
173. Oku, Y.; Nishiya, N.; Shito, T.; Yamamoto, R.; Yamamoto, Y.; Oyama, C.; Uehara, Y. Small molecules inhibiting the nuclear localization of YAP/TAZ for chemotherapeutics and chemosensizers against breast cancers. *FEBS Open Bio* **2015**, *5*, 542–549. [CrossRef]
174. Lindauer, M.; Hochhaus, A. Dasatinib. *Recent Results Cancer Res.* **2018**, *212*, 29–68.
175. Miyamoto, S.; Kakutani, S.; Sato, Y.; Hanashi, A.; Kinoshita, Y.; Ishikawa, A. Drug review: Pazopanib. *Jpn. J. Clin. Oncol.* **2018**, *48*, 503–513. [CrossRef]
176. Hayashi, K.; Nakazato, Y.; Morito, N.; Sagi, M.; Fujita, T.; Anzai, N.; Chida, M. Fluvastatin is effective against thymic carcinoma. *Life Sci.* **2020**, *240*, 117110. [CrossRef]
177. Giraud, J.; Molina-Castro, S.; Seeneevassen, L.; Sifré, E.; Izotte, J.; Tiffon, C.; Staedel, C.; Boeuf, H.; Fernandez, S.; Barthelemy, P.; et al. Verteporfin targeting YAP1/TAZ-TEAD transcriptional activity inhibits the tumorigenic properties of gastric cancer stem cells. *Int. J. Cancer* **2020**, *146*, 2255–2267. [CrossRef]
178. Sallam, Y.T.; Zhang, Q.; Pandey, S.K. Cortically based cystic supratentorial RELA fusion-positive ependymoma: A case report with unusual presentation and appearance and review of literature. *Radiol. Case Rep.* **2020**, *15*, 2495–2499. [CrossRef]
179. Gessi, M.; Giagnacovo, M.; Modena, P.; Elefante, G.; Gianno, F.; Buttarelli, F.R.; Arcella, A.; Donofrio, V.; Diomedi Camassei, F.; Nozza, P.; et al. Role of immunohistochemistry in the identification of supratentorial C11ORF95-RELA fused ependymoma in routine neuropathology. *Am. J. Surg. Pathol.* **2019**, *43*, 56–63. [CrossRef]
180. Tauziède-Espariat, A.; Siegfried, A.; Nicaise, Y.; Kergrohen, T.; Sievers, P.; Vasiljevic, A.; Roux, A.; Dezamis, E.; Benevello, C.; Machet, M.C.; et al. Supratentorial non-RELA, ZFTA-fused ependymomas: A comprehensive phenotype genotype correlation highlighting the number of zinc fingers in ZFTA-NCOA1/2 fusions. *Acta Neuropathol. Commun.* **2021**, *9*, 135. [CrossRef]
181. Parker, M.; Mohankumar, K.M.; Punchihewa, C.; Weinlich, R.; Dalton, J.D.; Li, Y.; Lee, R.; Tatevossian, R.G.; Phoenix, T.N.; Thiruvenkatam, R.; et al. C11orf95-RELA fusions drive oncogenic NF-κB signalling in ependymoma. *Nature* **2014**, *506*, 451–455. [CrossRef]
182. Zschernack, V.; Jünger, S.T.; Mynarek, M.; Rutkowski, S.; Garre, M.L.; Ebinger, M.; Neu, M.; Faber, J.; Erdlenbruch, B.; Claviez, A.; et al. Supratentorial ependymoma in childhood: More than just RELA or YAP. *Acta Neuropathol.* **2021**, *141*, 455–466. [CrossRef]
183. Tomomasa, R.; Arai, Y.; Kawabata-Iwakawa, R.; Fukuoka, K.; Nakano, Y.; Hama, N.; Nakata, S.; Suzuki, N.; Ishi, Y.; Tanaka, S.; et al. Ependymoma-like tumor with mesenchymal differentiation harboring C11orf95-NCOA1/2 or -RELA fusion: A hitherto unclassified tumor related to ependymoma. *Brain Pathol.* **2021**, *31*, e12943. [CrossRef]
184. Tamai, S.; Nakano, Y.; Kinoshita, M.; Sabit, H.; Nobusawa, S.; Arai, Y.; Hama, N.; Totoki, Y.; Shibata, T.; Ichimura, K.; et al. Ependymoma with C11orf95-MAML2 fusion: Presenting with granular cell and ganglion cell features. *Brain Tumor Pathol.* **2021**, *38*, 64–70. [CrossRef]

185. Zheng, T.; Ghasemi, D.R.; Okonechnikov, K.; Korshunov, A.; Sill, M.; Maass, K.K.; Benites Goncalves da Silva, P.; Ryzhova, M.; Gojo, J.; Stichel, D.; et al. Cross-Species Genomics Reveals Oncogenic Dependencies in ZFTA/C11orf95 Fusion–Positive Supratentorial Ependymomas. *Cancer Discov.* **2021**, *11*, 2230–2247. [CrossRef]
186. Kupp, R.; Ruff, L.; Terranova, S.; Nathan, E.; Ballereau, S.; Stark, R.; Sekhar Reddy Chilamakuri, C.; Hoffmann, N.; Wickham-Rahrmann, K.; Widdess, M.; et al. ZFTA Translocations Constitute Ependymoma Chromatin Remodeling and Transcription Factors. *Cancer Discov.* **2021**, *11*, 2216–2229. [CrossRef]
187. Ozawa, T.; Arora, S.; Szulzewsky, F.; Juric-Sekhar, G.; Miyajima, Y.; Bolouri, H.; Yasui, Y.; Barber, J.; Kupp, R.; Dalton, J.; et al. A De Novo Mouse Model of C11orf95-RELA Fusion-Driven Ependymoma Identifies Driver Functions in Addition to NF-κB. *Cell Rep.* **2018**, *23*, 3787–3797. [CrossRef]
188. Ozawa, T.; Kaneko, S.; Szulzewsky, F.; Qiao, Z.; Takadera, M.; Narita, Y.; Kondo, T.; Holland, E.C.; Hamamoto, R.; Ichimura, K. C11orf95-RELA fusion drives aberrant gene expression through the unique epigenetic regulation for ependymoma formation. *Acta Neuropathol. Commun.* **2021**, *9*, 36. [CrossRef]
189. Didonato, J.A.; Mercurio, F.; Karin, M. NF-κB and the link between inflammation and cancer. *Immunol. Rev.* **2012**, *246*, 379–400. [CrossRef] [PubMed]
190. Perkins, N.D. The diverse and complex roles of NF-κB subunits in cancer. *Nat. Rev. Cancer* **2012**, *12*, 121–132. [CrossRef]
191. Arabzade, A.; Zhao, Y.; Varadharajan, S.; Chen, H.-C.; Jessa, S.; Rivas, B.; Stuckert, A.J.; Solis, M.; Kardian, A.; Tlais, D.; et al. ZFTA–RELA Dictates Oncogenic Transcriptional Programs to Drive Aggressive Supratentorial Ependymoma. *Cancer Discov.* **2021**, *11*, 2200–2215. [CrossRef]
192. Lötsch, D.; Kirchhofer, D.; Englinger, B.; Jiang, L.; Okonechnikov, K.; Senfter, D.; Laemmerer, A.; Gabler, L.; Pirker, C.; Donson, A.M.; et al. Targeting fibroblast growth factor receptors to combat aggressive ependymoma. *Acta Neuropathol.* **2021**, *142*, 339–360. [CrossRef]
193. Wang, L.; Han, S.; Yan, C.; Yang, Y.; Li, Z.; Yang, Z. The role of clinical factors and immunocheckpoint molecules in the prognosis of patients with supratentorial extraventricular ependymoma: A single-center retrospective study. *J. Cancer Res. Clin. Oncol.* **2021**, *147*, 1259–1270. [CrossRef]
194. Pauken, K.E.; Wherry, E.J. Overcoming T cell exhaustion in infection and cancer. *Trends Immunol.* **2015**, *36*, 265–276. [CrossRef]
195. Rausch, T.; Jones, D.T.W.; Zapatka, M.; Stütz, A.M.; Zichner, T.; Weischenfeldt, J.; Jäger, N.; Remke, M.; Shih, D.; Northcott, P.A.; et al. Genome sequencing of pediatric medulloblastoma links catastrophic DNA rearrangements with TP53 mutations. *Cell* **2012**, *148*, 59–71. [CrossRef] [PubMed]

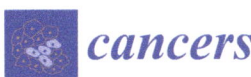

Review

Targeted Therapies for the Neurofibromatoses

Lauren D. Sanchez [1,†], Ashley Bui [2,†] and Laura J. Klesse [2,*]

1. Department of Pediatrics, Division of Neurology, UT Southwestern Medical Center, Dallas, TX 75235, USA; Lauren.Dengle@UTSouthwestern.edu
2. Department of Pediatrics, Division of Hematology/Oncology, UT Southwestern Medical Center, Dallas, TX 75235, USA; Ashley.Bui@UTSouthwestern.edu
* Correspondence: Laura.Klesse@UTSouthwestern.edu
† L.D.S. and A.B. contributed equally to this work.

Simple Summary: The neurofibromatoses—neurofibromatosis type 1, neurofibromatosis type 2, and schwannomatosis—are genetic tumor predisposition syndromes in which affected patients are at risk for the development of nerve-associated central and peripheral tumors. Patients often develop multiple tumors which can result in significant symptoms and morbidity. Treatment of the tumors associated with these disorders has evolved over the past decade, including significant work focused on inhibition of the signaling dysregulation and symptom minimization. This review outlines the most common tumor types associated with each of these syndromes and the current progress in therapeutic options.

Abstract: Over the past several years, management of the tumors associated with the neurofibromatoses has been recognized to often require approaches that are distinct from their spontaneous counterparts. Focus has shifted to therapy aimed at minimizing symptoms given the risks of persistent, multiple tumors and new tumor growth. In this review, we will highlight the translation of preclinical data to therapeutic trials for patients with neurofibromatosis, particularly neurofibromatosis type 1 and neurofibromatosis type 2. Successful inhibition of MEK for patients with neurofibromatosis type 1 and progressive optic pathway gliomas or plexiform neurofibromas has been a significant advancement in patient care. Similar success for the malignant NF1 tumors, such as high-grade gliomas and malignant peripheral nerve sheath tumors, has not yet been achieved; nor has significant progress been made for patients with either neurofibromatosis type 2 or schwannomatosis, although efforts are ongoing.

Keywords: neurofibromatosis; low grade glioma; plexiform neurofibroma; vestibular schwannoma

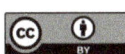

1. Introduction

Recent neurofibromatosis (NF)-focused clinical trials and consensus guidelines have highlighted the unique behavior and management needed for tumors which arise in this group of rare, genetic tumor predisposition syndromes. The neurofibromatoses are a group of three distinct genetic disorders which predispose one to the development of peripheral and central nervous system tumors and include neurofibromatosis type 1, neurofibromatosis type 2, and schwannomatosis. Although most of the tumors which arise are benign in nature, they are associated with significant clinical morbidity and the risks of malignant progression and mortality. No cure for any of the three NF disorders has been identified, and until recently, surgical resection of symptomatic tumors remained the only standard therapy. Treatment of the tumors associated with these disorders has evolved over the past decade, including significant work focused on inhibition of the signaling dysregulation and symptom minimization. Coordinated, multicenter trials have advanced the current understanding of the manifestations of NF and moved potential medical therapies more quickly through testing. In this review, we identify the most common tumors which arise in these patient populations and highlight recent therapeutic trials which leverage what is known about the aberrant cell signaling, particularly for neurofibromatosis type 1 and neurofibromatosis type 2.

2. Neurofibromatosis Type 1

Neurofibromatosis type 1 (NF1) is a common tumor predisposition syndrome, with an incidence estimated to be about 1 per 3000 individuals [1]. The most notable effects of NF1 involve the nervous system, but it is a multisystem disorder with a wide range of clinical manifestations. Individuals with NF1 typically manifest characteristic features, including café-au-lait macules, intertriginous freckling, and Lisch nodules (hamartomas of the iris) in childhood, but the disorder may not be recognized until later in many patients. Other common clinical manifestations include learning disabilities, characteristic osseous lesions, and a combination of benign and malignant central and peripheral nervous system tumors. It is from the most common tumor type in NF1, neurofibromas, that the syndrome derived its name. Neurofibromas are often grouped into two distinct entities, cutaneous neurofibromas and plexiform neurofibromas (PNs). Cutaneous neurofibromas are discrete dermal lesions associated with a single peripheral nerve, affecting almost all patients with NF1 by adulthood. PNs, however, are lesions involving multiple nerve fascicles or branches associated with significant morbidity and a risk of transforming into highly aggressive sarcomas known as malignant peripheral nerve sheath tumors (MPNSTs). Following neurofibromas, gliomas are the second most common tumor type in NF1. Optic pathway gliomas are the most common of these, but other gliomas, including high-grade gliomas, are also encountered. Individuals with NF1 are also at an increased risk for non-nervous system tumors, including but not limited to leukemia, pheochromocytoma, breast carcinoma, and gastrointestinal stromal tumors [2–9].

NF1 is an autosomal dominant disorder caused by inherited or de novo germline mutations of the *NF1* tumor suppressor gene located at chromosome 17q11.2, in most cases leading to a loss of function of the *NF1* gene product neurofibromin [1]. Neurofibromin, a large multifunctional protein, is expressed ubiquitously, especially during development, but it is found at highest levels in neurons, Schwann cells, and oligodendrocytes [10,11]. It is a GTPase-activating protein which acts as the common upstream molecule of several pathways, including the Ras/Raf/MEK/ERK signaling pathway and the interrelated mammalian target of rapamycin (mTOR) signaling pathway [12]. Through these pathways, among others, neurofibromin is involved in the regulation of fundamental cellular processes such as cell proliferation and growth. The loss of neurofibromin results in loss of regulation of these functions and allows increased cell growth and tumorigenesis [13]. Figure 1 summarizes the signaling cascades implicated in NF1 tumorgenicity. It is important to note that the specific pathway or mechanism through which this occurs varies depending on the tissue involved (i.e., in leukemic cells versus optic pathway gliomas) [14]. Furthermore, depending on the specific manifestation or tumor type, there may be additional requirements of the progenitor cells and microenvironment, including the need for a second hit and/or haploinsufficiency. For example, from genetically engineered mice, we have learned that haploinsufficiency of Schwann cells is not sufficient for the formation of a PN. A second hit causing inactivation of the *NF1* gene in Schwann cells is required, and haploinsufficiency of other cells in the surrounding microenvironment is additionally required for tumor formation [15].

These nuances have important implications for the treatment of the various manifestations of NF1. With a wide array of disease manifestations and the constellation of tumor types with varying pathogenesis, there is no singular treatment available. Management of the disorder has been mainly focused on routine screening and surveillance, with focused treatment of individual complications as they arise. Specifically, treatment of NF1-associated tumors with more conventional chemotherapy agents has been met with varying degrees of success. With improved understanding of the molecular pathogenesis of NF1 gained over the past decade, targeted treatments of tumors in NF1 have shown encouraging success. Here we will discuss the molecularly targeted approaches to some of the most common or clinically important tumors of NF1.

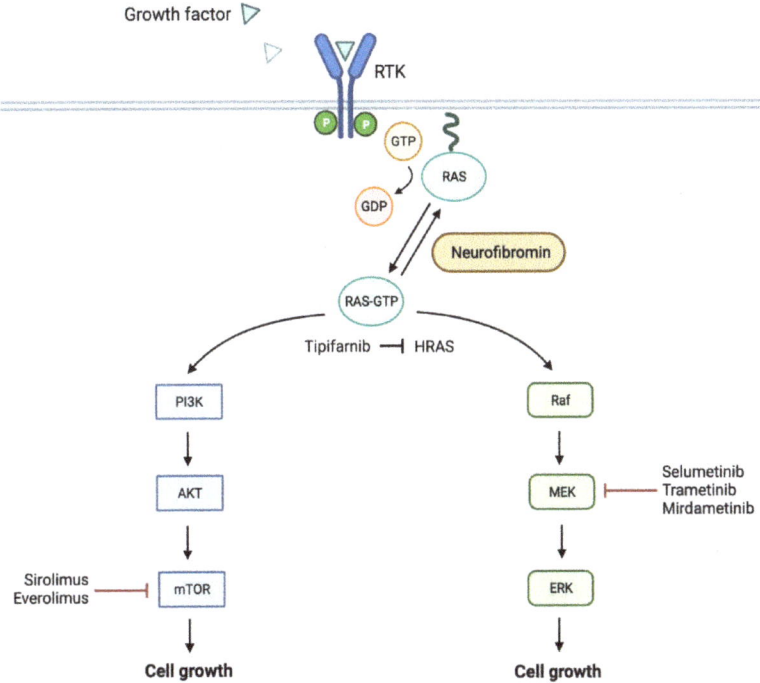

Figure 1. Schematic representation of the main NF1 associated signaling pathways with noted targeted therapies. RTK = receptor tyrosine kinase. Figure created with biorender.com (accessed on 19 October 2021).

2.1. Plexiform Neurofibromas

PNs occur in up to 50% of people with NF1 [16,17] and occur very rarely in absence of the disorder [18]. They appear to be congenital and tend to present and exhibit their most rapid growth during childhood [19]. PNs are benign peripheral nerve sheath tumors that grow along the length of nerves, often as distinct tumor masses, and can involve multiple fascicles and branches of a nerve [17]. Though histologically benign, PNs tend to be diffuse and infiltrative and can result in significant complications and morbidities, such as pain, impaired motor function, and disfigurement [20,21]. PNs also carry a risk of malignant transformation to the highly aggressive sarcoma MPNST, the leading cause of mortality and reduced life expectancy of patients with NF1 [22].

Histologically, PNs are composed of neoplastic Schwann cells lacking *NF1* gene expression and other cellular and noncellular components, such as *NF1*+/− fibroblasts, perineural cells, and mast cells embedded in a rich mucosubstance collagen matrix [23]. Loss of *NF1* gene expression in the neoplastic Schwann cells, subsequent impairment of neurofibromin-dependent Ras inactivation, and resultant Ras pathway dysregulation are the main cause of tumorigenesis in PNs [24]. However, this is not the complete story. Haploinsufficiency of other cells in the microenvironment, such as fibroblasts and mast cells, also contributes to the pathogenesis of these tumors [25,26]. Additional factors such as increased expression of growth factors and growth factor receptors may also impact tumorigenesis and growth [27,28].

Treatment options for PNs have historically been limited. Conventional cytotoxic chemotherapeutic agents have little effect on these slow-growing tumors. Given the risk of malignant transformation of the PN and the underlying predisposition to cancer in patients with NF1, radiation therapy is generally avoided [29,30]. Treatment of symptomatic lesions therefore has predominantly relied upon surgical debulking. Complete excision of a PN can be curative and this may be rendered increasingly possible via novel techniques such as surgery performed under fluorescein guidance as reported by Vetrano and colleagues [31]. Complete excision, however, is often not feasible due to extensive growth and invasion into surrounding tissues and the nerve itself, resulting in significant post-surgical complications. Tumor recurrence after surgery is also common [32]. The need for additional treatment options for these lesions has been long recognized. Early medication trials using nonspecific agents such as antihistamine, anti-inflammatory, antifibrotic, or antiangiogenic agents to impair the biological processes integral to PN progression had limited success [33–38]. More recently, pegylated interferon has demonstrated better results, with one study demonstrating doubling of the time to progression (TTP) in patients with active PNs compared to the placebo group [39]. However, the utility of interferon is limited by often intolerable side effects, and ideally, agents inducing a tumor response rather than just extending the time to progression are sought.

Continued advances in the understanding of the biology and molecular pathogenesis of PNs has led to molecularly targeted treatment approaches. While a marginal response or no response was documented in earlier trials, more recent interventions have been more successful. A first approach was targeted specifically at inhibition of Ras signaling. Ras is a GTPase which serves an integral role in normal cell survival, proliferation, and differentiation by transducing cell surface receptor responses to intracellular signaling molecules [40]. Dysregulation of the Ras signaling pathway is implicated in many tumor types. In a properly functioning cell expressing *NF1*, the *NF1* gene product neurofibromin functions as a negative regulator of Ras by accelerating hydrolysis from the active form Ras-GTP to the inactive form Ras-GDP. In NF1, loss of *NF1* expression leads to constitutive activation of the Ras pathway, which leads to tumorigenesis [41]. Blockade of this aberrant Ras signaling, therefore, is a rational target in the treatment of PNs [42]. Ras proteins in the Ras signaling pathway downstream of the defunct neurofibromin protein in NF1 require post-translational modification by farnesylation to be biologically active. The use of tipifarnib, a farnesyl transferase inhibitor, [43] in a randomized, double-blinded study treating children and young adults with NF1-related progressive PNs demonstrated tolerability of the drug but did not significantly increase TTP compared to placebo [44]. Notably, tipifarnib has been shown to effectively inhibit H-Ras farnesylation, but not other Ras proteins, N-Ras and K-Ras, which can undergo an alternate lipid modification [45]. In NF1-associated tumors, K-Ras is thought to be the predominant isoform involved, potentially underlying the poor clinical result in this trial.

An alternative signaling pathway that has been targeted is the mammalian target of rapamycin (mTOR) pathway, also demonstrated to be integral to cell survival, proliferation, and differentiation [46]. Akin to its role in the Ras pathway, neurofibromin plays a role in regulation of the mTOR pathway, and the mTOR pathway is constitutively activated in *NF1*-deficient cells and tumors [47]. mTOR signaling is upregulated in many cancers, and the mTOR kinase central to the pathway has been a successful target of other cancer treatments, including in the treatment of subependymal giant cell astrocytomas (SEGAs) in another Ras pathway disorder, tuberous sclerosis complex (TSC) [48]. mTOR was named for its susceptibility to the macrolide compound rapamycin, as rapamycin, in complex with another protein, inhibits the function of mTOR [49]. Rapamycin (also known as sirolimus) was trialed in NF1 for both non-progressive and progressive inoperable NF1-associated PNs but had limited success (NCT00634270). In patients with non-progressive PNs, no objective radiographic responses were demonstrated [50]. In patients with progressive PNs, a modest increase of 4 months in TTP was noted with without significant or frequent toxicity in a subset of patients [50]. Everolimus, another mTOR inhibitor, and pexidartinib, an inhibitor of a tyrosine kinase in the mTOR signaling pathway, have also been studied without much success [51,52]. Everolimus, in particular, was associated with significant adverse effects [53].

Conversely, the use of mitogen-activated protein kinase (MAPK) inhibitors has demonstrated significant responses and activity—a clear major advancement in clinical treatment for these patients. In the Ras/MAPK pathway, activation of Ras results in sequential activation of RAF kinase, MEK, and MAPK (ERK), respectively. MAPK acts as a regulator for several transcription factors, thereby acting as a regulator of the transcription of genes important in the cell cycle [42]. MEK inhibition has excitingly proven to be beneficial in the treatment of NF1-associated PNs. In 2016, a phase 1 study reported initial evidence of volumetric shrinkage of PNs in children who received the selective MEK inhibitor, selumetinib [54]. This was followed with a phase 2 study, published in 2020, which confirmed the previously reported radiographic response of >20% volumetric shrinkage. In addition to a sustained tumor response for 1 year or longer, 68% of the patients had some degree of clinical improvement in at least one PN-related complication, such as pain or limitation in physical functioning [55]. The therapy had an acceptable safety profile, with the most common adverse events including gastrointestinal symptoms (nausea, vomiting, and diarrhea), an asymptomatic increase in the creatine phosphokinase level, acneiform rash, and paronychia [55,56]. In response to these studies, selumetinib was granted FDA approval in 2020 for patients $\geq$2–18 years old with NF1 and symptomatic, inoperable PNs. The success of this therapy has spurred additional trials using selumetinib in adult patients with NF1-associated PNs, and trials utilizing alternative MEK inhibitiors such as trametinib, binimetinib, and mirdimetinib. These trials, some completed and some ongoing, have had subtle differences and varying degrees of efficacy, but as a group have shown remarkable success [57]. Limitations to the usage of MEK inhibitors in the treatment of PNs are not inconsequential and include a minimal tumor response often appreciated by conventional imaging, no complete responses obtained, a third of patients do not respond, and administration of the drug appears to be required over extended time periods, as PNs often become progressive after cessation. Therefore, although very exciting as a new medical therapy for NF1-associated PNs, ongoing work is clearly needed.

The use of tyrosine kinase inhibitors, specifically cabozantinib, has demonstrated activity as well and warrants ongoing investigation. This approach targets the critical role of the tumor microenvironment (TME) in PN formation. A previous study using imatinib mesylate, another tyrosine kinase inhibitor, to treat PNs showed modest success, but primarily in small tumors [58]. Cabozantinib, on the other hand, has demonstrated more success. Cabozantinib is a multiple tyrosine kinase inhibitor which, in preclinical and translational studies, modulated key kinases in the TME in *Nf1*-mutant mice and reduced the PN tumor burden in these mice [59]. Based on this rationale, adolescents and adults with NF1 and progressive or symptomatic unresectable PNs were enrolled in a phase 2 clinical trial for treatment with cabozantinib. In this study, 42% of participants achieved a partial response (PR, defined as $\geq$20% reduction in tumor lesion volume as assessed by MRI), and patients with PR had significant reductions in tumor pain intensity and pain interference in daily life. The medication was reasonably well tolerated, though a significant portion of patients did discontinue it due to low-grade adverse effects [59]. The response rate in this trial was the best rate seen thus far in adults, and future data from treatment of pediatric patients with cabozantinib and adult patients with selumetinib may better allow for comparisons of response to the two agents. Overall, these trials demonstrate monumental potential in another class of agents that are efficacious at increasing TTP, decreasing tumor size, and inducing a clinical benefit in patients with previously poorly remediable tumors. Combination strategies could potentially have even further benefits; investigation into the use of cabozantinib in combination with an MEK inhibitor is planned. With the knowledge gained through these endeavors over the past decade and the success of these two molecularly targeted approaches, a promising era in the treatment of NF1-associated PN has been entered.

2.2. Malignant Peripheral Nerve Sheath Tumors

PNs develop from any peripheral nerve branch or bundle and carry a risk of malignant transformation into an aggressive soft tissue sarcoma, or malignant peripheral nerve sheath tumor (MPNST) [60]. MPNST occurs in patients with and without NF1 but may be associated with worse outcomes in the former group [61]. In NF1, these high-grade tumors can occur sporadically but more often arise from a pre-existing PN. Patients with NF1 have an approximately 10–15% lifetime risk of MPNSTs [61–63]. MPNST is frequently associated with distant metastatic disease and local recurrence [64]. Risk factors for developing MPNST include whole body PN burden, presence of nodular or atypical lesions, prior radiation therapy, and *NF1* microdeletions [61].

The clinical presentation of MPNST is heterogeneous depending on tumor size and location, but patients with severe or refractory pain, new neurologic deficits, rapid growth, or hardening consistency of an existing PN warrant radiologic evaluation [62]. While MRI can be used to determine the location and extent of the tumor and may indicate changes, ^{18}F-fluorodeoxyglucose (FDG)-PET scan has been demonstrated to better distinguish between benign versus malignant tumor, as MPNST will demonstrate increased FDG uptake [62,63]. This can be particularly useful in the setting of a smaller malignant transformation in a larger PN to help direct surgical intervention.

In addition to the prerequisite biallelic inactivation of *NF1*, other somatic alterations contribute to the cancerous behavior of these tumors. Inactivation of other tumor suppressor genes, such as *TP53*, *CDKN2A/B*, *PTEN*, and the polycomb repressor complex 2 (PRC2, containing *EED* and *SUZ12*), and the amplification of growth-promoting genes, such as *EGFR* and *PDGFR*, have been documented [65,66]. Interestingly, alterations in *NF1*, *CDKN2A/B*, and the PRC2 genes are frequently found concurrently in non-NF1-associated MPNST as well, supporting the notion that sequential inactivation of these genes drives the malignant evolution of tumors [66].

Ultimately, disease progression from PN to MPNST involves the stepwise acquisition of additional genetic mutations and chromosomal rearrangements. Atypical neurofibromas (ANs) are indolent, premalignant, nodular lesions that develop from and/or within PNs. A subset of these tumors can be further classified as atypical neurofibromatous neoplasms of uncertain biologic potential (ANNUBP), which share more histologic features with MPNST [67,68]. Deletion in the *CDKN2A/B* gene appears to be the first step in disease progression [69]. Mutations in *SMARCA2* have also been identified, though their role in malignant transformation is not yet known. While not all ANs will fulfill their malignant potential, the approach to treatment involves surgical resection followed by clinical surveillance given the significant risks associated with MPNST [60,70].

Therapeutic options for MPNST remain limited. To date, surgery is the only curative option, though similarly to PNs, this is often limited by the invasive nature of the tumor and frequent involvement of vital surrounding structures [61,66,71]. The goal of surgical resection is complete excision with negative margins if feasible. Significant postoperative morbidity, however, with loss of sensory and/or motor function, particularly when major nerves are involved, is often seen and therefore supports a more cautious surgical approach that removes as much tumor as safely possible while attempting to preserve neurological functions and thus, quality of life [71,72]. Radiation, which again is typically avoided in patients with cancer predisposition syndromes, can be used for local control though it has been observed to delay the time to disease recurrence but not death [62]. Historically, MPNST has not demonstrated a clear response to systemic chemotherapy, but for certain individuals, neoadjuvant agents such as doxorubicin and ifosfamide, which are often used in the treatment of other sarcomas, may be used to shrink the tumor and optimize the feasibility of a gross total surgical resection [64].

Given its aggressive nature, MPNST is frequently associated with difficulty in achieving local control, and thus a poor prognosis. It represents a major cause of morbidity and mortality in patients with NF1 [62,64]. As with PNs and other clinical manifestations of NF1, increased understanding of molecular drivers in MPNST and expanded use of targeted therapies such as MEK inhibitors have paved the way for new therapeutic approaches. Current clinical trials for MPNST include a phase 2 study combining selumetinib and sirolimus for MEK and mTOR inhibition, respectively (NCT03433183). There are several studies combining mTOR inhibitors with other forms of targeted therapy (NCT01661283, NCT02008877, NCT02584647, NCT02601209). The emerging use of immunotherapy has also been integrated into early phase studies, including immune checkpoint inhibitor therapy (nivolumab, a PD-1 inhibitor, and ipilimumab, a CTLA-4 inhibitor [NCT02834013]; pembrolizumab with APG-115 [NCT03611868]); chimeric antigen receptor T-cells targeting EGFR (NCT03618381); and vaccine therapy (NCT02700230). Continued advances in genetic and molecular profiling are expected to provide new insights into tumor development and hopefully, translate to improved methods of detection, diagnosis, and treatment.

2.3. Low-Grade Gliomas

Low-grade gliomas (LGGs) are the most common intracranial tumors in NF1 [73]. The vast majority of these are pilocytic astrocytomas, World Health Organization (WHO) grade I tumors. They can occur almost anywhere in the brain but are most commonly found in the optic pathways or the brainstem [73]. Optic pathway gliomas (OPGs) can affect the optic nerves, chiasm, post-chiasmatic tracts, or radiations, and they can extend to the hypothalamus. They occur in 15–20% of patients with NF1 and typically present prior to 7 years of age [74]. Compared to the general population, NF1-associated OPGs tend to have a more benign course [75]. At least half of OPGs remain asymptomatic [76]. When symptoms do occur, patients can present with strabismus, ptosis, proptosis, pain, pupillary changes, vision changes, hypothalamic disturbances, and rarely, hydrocephalus. In the absence of symptoms, or even in mildly symptomatic cases, intervention for these tumors is most often unnecessary. There are no clear prognostic features to guide when intervention is needed, but suggested risk factors for progression include female sex, age of presentation less than 2 years or greater than 8–10 years, or tumor location in the post-chiasmatic optic pathway [77–79].

Like PNs and other solid tumors, OPGs are products of neoplastic cells with contributions from the TME. NF1-associated OPGs arise from glioma stem cells and astrocytes with bi-allelic inactivation of the *NF1* gene in a microenvironment of stromal cells including microglia, neurons, and endothelial cells haploinsufficient for *NF1*. As with PNs, these haploinsufficient cells are required for tumorigenesis [80]. It is the lack of negative regulation of the Ras signaling pathway by neurofibromin and aberrant signal transduction through the Raf/MEK/MAPK and mTOR signaling pathways, which underlies the development of OPGs [47,81].

Given their indolent course and low risk of progression, observation of OPGs in asymptomatic patients is often the preferred approach to management. Screening MRIs are not recommended, as, in the absence of clinical findings, detection of OPGs on MRI is unlikely to change management [82]. Standard screening in patients with NF1 for OPGs includes annual eye exams by an experienced pediatric ophthalmologist for all patients less than 10 years of age, then at least every two years until 18 years of age [83]. In addition, children with NF1 should undergo yearly height and weight measurements screening for precocious puberty or other evidence of hypothalamic dysfunction [83]. MRI is indicated in children with screening findings suggestive of OPG or potentially in children in whom reliable screening cannot be performed. Once an OPG is identified, increased ophthalmologic evaluation and MRI evaluations are indicated, though there is no consensus on timing interval [83]. MRI progression and visual outcomes do not clearly correlate; therefore, radiographic progression alone is often not an indication for therapy in NF1 patients [84]. When intervention is required, options remain focused on chemotherapy. Surgery may have a role when vision has already been lost in the affected eye or to treat specific ophthalmologic issues such as corneal exposure, but otherwise surgery is avoided as the goal of therapy is to maintain vision [83]. Radiation therapy to the tumor in this population is generally avoided due to the risk of secondary malignancy and the risk of moyamoya syndrome in patients with NF1 [85]. When indicated, first-line therapy for NF1-associated OPG is typically conventional cytotoxic chemotherapy, most often with carboplatin and vincristine [86]. Chemotherapy is effective at halting tumor progression in the majority of cases, but this may come with substantial systemic side effects [87]. Excitingly, OPGs have also shown encouraging response to MEK inhibition. In a phase 2 study treating patients with NF1-associated pediatric LGGs with selumetinib, 40% of patients achieved a sustained partial response, 96% of patients had 2 years of progression free survival, and the medication was overall well tolerated during the study [88]. Given this robust result, a phase 3 non-inferiority trial by the Children's Oncology Group is now underway, comparing carboplatin and vincristine to selumetinib monotherapy (NCAT03871257).

2.4. High-Grade Gliomas

While LGGs affecting the optic pathway and other intracranial structures predominate, patients with NF1 also have an estimated fifty-fold increased risk of developing high-grade gliomas (HGGs) compared to unaffected individuals [66,89,90]. HGGs, which include glioblastoma, anaplastic astrocytoma, and other histologic subtypes, typically present after the age of 10 years with most cases occurring in adulthood [66,89,90]. These tumors tend to affect the cerebral hemispheres and are more likely to be symptomatic than low-grade tumors [60,91].

Advances in molecular profiling and the overall understanding of tumor biology support the morphologic evolution from LGGs to HGGs with accumulation of additional somatic mutations [92]. In addition to the germline *NF1* mutation, a somatic mutation of the second *NF1* allele is common but not required for tumorigenesis. Based on genomic analysis of 59 NF1-associated glioma samples from pediatric and adult patients, HGGs were frequently found to have higher mutational burdens with abnormalities in *TP53* and *CDKN2A*, along with inactivation of *ATRX*, which appears to correlate with more aggressive clinical behavior [89,90]. DNA methylation is an emerging factor in the classification of brain tumors and potentially in NF1-associated gliomas as well [92]. Notably, hallmark mutations in the *IDH* genes or H3.3 histone genes which are found in sporadic pediatric gliomas have not been identified in NF1-associated HGGs [91,93].

The current treatment approach remains similar to that of sporadic cases, centering around surgical resection, adjuvant radiation, and chemotherapy such as temozolomide [62,91]. Though data are limited, largely by the rarity of the diagnosis, HGGs carry a poor prognosis with an overall survival of 50–60 weeks in adults and only slightly better in children [93,94].

3. Neurofibromatosis Type 2

Neurofibromatosis type 2 (NF2) is less common than NF1, affecting 1 in 25,000 individuals worldwide [95]. Individuals with NF2 are at risk for a variety of nervous system tumors including peripheral and central schwannomas, particularly vestibular schwannomas (affecting cranial nerve VIII), multiple meningiomas, and ependymomas. Affected individuals are also at risk for ocular manifestations such as juvenile posterior subcapsular cataracts and epiretinal membranes which can affect vision. Most of the tumors associated with NF2 are histologically benign in appearance but are clearly associated with significant patient morbidity given their number and often persistent growth over time. Malignant transformation of tumors is typically not seen, except in instances where patients have undergone prior irradiation [96,97].

NF2 is the result of a pathologic variant in the *NF2* gene, and the pathogenic variants result in loss of function of merlin, the protein product of the *NF2* gene. A member of the ERM (erzin/radixin/moesin) family of scaffolding proteins, merlin has been implicated in several cell signaling cascades, including the Ras/MAPK, FAK/SRC, PI3K/AKT and the HIPPO signaling cascades (Figure 2). The specific pathways involved in the development of the tumors in NF2 have not been clearly delineated. Loss of heterozygosity of *NF2* is required for tumor development, in keeping with its known tumor suppressor function, but other cooperating mutations may be necessary [98]. Patients with truncating mutations in the *NF2* gene often present with more severe disease at younger ages while patients with missense mutations will often have a milder course with tumors which are slower to progress [99]. NF2 is inherited in an autosomal dominant manner, however, 50% of newly diagnosed patients represent de novo mutations. Of these proband patients, a significant number will be mosaic for the *NF2* pathologic variant and may not be able to be identified by blood genetic testing even when they met the diagnostic criteria [100]. The Manchester Criteria for NF2 remains the standard for clinical diagnosis and was most recently updated in 2017 to exclude *LZTR1* pathologic variants [101]. The clinical diagnostic criteria include bilateral vestibular schwannomas (prior to age 70); or a known first-degree family member with NF2 and either a unilateral vestibular schwannoma or two or more meningiomas, cataracts, schwannomas, or cerebral calcifications. Alternatively, the diagnosis can also be made with a documented *NF2* pathologic variant along with either a unilateral vestibular schwannoma or two other distinct tumors. Surgical resection of the tumor, when feasible, remains the mainstay of therapy for the majority of patients with NF2, with the goal of minimizing tumor-associated symptoms. Given the work to identify the signaling cascades involved in the development of NF2-associated tumors, however, a number of clinical trials aimed at identifying a potential medical therapy have been undertaken with varied success.

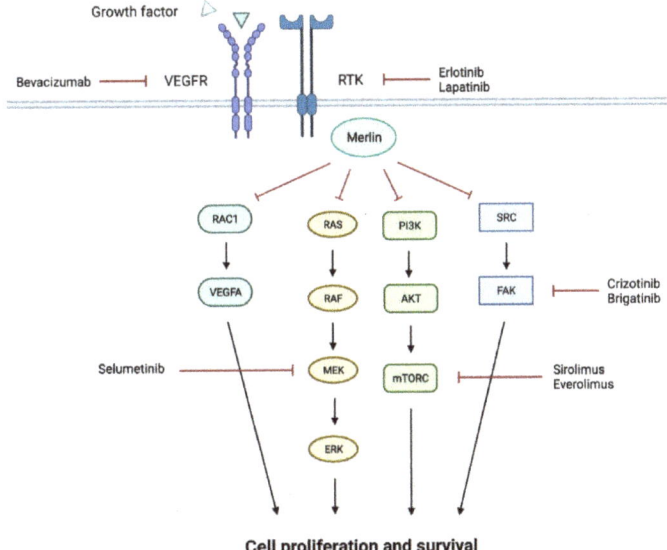

Figure 2. Simplified schema of the signaling pathways implicated in tumor formation with loss of merlin, the protein product of *NF2*. Therapies utilized to target these activated pathways are noted. This figure was created with Biorender.com (accessed on 19 October 2021).

3.1. Vestibular Schwannomas

Vestibular schwannomas are the most common intracranial tumor in patients with NF2, affecting up to 90% of individuals and are a significant cause of morbidity. Bilateral vestibular schwannomas are classically associated with a diagnosis of NF2, although bilateral disease may not be present at diagnosis in all patients [102]. Vestibular schwannomas arise from either branch of cranial nerve VIII and can lead to hearing loss, vestibular dysfunction, facial nerve palsies and ultimately brainstem compression. Patients with NF2 have been demonstrated to have numerous tumor nodules along the nerve, indicating that vestibular schwannomas in this population are likely composed of multiple tumor nodules instead of one discrete tumor, thereby complicating surgical resection. The size of the vestibular schwannoma does not correlate with hearing loss, supporting alternative mechanisms besides tumor compression of the nerve as the etiology of hearing loss [103,104].

Overall, the primary goal of therapy is to attempt to prolong functional hearing for as long as feasible. Therefore, surgical resection of NF2-associated vestibular schwannomas is usually considered in the setting of hearing sparing surgery, for progressive tumors once hearing has been lost or in the setting of any brainstem compression [105]. The use of radiation therapy (radiosurgery), a common therapy for sporadic vestibular schwannomas, has declined in patients with NF2. Although radiation therapy does result in tumor growth control, it has been associated with a small risk of malignant transformation [97] and poor hearing outcomes with less than half of patients demonstrating preserved hearing at 5 years [106,107]. At this time, there are limited data on the use of proton-based radiation therapy for NF2-associated vestibular schwannomas, although it is not likely to be significantly different than conventional or radiosurgery-based approaches in terms of hearing preservation. Given these limited options, the identification of medical therapy which cannot only control tumor growth but preserve hearing function has been a high priority for the NF2 care community. Conventional chemotherapy has not been demonstrated to be effective for NF2-associated vestibular schwannomas, and therefore many trials have focused on inhibition of potential NF2-associated molecular pathways. Table 1 summarizes several recent NF2-associated vestibular schwannoma clinic trials including the agents utilized, primary outcomes, enrollment, and results. Bevacizumab has been overall the most successfully utilized and reported, but several agents have demonstrated some preliminary activity.

One of the earliest signaling cascades to be identified as a potential therapeutic target was the mammalian target of rapamycin complex 1 (mTORC1). Loss of merlin results in activation of mTORC1 signaling and resultant cell growth [108]. Inhibition of mTORC1 by rapamycin resulted in decreased growth of merlin deficient Schwann cells both in vitro and in vivo in preclinical testing [109]. Two phase 2 clinical trials with the rapamycin analog, everolimus, were undertaken. Neither study demonstrated a radiographic response (tumor shrinkage of >20%) or hearing improvement in patients with NF2-associated vestibular schwannomas [110]. Time to radiographic progression of the vestibular schwannomas was improved, however, from a median of 4.2 months to more than 12 months [111]. Subsequent evaluation of tumor tissue from a phase 0 trial with everolimus indicated incomplete inhibition of the target pathway in the tumor even when blood levels were adequate, which may explain the minimal clinical response [112].

Lapatinib, an oral epidermal growth factor receptor (EGFR) and Erb2 inhibitor, has also demonstrated activity in NF2. Lapatinib was identified for potential use for NF2-associated vestibular schwannomas due to increased expression of both EGFR and Erb2 in tumor tissue and inhibited proliferation in schwannoma cell lines [113]. A phase 2 clinical trial of lapatinib in patients with NF2 and progressive vestibular schwannomas was undertaken with a primary tumor response endpoint of >15% volumetric reduction. Twenty-one patients were enrolled with 17 of them evaluable for radiographic response. Four of the 17 (23.5%) had tumor volumetric shrinkage of 15.7–23.9% over the therapy course with one response durable beyond 9 months. Hearing was assessed as a secondary aim and 4 of 13 patients (30%) had improvement in word recognition scores [114]. Overall, lapatinib was well tolerated in this patient population and demonstrated some activity. Although no future trials are currently planned with lapatinib, it remains a potential agent for use in NF2-associated vestibular schwannomas.

Table 1. Recent clinical trials assessing targeted therapy for NF2-associated vestibular schwannomas with intended targets, phases of therapy, endpoints, and references.

Drug Name	Therapy Target	Phase Trial/Number of Patients Enrolled	Notable Endpoints	Further Studies Planned	References
Erlotinib	Epidermal Growth Factor Receptor (EGFR)	Phase 2–10 Patients	3/10 with minimal radiographic response	No	Plotkin et al., 2010 [115]
Everolimus	Mammalian Target of Rapamycin (mTOR)	Phase 2–9 Patients	No radiographic or hearing responses. Prolonged time to progression	No	Karajannis et al., 2014 [110]; Goutagny et al., 2015 [111]
Lapatinib	EGFR and Erb2	Phase 2–21 patients (17 evaluable)	4/17 with >15% size reduction 4/13 with improved hearing	Unclear	Karajannis et al., 2012 [114]
Bevacizumab	Vascular Endothelial Growth Factor Receptor (VEGFR)	Phase 2, multiple studies (>100 patients reported)	RR in 41% Hearing improvement in 20% TTP improvement	No	Lu et al., 2019 [116]; Plotkin et al., 2012 [117]; 2019 [118]; Blakeley et al., 2016 [119]
Crizotinib/Brigatinib	Focal Adhesion Kinase (FAK1)	Phase 2, ongoing	Volumetric response as primary aim, hearing secondary	Ongoing	N/A

Aspirin as a modulator of growth of vestibular schwannomas has conflicting reports of efficacy. Vestibular schwannomas, including NF2-associated vestibular schwannomas, have been noted to express COX-2, and the degree of expression correlates with proliferation, indicating that COX-2 inhibition with aspirin might be a viable therapeutic [120]. Initial retrospective analysis of patients with sporadic vestibular schwannomas on aspirin for other indications indicated slower growth rates for those on aspirin [121]. More recent retrospective studies have not supported this correlation, and currently compelling data to recommend aspirin therapy for patients have not been reported [122,123]. To better define a potential role for aspirin, a phase 2 clinical trial for both NF2 and sporadic tumors is currently ongoing (NCT03079999).

The most successful and well reported medical therapy to date for patients with progressive or symptomatic vestibular schwannomas is bevacizumab. Prior work demonstrated increased vascular endothelial growth factor (VEGF) expression in NF2-associated vestibular schwannomas, and initial studies utilizing bevacizumab demonstrated both decreased tumor volume and hearing improvement in a subset of patients [117,119]. Overall, a recent meta-analysis reviewing eight studies covering 161 patients reported both prolonged time to tumor progression and to hearing loss [116]. Bevacizumab is currently considered the first line medical therapy for NF2-associated vestibular schwannomas in the setting of either hearing decline or tumor progression. Of note, pediatric patients may receive less benefit from bevacizumab than do older patients, and there is no clear benefit to the higher dose of 10 mg/kg than the lower doses of 5–7.5 mg/kg every 3 weeks [118]. As the duration of therapy may need to be prolonged, lower dosing regimens may be preferred as they may have a lower risk of toxicities, particularly renal impairment [124].

Both identification of novel potential therapeutic agents and clinical trials are ongoing for vestibular schwannomas. Two trials are currently ongoing to assess the impact of inhibition of alternative NF2-associated signaling cascade molecules such as focal adhesion kinase 1 (FAK1) and EphA2 by utilizing the FDA-approved ALK inhibitors, crizotinib and brigatinib. Crizotinib was identified via drug screening in a preclinical *NF2*-deficient cell line and xenograph testing [125]. Crizotinib inhibited tumor formation by inhibition of focal adhesion kinase 1 (FAK1) and is current being tested in a phase 2 trial for progressive NF2-associated vestibular schwannomas (NCT04283669). Brigatinib was identified as a potential therapeutic target for both meningiomas and vestibular schwannomas as part of a coordinated high throughput screen and in vivo mouse modeling/xenograph testing [126]. Brigatinib inhibits several tyrosine kinases including EphA2 and FAK1 and is also currently undergoing phase 2 clinical testing (NCT04374305). A second signaling pathway currently undergoing clinical trial evaluation is the Ras/extracellular signal-regulated kinase (ERK) cascade with inhibition of MEK [127]. Loss of merlin has been associated with activation of the Ras/ERK signaling cascade. In a mouse model, inhibition of this activation with MEK inhibitors resulted in decreased growth of schwannoma cells and decreased tumor burden and average tumor size [128]. A phase 2 trial of the MEK inhibitor, selumetinib, for progressive NF2-associated tumors is currently ongoing (NCT03095248).

3.2. Meningiomas

Meningiomas are the second most common tumor identified in patients with NF2, found intracranially in approximately 45–80% of patients and in the spinal axis in 20%. The development of multiple meningiomas is a hallmark of the disease [129,130]. Loss of *NF2* or instability of chromosome 22 is a frequent feature of sporadic meningiomas as well [131]. Surgical resection continues to be the mainstay of therapy for progressive or symptomatic tumors. Radiation and radiosurgery have also been utilized, but long-term outcome measures have been limited. As with vestibular schwannomas, therapeutic trials have leveraged known NF2 signaling cascades but with only limited success. Unlike NF2-associated vestibular schwannomas, bevacizumab has been demonstrated to have limited benefit, with only a subset of patients demonstrating radiographic response which appears to be of limited duration [132,133]. Retrospective analysis of 8 patients with meningiomas treated on the lapatinib trial for progressive vestibular schwannomas demonstrated slower volumetric growth rates of the meningioma while on the medication when compared to off therapy [134]. Analysis of 6 meningiomas in patients with NF2 who were treated with everolimus for progressive vestibular schwannomas showed prolonged time to progression of the meningiomas from 5.5 months pretreatment to more than 12 months on therapy. No tumor shrinkage was seen [111]. The combination of bevacizumab and everolimus for recurrent meningiomas, though not specifically in patients with NF2, resulted in stable disease for the majority of patients and performed similarly to bevacizumab alone [135]. The phase 2 CEVOREM trial for recurrent meningiomas utilizing everolimus and octreotide, given the strong expression of the sst2 somatostatin receptor in meningiomas, also included patients with NF2. This study reported a decrease in median growth rates of the meningioma from 16.6% over 3 months prior to study inclusion to 0.02% in the first 3 months and 0.48% in the second [136]. A recent trial utilizing the dual mTORC1/mTORC2 inhibitor AZD2014 for patients with NF2 with progressive or symptomatic meningiomas had a significant number of patients withdraw prior to study completion due to intolerable side effects (NCT02831257). Clearly, further research is necessary for this group of patients.

3.3. Ependymomas

Development of ependymomas, particularly in the cervical cord or cervicomedullary junction, is also a common finding in patients with NF2, and multiple ependymomas are found in over 50% of patients [137]. The majority of ependymomas associated with NF2 appear to be asymptomatic and exhibit indolent growth. Therefore, a conservative management approach with observation is usually taken. Symptoms develop in approximately 20% of patients with NF2. In these patients, surgical resection, if feasible without significant morbidity, is the primary therapy approach and may be associated with improved neurologic outcome [138]. For patients with symptomatic tumors and no surgical options, bevacizumab has been reported to improve symptoms and has also been shown to lead to radiographic response in some [139,140]. Given their limited morbidity for the majority of patients, fewer therapeutic clinical trials have focused on NF2-associated ependymomas.

4. Schwannomatosis

Schwannomatosis is less common, less well studied, and less well understood compared to NF1 and NF2. The general incidence for schwannomatosis is 1 in 40,000, and most patients are diagnosed in their third and fourth decades of life. Schwannomotosis is characterized by the development of multiple non-intradermal schwannomas, and in 5% of patients, meningiomas. Patients with schwannomatosis often present with neurological symptoms—classically chronic pain, which can be either focal or diffuse. Although there is a phenotypic overlap with NF2, two distinct genes have been identified for schwannomatosis, *SMARCB1* and *LZTR1*. These are inherited in an autosomal dominant fashion but with incomplete penetrance, and less than 20% of patients have a known family history of the disease. At this time, there is no medical therapy for the treatment of the tumors associated with schwannomatosis. Therapy is often focused on treatment of the associated pain, typically with gabapentin and/or tricyclic antidepressants. Surgical resection can also be utilized for uncontrolled pain, with the goal of preserving neurologic function. The size of the schwannoma does not appear to correlate with degree of pain, although patients with *LZTR1* pathologic variants have been reported to have increased pain. Current clinical trials focus on pain management, with one study utilizing tanezumab, a monoclonal antibody to nerve growth factor (NGF), as NGF has been implicated as a mediator of pain (NCT04163419). Hopefully, as research progresses in this poorly understood disease, more therapies will be identified.

5. Conclusions

Patients with neurofibromatosis are at clear risk for tumor development and subsequent associated morbidity and mortality. While malignant NF-associated tumors, particularly MPNSTs and HGGs in NF1, exhibit clinical behavior similar to their sporadic counterparts, the benign NF-associated lesions often have a distinct, potentially more indolent natural history. This clinical behavior, coupled with the risk of developing multiple tumors over time, has shifted the focus to symptomatic treatment for the majority of these tumors. When symptomatic, however, therapeutic options remain quite limited. With only one FDA-approved therapy for NF1, no approved therapies for NF2 or schwannomatosis, and significant limitations to conventional therapeutic options in general, novel agents are greatly needed. In this review, we have focused on the identification of molecularly targeted therapies which leverage the known signaling aberrations associated with each of these disorders. Although progress has been made, the need for more tumor-directed therapies with tolerable short and long-term toxicities is clear. Given the complexity of the signaling pathways involved, it is probable that combination therapy will be necessary—although concern arises about therapy-related toxicities given the likely need for prolonged therapy.

Additionally, the NF community has made a more coordinated approach to collaborate and accelerate therapy recommendations and develop more clinical trials. Several consortia have formed to design consensus recommendations and identify targets to streamline NF-focused clinical trials. Since 2006, the Department of Defense, as part of the Congressionally Mandated Research Program, has supported a National Neurofibromatosis Clinical Trials Consortium (NFCTC). The NFCTC is focused on designing and performing clinical trials for NF patients. To date, the NFCTC has undertaken 15 trials: 4 focused on PNs, 3 on LGGs, 4 on MPNSTs, and 2 for NF2-associated vestibular schwannomas. The consortium currently has 15 primary sites and 10 affiliate sites across the United States and one in Australia. The Children's Tumor Foundation has likewise supported a Neurofibromatosis Preclinical Consortium to consistently evaluate potential therapeutic targets. Utilizing genetically engineered mouse models of tumor specific manifestations of both NF1 and NF2, and appropriate cell lines, the preclinical consortium has focused on screening and testing potential therapeutic options of reach tumor type. To date, mouse (and some zebrafish) models of MPNSTs, PNs, and OPGs have been developed for NF1 while a vestibular schwannoma model has been developed for NF2 [141–143]. Although rodent model systems have been extremely beneficial for understanding the mechanisms of tumor formation, they have been less consistent as models for the multiple manifestations of disease or as preclinical tests of potential therapeutic targets. To improve the translatability of findings to clinical use, more recent efforts have focused on development of more relevant animal modeling systems, such as a minipig NF1 model, or on more in-depth analysis of human-derived tumors for target identification [144,145]. Included in these efforts are the Children's Tumor Foundation developed series of Synodos programs: collaborations between multidisciplinary team members focused on identifying potential therapeutic targets and bringing novel therapeutics forward in an open data sharing approach. Four groups have been formed to date and include (1) a group focused on identification of molecular targets in NF1-associated gliomas by sequencing analysis of patient samples, (2) a group trying to accelerate preclinical testing in NF1 by development of a minipig model of NF1, a closer to human model system, (3) a group trying to identify therapies for NF2-associated complications by utilizing both cell and animal model systems for screening (which identified Brigitinib as a potential therapy), and (4) a group focused on improving therapy for schwannomatosis by undertaking molecular analysis of patient-derived tumors. The overall goal of this program is acceleration of drug discovery and translation to clinical trials.

Given the complexity of NF-associated tumors, including their unique natural histories and indications for therapy, the standard imaging response, i.e., tumor shrinkage, has been recognized as potentially not an ideal representation of agent efficacy or clinical improvement in this patient population. In response, an international group was formed in 2011—the Response Evaluation in Neurofibromatosis and Schwannomatosis (REiNS) International Collaboration, with the goal of identifying improved endpoints, particularly for clinical trial design, which better reflect the clinical need in this patient population. The group currently includes seven working groups, five of which are focused on outcome measures, including tumor imaging, functional, visual, patient reported, and neurocognitive outcomes. The other two groups examine whole body MRI and disease biomarkers. REiNS has published several recommendations regarding NF-associated outcome measures—such as visual acuity for OPGs and volumetric imaging for PNs—for trials to give better consideration to long term clinical benefits [146,147].

Overall, therapeutic approaches to NF-associated tumors cannot simply be modeled after sporadic counterparts, particularly for the benign tumors associated with these disorders. The unique role of the microenvironment in tumor development, the window of risk during development, and the risk for the formation of multiple tumors require a unique clinical response which prioritizes clinical outcomes and symptom management. This need has resulted in numerous clinical trials aimed not only at tumor control but evaluation of clinically relevant outcome measures such as pain, hearing, and functional outcomes. Ongoing research into the aberrant signaling cascades and the interactions of these cascades will continue to identify potential therapeutic targets which may improve patient outcomes. A landmark FDA-approved therapy has been achieved for NF1-associated PNs, but similar success for NF2 and schwannomatosis is still needed.

Author Contributions: Conceptualization, L.J.K. software, L.J.K. and A.B.; validation, L.D.S., A.B. and L.J.K.; writing—original draft preparation, L.D.S., A.B. and L.J.K. writing—review and editing, L.D.S., A.B. and L.J.K.; visualization, L.D.S., A.B. and L.J.K.; supervision, L.J.K.; project administration, L.J.K.; funding acquisition, L.J.K. All authors have read and agreed to the published version of the manuscript.

Funding: This research received no external funding. L.J.K is supported by the Dedman Family Scholar in Clinical Care.

Conflicts of Interest: L.J.K. has served on a medical advisory board for AstraZeneca.

References

1. Friedman, J.M. Epidemiology of neurofibromatosis type 1. *Am. J. Med. Genet.* **1999**, *89*, 1–6. [CrossRef]
2. Shannon, K.M.; O'Connell, P.; Martin, G.A.; Paderanga, D.; Olson, K.; Dinndorf, P.; McCormick, F. Loss of the normal NF1 allele from the bone marrow of children with type 1 neurofibromatosis and malignant myeloid disorders. *N. Engl. J. Med.* **1994**, *330*, 597–601. [CrossRef] [PubMed]
3. Stiller, C.A.; Chessells, J.M.; Fitchett, M. Neurofibromatosis and childhood leukaemia/lymphoma: A population-based UKCCSG study. *Br. J. Cancer* **1994**, *70*, 969–972. [CrossRef] [PubMed]
4. Seminog, O.O.; Goldacre, M.J. Risk of benign tumours of nervous system, and of malignant neoplasms, in people with neurofibromatosis: Population-based record-linkage study. *Br. J. Cancer* **2013**, *108*, 193–198. [CrossRef]
5. Zinnamosca, L.; Petramala, L.; Cotesta, D.; Marinelli, C.; Schina, M.; Cianci, R.; Giustini, S.; Sciomer, S.; Anastasi, E.; Calvieri, S.; et al. Neurofibromatosis type 1 (NF1) and pheochromocytoma: Prevalence, clinical and cardiovascular aspects. *Arch. Dermatol. Res.* **2011**, *303*, 317–325. [CrossRef]
6. Giuly, J.A.; Picand, R.; Giuly, D.; Monges, B.; Nguyen-Cat, R. Von Recklinghausen disease and gastrointestinal stromal tumors. *Am. J. Surg.* **2003**, *185*, 86–87. [CrossRef]
7. Takazawa, Y.; Sakurai, S.; Sakuma, Y.; Ikeda, T.; Yamaguchi, J.; Hashizume, Y.; Yokoyama, S.; Motegi, A.; Fukayama, M. Gastrointestinal stromal tumors of neurofibromatosis type I (von Recklinghausen's disease). *Am. J. Surg. Pathol.* **2005**, *29*, 755–763. [CrossRef]
8. Yantiss, R.K.; Rosenberg, A.E.; Sarran, L.; Besmer, P.; Antonescu, C.R. Multiple gastrointestinal stromal tumors in type I neurofibromatosis: A pathologic and molecular study. *Mod. Pathol.* **2005**, *18*, 475–484. [CrossRef]
9. Miettinen, M.; Fetsch, J.F.; Sobin, L.H.; Lasota, J. Gastrointestinal stromal tumors in patients with neurofibromatosis 1: A clinicopathologic and molecular genetic study of 45 cases. *Am. J. Surg. Pathol.* **2006**, *30*, 90–96. [CrossRef]
10. Daston, M.M.; Ratner, N. Neurofibromin, a predominantly neuronal GTPase activating protein in the adult, is ubiquitously expressed during development. *Dev. Dyn.* **1992**, *195*, 216–226. [CrossRef]
11. Daston, M.M.; Scrable, H.; Nordlund, M.; Sturbaum, A.K.; Nissen, L.M.; Ratner, N. The protein product of the neurofibromatosis type 1 gene is expressed at highest abundance in neurons, Schwann cells, and oligodendrocytes. *Neuron* **1992**, *8*, 415–428. [CrossRef]
12. Cimino, P.J.; Gutmann, D.H. Neurofibromatosis type 1. *Handb. Clin. Neurol.* **2018**, *148*, 799–811. [CrossRef]
13. Bergoug, M.; Doudeau, M.; Godin, F.; Mosrin, C.; Vallee, B.; Benedetti, H. Neurofibromin Structure, Functions and Regulation. *Cells* **2020**, *9*, 2365. [CrossRef] [PubMed]

14. Lauchle, J.O.; Kim, D.; Le, D.T.; Akagi, K.; Crone, M.; Krisman, K.; Warner, K.; Bonifas, J.M.; Li, Q.; Coakley, K.M.; et al. Response and resistance to MEK inhibition in leukaemias initiated by hyperactive Ras. *Nature* **2009**, *461*, 411–414. [CrossRef] [PubMed]
15. Zhu, Y.; Ghosh, P.; Charnay, P.; Burns, D.K.; Parada, L.F. Neurofibromas in NF1: Schwann cell origin and role of tumor environment. *Science* **2002**, *296*, 920–922. [CrossRef]
16. Mautner, V.F.; Asuagbor, F.A.; Dombi, E.; Funsterer, C.; Kluwe, L.; Wenzel, R.; Widemann, B.C.; Friedman, J.M. Assessment of benign tumor burden by whole-body MRI in patients with neurofibromatosis 1. *Neuro Oncol.* **2008**, *10*, 593–598. [CrossRef]
17. Korf, B.R. Plexiform neurofibromas. *Am. J. Med. Genet.* **1999**, *89*, 31–37. [CrossRef]
18. Ruggieri, M.; Huson, S.M. The clinical and diagnostic implications of mosaicism in the neurofibromatoses. *Neurology* **2001**, *56*, 1433–1443. [CrossRef]
19. Tucker, T.; Friedman, J.M.; Friedrich, R.E.; Wenzel, R.; Funsterer, C.; Mautner, V.F. Longitudinal study of neurofibromatosis 1 associated plexiform neurofibromas. *J. Med. Genet.* **2009**, *46*, 81–85. [CrossRef]
20. Gross, A.M.; Singh, G.; Akshintala, S.; Baldwin, A.; Dombi, E.; Ukwuani, S.; Goodwin, A.; Liewehr, D.J.; Steinberg, S.M.; Widemann, B.C. Association of plexiform neurofibroma volume changes and development of clinical morbidities in neurofibromatosis 1. *Neuro Oncol.* **2018**, *20*, 1643–1651. [CrossRef]
21. Nguyen, R.; Kluwe, L.; Fuenster, C.; Kentsch, M.; Friedrich, R.E.; Mautner, V.F. Plexiform neurofibromas in children with neurofibromatosis type 1: Frequency and associated clinical deficits. *J. Pediatr.* **2011**, *159*, 652–655.e652. [CrossRef] [PubMed]
22. Ratner, N.; Miller, S.J. A RASopathy gene commonly mutated in cancer: The neurofibromatosis type 1 tumour suppressor. *Nat. Rev. Cancer* **2015**, *15*, 290–301. [CrossRef] [PubMed]
23. Packer, R.J.; Gutmann, D.H.; Rubenstein, A.; Viskochil, D.; Zimmerman, R.A.; Vezina, G.; Small, J.; Korf, B. Plexiform neurofibromas in NF1: Toward biologic-based therapy. *Neurology* **2002**, *58*, 1461–1470. [CrossRef]
24. Ballester, R.; Marchuk, D.; Boguski, M.; Saulino, A.; Letcher, R.; Wigler, M.; Collins, F. The NF1 locus encodes a protein functionally related to mammalian GAP and yeast IRA proteins. *Cell* **1990**, *63*, 851–859. [CrossRef]
25. Kopelovich, L.; Rich, R.F. Enhanced radiotolerance to ionizing radiation is correlated with increased cancer proneness of cultured fibroblasts from precursor states in neurofibromatosis patients. *Cancer Genet. Cytogenet.* **1986**, *22*, 203–210. [CrossRef]
26. Ingram, D.A.; Yang, F.C.; Travers, J.B.; Wenning, M.J.; Hiatt, K.; New, S.; Hood, A.; Shannon, K.; Williams, D.A.; Clapp, D.W. Genetic and biochemical evidence that haploinsufficiency of the Nf1 tumor suppressor gene modulates melanocyte and mast cell fates in vivo. *J. Exp. Med.* **2000**, *191*, 181–188. [CrossRef]
27. Perosio, P.M.; Brooks, J.J. Expression of growth factors and growth factor receptors in soft tissue tumors. Implications for the autocrine hypothesis. *Lab. Investig.* **1989**, *60*, 245–253.
28. DeClue, J.E.; Heffelfinger, S.; Benvenuto, G.; Ling, B.; Li, S.; Rui, W.; Vass, W.C.; Viskochil, D.; Ratner, N. Epidermal growth factor receptor expression in neurofibromatosis type 1-related tumors and NF1 animal models. *J. Clin. Investig.* **2000**, *105*, 1233–1241. [CrossRef] [PubMed]
29. Gutmann, D.H.; Blakeley, J.O.; Korf, B.R.; Packer, R.J. Optimizing biologically targeted clinical trials for neurofibromatosis. *Expert. Opin. Investig. Drugs* **2013**, *22*, 443–462. [CrossRef]
30. Wentworth, S.; Pinn, M.; Bourland, J.D.; Deguzman, A.F.; Ekstrand, K.; Ellis, T.L.; Glazier, S.S.; McMullen, K.P.; Munley, M.; Stieber, V.W.; et al. Clinical experience with radiation therapy in the management of neurofibromatosis-associated central nervous system tumors. *Int. J. Radiat. Oncol. Biol. Phys.* **2009**, *73*, 208–213. [CrossRef]
31. Vetrano, I.G.; Acerbi, F.; Falco, J.; Devigili, G.; Rinaldo, S.; Messina, G.; Prada, F.; D'Ammando, A.; Nazzi, V. Fluorescein-guided removal of peripheral nerve sheath tumors: A preliminary analysis of 20 cases. *J. Neurosurg.* **2019**, *134*, 260–269. [CrossRef]
32. Needle, M.N.; Cnaan, A.; Dattilo, J.; Chatten, J.; Phillips, P.C.; Shochat, S.; Sutton, L.N.; Vaughan, S.N.; Zackai, E.H.; Zhao, H.; et al. Prognostic signs in the surgical management of plexiform neurofibroma: The Children's Hospital of Philadelphia experience, 1974–1994. *J. Pediatr.* **1997**, *131*, 678–682. [CrossRef]
33. Riccardi, V.M. Mast-cell stabilization to decrease neurofibroma growth. Preliminary experience with ketotifen. *Arch. Dermatol.* **1987**, *123*, 1011–1016. [CrossRef]
34. Riccardi, V.M. A controlled multiphase trial of ketotifen to minimize neurofibroma-associated pain and itching. *Arch. Dermatol.* **1993**, *129*, 577–581. [CrossRef] [PubMed]
35. Gupta, A.; Cohen, B.H.; Ruggieri, P.; Packer, R.J.; Phillips, P.C. Phase I study of thalidomide for the treatment of plexiform neurofibroma in neurofibromatosis 1. *Neurology* **2003**, *60*, 130–132. [CrossRef]
36. Gurujeyalakshmi, G.; Hollinger, M.A.; Giri, S.N. Pirfenidone inhibits PDGF isoforms in bleomycin hamster model of lung fibrosis at the translational level. *Am. J. Physiol.* **1999**, *276*, L311–L318. [CrossRef] [PubMed]
37. Iyer, S.N.; Gurujeyalakshmi, G.; Giri, S.N. Effects of pirfenidone on procollagen gene expression at the transcriptional level in bleomycin hamster model of lung fibrosis. *J. Pharmacol. Exp. Ther.* **1999**, *289*, 211–218.
38. Widemann, B.C.; Babovic-Vuksanovic, D.; Dombi, E.; Wolters, P.L.; Goldman, S.; Martin, S.; Goodwin, A.; Goodspeed, W.; Kieran, M.W.; Cohen, B.; et al. Phase II trial of pirfenidone in children and young adults with neurofibromatosis type 1 and progressive plexiform neurofibromas. *Pediatr. Blood Cancer* **2014**, *61*, 1598–1602. [CrossRef] [PubMed]
39. Jakacki, R.I.; Dombi, E.; Steinberg, S.M.; Goldman, S.; Kieran, M.W.; Ullrich, N.J.; Pollack, I.F.; Goodwin, A.; Manley, P.E.; Fangusaro, J.; et al. Phase II trial of pegylated interferon alfa-2b in young patients with neurofibromatosis type 1 and unresectable plexiform neurofibromas. *Neuro Oncol.* **2017**, *19*, 289–297. [CrossRef]
40. Satoh, T.; Kaziro, Y. Ras in signal transduction. *Semin. Cancer Biol.* **1992**, *3*, 169–177.

41. Cichowski, K.; Jacks, T. NF1 tumor suppressor gene function: Narrowing the GAP. *Cell* **2001**, *104*, 593–604. [CrossRef]
42. Weiss, B.; Bollag, G.; Shannon, K. Hyperactive Ras as a therapeutic target in neurofibromatosis type 1. *Am. J. Med. Genet.* **1999**, *89*, 14–22. [CrossRef]
43. End, D.W. Farnesyl protein transferase inhibitors and other therapies targeting the Ras signal transduction pathway. *Invest. New Drugs* **1999**, *17*, 241–258. [CrossRef]
44. Widemann, B.C.; Dombi, E.; Gillespie, A.; Wolters, P.L.; Belasco, J.; Goldman, S.; Korf, B.R.; Solomon, J.; Martin, S.; Salzer, W.; et al. Phase 2 randomized, flexible crossover, double-blinded, placebo-controlled trial of the farnesyltransferase inhibitor tipifarnib in children and young adults with neurofibromatosis type 1 and progressive plexiform neurofibromas. *Neuro Oncol.* **2014**, *16*, 707–718. [CrossRef] [PubMed]
45. Rowinsky, E.K.; Windle, J.J.; Von Hoff, D.D. Ras protein farnesyltransferase: A strategic target for anticancer therapeutic development. *J. Clin. Oncol.* **1999**, *17*, 3631–3652. [CrossRef] [PubMed]
46. Mendoza, M.C.; Er, E.E.; Blenis, J. The Ras-ERK and PI3K-mTOR pathways: Cross-talk and compensation. *Trends Biochem. Sci.* **2011**, *36*, 320–328. [CrossRef] [PubMed]
47. Dasgupta, B.; Yi, Y.; Chen, D.Y.; Weber, J.D.; Gutmann, D.H. Proteomic analysis reveals hyperactivation of the mammalian target of rapamycin pathway in neurofibromatosis 1-associated human and mouse brain tumors. *Cancer Res.* **2005**, *65*, 2755–2760. [CrossRef]
48. Franz, D.N.; Leonard, J.; Tudor, C.; Chuck, G.; Care, M.; Sethuraman, G.; Dinopoulos, A.; Thomas, G.; Crone, K.R. Rapamycin causes regression of astrocytomas in tuberous sclerosis complex. *Ann. Neurol.* **2006**, *59*, 490–498. [CrossRef]
49. Dutcher, J.P. Mammalian target of rapamycin inhibition. *Clin. Cancer Res.* **2004**, *10*, 6382S–6387S. [CrossRef]
50. Weiss, B.; Widemann, B.C.; Wolters, P.; Dombi, E.; Vinks, A.A.; Cantor, A.; Korf, B.; Perentesis, J.; Gutmann, D.H.; Schorry, E.; et al. Sirolimus for non-progressive NF1-associated plexiform neurofibromas: An NF clinical trials consortium phase II study. *Pediatr. Blood Cancer* **2014**, *61*, 982–986. [CrossRef]
51. Franz, D.N.; Belousova, E.; Sparagana, S.; Bebin, E.M.; Frost, M.; Kuperman, R.; Witt, O.; Kohrman, M.H.; Flamini, J.R.; Wu, J.Y.; et al. Efficacy and safety of everolimus for subependymal giant cell astrocytomas associated with tuberous sclerosis complex (EXIST-1): A multicentre, randomised, placebo-controlled phase 3 trial. *Lancet* **2013**, *381*, 125–132. [CrossRef]
52. Zehou, O.; Ferkal, S.; Brugieres, P.; Barbarot, S.; Bastuji-Garin, S.; Combemale, P.; Valeyrie-Allanore, L.; Sbidian, E.; Wolkenstein, P. Absence of Efficacy of Everolimus in Neurofibromatosis 1-Related Plexiform Neurofibromas: Results from a Phase 2a Trial. *J. Investig. Dermatol.* **2019**, *139*, 718–720. [CrossRef] [PubMed]
53. Boal, L.H.; Glod, J.; Spencer, M.; Kasai, M.; Derdak, J.; Dombi, E.; Ahlman, M.; Beury, D.W.; Merchant, M.S.; Persenaire, C.; et al. Pediatric PK/PD Phase I Trial of Pexidartinib in Relapsed and Refractory Leukemias and Solid Tumors Including Neurofibromatosis Type I-Related Plexiform Neurofibromas. *Clin. Cancer Res.* **2020**, *26*, 6112–6121. [CrossRef]
54. Dombi, E.; Baldwin, A.; Marcus, L.J.; Fisher, M.J.; Weiss, B.; Kim, A.; Whitcomb, P.; Martin, S.; Aschbacher-Smith, L.E.; Rizvi, T.A.; et al. Activity of Selumetinib in Neurofibromatosis Type 1-Related Plexiform Neurofibromas. *N. Engl. J. Med.* **2016**, *375*, 2550–2560. [CrossRef] [PubMed]
55. Gross, A.M.; Wolters, P.L.; Dombi, E.; Baldwin, A.; Whitcomb, P.; Fisher, M.J.; Weiss, B.; Kim, A.; Bornhorst, M.; Shah, A.C.; et al. Selumetinib in Children with Inoperable Plexiform Neurofibromas. *N. Engl. J. Med.* **2020**, *382*, 1430–1442. [CrossRef] [PubMed]
56. Klesse, L.J.; Jordan, J.T.; Radtke, H.B.; Rosser, T.; Schorry, E.; Ullrich, N.; Viskochil, D.; Knight, P.; Plotkin, S.R.; Yohay, K. The Use of MEK Inhibitors in Neurofibromatosis Type 1-Associated Tumors and Management of Toxicities. *Oncologist* **2020**, *25*, e1109–e1116. [CrossRef] [PubMed]
57. Gross, A.M.; Dombi, E.; Widemann, B.C. Current status of MEK inhibitors in the treatment of plexiform neurofibromas. *Childs Nerv. Syst.* **2020**, *36*, 2443–2452. [CrossRef]
58. Robertson, K.A.; Nalepa, G.; Yang, F.C.; Bowers, D.C.; Ho, C.Y.; Hutchins, G.D.; Croop, J.M.; Vik, T.A.; Denne, S.C.; Parada, L.F.; et al. Imatinib mesylate for plexiform neurofibromas in patients with neurofibromatosis type 1: A phase 2 trial. *Lancet Oncol.* **2012**, *13*, 1218–1224. [CrossRef]
59. Fisher, M.J.; Shih, C.S.; Rhodes, S.D.; Armstrong, A.E.; Wolters, P.L.; Dombi, E.; Zhang, C.; Angus, S.P.; Johnson, G.L.; Packer, R.J.; et al. Cabozantinib for neurofibromatosis type 1-related plexiform neurofibromas: A phase 2 trial. *Nat. Med.* **2021**, *27*, 165–173. [CrossRef]
60. Gutmann, D.H.; Ferner, R.E.; Listernick, R.H.; Korf, B.R.; Wolters, P.L.; Johnson, K.J. Neurofibromatosis type 1. *Nat. Rev. Dis. Primers* **2017**, *3*, 17004. [CrossRef]
61. Peltonen, S.; Kallionpaa, R.A.; Rantanen, M.; Uusitalo, E.; Lahteenmaki, P.M.; Poyhonen, M.; Pitkaniemi, J.; Peltonen, J. Pediatric malignancies in neurofibromatosis type 1: A population-based cohort study. *Int. J. Cancer* **2019**, *145*, 2926–2932. [CrossRef]
62. Hirbe, A.C.; Gutmann, D.H. Neurofibromatosis type 1: A multidisciplinary approach to care. *Lancet Neurol.* **2014**, *13*, 834–843. [CrossRef]
63. Evans, D.G.R.; Salvador, H.; Chang, V.Y.; Erez, A.; Voss, S.D.; Schneider, K.W.; Scott, H.S.; Plon, S.E.; Tabori, U. Cancer and Central Nervous System Tumor Surveillance in Pediatric Neurofibromatosis 1. *Clin. Cancer Res.* **2017**, *23*, e46–e53. [CrossRef] [PubMed]
64. Carli, M.; Ferrari, A.; Mattke, A.; Zanetti, I.; Casanova, M.; Bisogno, G.; Cecchetto, G.; Alaggio, R.; De Sio, L.; Koscielniak, E.; et al. Pediatric malignant peripheral nerve sheath tumor: The Italian and German soft tissue sarcoma cooperative group. *J. Clin. Oncol.* **2005**, *23*, 8422–8430. [CrossRef] [PubMed]

65. Laycock-van Spyk, S.; Thomas, N.; Cooper, D.N.; Upadhyaya, M. Neurofibromatosis type 1-associated tumours: Their somatic mutational spectrum and pathogenesis. *Hum. Genom.* **2011**, *5*, 623–690. [CrossRef]
66. Pemov, A.; Li, H.; Presley, W.; Wallace, M.R.; Miller, D.T. Genetics of human malignant peripheral nerve sheath tumors. *Neurooncol. Adv.* **2020**, *2*, i50–i61. [CrossRef] [PubMed]
67. Chaney, K.E.; Perrino, M.R.; Kershner, L.J.; Patel, A.V.; Wu, J.; Choi, K.; Rizvi, T.A.; Dombi, E.; Szabo, S.; Largaespada, D.A.; et al. Cdkn2a Loss in a Model of Neurofibroma Demonstrates Stepwise Tumor Progression to Atypical Neurofibroma and MPNST. *Cancer Res.* **2020**, *80*, 4720–4730. [CrossRef]
68. Miettinen, M.M.; Antonescu, C.R.; Fletcher, C.D.M.; Kim, A.; Lazar, A.J.; Quezado, M.M.; Reilly, K.M.; Stemmer-Rachamimov, A.; Stewart, D.R.; Viskochil, D.; et al. Histopathologic evaluation of atypical neurofibromatous tumors and their transformation into malignant peripheral nerve sheath tumor in patients with neurofibromatosis 1-a consensus overview. *Hum. Pathol.* **2017**, *67*, 1–10. [CrossRef]
69. Beert, E.; Brems, H.; Daniels, B.; De Wever, I.; Van Calenbergh, F.; Schoenaers, J.; Debiec-Rychter, M.; Gevaert, O.; De Raedt, T.; Van Den Bruel, A.; et al. Atypical neurofibromas in neurofibromatosis type 1 are premalignant tumors. *Genes Chromosomes Cancer* **2011**, *50*, 1021–1032. [CrossRef]
70. Pemov, A.; Hansen, N.F.; Sindiri, S.; Patidar, R.; Higham, C.S.; Dombi, E.; Miettinen, M.M.; Fetsch, P.; Brems, H.; Chandrasekharappa, S.C.; et al. Low mutation burden and frequent loss of CDKN2A/B and SMARCA2, but not PRC2, define premalignant neurofibromatosis type 1-associated atypical neurofibromas. *Neuro Oncol.* **2019**, *21*, 981–992. [CrossRef]
71. Martin, E.; Pendleton, C.; Verhoef, C.; Spinner, R.J.; Coert, J.H.; Flucke, U.E.; Slooff, W.B.M.; van Dalen, T.; van de Sande, M.A.; Grünhagen, D.J.; et al. Morbidity and Function Loss after Resection of Malignant Peripheral Nerve Sheath Tumors. *Neurosurgery* **2021**, nyab342. [CrossRef] [PubMed]
72. Lu, V.M.; Wang, S.; Daniels, D.J.; Spinner, R.J.; Levi, A.D.; Niazi, T.N. The clinical course and role of surgery in pediatric malignant peripheral nerve sheath tumors: A database study. *J. Neurosurg. Pediatr.* **2021**, *1*, 1–8. [CrossRef]
73. Campen, C.J.; Gutmann, D.H. Optic Pathway Gliomas in Neurofibromatosis Type 1. *J. Child Neurol.* **2018**, *33*, 73–81. [CrossRef] [PubMed]
74. Lewis, R.A.; Gerson, L.P.; Axelson, K.A.; Riccardi, V.M.; Whitford, R.P. von Recklinghausen neurofibromatosis. II. Incidence of optic gliomata. *Ophthalmology* **1984**, *91*, 929–935. [CrossRef]
75. Listernick, R.; Charrow, J.; Gutmann, D.H. Intracranial gliomas in neurofibromatosis type 1. *Am. J. Med. Genet.* **1999**, *89*, 38–44. [CrossRef]
76. Friedrich, R.E.; Nuding, M.A. Optic Pathway Glioma and Cerebral Focal Abnormal Signal Intensity in Patients with Neurofibromatosis Type 1: Characteristics, Treatment Choices and Follow-up in 134 Affected Individuals and a Brief Review of the Literature. *Anticancer Res.* **2016**, *36*, 4095–4121.
77. Fisher, M.J.; Loguidice, M.; Gutmann, D.H.; Listernick, R.; Ferner, R.E.; Ullrich, N.J.; Packer, R.J.; Tabori, U.; Hoffman, R.O.; Ardern-Holmes, S.L.; et al. Gender as a disease modifier in neurofibromatosis type 1 optic pathway glioma. *Ann. Neurol.* **2014**, *75*, 799–800. [CrossRef]
78. Creange, A.; Zeller, J.; Rostaing-Rigattieri, S.; Brugieres, P.; Degos, J.D.; Revuz, J.; Wolkenstein, P. Neurological complications of neurofibromatosis type 1 in adulthood. *Brain* **1999**, *122 Pt 3*, 473–481. [CrossRef]
79. Zeid, J.L.; Charrow, J.; Sandu, M.; Goldman, S.; Listernick, R. Orbital optic nerve gliomas in children with neurofibromatosis type 1. *J. AAPOS* **2006**, *10*, 534–539. [CrossRef]
80. Gutmann, D.H.; McLellan, M.D.; Hussain, I.; Wallis, J.W.; Fulton, L.L.; Fulton, R.S.; Magrini, V.; Demeter, R.; Wylie, T.; Kandoth, C.; et al. Somatic neurofibromatosis type 1 (NF1) inactivation characterizes NF1-associated pilocytic astrocytoma. *Genome Res.* **2013**, *23*, 431–439. [CrossRef]
81. Gutmann, D.H.; Giordano, M.J.; Mahadeo, D.K.; Lau, N.; Silbergeld, D.; Guha, A. Increased neurofibromatosis 1 gene expression in astrocytic tumors: Positive regulation by p21-ras. *Oncogene* **1996**, *12*, 2121–2127. [PubMed]
82. King, A.; Listernick, R.; Charrow, J.; Piersall, L.; Gutmann, D.H. Optic pathway gliomas in neurofibromatosis type 1: The effect of presenting symptoms on outcome. *Am. J. Med. Genet. A* **2003**, *122A*, 95–99. [CrossRef]
83. Listernick, R.; Ferner, R.E.; Liu, G.T.; Gutmann, D.H. Optic pathway gliomas in neurofibromatosis-1: Controversies and recommendations. *Ann. Neurol.* **2007**, *61*, 189–198. [CrossRef] [PubMed]
84. Fisher, M.J.; Loguidice, M.; Gutmann, D.H.; Listernick, R.; Ferner, R.E.; Ullrich, N.J.; Packer, R.J.; Tabori, U.; Hoffman, R.O.; Ardern-Holmes, S.L.; et al. Visual outcomes in children with neurofibromatosis type 1-associated optic pathway glioma following chemotherapy: A multicenter retrospective analysis. *Neuro Oncol.* **2012**, *14*, 790–797. [CrossRef] [PubMed]
85. Ullrich, N.J.; Robertson, R.; Kinnamon, D.D.; Scott, R.M.; Kieran, M.W.; Turner, C.D.; Chi, S.N.; Goumnerova, L.; Proctor, M.; Tarbell, N.J.; et al. Moyamoya following cranial irradiation for primary brain tumors in children. *Neurology* **2007**, *68*, 932–938. [CrossRef]
86. Packer, R.J.; Lange, B.; Ater, J.; Nicholson, H.S.; Allen, J.; Walker, R.; Prados, M.; Jakacki, R.; Reaman, G.; Needles, M.N.; et al. Carboplatin and vincristine for recurrent and newly diagnosed low-grade gliomas of childhood. *J. Clin. Oncol.* **1993**, *11*, 850–856. [CrossRef]
87. Ater, J.L.; Zhou, T.; Holmes, E.; Mazewski, C.M.; Booth, T.N.; Freyer, D.R.; Lazarus, K.H.; Packer, R.J.; Prados, M.; Sposto, R.; et al. Randomized study of two chemotherapy regimens for treatment of low-grade glioma in young children: A report from the Children's Oncology Group. *J. Clin. Oncol.* **2012**, *30*, 2641–2647. [CrossRef]

88. Fangusaro, J.; Onar-Thomas, A.; Young Poussaint, T.; Wu, S.; Ligon, A.H.; Lindeman, N.; Banerjee, A.; Packer, R.J.; Kilburn, L.B.; Goldman, S.; et al. Selumetinib in paediatric patients with BRAF-aberrant or neurofibromatosis type 1-associated recurrent, refractory, or progressive low-grade glioma: A multicentre, phase 2 trial. *Lancet Oncol.* **2019**, *20*, 1011–1022. [CrossRef]
89. Nix, J.S.; Blakeley, J.; Rodriguez, F.J. An update on the central nervous system manifestations of neurofibromatosis type 1. *Acta Neuropathol.* **2020**, *139*, 625–641. [CrossRef]
90. D'Angelo, F.; Ceccarelli, M.; Garofano, L.; Zhang, J.; Frattini, V.; Caruso, F.P.; Lewis, G.; Alfaro, K.D.; Bauchet, L.; Berzero, G.; et al. The molecular landscape of glioma in patients with Neurofibromatosis 1. *Nat. Med.* **2019**, *25*, 176–187. [CrossRef]
91. Costa, A.A.; Gutmann, D.H. Brain tumors in Neurofibromatosis type 1. *Neurooncol. Adv.* **2019**, *1*, vdz040. [CrossRef]
92. Packer, R.J.; Iavarone, A.; Jones, D.T.W.; Blakeley, J.O.; Bouffet, E.; Fisher, M.J.; Hwang, E.; Hawkins, C.; Kilburn, L.; MacDonald, T.; et al. Implications of new understandings of gliomas in children and adults with NF1: Report of a consensus conference. *Neuro Oncol.* **2020**, *22*, 773–784. [CrossRef]
93. Lobbous, M.; Bernstock, J.D.; Coffee, E.; Friedman, G.K.; Metrock, L.K.; Chagoya, G.; Elsayed, G.; Nakano, I.; Hackney, J.R.; Korf, B.R.; et al. An Update on Neurofibromatosis Type 1-Associated Gliomas. *Cancers* **2020**, *12*, 114. [CrossRef] [PubMed]
94. Huttner, A.J.; Kieran, M.W.; Yao, X.; Cruz, L.; Ladner, J.; Quayle, K.; Goumnerova, L.C.; Irons, M.B.; Ullrich, N.J. Clinicopathologic study of glioblastoma in children with neurofibromatosis type 1. *Pediatr. Blood Cancer* **2010**, *54*, 890–896. [CrossRef]
95. Evans, D.G.; Moran, A.; King, A.; Saeed, S.; Gurusinghe, N.; Ramsden, R. Incidence of vestibular schwannoma and neurofibromatosis 2 in the North West of England over a 10-year period: Higher incidence than previously thought. *Otol. Neurotol.* **2005**, *26*, 93–97. [CrossRef]
96. King, A.T.; Rutherford, S.A.; Hammerbeck-Ward, C.; Lloyd, S.K.; Freeman, S.R.; Pathmanaban, O.N.; Kellett, M.; Obholzer, R.; Afridi, S.; Axon, P.; et al. Malignant Peripheral Nerve Sheath Tumors are not a Feature of Neurofibromatosis Type 2 in the Unirradiated Patient. *Neurosurgery* **2018**, *83*, 38–42. [CrossRef] [PubMed]
97. Maniakas, A.; Saliba, I. Neurofibromatosis type 2 vestibular schwannoma treatment: A review of the literature, trends, and outcomes. *Otol. Neurotol.* **2014**, *35*, 889–894. [CrossRef]
98. Woods, R.; Friedman, J.M.; Evans, D.G.; Baser, M.E.; Joe, H. Exploring the "two-hit hypothesis" in NF2: Tests of two-hit and three-hit models of vestibular schwannoma development. *Genet. Epidemiol.* **2003**, *24*, 265–272. [CrossRef] [PubMed]
99. Halliday, D.; Emmanouil, B.; Pretorius, P.; MacKeith, S.; Painter, S.; Tomkins, H.; Evans, D.G.; Parry, A. Genetic Severity Score predicts clinical phenotype in NF2. *J. Med. Genet.* **2017**, *54*, 657–664. [CrossRef]
100. Kluwe, L.; Mautner, V.; Heinrich, B.; Dezube, R.; Jacoby, L.B.; Friedrich, R.E.; MacCollin, M. Molecular study of frequency of mosaicism in neurofibromatosis 2 patients with bilateral vestibular schwannomas. *J. Med. Genet.* **2003**, *40*, 109–114. [CrossRef]
101. Smith, M.J.; Bowers, N.L.; Bulman, M.; Gokhale, C.; Wallace, A.J.; King, A.T.; Lloyd, S.K.; Rutherford, S.A.; Hammerbeck-Ward, C.L.; Freeman, S.R.; et al. Revisiting neurofibromatosis type 2 diagnostic criteria to exclude LZTR1-related schwannomatosis. *Neurology* **2017**, *88*, 87–92. [CrossRef]
102. Baser, M.E.; Makariou, E.V.; Parry, D.M. Predictors of vestibular schwannoma growth in patients with neurofibromatosis Type 2. *J. Neurosurg.* **2002**, *96*, 217–222. [CrossRef]
103. Badie, B.; Pyle, G.M.; Nguyen, P.H.; Hadar, E.J. Elevation of internal auditory canal pressure by vestibular schwannomas. *Otol. Neurotol.* **2001**, *22*, 696–700. [CrossRef]
104. Roosli, C.; Linthicum, F.H., Jr.; Cureoglu, S.; Merchant, S.N. Dysfunction of the cochlea contributing to hearing loss in acoustic neuromas: An underappreciated entity. *Otol. Neurotol.* **2012**, *33*, 473–480. [CrossRef]
105. Blakeley, J.O.; Evans, D.G.; Adler, J.; Brackmann, D.; Chen, R.; Ferner, R.E.; Hanemann, C.O.; Harris, G.; Huson, S.M.; Jacob, A.; et al. Consensus recommendations for current treatments and accelerating clinical trials for patients with neurofibromatosis type 2. *Am. J. Med. Genet. A* **2012**, *158A*, 24–41. [CrossRef]
106. Mathieu, D.; Kondziolka, D.; Flickinger, J.C.; Niranjan, A.; Williamson, R.; Martin, J.J.; Lunsford, L.D. Stereotactic radiosurgery for vestibular schwannomas in patients with neurofibromatosis type 2: An analysis of tumor control, complications, and hearing preservation rates. *Neurosurgery* **2007**, *60*, 460–468. [CrossRef] [PubMed]
107. Phi, J.H.; Paek, S.H.; Chung, H.T.; Jeong, S.S.; Park, C.K.; Jung, H.W.; Kim, D.G. Gamma Knife surgery and trigeminal schwannoma: Is it possible to preserve cranial nerve function? *J. Neurosurg.* **2007**, *107*, 727–732. [CrossRef] [PubMed]
108. James, M.F.; Han, S.; Polizzano, C.; Plotkin, S.R.; Manning, B.D.; Stemmer-Rachamimov, A.O.; Gusella, J.F.; Ramesh, V. NF2/merlin is a novel negative regulator of mTOR complex 1, and activation of mTORC1 is associated with meningioma and schwannoma growth. *Mol. Cell Biol.* **2009**, *29*, 4250–4261. [CrossRef] [PubMed]
109. Giovannini, M.; Bonne, N.X.; Vitte, J.; Chareyre, F.; Tanaka, K.; Adams, R.; Fisher, L.M.; Valeyrie-Allanore, L.; Wolkenstein, P.; Goutagny, S.; et al. mTORC1 inhibition delays growth of neurofibromatosis type 2 schwannoma. *Neuro Oncol.* **2014**, *16*, 493–504. [CrossRef] [PubMed]
110. Karajannis, M.A.; Legault, G.; Hagiwara, M.; Giancotti, F.G.; Filatov, A.; Derman, A.; Hochman, T.; Goldberg, J.D.; Vega, E.; Wisoff, J.H.; et al. Phase II study of everolimus in children and adults with neurofibromatosis type 2 and progressive vestibular schwannomas. *Neuro Oncol.* **2014**, *16*, 292–297. [CrossRef] [PubMed]
111. Goutagny, S.; Raymond, E.; Esposito-Farese, M.; Trunet, S.; Mawrin, C.; Bernardeschi, D.; Larroque, B.; Sterkers, O.; Giovannini, M.; Kalamarides, M. Phase II study of mTORC1 inhibition by everolimus in neurofibromatosis type 2 patients with growing vestibular schwannomas. *J. Neurooncol.* **2015**, *122*, 313–320. [CrossRef]

112. Karajannis, M.A.; Mauguen, A.; Maloku, E.; Xu, Q.; Dunbar, E.M.; Plotkin, S.R.; Yaffee, A.; Wang, S.; Roland, J.T.; Sen, C.; et al. Phase 0 Clinical Trial of Everolimus in Patients with Vestibular Schwannoma or Meningioma. *Mol. Cancer Ther.* **2021**, *20*, 1584–1591. [CrossRef]
113. Ammoun, S.; Cunliffe, C.H.; Allen, J.C.; Chiriboga, L.; Giancotti, F.G.; Zagzag, D.; Hanemann, C.O.; Karajannis, M.A. ErbB/HER receptor activation and preclinical efficacy of lapatinib in vestibular schwannoma. *Neuro Oncol.* **2010**, *12*, 834–843. [CrossRef]
114. Karajannis, M.A.; Legault, G.; Hagiwara, M.; Ballas, M.S.; Brown, K.; Nusbaum, A.O.; Hochman, T.; Goldberg, J.D.; Koch, K.M.; Golfinos, J.G.; et al. Phase II trial of lapatinib in adult and pediatric patients with neurofibromatosis type 2 and progressive vestibular schwannomas. *Neuro Oncol.* **2012**, *14*, 1163–1170. [CrossRef] [PubMed]
115. Plotkin, S.R.; Halpin, C.; McKenna, M.J.; Loeffler, J.S.; Batchelor, T.T.; Barker, F.G., II. Erlotinib for progressive vestibular schwannoma in neurofibromatosis 2 patients. *Otol. Neurotol.* **2010**, *31*, 1135–1143. [CrossRef]
116. Lu, V.M.; Ravindran, K.; Graffeo, C.S.; Perry, A.; Van Gompel, J.J.; Daniels, D.J.; Link, M.J. Efficacy and safety of bevacizumab for vestibular schwannoma in neurofibromatosis type 2: A systematic review and meta-analysis of treatment outcomes. *J. Neurooncol.* **2019**, *144*, 239–248. [CrossRef] [PubMed]
117. Plotkin, S.R.; Merker, V.L.; Halpin, C.; Jennings, D.; McKenna, M.J.; Harris, G.J.; Barker, F.G., II. Bevacizumab for progressive vestibular schwannoma in neurofibromatosis type 2: A retrospective review of 31 patients. *Otol. Neurotol.* **2012**, *33*, 1046–1052. [CrossRef] [PubMed]
118. Plotkin, S.R.; Duda, D.G.; Muzikansky, A.; Allen, J.; Blakeley, J.; Rosser, T.; Campian, J.L.; Clapp, D.W.; Fisher, M.J.; Tonsgard, J.; et al. Multicenter, Prospective, Phase II and Biomarker Study of High-Dose Bevacizumab as Induction Therapy in Patients with Neurofibromatosis Type 2 and Progressive Vestibular Schwannoma. *J. Clin. Oncol.* **2019**, *37*, 3446–3454. [CrossRef] [PubMed]
119. Hong, B.; Krusche, C.A.; Schwabe, K.; Friedrich, S.; Klein, R.; Krauss, J.K.; Nakamura, M. Cyclooxygenase-2 supports tumor proliferation in vestibular schwannomas. *Neurosurgery* **2011**, *68*, 1112–1117. [CrossRef]
120. Kandathil, C.K.; Cunnane, M.E.; McKenna, M.J.; Curtin, H.D.; Stankovic, K.M. Correlation between Aspirin Intake and Reduced Growth of Human Vestibular Schwannoma: Volumetric Analysis. *Otol. Neurotol.* **2016**, *37*, 1428–1434. [CrossRef]
121. Hunter, J.B.; O'Connell, B.P.; Wanna, G.B.; Bennett, M.L.; Rivas, A.; Thompson, R.C.; Haynes, D.S. Vestibular Schwannoma Growth with Aspirin and Other Nonsteroidal Anti-inflammatory Drugs. *Otol. Neurotol.* **2017**, *38*, 1158–1164. [CrossRef] [PubMed]
122. Ignacio, K.H.D.; Espiritu, A.I.; Diestro, J.D.B.; Chan, K.I.; Dmytriw, A.A.; Omar, A.T., II. Efficacy of aspirin for sporadic vestibular schwannoma: A meta-analysis. *Neurol. Sci.* **2021**. [CrossRef] [PubMed]
123. Blakeley, J.O.; Ye, X.; Duda, D.G.; Halpin, C.F.; Bergner, A.L.; Muzikansky, A.; Merker, V.L.; Gerstner, E.R.; Fayad, L.M.; Ahlawat, S.; et al. Efficacy and Biomarker Study of Bevacizumab for Hearing Loss Resulting from Neurofibromatosis Type 2-Associated Vestibular Schwannomas. *J. Clin. Oncol.* **2016**, *34*, 1669–1675. [CrossRef] [PubMed]
124. Morris, K.A.; Golding, J.F.; Blesing, C.; Evans, D.G.; Ferner, R.E.; Foweraker, K.; Halliday, D.; Jena, R.; McBain, C.; McCabe, M.G.; et al. Toxicity profile of bevacizumab in the UK Neurofibromatosis type 2 cohort. *J. Neurooncol.* **2017**, *131*, 117–124. [CrossRef] [PubMed]
125. Troutman, S.; Moleirinho, S.; Kota, S.; Nettles, K.; Fallahi, M.; Johnson, G.L.; Kissil, J.L. Crizotinib inhibits NF2-associated schwannoma through inhibition of focal adhesion kinase 1. *Oncotarget* **2016**, *7*, 54515–54525. [CrossRef]
126. Chang, L.S.; Oblinger, J.L.; Smith, A.E.; Ferrer, M.; Angus, S.P.; Hawley, E.; Petrilli, A.M.; Beauchamp, R.L.; Riecken, L.B.; Erdin, S.; et al. Brigatinib causes tumor shrinkage in both NF2-deficient meningioma and schwannoma through inhibition of multiple tyrosine kinases but not ALK. *PLoS ONE* **2021**, *16*, e0252048. [CrossRef]
127. Morrison, H.; Sperka, T.; Manent, J.; Giovannini, M.; Ponta, H.; Herrlich, P. Merlin/neurofibromatosis type 2 suppresses growth by inhibiting the activation of Ras and Rac. *Cancer Res.* **2007**, *67*, 520–527. [CrossRef]
128. Fuse, M.A.; Dinh, C.T.; Vitte, J.; Kirkpatrick, J.; Mindos, T.; Plati, S.K.; Young, J.I.; Huang, J.; Carlstedt, A.; Franco, M.C.; et al. Preclinical assessment of MEK1/2 inhibitors for neurofibromatosis type 2-associated schwannomas reveals differences in efficacy and drug resistance development. *Neuro Oncol.* **2019**, *21*, 486–497. [CrossRef]
129. Goutagny, S.; Bah, A.B.; Henin, D.; Parfait, B.; Grayeli, A.B.; Sterkers, O.; Kalamarides, M. Long-term follow-up of 287 meningiomas in neurofibromatosis type 2 patients: Clinical, radiological, and molecular features. *Neuro Oncol.* **2012**, *14*, 1090–1096. [CrossRef] [PubMed]
130. Smith, M.J.; Higgs, J.E.; Bowers, N.L.; Halliday, D.; Paterson, J.; Gillespie, J.; Huson, S.M.; Freeman, S.R.; Lloyd, S.; Rutherford, S.A.; et al. Cranial meningiomas in 411 neurofibromatosis type 2 (NF2) patients with proven gene mutations: Clear positional effect of mutations, but absence of female severity effect on age at onset. *J. Med. Genet.* **2011**, *48*, 261–265. [CrossRef]
131. Clark, V.E.; Harmanci, A.S.; Bai, H.; Youngblood, M.W.; Lee, T.I.; Baranoski, J.F.; Ercan-Sencicek, A.G.; Abraham, B.J.; Weintraub, A.S.; Hnisz, D.; et al. Recurrent somatic mutations in POLR2A define a distinct subset of meningiomas. *Nat. Genet.* **2016**, *48*, 1253–1259. [CrossRef] [PubMed]
132. Alanin, M.C.; Klausen, C.; Caye-Thomasen, P.; Thomsen, C.; Fugleholm, K.; Poulsgaard, L.; Lassen, U.; Mau-Sorensen, M.; Hofland, K.F. Effect of bevacizumab on intracranial meningiomas in patients with neurofibromatosis type 2—A retrospective case series. *Int. J. Neurosci.* **2016**, *126*, 1002–1006. [CrossRef] [PubMed]
133. Nunes, F.P.; Merker, V.L.; Jennings, D.; Caruso, P.A.; di Tomaso, E.; Muzikansky, A.; Barker, F.G., II; Stemmer-Rachamimov, A.; Plotkin, S.R. Bevacizumab treatment for meningiomas in NF2: A retrospective analysis of 15 patients. *PLoS ONE* **2013**, *8*, e59941. [CrossRef]

134. Osorio, D.S.; Hu, J.; Mitchell, C.; Allen, J.C.; Stanek, J.; Hagiwara, M.; Karajannis, M.A. Effect of lapatinib on meningioma growth in adults with neurofibromatosis type 2. *J. Neurooncol.* **2018**, *139*, 749–755. [CrossRef]
135. Shih, K.C.; Chowdhary, S.; Rosenblatt, P.; Weir, A.B., III; Shepard, G.C.; Williams, J.T.; Shastry, M.; Burris, H.A., III; Hainsworth, J.D. A phase II trial of bevacizumab and everolimus as treatment for patients with refractory, progressive intracranial meningioma. *J. Neurooncol.* **2016**, *129*, 281–288. [CrossRef]
136. Graillon, T.; Sanson, M.; Campello, C.; Idbaih, A.; Peyre, M.; Peyriere, H.; Basset, N.; Autran, D.; Roche, C.; Kalamarides, M.; et al. Everolimus and Octreotide for Patients with Recurrent Meningioma: Results from the Phase II CEVOREM Trial. *Clin. Cancer Res.* **2020**, *26*, 552–557. [CrossRef]
137. Plotkin, S.R.; O'Donnell, C.C.; Curry, W.T.; Bove, C.M.; MacCollin, M.; Nunes, F.P. Spinal ependymomas in neurofibromatosis Type 2: A retrospective analysis of 55 patients. *J. Neurosurg. Spine* **2011**, *14*, 543–547. [CrossRef] [PubMed]
138. Kalamarides, M.; Essayed, W.; Lejeune, J.P.; Aboukais, R.; Sterkers, O.; Bernardeschi, D.; Peyre, M.; Lloyd, S.K.; Freeman, S.; Hammerbeck-Ward, C.; et al. Spinal ependymomas in NF2: A surgical disease? *J. Neurooncol.* **2018**, *136*, 605–611. [CrossRef] [PubMed]
139. Farschtschi, S.; Merker, V.L.; Wolf, D.; Schuhmann, M.; Blakeley, J.; Plotkin, S.R.; Hagel, C.; Mautner, V.F. Bevacizumab treatment for symptomatic spinal ependymomas in neurofibromatosis type 2. *Acta Neurol. Scand.* **2016**, *133*, 475–480. [CrossRef]
140. Snyder, M.H.; Ampie, L.; DiDomenico, J.D.; Asthagiri, A.R. Bevacizumab as a surgery-sparing agent for spinal ependymoma in patients with neurofibromatosis type II: Systematic review and case. *J. Clin. Neurosci.* **2021**, *86*, 79–84. [CrossRef]
141. Brossier, N.M.; Carroll, S.L. Genetically engineered mouse models shed new light on the pathogenesis of neurofibromatosis type I-related neoplasms of the peripheral nervous system. *Brain Res. Bull.* **2012**, *88*, 58–71. [CrossRef]
142. Gehlhausen, J.R.; Park, S.J.; Hickox, A.E.; Shew, M.; Staser, K.; Rhodes, S.D.; Menon, K.; Lajiness, J.D.; Mwanthi, M.; Yang, X.; et al. A murine model of neurofibromatosis type 2 that accurately phenocopies human schwannoma formation. *Hum. Mol. Genet.* **2015**, *24*, 1–8. [CrossRef] [PubMed]
143. Chen, J.; Landegger, L.D.; Sun, Y.; Ren, J.; Maimon, N.; Wu, L.; Ng, M.R.; Chen, J.W.; Zhang, N.; Zhao, Y.; et al. A cerebellopontine angle mouse model for the investigation of tumor biology, hearing, and neurological function in NF2-related vestibular schwannoma. *Nat. Protoc.* **2019**, *14*, 541–555. [CrossRef]
144. Williams, K.B.; Largaespada, D.A. New Model Systems and the Development of Targeted Therapies for the Treatment of Neurofibromatosis Type 1-Associated Malignant Peripheral Nerve Sheath Tumors. *Genes* **2020**, *11*, 477. [CrossRef] [PubMed]
145. Isakson, S.H.; Rizzardi, A.E.; Coutts, A.W.; Carlson, D.F.; Kirstein, M.N.; Fisher, J.; Vitte, J.; Williams, K.B.; Pluhar, G.E.; Dahiya, S.; et al. Genetically engineered minipigs model the major clinical features of human neurofibromatosis type 1. *Commun. Biol.* **2018**, *1*, 158. [CrossRef]
146. Dombi, E.; Ardern-Holmes, S.L.; Babovic-Vuksanovic, D.; Barker, F.G.; Connor, S.; Evans, D.G.; Fisher, M.J.; Goutagny, S.; Harris, G.J.; Jaramillo, D.; et al. Recommendations for imaging tumor response in neurofibromatosis clinical trials. *Neurology* **2013**, *81*, S33–S40. [CrossRef]
147. Fisher, M.J.; Avery, R.A.; Allen, J.C.; Ardern-Holmes, S.L.; Bilaniuk, L.T.; Ferner, R.E.; Gutmann, D.H.; Listernick, R.; Martin, S.; Ullrich, N.J.; et al. Functional outcome measures for NF1-associated optic pathway glioma clinical trials. *Neurology* **2013**, *81*, S15–S24. [CrossRef] [PubMed]

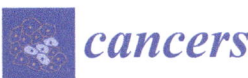

Review

Therapeutic Targets in Diffuse Midline Gliomas—An Emerging Landscape

Elisha Hayden [1], Holly Holliday [1,2], Rebecca Lehmann [1,2], Aaminah Khan [1], Maria Tsoli [1,2], Benjamin S. Rayner [1,2] and David S. Ziegler [1,2,3,*]

[1] Children's Cancer Institute, Lowy Cancer Research Centre, UNSW Sydney, Kensington 2052, Australia; ehayden@ccia.org.au (E.H.); HHolliday@ccia.org.au (H.H.); RLehmann@ccia.org.au (R.L.); AKhan@ccia.org.au (A.K.); mtsoli@ccia.org.au (M.T.); brayner@ccia.org.au (B.S.R.)

[2] School of Women's and Children's Health, Faculty of Medicine, University of New South Wales, Kensington 2052, Australia

[3] Kids Cancer Centre, Sydney Children's Hospital, Randwick 2031, Australia

* Correspondence: d.ziegler@unsw.edu.au; Tel.: +61-2-9382-1730; Fax: +61-2-9382-1789

Simple Summary: Diffuse midline gliomas (DMGs) remain one of the most devastating childhood brain tumour types, for which there is currently no known cure. In this review we provide a summary of the existing knowledge of the molecular mechanisms underlying the pathogenesis of this disease, highlighting current analyses and novel treatment propositions. Together, the accumulation of these data will aid in the understanding and development of more effective therapeutic options for the treatment of DMGs.

Abstract: Diffuse midline gliomas (DMGs) are invariably fatal pediatric brain tumours that are inherently resistant to conventional therapy. In recent years our understanding of the underlying molecular mechanisms of DMG tumorigenicity has resulted in the identification of novel targets and the development of a range of potential therapies, with multiple agents now being progressed to clinical translation to test their therapeutic efficacy. Here, we provide an overview of the current therapies aimed at epigenetic and mutational drivers, cellular pathway aberrations and tumor microenvironment mechanisms in DMGs in order to aid therapy development and facilitate a holistic approach to patient treatment.

Keywords: diffuse midline gliomas; molecular targets; potential therapy development

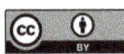

1. Introduction

Diffuse midline gliomas (DMG), including diffuse intrinsic pontine gliomas (DIPGs), are aggressive central nervous system (CNS) pediatric tumours located in the brainstem, thalamus, spinal cord and cerebellum [1,2]. Their prognosis is dismal and patients have a five-year survival of less than 1% due to their high level of resistance to current standard therapies, with no significant improvement in the treatment or prognosis of DMGs having occurred in more than three decades [3]. DMG tumours typically display no contrast enhancement by magnetic resonance imaging (MRI), suggesting an intact blood–brain barrier (BBB) that impedes further the delivery of therapeutic agents [4]. As such, new and innovative treatment strategies are urgently needed to counter these devastating tumours. To facilitate research, a greater understanding of the underlying molecular mechanisms that promote DMG tumour growth is required. Approximately 80% of DMGs harbour lysine-to-methionine substitutions at position 27 in Histone 3 genes encoding H3.3 (*H3F3A*), and to a lesser extent H3.1 (*HIST1H3B*), collectively referred to as H3K27M [5–7]. In 2016 the World Health Organization (WHO) classified all gliomas harbouring the H3K27M mutant as a new entity, a "Diffuse Midline Glioma H3 K27M-mutant" [1]. Subsequent functional studies demonstrated that the H3K27M mutation drives DMG growth, suggesting that this epigenetic dysregulation is the key promotor of DMG tumorigenesis through the global reduction in the repressive epigenetic mark H3K27me3 [8–10]. In 2021 the WHO further classified the inclusion of a subset of DMGs that lack the H3K27M mutation but exhibit a global loss of tri-methylation [2], potentially mediated by the overexpression of EZH inhibitory protein (EZHIP) which functionally acts as a K27M-like inhibitor of polycomb repressive complex 2 (PRC2) [11]. Collectively, these tumors have now been termed "diffuse midline glioma, H3 K27-altered". Combined, this knowledge has resulted in research focussed on the development of pharmacological inhibitors designed to regulate these epigenetic mechanisms by particularly targeting epigenetic modifiers, including methyltransferase activity [12,13], demethylases [14,15], acetylation [16], chromatin readers and writers [17–19], and histone chaperones [20,21]. It is also becoming increasingly apparent that there exists a link between DMG cell metabolism and the underlying activation status of key epigenetic marks in DMGs, resulting in novel DMG targets involving metabolic pathway regulation [22–24]. Furthermore, the developed understanding of DMG tumour biology has also revealed additional novel therapeutic targets within the tumour microenvironment, particularly within the regulation of the immune system [25,26] and the interplay of DMG tumours with neuronal cells [27]. This comprehensive review summarises the current understanding of DMG biology in relation to therapeutic targets in preclinical development and proposes further research avenues to highlight novel mechanisms capable of being manipulated for the treatment of DMGs.

2. Targeting Epigenetic Mechanisms in DMGs

Since the discovery of the importance of the H3K27M mutation to DMG tumorigenicity a plethora of inhibition studies within this disease setting have been undertaken, summarised in Table 1. The H3K27M mutation causes broad epigenetic reprogramming through the inhibition of PRC2, which deposits the repressive histone mark H3K27me3. This results in global H3K27 hypomethylation in all histone H3 variants and is central to DMG oncogenesis [5–7,28,29]. Restoring H3K27me3, therefore, is a key therapeutic strategy to reduce DMG tumorigenicity, and targeting the enzymes that erase this mark—histone demethylases—is one such way to achieve this. The demethylation of H3K27me3 is catalysed by the lysine demethylase 6 (KDM6) subfamily of demethylases, consisting of JMJD3 and UTX [30]. Confirmation of their role in DMGs was obtained through the use of GSKJ4, a pro-drug for GSKJ1, which is a potent and selective pharmacological inhibitor of JMJD3 and UTX [31]. Hashizume et al. found that GSKJ4 treatment in vitro increased H3K27me3 levels and reduced cell viability as well as clonogenicity in H3K27M-mutant DIPG cells but not H3-WT DMGs or normal astrocytes [32]. The genetic depletion of JMJD3, but not UTX, was able to phenocopy GSKJ4 treatment, indicating that JMJD3 is the enzyme target responsible for demethylating H3K27me3 in DMGs [32].

Similarly, GSKJ4 treatment significantly extended survival in two H3K27M-mutant DMG PDX models but had no effect in an H3-WT glioma PDX model. The active derivative of the drug, GSKJ1, was detected in the brainstem of non-tumour-bearing mice, confirming BBB penetration of the drug [32]. Delving further into the transcriptional consequences of GSKJ4, Hashizume et al. found that treatment decreased the chromatin accessibility and expression of genes involved in DNA double-strand break repair, such as *PCNA* and *XRCC1*. Moreover, GSKJ4 was able to enhance radiation-induced DNA damage and subsequent apoptosis in H3K27M-mutant DIPGs both in vitro and in vivo [33]. Building upon these findings, combining GSKJ4 with APR-246, an inhibitor of mutant TP53, further enhanced radiosensitivity in vitro [34]. GSKJ4 is not yet in clinical development due to challenges associated with the rapid conversion of the pro-drug into its active form, which has restricted cell permeability due to its high polarity, indicating that efforts should be therefore focused on increasing the stability of GSKJ4 in vivo if it were to progress from a potential to a beneficial treatment for DMGs.

Table 1. Summary of inhibition studies targeting epigenetic mechanisms in DMGs.

Epigenetic Drug Category	Drugs	Target	References
H3K27 demethylase inhibitor	GSKJ4/GSKJ1	JMJD3	[15,33,34]
EZH2 (H3K27 histone methyltransferase) inhibitor	EPZ6438 (Tazemetostat), GSK343	EZH2	[13,17,35]
BMI1 (H2AK119 ubiquitinase) inhibitor	PTC209, PTC028 and PTC596	BMI1	[36–38]
HDAC inhibitor	Panobinostat	HDACs	[16,39]
BET inhibitor	JQ1	BRD4	[17,19,40,41]
Curaxin	CBL0137	FACT	[21]
DNA demethylating agent	5-azacytidine	DNMTs	[42]
Epigenetic Drug Combination			
HDACi + H3K27 demethylase inhibitor	Panobinostat + GSKJ4/1	HDACs + JMJD3	[16]
HDACi + BETi	Panobinostat + JQ1	HDACs + BRD4	[40]
HDACi + CDK7i	Panobinostat + THZ1	HDACs + CDK7/9	[40]
HDACi + demethylating agent	Panobinostat + 5-azacytidine	HDACs + DNMTs	[42]
HDAC + Curaxin	Panobinostat + CBL0137	HDACs + FACT	[21]
BETi + CDK7i	JQ1 + THZ1	BRD4 + CDK7/9	[40]
BETi + EZHi	JQ1 + EPZ6468	BRD4 + EZH2	[43]
BETi + HATi	JQ1 + ICG-001	BRD4 + CBP	[44]
HDACi + H3K4me1 histone demethylase inhibitor	Corin	HDACs + LSD1	[45]

Importantly, the inhibition of PRC2 by H3K27M is not equivalent to complete PRC2 loss of function, and despite a global reduction in H3K27me3 in DIPGs PRC2 and its product, H3K27me3, persist at hundreds of genomic loci. This occurs at CpG islands, high-affinity PRC2 binding sites thought to be "strong" PRC2 targets [12,13,17]. Genes that remain epigenetically silenced in DIPGs by PRC2 include *CDKN2A*, encoding the cell cycle inhibitor p16, and neuronal differentiation genes [13,17]. Enhancer of zeste homolog 2 (EZH2) is the histone methyltransferase catalytic subunit of PRC2. Targeting residual PRC2 activity with EZH2 inhibitors to switch on tumour suppressor and pro-differentiation genes is another plausible avenue for DMG treatment. Indeed, treatment of multiple DMG cell lines with the EZH2 inhibitors GSK343 and EPZ6438 reduced H3K27me3 at the *CDKN2A* locus and reactivated the expression of p16, accompanied by a reduction in the proliferation and induction of cellular senescence [13]. Importantly, H3-WT glioblastoma (GBM) lines, or those with G34R mutations, were not affected by EZH2 inhibitors, demonstrating the specific H3K27M context required for EZH2 inhibitor efficacy [13]. In contrast, Wiese et al. found no cytotoxic effect of EPZ6438 in DIPG models regardless of H3K27M status [35]. This discrepancy could be due to different time points selected for their proliferation assays (15 days versus 3 days). The genetic knockout of EZH2 prolonged survival when H3K27M mouse tumour cells were orthotopically transplanted, demonstrating that EZH2 activity is required for tumour growth in vivo [13]. In agreement, the knockdown of other core components of the PRC2 complex, EED and SUZ12, reduced the growth and survival of human DIPG cells in vitro [17]. This was mediated via p16 de-repression in the SF8628 model, but not for SU-DIPG-VI cells, indicating that p16-independent mechanisms are also important for PRC2-mediated tumorigenesis.

The above studies demonstrate therapeutic potential for targeting residual PRC2 activity in H3K27M-mutant DIPGs. EPZ6438 (Tazemetostat) is currently being trialled in other solid tumours such as pediatric sarcomas (NCT02601937) and lymphoma (NCT01897571). However, there are limited data on the activity of EZH2 inhibitors in animal models of DIPGs due to their poor BBB penetration. While brain delivery of EZH2 inhibitors can be improved by co-administration of the drug efflux transporter inhibitor elacridar, its clinical development has been discontinued [46]. Further pre-clinical testing in orthoptic mouse models is required before EZH2 inhibitors can be considered for clinical applications in DMG.

Polycomb repressive complex 1 (PRC1) is another repressive polycomb complex which plays critical roles during embryonic development and catalyses the ubiquitination of histone H2A at lysine 119 (H2AK119ub) [47]. BMI1 is a core component of PRC1 and acts as an oncogene in several cancers, including DMGs, where it promotes self-renewal and stem cell maintenance [36,37]. Expression of BMI1 and its associated mark, H2AK119ub, is upregulated in DIPGs compared to normal pons [37]. BMI1 expression is directly regulated by H3K27M, as ectopic expression of the oncohistone in H3-WT cells caused increased BMI1 and H2AK119ub levels and increased proliferation, while the inverse was observed when WT H3.3 was expressed in H3K27M-mutant DMG cells. This was reflected on the chromatin level, where the removal of H3K27M increased H3K27me3 at the *BMI1* locus [37]. Targeting BMI1 with small-molecule inhibitors PTC209 and PTC028 was effective against H3K27M-mutant DIPG models in vitro and in vivo, reducing global BMI1 chromatin binding. However, long-term drug exposure resulted in recurrence due to an accumulation of secretory senescent cells. Combining the BMI1 inhibitor PTC028 (oral gavage 12.5 mg/kg) with the BH3 protein mimetic obatoclax (IP 3 mg/kg) significantly increased survival time compared to BMI1 inhibition alone in an orthotopic DMG PDX model, mediated through the clearing of residual senescent DMG cells by obatoclax. The inhibition of BMI1 with another drug, PCT596, was also shown to be effective both in vitro and in vivo [38]. A clinical trial for PTC596 in DMG and HGG patients is currently recruiting (NCT03605550). Given the recent data revealing the potentially pro-tumorigenic activity of prolonged BMI1 inhibition, caution will be needed in clinical translation and the selection of dosing schedules.

H3K27M-mutant DMGs have elevated levels of H3K27ac, an active epigenetic mark found at the promoters and enhancers of actively transcribed genes [28]. The enzymes responsible for writing and erasing histone acetylation are histone acetyltransferases (HATs) and histone deacetylases (HDACs), respectively. Histone acetylation is read by the bromodomain and extra terminal (BET) family of proteins, including BRD4. HDAC inhibitors are perhaps the most studied mode of epigenetic-targeted therapy in DMGs. These drugs increase histone acetylation by targeting enzymes that remove the mark. Grasso et al. identified HDAC inhibitors from a targeted drug screen performed across a panel of human DIPG cultures. Panobinostat, a pan-HDAC inhibitor, was selected for follow-up due to its higher potency compared to other HDAC inhibitors [16]. Panobinostat treatment caused a dose-dependent increase in histone acetylation and, unexpectedly, a partial rescue of H3K27me3. Panobinostat displayed in vitro efficacy, reducing DMG cell proliferation and inducing cell death, and was also efficacious in vivo in both H3K27M-mutant and H3-WT DMG models when delivered systemically (IP 20 mg/kg once a week for 4 weeks), reaching doses in the brain higher than in vitro IC50. However, when surviving mice were re-challenged with panobinostat, DMG tumours were found to be resistant, highlighting a need for combination therapies [16]. In another study, panobinostat at the same dose was not well-tolerated over an extended treatment, resulting in significant toxicity and no survival benefit [39]. Similarly a phase I trial of panobinostat in DMGs has shown significant toxicity, limiting dose escalation with no efficacy yet demonstrated [9]. Together these data suggest that although panobinostat may have some anti-DMG activity it is limited by a narrow therapeutic window, suggesting that combination therapies may be needed to lead to clinical efficacy.

Given that H3K27ac is already elevated in DMGs, it seems counter-intuitive that further elevation of it through HDAC inhibition can reduce DMG growth. There are two suggested explanations for this, which are not necessarily mutually exclusive. In the first, panobinostat-mediated poly-acetylation of residues nearby the mutated K27M residue disrupt the repression of PRC2, thereby restoring H3K27me3 and diminishing DMG growth [16,48]. In the second, panobinostat causes histone hyperacetylation and aberrant transcription of endogenous retroviruses, triggering an interferon response which sensitises cells to the innate immune system [42]. Panobinostat has been tested in combination with a suite of other epigenetic-targeted therapies in DIPGs. The histone demethylase inhibitor GSKJ4 demonstrated in vitro synergy with panobinostat [16], warranting further in vivo testing and mechanistic studies. The disruption of oncogenic transcription using either THZ1 or JQ1 was also synergistic with panobinostat in vitro [40]. CDK7, the target of THZ1, phosphorylates RNA polymerase II (Pol II); this is required for transcription. Mechanistically, THZ1 and panobinostat reduced H3K27ac at super-enhancer-associated genes fundamental to DMG biology, such as those important for communication with neurons in the microenvironment [40,49]. Importantly, panobinostat-resistant cells also became resistant to BET inhibitor JQ1, likely due to their shared transcriptional targets [40]. Krug et al. found that the combination of panobinostat with the DNA demethylating agent 5-azacytidine prolonged survival in two DMG PDX models [42]. Finally, another potent panobinostat combination is with CBL0137, which targets the histone chaperone facilitates chromatin transcription (FACT) [21], discussed in more detail below.

Bifunctional inhibitors are an innovative approach for the simultaneous targeting of epigenetic modifiers. Corin is one such example of these hybrid drugs, derived from the HDAC inhibitor entinostat and an LSD1 inhibitor [45]. LSD1 demethylates the active enhancer mark H3K4me1. LSD1 inhibitors have also recently been suggested to enhance immune sensitivity in DMGs [50]. Corin treatment increased H3K27ac, H3K4me1 and H3K27me3, reduced proliferation and induced apoptosis as well as neuronal differentiation in vitro, and reduced DMG PDX growth when delivered by convection-enhanced delivery (CED) [45]. Thus, HDAC inhibitors hold promise as future DMG therapeutics, especially in combination with other epigenetic drugs.

The bromodomain and extra-terminal (BET) family of proteins, consisting of BRD2, BRD3, BRD4 and BRDT, are chromatin readers and positive regulators of transcription. BET proteins bind to acetylated histones via their bromodomains and recruit the transcription elongation complex to promote Pol-II-mediated transcription of oncogenes such as *MYC* [51,52]. BRD4 is the predominant, and consequently most studied, member of the BET family of proteins [52]. In DMGs, H3K27M forms heterotypic nucleosomes with H3K27ac which are bound by BRD4 at super-enhancers, large clusters of enhancers with high levels of transcription factor binding, controlling the expression of cell identity genes [17]. Genes associated with BRD4-bound super-enhancers in cancer are enriched for oncogenic drivers [18]. Consequently, DMG cells are particularly vulnerable to transcriptional disruption using BET inhibitors [40].

JQ1, a well-studied BET inhibitor that competitively binds to bromodomains [53], is a potent inhibitor of DMG growth in vitro [17,19,40]. H3K27M-mutant cell lines were more sensitive to JQ1 than H3-WT glioblastoma cells [17]. JQ1 caused growth arrest, in part by reducing *MYC* transcription, but its effects on apoptosis were minimal [17,40]. Rather, this drug increased the expression of mature neuronal marker genes (*TUJ1* and *MAP2*) and induced neuronal-like morphological changes, suggesting that JQ1 is a differentiation therapy in DIPG [17]. Mechanistically, BET inhibition resulted in an overall shutdown of transcription [17] and reduced promoter–enhancer looping at tumour-specific genes (e.g., *OLIG2* and *SOX6*) [41]. The genetic depletion of BRD4 resulted in a stark decrease in tumour growth and improved survival when xenografted into mice [40], demonstrating the dependence of DIPG tumours on BRD4. Consistently, treatment of orthoptic DMG PDXs with JQ1 (IP 50 mg/kg daily for 10 days) reduced tumour burden and significantly extended survival [17]. However, when other BET inhibitors were tested, namely iBET762 and OTX015, they were less potent than JQ1 in vitro and were not able to achieve sufficient levels in the brain [40].

One of the key advantages of synergistic combination therapies is that the dose of each monotherapy can be reduced, potentially circumventing the drug delivery issues seen with BET inhibitors. Several BET inhibitor combinations have been explored in DMGs. Nagaraja et al. combined JQ1 with both panobinostat (HDAC inhibitor) and THZ1 (CDK7 inhibitor) and observed synergy with both epigenetic drugs in three human DMG cultures in vitro. However, as mentioned above, DMG cells had shared resistance to both panobinostat and JQ1 due to their similar transcriptional targets [40]. The combination of JQ1 and

EZH2 inhibitor EPZ6438 blocked proliferation, increased apoptosis and extended survival in a mouse model of DMGs [43]. Given the poor BBB penetration of EPZ6438 [46], it is surprising that this drug was able to reduce tumour burden. Further preclinical testing of dual BET and EZH2 targeting is required to see if this promising result is consistent across additional DMG models, including human-derived models. Finally, JQ1 has been combined with ICG-001, which targets CREB-binding protein (CBP)—a histone acetyltransferase (HAT) that also interacts with other transcriptional regulators, such as BRD4 itself [44]. JQ1 and ICG-001 reduced in vitro proliferation, self-renewal and migration, and increased radiosensitivity [44]. While ICG-001 has not yet been tested in orthotopic models, this drug is interesting proposed to increase BBB permeability by targeting endothelial cells [54]. Therefore, co-treatment with ICG-001 may both improve the delivery of, as well as synergise with, JQ1.

While the effect of JQ1 on DMGs has been immensely beneficial for understanding the biology of BET proteins and establishing BET inhibition as an anti-cancer strategy, this compound has a poor pharmacokinetic profile. Other BET inhibitors, including OTX015, CPI-0610 and iBET762, have been tested in clinical trials for a variety of cancers (see [55] for a comprehensive review). It is important to acknowledge that significant toxicities such as gastrointestinal disorders, anaemia and thrombocytopenia were reported in some of these trials, stressing the need to find potent synergies and to define predictive biomarkers of response.

The FACT histone chaperone complex is important for maintaining nucleosome stability and the local recycling of histones during transcription, replication and repair [56,57]. It is required in large amounts in transcriptionally active cells, with higher expression in cancer and stem cells compared to normal, differentiated cells [58,59]. Accordingly, cancer cells are exquisitely sensitive to curaxins, which are indirect inhibitors of the FACT complex. Curaxins are derived from anti-malarial quinacrine drugs and have been screened for their ability to simultaneously activate p53 and suppress NF-κB-mediated transcription without causing genotoxicity [20]. Their proposed mechanism is through DNA intercalation and the subsequent unfolding of nucleosomes, causing FACT to become trapped in chromatin and thereby depleting the pool of functionally active soluble FACT [20,59,60]. CBL0137 is the lead curaxin in clinical development due to its high stability and water solubility [20].

It has recently been found that DMG growth is inhibited by targeting FACT with CBL0137 or by the shRNA-mediated knockdown of FACT subunits SPT16 and SSRP1. CBL0137 had higher efficacy in H3K27M mutants compared to H3-WT models and minimal toxicity to normal cells, which express much lower levels of FACT [21]. CBL0137 administered as a single agent (IV 50 mg/kg once a week for 4 weeks or 20 mg/kg 5 days on/2 days off for 3 weeks) significantly extended the survival of mice bearing orthotopic DIPG tumours; the drug reached clinically relevant doses in the brain [21]. Importantly, FACT directly interacts with H3K27M and FACT inhibition increased H3K27me3, indicating that FACT is required for H3K27M's oncogenic effects [21]. In support of this, the depletion of FACT can scramble histone positioning due to the loss of local nucleosome recycling [61,62]. It seems that FACT is required for maintaining H3K27M on chromatin; inhibition with CBL0137 causes H3K27M to be ejected or mis-localised, removing its downstream epigenetic effects. Furthermore, CBL0137 potently synergised with panobinostat both in vitro and in vivo and was accompanied by an increase in both H3K27me3 and H3K27ac [21]. Further investigation will be important for dissecting the precise genomic loci affected by these epigenetic therapies. In addition, combination treatment suppressed the expression of cell cycle genes (e.g., *E2F1* and *CDK4*) and oligodendrocyte developmental genes (e.g., *ASCL1* and *LINGO1*) [21]. Such lineage genes are known to be regulated by super-enhancers in DMGs and are disrupted by treatment with panobinostat [40]. It is therefore possible that CBL0137 exacerbates the effects of panobinostat on the super-enhancer landscape in DIPGs. CBL0137 has recently completed phase I clinical trials in adults with recurrent solid tumours and was found to be well-tolerated as well as exhibit preliminary anti-tumour activity (NCT01905228) [63]. Excitingly, this drug is due to enter a phase I/II trial (NCT04870944) in paediatric cancer patients, with activity to be tested in a DMG expansion cohort.

In addition to histone hypomethylation in H3K27M-mutant DMGs, these tumours are also characterised by global DNA hypomethylation, which is thought to contribute to the highly characteristic gene expression program in DIPGs [29,64]. Genome-wide methylation profiling in GBMs revealed that H3K27M GBMs had a distinct methylome to H3-WT GBMs, with differential methylation of genes involved in neuronal development [64,65]. Given the intimate link between H3K27me3 and DNA methylation [66], it follows that H3K27M, which hinders H3K27me3, would also impact DNA methylation. DNA methylation primarily occurs on the fifth position of cytosine (5-methylcytosine; 5mC) in the CpG sequence context and is generally associated with gene silencing [67,68]. DNA methylation is mediated by DNA methyltransferase (DNMT) enzymes [68]. DNA demethylating agents, such as 5-azacytidine (5-aza) and decitabine, are nucleoside analogues that target DNMT activity. Treatment with 5-aza improved survival in two DMG PDX models as a single agent (IP 3 mg/kg 5 days on/2 days off for 4 weeks), and its efficacy was further enhanced when combined with panobinostat (IP 10 mg/kg) [42]. The mechanism involved further loss of DNA methylation and, similar to HDAC inhibition, subsequent de-repression of silent endogenous retroviruses, triggering an interferon response and viral mimicry [42]. Testing 5-aza and panobinostat in immunocompetent mouse models is warranted to investigate if this translates to an augmented immune response. DNA-demethylating agents are commonly used in chronic myelomonocytic leukaemia (CMML), acute myeloid leukaemia (AML) and myelodysplastic syndrome, and are currently in clinical trials in solid tumours, including adult HGGs (NCT03666559).

The active removal of DNA methylation involves ten-eleven translocation (TET) enzymes, which catalyse the conversion of 5 mC into 5-hydroxymethylcososine (5hmC) [69]. Thymine DNA glycosylases and base excision repair machinery further process and excise 5 hmC to restore unmethylated cytosines [70]. DMG tumours have elevated mRNA expression of *TET1* and *TET3* compared to a patient-matched normal brain in addition to increased levels of 5 hmC compared to paediatric GBMs [71]. These findings hint that active DNA demethylation by TET enzymes contributes to DMGs' hypomethylated signature and pathological gene expression. In addition, similar to histone demethylase enzymes, TET enzymes are dependent on the metabolic intermediate α-KG as a co-factor. It is therefore possible that the increased α-KG levels in DMGs [22] fuel TET-mediated DNA demethylation to maintain a hypomethylated genome. Thus, targeting TET enzymes to restore DNA methylation may represent a novel avenue of treatment for DMGs. The TET inhibitor Bobcat339 has recently been synthesised as a tool compound for understanding TET biology and is a promising starting point for the development of therapeutic inhibitors of DNA demethylation [72].

Similarly, investigation into the RNA polymerase II (RNAPII) transcriptional machinery has gained traction in recent years [18,73]. This includes targeting CDK7 in order to prevent RNAPII phosphorylation and subsequent transcription initiation, with the CDK7 inhibitor THZ1 having been shown to suppress tumour growth in orthotopic DMG orthotopic [74]. More recently, CDK9 suppression has demonstrated anti-tumour effects in DMG models [75]. As an integral component of the super elongation complex (SEC), CDK9 kinase regulates the RNA polymerase II proximal pausing mechanism. The SEC is vital for cellular differentiation and development and can be misregulated in states of cellular transformation [76]. Suppressing aberrant SEC signalling in DMG cells was found to induce neuroglial differentiation with increases observed in GFAP, NGFR and NRN expression [75].

Targeting transcriptional elongation has been particularly efficacious in enhancer-driven malignancies where MYC aberrations are commonplace. Suppressing CDK7 and CDK9 activity has been known to substantially reduce MYC expression and downregulate MYC target genes in T cell acute lymphoblastic leukaemia, mixed-lineage leukaemia, neuroblastomas and small-cell lung cancers [77,78]. Interestingly however, SEC suppression exerts uniform anti-proliferative effects across DMG tumour subtypes irrespective of MYC expression [75]. However, translating these inhibitors into the clinic for DMGs may be challenging. Despite global changes in H3K27 posttranslational modifications transcriptomic changes are relatively restricted in DMG tumours [8]. Furthermore, BBB penetrance remains a significant hurdle for current transcription elongation inhibitors [75,79]. Precise understanding into the nature of off-target effects and effective drug design is critical for validating transcription elongation inhibition as a potential therapy for DMGs [77,78,80].

3. Targeting Cell Metabolism in DMGs

Targeting DMG metabolism is evolving as a potential treatment strategy, spurred on by the discovery of distinct links between metabolic reprogramming, mitochondrial dysfunction, and heightened levels of oxidative stress in DMG tumours, with significant advances also made in recent years in the understanding of the interplay between the DMG epigenome and metabolism. For example, glycolytic enzymes such as pyruvate kinase M2 (PKM2) have been implicated in H3K9 acetylation, causing a chromatin open state at *CCND1* (cyclin D1) and c-*Myc* loci, consistent with their subsequent activation [81]. PKM2 catalyses the rate-limiting step of glycolysis, shunting glucose metabolism away from oxidative phosphorylation towards anaerobic glycolysis and lactate production in tumour cells, a key feature during cancer development and progression. The depletion of PKM2 with regulatory microRNAs (miRNAs), long non-coding RNAs (lncRNAs) and circular RNAs (circRNAs) has yielded promising results in in vitro models of GBMs [82]. PKM2 expression, but not activity, is regulated in a grade-specific manner in gliomas, but changes in both PKM activity and PKM2 expression contribute to the growth of GBMs. The knockdown of PKM1/2 activated AMP-activated protein kinase (AMPK1) and suppressed viability in lung carcinoma cell lines [83]. AMPK1 plays an important role in maintaining H3K27 methylation deficiency. AMPK1 has been shown to directly target EZH2, disrupting the EZH2-dependent methylation of H3K27 and consequently PRC2 activity [13,84]. Furthermore, studies have shown that AMPK1 has a role in maintaining H3K27 methylation deficiency. AMPK1 has been shown to directly target EZH2, disrupting the EZH2-dependent methylation of H3K27 and consequently PRC2 activity [13,84]. Indeed, preclinical studies have demonstrated AMPK1 induction to suppress glycolysis through mTOR signalling, which was able to decrease tumour burden in DMG orthografts [23]. Additionally, pyruvate dehydrogenase kinase (PDK1) inhibition reverses the conversion of pyruvate into acetyl-CoA, uncoupling glycolysis from oxidative phosphorylation. It has been shown that simultaneous AMPK1 activation and PDK1 suppression is able to repress the glycolytic phenotype and enhance DIPG radiosensitisation within in vitro and DIPG orthograft models [85].

In a recent study, Chung et al. discovered that DIPG cells had enhanced glycolysis and tricarboxylic acid (TCA) cycle metabolism, resulting in elevated levels of α-ketoglutarate (α-KG). Targeting the metabolic enzymes that produce α-KG with the glutamine antagonist JHU-83 (oral gavage 20 mg/kg) and an IDH1 inhibitor (IP 10 mg/kg) increased survival in two orthotopic human DIPG PDX models [22]. α-KG has been well-documented as an important co-factor of JMJD3. Mechanistically, JMJD3 metabolizes α-KG to succinate, while demethylating H3K27me3. Inbuilt redundancies through the activity of hexokinase, WT IDH1 and glutamate dehydrogenase (GDH), which are heterogeneously expressed in both H3.3K27 and H3.1K27 DMG cells, may also serve as potential targets for therapeutic development. This work highlights the intimate relationship between metabolic and epigenetic mechanisms, indicating that disrupting metabolic pathways is an innovative strategy to deplete the essential co-factors required for maintaining H3K27 hypomethylation in DMGs.

Likewise, polyamines have been investigated in aggressive cancers as they play a pivotal role in multiple cellular processes and facilitate rapid cell proliferation. The intracellular concentration of polyamine is tightly regulated through biosynthetic and catabolic pathways as well as the uptake of polyamines from the microenvironment [86]. It has recently been shown that the polyamine pathway is not only upregulated within the setting of DMGs, but that combination treatment with the polyamine synthesis inhibitor difluoromethylornithine (DFMO) coupled with the polyamine transport inhibitor AMXT 1501 leads to a significant depletion of polyamine levels, resulting in a reduction in cell proliferation, clonogenic potential and cell migration, concurrent with the induction of apoptosis in DIPG neurosphere cultures. Furthermore, the combination of DFMO with AMXT 1501 significantly enhanced the survival of three orthotopic models of DMGs, further combining effectively with irradiation [24], with a treatment regime of DFMO and AMXT 1501 in combination currently being tested in an adult phase I clinical trial (NCT03536728) and a phase I trial in pediatric DMGs currently in development.

4. Targeting Cellular Signalling Pathways in DMGs

Since DMG tumours exhibit irregular activation of growth-factor-receptor-mediated signal transduction pathways, utilising drugs that target these pathways is a logical tactic. In vitro and in vivo studies have verified the efficacy of tyrosine kinase inhibitors, such as dasatinib, in diminishing tumour proliferation and inhibiting *PDGFRA* activity [87]. Phase I studies of PDGFR pathway inhibition by imatinib [88] and dasatinib [89], VEGFR2 inhibition by vandetinib [90] and EGFR inhibition by gefitinib [91] as well as erlotinib [92] revealed the safety of using these drugs in children and provided doses for future phase II studies. However, these inhibitors failed to show a clinical benefit when tested in further trials. Phase II trials for dasatinib (NCT00423735) and imatinib did not show clinically meaningful anti-tumour activity against recurrent adult GBMs [93,94]. The BIOMEDE trial was a clinically adaptive trial where DMG tumours from patients in Australia, Europe and the UK were specifically tested against three approved inhibitors targeting EGFR (erlotinib), mTOR (everolimus) or PDGFR (dastanib) for efficacy and in combination with standard radiotherapy followed by maintenance therapy (NCT02233049). However, there was no benefit observed, as measured by overall survival, with any of the drugs and this study was discontinued due to toxicity in 15%, 2% and 13% of patients, respectively [95].

Growth factor receptors are receptor tyrosine kinases (RTKs), and their downstream activity is facilitated through the activation of the specific RTK. RTK-dependent mitogenic activation plays a vital role in proliferation, invasiveness, cell survival and chemo- as well as radioresistance in a variety of cancers, including DMGs (Figure 1). DMG tumours regularly display focal amplifications in PDGFRA and EGFR accompanied by amplifications in KIT, KDR, EGFR and MET [96–98]. In vitro RTK suppression yielded promising results, although multikinase inhibition was more efficacious than specific-kinase inhibition, with only multi-kinase inhibitors such as dasatinib and crizotinib having thus far been shown to be effective [16,99]. Despite these positive results, both single- and multitargeted RTK inhibitors have failed to achieve relevant antitumor effects in vivo, ultimately failing to confer a survival benefit in phase I and II clinical trials relevant to DMGs [90,100]. The reasons behind the failure to target RTKs has been linked to the in-built redundancies in growth signalling pathways, tumoral heterogeneity, multidrug efflux transporters and the lack of specific and BBB-penetrant inhibitors [97,101]. Indeed, combination therapy regimes using dasatinib combined with cabozantinib, targeting hyperactive c-Met expression, demonstrated synergism against cultured DIPG neurospheres [87]. It is evident that there is still promise in the use of RTK inhibitors in treating paediatric malignancies with hyperactive RTK signalling. For example, the NCT03352427 study is investigating combination strategies that combine dasatinib with the mTOR inhibitor everolimus in DMG patients.

The PI3K/AKT/mTOR intracellular signalling pathway is important in regulating the cell cycle, with mTOR activity, a common target for cancer therapeutics, being frequently upregulated across multiple cancer types. Growth factors, neurotransmitters and hormones are all able to activate the mTOR pathway through their specific RTKs and G-protein-coupled receptors (GPCRs) [102]. The first identified mTOR inhibitor, rapamycin, acts by binding to FK506-binding protein (FKBP) 12, forming a complex which then binds to mTOR, resulting in the downstream inhibition of the mTORC1 pathway [103].

Several analogues have since been developed due to the poor water solubility and pharmacokinetics of rapamycin. Two of these therapeutics, temsirolimus and everolimus, are currently available in the clinic, with temsirolimus approved for use in advanced renal cell carcinoma and everolimus for a range of non-CNS tumours in addition to subependymal giant-cell astrocytomas, which are benign tumours largely associated with tuberous sclerosis [104,105].

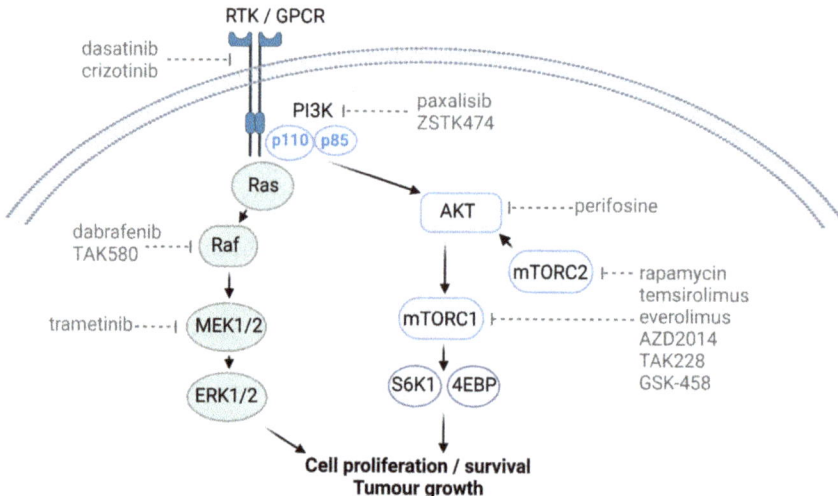

Figure 1. Therapeutic targets of RTK activation and PI3K/AKT/mTOR signalling pathways in DMG. Receptor tyrosine kinases (RTK) and/or G-protein-coupled receptors (GPCRs) are activated by a variety of growth factors, neurotransmitters and hormones, including insulin, brain-derived neurotropic factor, glutamate and cannabinoids (reviewed in [102]). Receptor activation recruits the intracellular association of the phosphatidylinositol 3-kinase (PI3K) regulatory (p85) and catalytic (p110) subunits. The subsequent engagement of Ras results in the activation of the Raf–mitogen-activated protein kinase kinase (MEK)–extracellular signal-regulated kinase (ERK) 1/2 pathway. Alternately, RTK-induced PI3K activation promotes AKT signalling involving the mechanistic target of the rapamycin (mTORC1/2) pathway. The triggering of these pathways initiates a variety of signals that promote DMG tumour cell proliferation, survival and tumour growth. A range of inhibitory compounds, shown in grey with dotted lines indicating specific mechanistic targets, have been tested within the setting of DMGs.

The PI3K/AKT/mTOR pathway has been identified as a promising target for therapeutics for DMGs due to its frequent dysregulation. Up to 50% of DMGs harbour mutations in genes upstream of mTOR, most prominently *PDGFRA*, *MET* and *IGFR1*, but also *EGFR*, *ERBB4*, *HGF*, *IGF2*, *KRAS*, *NF1*, *AKT1*, *AKT3*, *PTEN* and *PIK3CA*, leading to pathway overactivity [96,106,107]. PI3Ks are a family of intracellular signal transducers, consisting of three subunits: p85 regulatory subunit, p55 regulatory subunit and p110 catalytic subunit [108]. PI3Ks transmit signals from activated G-protein-coupled receptors and receptor tyrosine kinases, activating the downstream AKT pathway and subsequently mTOR signalling. mTOR is a serine/threonine protein kinase composed of two distinct complexes which differ in components, substrate specificity and downstream regulation: mTORC1, composed of mTOR, raptor, GβL and deptor, and mTORC2, composed of mTOR, rictor, GβL, PRR5, deptor and SIN1 [109,110]. mTORC1 exerts its downstream actions primarily through the phosphorylation of two proteins: p70S6 kinase 1 (S6K1) and eIF4E binding protein (4EBP). 4EBP and S6K1 are independent of one another, exerting their action on downstream substrates through distinctive approaches [111]. mTORC1 ultimately is involved in regulating the balance between anabolism and catabolism, promoting cell growth and glucose metabolism whilst suppressing autophagy, lysosomal biogenesis and proteasome activation [111–117]. mTORC2 acts via multiple mechanisms, including serine/threonine phosphorylation, the subsequent activation of AKT and the phosphorylation of members of the AGC family of protein kinases (PK), most notably from the PKA, PKB, PKC and SGK families [111,118,119]. mTORC2 activation results in increased cell migration and cytoskeletal rearrangement, decreased apoptosis and changes in glucose metabolism as well as ion transport [111].

While PI3K/AKT/mTOR inhibitors provide an attractive option for therapy, they are likely to be most effective when administered in combination with a second therapeutic due to the traditionally poor response of DMGs to single therapies (Figure 1). Indeed, temsirolimus has shown significantly increased efficacy against DMGs in vitro when combined with the mitochondrial protein adenine nucleotide translocase (ANT) inhibitor PENAO (4-(N-(Spenicillaminylacetyl)-amino)phenylarsonous acid), exhibiting increased apoptosis, decreased PI3K and mTOR signalling in addition to disrupted mitochondrial integrity in comparison to single-agent-treated cells. Unfortunately, these same promising results could not be recapitulated in vivo [23]. Similarly, PI3K/AKT and MEK/ERK inhibitors have been identified as a promising potential combination therapeutic for DMGs, with combination treatment resulting in a synergistic decrease in cell viability and an increase in apoptosis in comparison to single therapeutics in vitro [120,121]. Furthermore, PI3K/AKT inhibition with ZSTK474 and MEK/ERK inhibition with trametinib in combination reduced tumor burden compared to either agent alone; furthermore, median survival was significantly extended from 35 days in the vehicle controls to 47 days in mice treated with the combination therapy [121]. Combination targeting of PI3K/AKT/mTOR and HDAC has also shown efficacy in DMGs, with the dual PI3K/HDAC inhibitor CUDC-907 having been shown to decrease PI3K signalling and inhibit HDAC function in DMG and HGG cells in vitro. CUDC-907 was also identified as a radiosensitiser, with dual application of CUDC-907 and irradiation treatment resulting in a synergistic decrease in cell viability in vitro and a synergistic increase in animal survival [122]. A phase I clinical trial for CUDC-907 is currently underway for patients with DIPG (NCT03893487). Dual-targeting of the mTOR and CDK4/6 pathways has also been identified as a potential therapeutic option for DMGs [123], as discussed further below.

It has been recognised that mTORC1 inhibition can result in the detrimental upregulation of mTORC2, associated with increased tumor cell proliferation, migration and metabolism [111,123]. Subsequently, therapeutics capable of simultaneously targeting both mTORC complexes are considered advantageous. The dual mTORC1/2 inhibitor AZD2014 has shown significant efficacy against DMGs in vitro, being more efficacious than the mTORC1 inhibitor everolimus [124]. Another mTORC1/2 inhibitor, sapanisertib (TAK228), successfully suppressed DMG cell growth and invasion in vitro, and increased the survival of an orthotopic DMG model [125]. The addition of irradiation has been shown to further improve the response of dual mTORC1/2 inhibitors against DMGs, whilst the dual mTORC1/2 inhibitor GSK-458 was found to target DMG cells with stem-like cell qualities both in vitro and in vivo [124–126].

To date, two drugs targeting the PI3K/AKT/mTOR pathway have published results from DMG clinical trials: perifosine and temsirolimus [127,128]. As a monotherapy, the AKT inhibitor perifosine was found to be well-tolerated in children with DIPGs and other paediatric CNS and solid tumours at all tested doses (between 25 mg/m^2/day and 125 mg/m^2/day). Unfortunately, perifosine did not show significant efficacy in this trial, with the highest perifosine dose resulting in progressive disease in five of the six treated patients, across a range of pediatric CNS and solid tumours. Furthermore, two of the three DMG patients enrolled across the study exhibited progressive disease [127]. The combination therapy of perifosine and temsirolimus was arguably more successful, with all five DMG patients treated exhibiting stable disease at the first evaluation. However, across the study, which included patients with a range of recurrent or refractory solid brain tumours, including DIPGs, no significant responses were observed to the treatment [128]. The potential for therapeutically targeting the PI3K/AKT/mTOR signalling pathway in DMGs is evident, with several clinical trials currently underway. These include a monotherapy trial for paxalisib, a PI3K inhibitor (NCT03696355), a dual combination therapy trial of paxalisib and ONC201, a dopamine receptor D2 antagonist (NCT05009992), and temsirolimus combined with the HDAC inhibitor vorinostat, together with irradiation (NCT02420613).

The activation of the PI3K/AKT/mTOR pathway is able to modulate TGFβ signalling in cancer [129]. The TGFβ superfamily is composed primarily of two distinct pathways involving TGFβ- and BMP-mediated signalling. The TGFβ pathway has known tumour suppressor properties, inhibiting cell growth and promoting apoptosis. The identification of mutations in components of the TGFβ pathway, such as *TGFBR2*, *SMAD2*, *SMAD3*, *SMAD4* and *ENG*, demonstrate the tumour suppressor role this pathway can play [130–133]. However, paradoxically, it can also act as a tumour promotor, enhancing tumour growth, invasion and metastasis [134]. TGFβ is especially associated with the epithelial-to-mesenchymal transition (EMT), a process associated with invasion, migration, metastasis and drug resistance [135,136]. BMP has a similarly paradoxical role in tumour suppression. Several BMP ligands are upregulated in a range of cancers, with BMPs able to stimulate tumour migration and invasion [137–140]. However, there is also evidence that BMP plays a suppressive role in tumorigenesis through several SMAD-independent pathways [141–144].

Both the TGFβ and BMP pathways signal through serine/threonine kinase receptors, resulting in downstream signalling through SMADs. Two distinct SMAD pathways are upregulated by the TGFβ superfamily: TGFβ ligands activate SMAD2/3 signalling whilst BMP ligands activate SMAD1/5/8 signalling [145]. These two distinct pathways result in upregulation in a wide range of genes involved in cell fate determination, cell cycle arrest, apoptosis and actin rearrangements [145]. The BMP pathway in particular is closely associated with DMGs. Mutations in *ACVR1*, which encodes a BMP type I receptor, activin-receptor-like kinase 2 (ALK2), are present up to 30% of DIPG patients [96,107,146,147]. ALK2 binds both BMP ligands, which activate the SMAD1/5/8 pathway, and activin A, which activates the SMAD2/3 pathway. *ACVR1* mutations result in hyperactivity in response to BMP ligands and constitutive BMP signalling, independent of ligand binding [148–150]. Furthermore, activin A promotes SMAD1/5/8 signalling in *ACVR1* mutated cells at even low ligand concentrations as a result of activin A forming ACVR2A/B–ACVR1R206H complexes [151–154]. *ACVR1* mutations in DMGs are associated with upregulated SMAD1/5/8 signalling and increases in cell proliferation, indicating an oncogenic role for the BMP pathway in this context [107,151,155]. Interestingly, *ACVR1* mutations appear to be unique to DMG tumors and are not present in other cancers; however, they are closely associated with the genetic condition fibrodysplasia ossificans progressive (FOP). FOP is a rare skeletal malformation disorder which results in aberrant, episodic heterotopic ossification (HO) of muscles, tendons and ligaments [156]. The progressive HO causes a range of skeletal pathologies, ultimately resulting in early death [157]. FOP is caused by mutations in *ACVR1*, primarily at residue 206 (R206H), which results in the classical, most severe phenotype [158]. Less common mutations are at the 258, 328 and 356 residues, resulting in a milder FOP phenotype [159–161]. Interestingly, the same mutations are observed in DMGs, with the R206H mutation shown to exhibit the most potent tumor phenotype. However, patients with FOP are at no greater risk of DMGs (or any other cancers), indicating that *ACVR1* mutations alone are not sufficient for tumorigenesis [146,147,151,155]. Previous work has identified a strong association between *ACVR1* mutation and the H3.1K27M mutation [96,107,146,147,151]. In addition, *ACVR1*-mutant DMGs exhibit a significant increase in mutations in PI3K-pathway-associated genes, whilst alterations to the TP53 pathway were less common [107,146,151].

The first small-molecule inhibitor of ALK2 that was identified was dorsomorphin, a compound capable of "dorsalising" zebrafish embryos and inhibiting BMP signalling [162]. Subsequently, further inhibitors based on the dorsomorphin pyrazolo[1,5-a]pyrimidine scaffold have been developed for use in both FOP and DMGs. A recent study examined eleven potential ALK2 inhibitors against DMGs, including compounds related to the dorsomorphin scaffold, pyridine compounds and drugs with reported anti-ALK2 activity. Nine compounds displayed efficacy against both *ACVR1*-mutant and *ACVR1*-wild-type

DIPG cells, with very little selectivity for mutational status evident. In contrast, the two compounds tested in vivo, the pyrazolo[1,5-a]pyrimidine compound, LDN-193189, and the pyridine compound, LDN-214117, were only able to extend survival in an *ACVR1* (R206H)-mutant PDX model, with no improvement in survival seen in the *ACVR1*-wild-type PDX. However, it should be noted that whilst statistically significant the increase in survival was only modest, with both drugs increasing survival by 15 days [151]. The in vitro efficacy of LDN-193189 in DMGs has been observed by others, with some evidence of improved efficiency in *ACVR1*-mutant cells above those of the wild type; in contrast, another study into LDN-214117 found no significant effect on DMGs in vitro [107,153,155]. However, several analogues of LDN-214117 have been developed which exhibit a profile with increased potency, selectivity and BBB permeability. Preliminary studies have shown that they are efficacious against DMG cell lines, with some selectivity for *ACVR1*-mutant cultures [163]. A further analogue, M4K2127, has been identified as highly BBB-penetrable, including into the pons region of the brainstem [164]. Another ALK2 inhibitor, LDN-212854, a pyrazolo[1,5-a]pyrimidine compound, has also shown efficacy for DMGs, demonstrating sensitivity for *ACVR1*-mutant human DMG cell cultures in vitro. Furthermore, LDN-212854 was found to improve survival in a Nestin tv-a; p53fl/fl mouse model expressing *ACVR1* (R206H), H3.1K27M, PDGFA and Cre. However, similar to LDN-214117 this increase was only modest, with an eight-day increase in survival [155]. This work into ALK2 inhibitors is still at an early stage in DMGs. The preliminary results show that this area could be promising for developing new therapeutics; however, due to the varied results and few in vivo studies evident to date, more work is required in this field.

Several analogues of the currently used ALK2 inhibitors have been developed in attempts to increase and improve their potency, selectivity, BBB permeability and pharmacokinetic properties, although to date not all have been tested in DMG cells or PDX models. A modified structure of LDN-214117, known as M4K2149, has been developed and identified as a more potent inhibitor. M4K2149 analogues have also been developed with increased selectivity for ALK2, increased permeability and improved pharmacokinetic properties [165]. Analogues based on the pyridine compound K02288 have shown improved potency with increased cytotoxicity evident against HEPG2 cells derived from hepatocellular carcinoma. Interestingly, analogue cytotoxicity did not correlate with BMP signalling inhibition capacity [166]. Another area of focus has been inhibitors with an imidazo[1,2-a]pyridine scaffold, with a range of inhibitors identified with improved potency and PK properties [167]. It will be of interest to determine if these analogues are effective in DMG in vitro and in vivo models in the future.

Some surprising inhibitors of ACVR1/ALK2 have been identified. Binding between a MEK1/2 inhibitor, E6201 and ALK2 has identified E6201 as a potential BMP pathway inhibitor. This hypothesis was supported by its ability to dose-dependently inhibit BMP signalling in vitro and prolong DMG PDX survival in vivo [168]. OKlahoma Nitrone-007 (OKN-007) is an anti-cancer agent which acts through multiple mechanisms, including as an anti-angiogenic, GLUT-1 inhibitor and SULF2 enzyme activity inhibitor [169,170]. However, OKN-007 was also found to significantly reduce the expression of ALK2 in a DMG PDX model whilst also reducing tumor growth and increasing apoptosis, providing a promising potential therapeutic [171]. Due to the prevalence of the *ACVR1*-activating mutations in DMGs the BMP family has been the primary target of focus for DMG therapeutics, with little investigation into the TGFβ pathway. However, a recent study identified that the TβRI inhibitors EW7197 (vactosertib), LY3200882 and LY2157299 (galunisertib) were all effective in reducing DMG cell viability, with a further synergistic response seen with the addition of the HDAC inhibitor GSK-J4. Interestingly, these effects were most prominent in *ACVR1*-wild-type lines, with no response seen in the *ACVR1*-G328V-mutant DIPG line. It has been suggested that the constitutively activating *ACVR1* G328V mutation may suppress the TβRI pathway, thereby reducing the inhibitory efficacy of therapeutics [172]. Therefore, TβRI inhibitors may be a potential therapeutic option for *AVCR1*-wild-type DIPGs. Unfortunately, the effects of these drugs on downstream signalling in DIPG cells was not examined; this would be valuable due to the complex role of TGFβ signalling in cancer. The authors of this work suggest that the suppression of TβRI by the constitutively activating *ACVR1* mutation may contribute to the longer survival seen in DMG patients with *ACVR1* mutations, as it has been previously proposed that the increased kinase activity of mutant *ACVR1* may be involved in this phenomenon [107,146,172].

The ubiquitin–proteasome system (UPS), through the activity of several E3 ubiquitin ligases, plays a crucial role in the recognition and degradation of TGFβ family receptors, including SMAD components and their interacted proteins, to regulate TGFβ family signalling [173]. Additionally, the UPS pathway plays a critical role in facilitating neurogenesis and the growth of cerebellar granule cell precursors during brain development [174,175], with deregulation in the UPS being a well-known hallmark in a variety of CNS malignancies, including medulloblastoma and adult GBMs [176,177]. Ubiquitination by ligases, such as E3 ubiquitin ligase, play an integral role in the proteostasis of oncogenes and tumour suppressors, and subsequently regulate proliferation, DNA repair and apoptosis [174,178,179]. Furthermore, aberrations in E3 ligases dysregulate Shh and Wnt signalling, both of which result in medulloblastoma progression [177,180]. UPS suppression in medulloblastoma cell lines causes the activation of cell cycle checkpoints, with increases in the levels of cyclin-dependent kinase inhibitors p21 and p16 [181]. BBB-penetrant proteasomal inhibitors such as marizomib have demonstrated potent in vivo antitumor effects in orthotopic xenograft models of human GBMs and DIPGs [176,182]. A phase III study is now open for patients newly diagnosed with GBMs to study marizomib's impact on overall survival (NCT03345095), with paediatric trials examining the use of proteasome inhibitors as a monotherapy versus a combination therapy for CNS tumours (NCT01132911 and NCT00994500) still ongoing.

Similarly, there is evidence that aberrations in the UPS, through E3 ligase dysregulation [183], extend to the Notch signalling pathway, itself also involved in cell proliferation, differentiation and survival, as well as being one of the most commonly activated signalling pathways in cancer [184], including DMGs [19]. Notch signalling is essential for maintaining stem-cell-ness, with the presence of quiescent stem-like cells in DMG tumours driving resistance to standard therapies and radiation [185–187]. In light of this, Notch inhibition with the γ-secretase inhibitor MRK003 has been shown to enhance radiotherapy-induced apoptosis in H3-K27M DIPG cells [19], with a co-dependency shown between H3K27me hypomethylation and Notch-mediated stemness in DIPGs in addition to the inhibition of key Notch pathway effectors ASCL1 and RBPJ demonstrating significant anti-tumour effects [188].

Studies have identified a potential role for cannabinoids in the regulation of the mTOR pathway, with cannabinoid-dependent increases in ceramide levels associated with the sustained activation of the Raf-1/MEK/ERK signalling cascade and the subsequent production of damaging cellular ROS and ER stress [189,190], culminating in the inhibition of Akt/mTORC1, triggering cell cycle arrest, autophagy and apoptosis [191]. The cannabinoids Δ9-tetrahydrocannabinol (THC) and cannabidiol (CBD) have been shown to possess some efficacy as potential therapeutic agents against adult brain tumours, particularly GBM (reviewed in [192]), acting via the G-protein-coupled cannabinoid receptors type 1 and 2 (CB1R and CB2R [193]. Compared to normal brain tissues, both low- and high-grade human gliomas are known to have increased CB2R expression on tumour cells, invading microglia/macrophages and endothelial cells of the tumour blood vessels [194–196]. However, the expression or abundance of CB1R or CB2R and their relevance in DMG biology is unknown [197], with the effects of cannabinoids within the pediatric setting, generally, remaining relatively understudied (reviewed in [198]). From the limited available data, Andradas et al. have recently demonstrated that THC and CBD exert cytotoxic activity against a range of paediatric medulloblastoma and ependymoma cell lines [193]. Here, it was determined that treatment with THC and CBD had variable effects on ROS production and the activation of MAPK or mTOR signalling in vitro, with no discernible benefit shown by either of the compounds within a pediatric medulloblastoma mouse xenograft model, alone or in combination with cyclophosphamide, one of the major chemotherapeutics used in clinical treatment. Taken together, the lack of therapeutic efficacy thus far demonstrated coupled with potential toxicity concerns [199] indicates that more research and beneficial evidence are required for cannabinoids to be a viable therapeutic option in DMGs.

5. Targeting the Cell Cycle and DNA Repair Mechanisms in DMGs

Aberrant cell signalling, leading to the constitutive initiation of the cell cycle and increased proliferation, is a hallmark of many cancers (reviewed recently in Matthews 2021) [200], including DMGs, presenting further potential therapeutic targets. For example, the cyclin-dependent kinase (CDK) 4/6 pathway is involved in the tight regulation of the cell cycle through mediation of the G1–S phase transition (Figure 2). Following CDK4/6 binding to cyclin D, the complex then phosphorylates the Rb protein. Phosphorylated Rb is unable to bind the E2F transcription factor, increasing its availability and thus downstream signalling [201]. Genes regulated by E2F include those involved in the cell cycle, DNA replication and mitosis [14]. The involvement of CDK4/6 in the cell cycle provides a key target for cancer therapeutics, with the pathway commonly targeted in breast cancer and three therapeutics currently approved for use in the clinic: palbociclib, ribociclib and abemaciclib. All three drugs target CDK4 and CDK6, with abemaciclib also being able to inhibit CDK9 [202]. The CDK4/6 pathway has been identified as a promising potential therapeutic target for DMGs due to its frequent dysregulation: approximately 30% of DMGs carry amplifications in genes involved in Rb signalling, including *CDK4*, *CDK6*, *CCND1*, *CCND2* and *CCND3* [106]. A study of more than 1000 cases of DMGs and pediatric HGGs identified co-segregation of the H3.3K27M mutation and G1–S phase dysregulation [203]. In contrast to other HGGs, deletions in *CDKN2A/B*, encoding the p16INK4A and p15INK4B tumour suppressors, are rare in DMGs; however, it has been shown that *CDKN2A* is epigenetically silenced due to the H3K27M mutation [106,203,204].

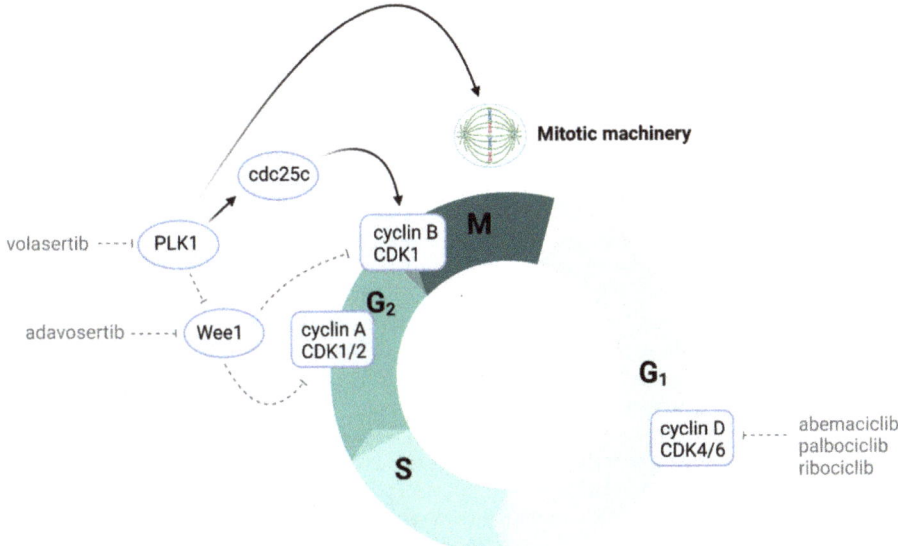

Figure 2. Cell-cycle-dependent therapeutic targets in DMGs. Constitutive expression and heightened activation of the cell cycle is a hallmark of DMGs. A range of inhibitory compounds, shown in grey with dotted lines indicating specific mechanistic targets, have been tested within the setting of DMGs. These include the cell cycle G1 phase, cyclin-dependant kinase 4 and 6 (CDK4/6) inhibitors abemaciclib, palbociclib and ribociclib, as well as inhibition through the targeting of molecules PLK1 and Wee1 to halt the cell cycle in the G2/M phase.

Whilst single therapeutic treatments have had little success in DMGs, CDK4/6 inhibitors have shown some efficacy as single agents pre-clinically. The CDK4/6 inhibitor palbociclib successfully reduced DMG cell proliferation in vitro and increased DMG PDX survival [205–207]. However, these effects have not been translated into the clinic; whilst both palbociclib and ribociclib have been well-tolerated by DIPG patients, phase I trials for both drugs have shown little survival benefit [208,209]. This was to some extent predicted by the preclinical data, which indicated that the in vivo doses of palbociclib required to achieve single-agent activity were not clinically achievable [210]. A phase I trial is currently underway for abemaciclib for patients with DMGs (NCT02644460). CDK4/6 inhibitors have shown the greatest efficacy when used in combination with secondary therapeutics. For example, a preclinical trial using PD-0332991 (PD), a CDK4/6 inhibitor, that induces cell cycle arrest both in vitro and in vivo in high-grade brainstem glioma cell lines enhanced survival when used in combination with radiotherpy in a genetically engineered, PDGF-B overexpressing, Ink4a-ARF and p53 deficient brainstem glioma mouse model [205]. Similarly, both irradiation and the EGFR inhibitor erlotinib were able to improve the efficacy of palbociclib in vivo [205,206]. A genome-wide analysis has previously identified 21% of DMGs with co-amplifications of the CDK4/6 and PI3K/AKT/mTOR pathway, providing an ideal dual target for combination therapy [106]. In addition, a study on glioblastomas found that mTOR inhibitors were able to reverse the increased mTOR signalling triggered by CDK4/6 inhibitors, with this compensatory relationship suggesting a promising potential combination therapy [211]. Subsequently, the dual inhibition of CDK4/6 and mTOR has shown promise for DMGs, with a combination treatment with palbociclib and the mTOR inhibitor temsirolimus synergistically reducing DMG cell proliferation in vitro [123]. Interestingly, palbociclib did not have any significant direct effects on mTOR signalling as a single agent in DMGs, in contrast to its actions on mTOR observed in glioblastomas [123,211]. Several phase I clinical trials investigating the efficacy of the dual combination of ribociclib and the mTOR inhibitor everolimus are currently underway for children with DMG and other HGGs (NCT03387020; NCT03355794). Determining if the synergistic effects observed in the lab can be translated into the clinic will be imperative.

It has been established that DMG tumours have aberrations in components of the DNA damage response (DDR) [212], which are coupled with the propensity of H3K27M mutations to lead to highly unstable genomes [96]. It is well-known that germline mutations in homologous recombination genes, for example *BRCA1/2*, predispose individuals to breast and ovarian cancer, and that these mutations are synthetic lethal with poly(ADP-ribose) polymerase (PARP) inhibition [213,214]. PARP binds to single-strand breaks to facilitate DNA repair; PARP inhibition results in an accumulation of double-strand breaks which cannot be repaired in homologous recombination (HR)-deficient cells, resulting in cell death [213]. PARP inhibitors are currently FDA-approved for *BRCA1/2*-mutant breast, prostate and ovarian cancer. It is now emerging that HR deficiency is apparent in a subset of DMG patients. Multiple members of the pathway undergo a loss of heterozygosity (LOH) or are deleted in DMGs, including *BRCA1*, *BRCA2*, *RAD50* and *RAD51L1* [215]. Furthermore, a recent integrated genomic analysis found that genetic alterations in DNA repair genes (including HR genes) were found in ~61% of DMGs [203]. These findings highlight HR-mediated DNA repair as a potential therapeutic target in DMGs. PARP1 was found to be expressed in DMG patient samples and cell lines, and DMG cells were sensitive to PARP inhibition with nirapirib [216]. Nirapirib reduced the rate of DNA repair and sensitised DMG cells to radiation [216]. Moreover, gain-of-function mutations in protein phosphatase 1D (*PPM1D*), a negative regulator of the DDR, were found in up to 29% of DMGs [217]. The inhibition of PPM1D sensitised *PPM1D*-mutant DMG cells to the PARP inhibitor olaparib, likely due to impaired HR-mediated repair [218]. Therefore, targeting DNA repair using PARP inhibitors may be a feasible strategy for HR-deficient DMG tumours.

Cell cycle progression is intricately linked to DNA repair and DDR activation, with DMG tumours relying on G1–S and G2–M checkpoint activation and arrest to halt cell cycle progression in order to allow time for DNA repair to take place [205,212]. Mutations in *TP53*, found in 42–77% of DMGs, have been hypothesized to be primary driver of radioresistance by relieving the TP53-mediated inhibitory control over the homologous recombination (HDR) activity, which primarily occurs during the G2 phase [219,220]. Moreover, *PPM1D* mutations are known to inactivate checkpoint kinases ataxia-telangiectasia mutated (ATM) and checkpoint kinases 1/2 (Chk1/2), impairing the initiation of the DDR after radiotherapy [218]. Given their role as a vital conduit, connecting the DDR to cell cycle machinery, targeting Chk1/Chk2 and ATM has been investigated as a therapeutic strategy [221,222]. Chk1 and Chk2 mediate TP53 activation and subsequently the facilitation of the DDR [220]. Chk1 inhibition with the Chk1-specific inhibitor prexasertib (LY2606368) exacerbated the anti-tumor effects of radiotherapy and suppressed RT-activated G1–S and G2–M checkpoint activation, allowing for DNA replication and mitosis to take place uninhibited. Moreover, radiosensitisation with prexasertib was particularly effective in *TP53*-mutant H3K27M cells but not in *TP53*-wild-type cells, where the latter remained arrested in G1 [220]. However, there are still challenges in translating the therapeutic potential of Chk1 inhibition into the clinic. A phase I clinical trial (NCT02808650) that investigated prexasertib in paediatric patients with recurrent or refractory solid and CNS tumours did not show any objective responses, indicating that it was well-tolerated [223].

Chk1/2 are known to target key players in G2/M progression: Wee1 and polo-like kinase 1 (PLK1), both of which are found to be overexpressed and have themselves been targets of investigation in recent years [212]. Wee1 is a serine/threonine checkpoint kinase that acts as a gatekeeper of cell cycle progression. Following DNA damage, Wee1 is activated by Chk1/2, triggering G2–M checkpoint activation. Wee1 phosphorylation and subsequent degradation by PLK1 relieves Wee1's inhibitory control over cyclin-dependent kinase 1 (CDK1) at the G2/M checkpoint, enabling the CDK1/cyclin B complex to drive the G2–M transition [224]. Werbrouck et al. identified a synthetic lethal interaction between RT and the knockdown of Wee1 and PLK1 in TP53-mutant H3-K27M DMG cells [220]. Targeting Wee1 with the small-molecule inhibitor adavosertib (MK1775/AZD1775) attenuated radiotherapy-induced G2/M arrest, forced mitotic entry in DMG cells and exerted anti-tumor effects in DMG orthografts [225,226]. However, Wee1 is also thought to directly exert DNA damage irrespective of its effect on the cell cycle, although the underlying mechanisms are unclear [226]. Interestingly, both CDK1 and Wee1 are known to phosphorylate EZH2 and facilitate its ubiquitination [227,228], although this interplay between epigenetic regulation and cell cycle mechanisms is yet to be fully explored. The NCT01922076 trial is currently assessing the safety, toxicity and MTD of concurrent adavosertib treatment with radiotherapy in DMG patients.

PLK1 is a key regulator of the G2–M transition and mediates centrosome maturation, spindle assembly mitotic entry, the metaphase-to-anaphase transition and cytokinesis [229,230]. PLK1 exerts its effects on the G2–M transition via the activation of the M-phase inducer phosphatase 3 (CDC25C), which subsequently dephosphorylates and activates the CDK1/cyclin B complex [231]. In addition, PLK1 drives mitotic entry via Wee1 degradation, which relieves Wee1's inhibitory control over CDK1 [232]. The forced mitotic entry caused by PLK1-mediated Wee1 degradation is thought to play an important role in cell recovery following DNA damage and G2 arrest [228]. However, functional TP53 is known to attenuate PLK1-inhibition-induced cytotoxicity by activating the DDR via ATM and ATR as well as permitting centrosome separation in colon carcinoma cell models [233]. As such, the extent to which TP53 modulates sensitivity to PLK1 inhibitors requires further investigation in DIPG cell line models.

The therapeutic impact of targeting PLK1 is relatively unknown in paediatric gliomas, with only one study describing the in vitro efficacy of direct PLK1 inhibition in DMGs [234]. Here, it was found that the targeting of PLK1 with the PLK1 selective inhibitor volasertib (BI 6727) exerted anti-tumour effects against a range of cultured DMG cell lines, with PLK1 inhibition leading to significant G2-to-M-phase cell cycle arrest and H3.1K27M-mutant

DMG cell lines showing more sensitivity than their H3.3K27M counterparts. It was further shown that the inhibition of PLK1 with volasertib acted to sensitise DMG cells to the effects of irradiation [234], further highlighting PLK1as a therapeutic target beyond its role in cell cycle progression towards a further role in DNA damage repair mechanisms.

6. Activating the Immune Response as a Potential Therapeutic Option in DMGs

Examination of the differences between the immune profiles of both pediatric HGGs and DMGs has demonstrated that DMGs typically have higher leukocyte chemo-attractant expression, with immune cells constituting a large portion of the cells within the DMG tumour mass. However, the immune environment in DMGs is largely non-inflammatory, with a low adaptive immune response and decreased infiltration of natural killer (NK) cells (reviewed in [235]). Of the immune cells present, bone-marrow-derived macrophages (BMDMs), over microglia, are the predominant tumour-associated macrophages/microglia (TAM) subpopulation in DMGs [25]; it has been established that human DMG samples express high levels of the pan-macrophage markers CD11b, CD45 and CD68 concurrently with increased expression of the M2 marker CD163 [236], confirming that high expression of chemo-attractants results in the enhanced infiltration of, in particular, alternatively activated macrophages within this disease setting. Despite this knowledge, therapeutic targeting of non-tumour-infiltrating cell types, including TAMs, has only recently begun to be investigated.

Macrophages retain an inherent plasticity, capable of being polarised to either a classically activated, proinflammatory M1 or an alternatively activated M2 phenotype depending entirely on the inflammatory environment encountered (Figure 3). It is this very plasticity that makes macrophages a prime therapeutic target in many forms of cancer. Classically activated macrophages assume the M1 phenotype, which is characterised by an increased expression of the STAT1 signalling pathway and iNOS activation [237]. These cells are capable of stimulating an antitumor immune response through presenting antigens to adaptive immune cells, producing proinflammatory cytokines such as IL-1β, IL-6, IL-12 and TNFα in addition to chemotactic factors such as IL-8 and MCP-1 [238,239], as well as by phagocytosing tumour cells [240,241]. In comparison, alternatively activated M2 macrophages are characterised by the activation of the STAT3 pathway, resulting in the expression of the scavenger receptors CD163, CD204 and CD206 [242], as well as the production of immunosuppressive cytokines, including predominately Arg-1 [243], TGF-β [244] and IL-10 [245].

In support of the consensus that DMGs have been historically considered "immune cold" with respect to infiltrating leukocytes, Lin et al. have subsequently demonstrated that, compared to the situation in GBMs, there exists a low intrinsic inflammatory signature that contributes to the non-inflammatory phenotype of DMG TAMs [26]. Here, building on the earlier obtained data [236], pre-ranked gene-set enrichment analysis on DMG TAMs found that there were no significant increases in either M1- or M2-defined gene sets, with the authors concluding that DMG TAMs do not easily fit into a strict M1 or M2 classification [26]. These results mirror data collected from studies within the setting of gliomas [246] and GBMs [247]. Within these disease settings, the majority of TAMs, and likewise microglia, as well as macrophages isolated from normal brain regions could not be categorised into individual polarisation phenotypes. Indeed, comparative profiling of TAMs with matched controls, including circulating blood monocytes, non-polarised M0 and polarised M1 or M2 macrophages, indicate that macrophages that have infiltrated into GBM tumour tissue exhibit a continuum state more consistently resembling an undifferentiated M0 macrophage state [247], with similar results demonstrated in gliomas [246]. From these data, as well as those generated from a previous preliminary study [248], comprehensive analysis found that GBM TAMs also express comparatively lower levels of the M2 markers CD163, TGFβ and IL-10 compared to control macrophage populations specifically polarised to an M2 phenotype despite demonstrating increased activation of the STAT3 signalling pathway, a characteristic indicative of an M2 phenotype [247]. Additionally, the authors here also demonstrated that GBM TAMs express lower levels of the M1 markers IL-1β and IL-6 relative to control M1-polarised macrophages [247,248].

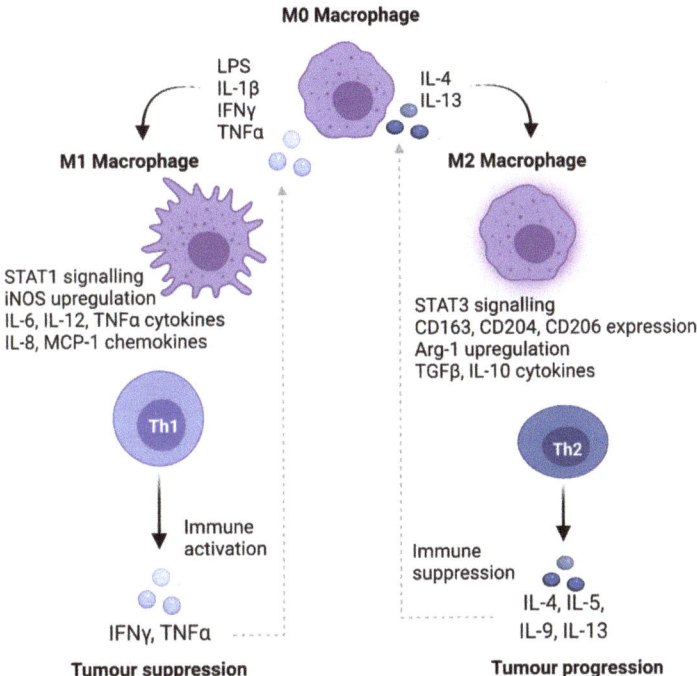

Figure 3. The role of macrophage phenotype and immune system signalling in DMGs. Macrophages are the predominant immune cell within the DMG microenvironment, where they exhibit a basal M0 phenotype. M0 macrophages are capable of being polarised to either a classically activated, proinflammatory M1 or an alternatively activated M2 phenotype depending entirely on the inflammatory environment encountered. Macrophages are transformed into an M1 phenotype by exposure to proinflammatory LPS, IL-1β, IFNγ or TNFα, which activates STAT1 signalling and therefore upregulates iNOS expression and the release of cytokines such as IL-6, IL-12 and TNFα along with increased production of chemokines such as IL-8 and MCP-1. Alternately, macrophages are polarised to an M2 phenotype following exposure to the cytokines IL-4 and IL-13, inducing STAT3 signalling and therefore the upregulation of cell surface markers CD 163, CD204 and CD206 as well as the release of Arg-1, TGFβ and IL-10. The activation of M1 macrophages promotes immune activation through the Th1 T cell response and subsequent release of proinflammatory IFNg and TNFa, leading to DMG tumour suppression and ongoing macrophage M1 activation. In contrast, M2 macrophages suppress the immune response through Th2 T cell activation, promoting DMG progression through establishing a tumour microenvironment which favours M2 macrophage polarisation.

Taken together, these results suggest the complex nature of TAMs in general but overall confirm that within these disease settings there exists a low inflammatory state, with the propensity of TAMs to exhibit a primarily M0 basal phenotype. Indeed, authors of these studies concluded that the thorough elucidation and identification of the mechanisms and pathways associated with an M0 macrophage phenotype alignment provide the basis for the development of macrophage-targeted therapeutic strategies focussed on propelling TAMs from this evident M0 towards an M1 inflammatory phenotype [247], thereby promoting the T cell Th1 proinflammatory cytokine immune response, resulting in tumour suppression [249]. As it is known that there is minimal active T cell infiltrate within DMGs [26], promoting the immune response by targeting M1 macrophage phenotype activation mechanisms would result in greater tumour regression and clearance.

There are a number of potential DMG therapeutics that target diverse cellular processes including the cell cycle, metabolism and epigenetic mechanisms that have the concurrent ability to modulate the macrophage phenotypic switch towards an M1-dominant TAM population, required to assist in tumour clearance. For example, the mTOR signalling pathway plays a central role in the metabolic programming of TAMs [250]; downstream of mTOR activation the activation of STAT3 negatively regulates the macrophage-derived anti-tumor immune response [251] by conferring an M2 phenotype [242]. In addition to having a directly positive effect against DMG cells [124], targeting of macrophage mTOR activity with rapamycin has been shown to stimulate macrophages towards an M1 phenotype, contributing to an overall anti-tumour effect within the setting of GBMs [252]. Similarly, in gliomas, a gain-of-function mutation in STAT3 results in increased immunosuppression and heightened tumour invasion, whilst within the setting of DMGs specifically it is known that STAT3 is elevated. In confirmation of its role in DMGs, exposure to the JAK2-specific STAT3 inhibitor AG490 resulted in decreased DMG cell invasion, migration and viability, whilst sensitising DMG cells to radiation by interfering with DNA damage repair mechanisms [253]. Whilst these studies did not extend to in vivo analysis of DMG tumorgenicity in response to AG490 therapy, it is interesting to note that it is also known that the STAT3 inhibitor AG490 is able to abrogate M2 macrophage polarisation. For example, within the setting of multiple myeloma, exposure to AG490 drives macrophages from an alternatively activated state, previously invoked by being co-cultured with tumour cells, towards an inflammatory phenotype. This was evidenced by the decreased expression of M2 markers Arg-1, CD163 and CD206 that was concurrent with a significant elevation in TNFα expression, characteristic of an M1 phenotypic switch, demonstrating the dual role that STAT3 inhibition may play within this disease setting [254].

Likewise, PLK1 is a key regulator of the cell cycle that demonstrates heightened expression in DMGs, making it an attractive therapeutic target. Indeed, targeting of PLK1 with volasertib demonstrates anti-tumour effects against DMG cell lines in vitro, where it leads to significant cell cycle arrest and apoptosis [234]. Highly expressed PLK1 promotes TNFα-stimulated gene 6 (TSG6) signalling and enhances an invasive phenotype in lung cancer cells [255], with TSG6 activation preventing the macrophage expression of proinflammatory M1 markers such as iNOS, IL-6, TNFα and IL-1β while increasing the expression of anti-inflammatory M2 markers such as CD206, IL-4 and IL-10 [256]. These results suggest that targeting PLK1 may also invoke a favourable immune response capable of enhancing tumour clearance. However, it has also been shown within a THP-1 monocytic cell line model of macrophage function that PLK1 inhibition, mediated via the PLK1 inhibitor GW843682X, significantly decreased lipopolysaccharide (LPS)-induced TNFα mRNA expression in a dose-dependent manner. The authors here attributed this apparent decrease in the M1 macrophage response to LPS stimulation to the inhibition of the MAPK and NFKβ signalling pathways by the PLK1 inhibitor [257]. Whilst the role of PLK1 in DMGs within an in vivo setting is yet to be functionally determined, the non-inflammatory tumour microenvironment within this setting would support the absence of macrophage toll-like receptor 4 (TLR-4) engagement, required for LPS-induced signalling [258] within the macrophage cell model used above [257].

The consistently inactivated state of TAM TLR-4 signalling may itself present a viable therapeutic target in DMGs. As an example of how this may be effective, it has been demonstrated that TLR-4 activation, using the chemotherapeutic agent paclitaxel, was able to polarise immunosuppressed M2 macrophages towards an M1 state, with their inflammatory activation able to inhibit tumour progression in both breast cancer and melanoma models, with TAMs isolated from tumour-bearing mice treated with paclitaxel exhibiting an increase in M1 phenotype iNOS, IL-6 and IL-12 expression concurrent with decreased M2 phenotype expression of CD206 and Arg-1 [259]. Whilst paclitaxel has been reported to display limited efficacy when previously trialled as a radiosensitiser in DMGs [260], it may yet prove useful within this disease setting as a specific beneficial modulator of the macrophage inflammatory response.

Similarly, the targeting of polyamine synthesis and transport has been shown to be an effective therapeutic against DMG tumorgenicity whilst also being known to drive an M1 macrophage inflammatory state. Khan et al. [24] have shown that polyamine synthesis is upregulated in DMGs. When the rate-limiting enzyme in this process, ODC1, is targeted with DMFO treatment compensatory mechanisms are invoked that result in enhanced polyamine transport through upregulation in the cellular membrane transporter SLC3A2. Confirmation of the pivotal role the polyamine pathway plays in DMG tumorgenicity was subsequently ascertained, both in vitro and in vivo, through the dual-targeting of polyamine synthesis with a combined therapeutic regime using DFMO to target polyamine synthesis, coupled with the inhibition of polyamine transport using the compound AMXT 1501 [24]. Whilst the authors here did not seek to ascertain the inflammatory status within their mouse PDX DMG model following polyamine pathway targeting, a similar study within the setting of melanoma provides an informative indication. Alexander et al. [261] have targeted melanoma tumour growth in mice by treatment with DFMO combined with the polyamine transport inhibitor trimer PT1. In this study they found that this combination therapy concurrently decreased tumour growth whilst significantly increasing proinflammatory TNFα, IFNγ and MCP-1 cytokine and chemokine expression, concomitant with a significant reduction in the M2-polarised macrophage population [261]. These studies highlight that, although not routinely examined within the setting of DMGs, targeting pathways commonly expressed in tumours and infiltrating TAMs such as mTOR and STAT3 signalling or polyamine synthesis and transport may provide an additive effect that disrupts the cross-talk between immune and malignant cells, effectively reducing immunosuppression and promoting tumour sequestration and removal [262].

Epigenetic dysfunction resulting from H3K27M mutations are frequently observed in DMGs, with the targeting of epigenetic regulation and associated mechanisms offering viable treatment options (Table 1). For example, DMGs have been shown to be exquisitely sensitive to HDAC inhibition [16], with the specific role of HDACs in DMG epithelial-to-mesenchymal transition (EMT), which results in increased tumour invasiveness, being subsequently shown in [263]. In this latter study, treatment of DMG cultures with up to 200 nmol/L of the HDAC inhibitor panobinostat significantly decreased the protein expression of EMT transcription factors, including ZEB1 and SNAIL/SLUG. Furthermore, panobinostat exposure also led to a concomitant decrease in the expression of stem cell phenotype markers SOX2 and NESTIN, implicating a direct connection between the epigenetic regulation of both the mesenchymal and stem cell characteristics of DMGs [263]. SNAIL expression has been implicated in the modulation and secretion of cytokines that can influence the tumour immune infiltrate, with tumour-cell-specific SNAIL deletion within the setting of breast cancer causing a higher percent of TAMs to be polarised towards an M1 phenotype coupled with a decrease in the percent of M2 macrophages [264]. In support of this, the treatment of DMGs with panobinostat and the resultant histone hyperacetylation induces an interferon type I response. This results in the increased expression of interferon-stimulated genes, which can sensitise tumour cells to the innate immune system [42] by potentiating the activation of the M1 macrophages' response [265,266] and enhancing effector T cell differentiation [267].

Similarly, the use of the HDAC inhibitor trichostatin-A (TSA) at 0.5 μM/kg in mouse models of melanoma or breast cancer was shown to be dependent on an active immune system, with treatment shown to be beneficial in C57BL/6 mice but have no effect in athymic nude mice. TAMs isolated from C57BL/6 mouse tumour models treated with TSA exhibited decreased expression of the M2 markers Arg-1 and CD206, with heightened expression of the M1 markers iNOS and IL-6 [268]. Furthermore, the authors here conclude that TAMs act as mediators of HDAC-inhibited immunomodulatory activity, directly leading to tumour suppression. In support of this, TAMs from TSA-treated mice were adoptively transferred to new tumour-bearing recipient mice. Compared to controls, inoculation with the TSA-modulated TAMs resulted in a significant decrease in tumour burden in the recipient mice, suggesting that HDAC inhibition epigenetically rewires macrophages into an M1 state, decreasing phenotypic plasticity and thereby stabilising their anti-tumour activity. This study went on to highlight the therapy-evasive nature of tumours, finding that TSA treatment, whilst effective at modulating TAM function, also increased programmed death ligand 1 (PD-L1) expression. PD-L1 expression is an immune evasion mechanism exploited by various malignancies and generally associated with poorer prognoses [269], including within DMGs where its expression is correlated with the extent of tumour-infiltrating lymphocytes [270,271]. In their study, Li et al. found that a dual-targeted approach was required in order to effectively combat tumour reoccurrence, combining TSA with anti-PD-L1 therapy to significantly enhance tumour reduction durability and prolong survival of tumour-bearing mice [268].

It is accepted that any potential DMG therapy regime would rely on a combination of treatment options tailored to the ongoing status of individual patients. The significance of the above study may therefore be in highlighting the potential therapeutic advantage of targeting epigenetic regulation in DMGs and the additive, cross-over effect such a strategy would have on the regulation of the immune response. It is known that the H3K27M mutation alters the methylation ability of EZH2 within the PRC2 complex, with this epigenetic mechanism having a profound impact on DMG/DIPG tumorgenicity. Whist directly targeting EZH2 in DIPG cells demonstrates limited efficacy, Keane and co-workers have recently demonstrated that EZH2 activity also regulates DIPG-induced microglia activation. Here, it was shown that the targeted siRNA knockdown of EZH2 resulted in a phenotypic switch of microglia towards an M1 state, indicated by the increased expression of iNOS [272]. This is consistent with the ability of EZH2 activation to repress the M1 macrophage inflammatory response, with the targeted inhibition of EZH2 by exposing macrophages to the EZH2 inhibitor UNC199 able to induce a dose-dependent increase in the LPS-induced expression of the M1 polarisation marker IL-6 [273]. These results suggest that EZH2 inhibition may exert its clinical benefit within the setting of DIPGs by targeting the tumour microenvironment rather than the tumour cells themselves, leading to a proinflammatory microglia and macrophage state that favours tumour clearance [272].

Taken together, these data suggest that beneficially modulating the immune response in parallel to, or combination with, DMG tumour targeting may work to enhance patient therapy, highlighting the need for a more holistic approach when evaluating potential treatment options for the disease. Additionally, there is a direct link between TAM phenotype status and subsequent T cell activation, which bears consequences for immunomodulatory therapy for brain tumours. Although the precise mechanisms in DMGs remain to be fully elucidated, it has been shown that GBM tumour cells recruit and polarise both macrophages and microglia to an M2 phenotype, resulting in the inhibition of T cell proliferation through the production of the immunosuppressive cytokines TGFβ and IL-10 [274], whilst also preventing the production of cytokines required to support activated tumour-specific CD8+ T, CD4+ Th1 and Th17 cells [247]. Mechanistically, GBM tumour cell kynurenine production activates the aryl hydrocarbon receptor (AHR) on TAMs, decreasing NFKβ signalling and thereby promoting an M2-like phenotype, leading to cytotoxic CD8+ T cell dysfunction [275]. Dysfunctional T cells are defined by the loss of effector function, including the loss of cytotoxicity and the decreased secretion of inflammatory cytokines such as TNFα and IFNγ [276] which, in turn, decrease M1 TAM polarisation, perpetuating the low inflammatory microenvironment characteristic of this disease. Further, the increased expression of Arg-1 by M2 macrophages is able to directly suppress T cell function within the microenvironment through the arginase-mediated depletion of arginine, which induces the down-regulation of the T cell CD3ζ chain [277]. It being the case that the activation domain of the CD3ζ chain is the major feature of the intracellular portion of the chimeric antigen receptor (CAR) of T cells, TAM overexpression of Arg-1 within the tumour microenvironment can be seen as a direct impediment for successful immunological targeting in DMGs using CAR T therapy.

In addition to targeting the upstream activation of the inflammatory response through modulation of the TAM phenotype switch, augmentation of T cell activation by employing

CAR T therapy is another potential therapeutic avenue aimed at beneficially altering the DMG tumour microenvironment. In CAR T therapy, peripherally circulating T cells are primed against antigens by ex vivo co-culturing with antigen-loaded dendritic cells or, alternately, are modified with a CAR gene, arming these cytolytic T cells with a receptor that can recognize a surface protein on tumour cells [276]. These cells are then expanded in culture before being infused into patients as an adoptive T cell transfer [278]. Using CAR T cells to deliver antibodies in this manner overcomes the inability of the antibodies alone to cross the BBB.

The primary hurdle to successful CAR T cell therapy is the engraftment of cells, involving both the sufficient migration of the transferred cells to within the tumour microenvironment and the sustained activation of their anti-tumour responses [276]. One approach to improve engraftment is the pre-conditioning of patients with chemotherapy to induce lymphopenia, with this approach currently in the recruitment stage of a phase I clinical trial within the setting of DMGs (NCT03396575). Another barrier to successful T cell therapy in DMGs is the lack of a sustained level of potency in the transferred T cells. The decreased efficacy of transferred T cells can be overcome through the concurrent therapeutic use of antibodies targeting immune checkpoints. Immune checkpoint molecules are frequently overexpressed during tumour development as a mechanism by which tumour cells are able to subvert the immune system response. A range of these molecules are known to be expressed within the tumour environment, including PD-L1/PD-1, cytotoxic T-lymphocyte antigen 4 (CTLA-4) [279], lymphocyte activation gene 3 (LAG-3) [280], B7-H3 [278] and indoleamine 2,3-dioxygenase (IDO) [281], although relatively few of them have been evaluated within the setting of DMGs as potential therapeutic targets [235]. For example, the disruption of the PD-L1/PD-1 immune inhibitory axis is known to be a mechanism by which other tumours evade the immune system [282]. In support of anti-PD-L1 therapy significantly enhancing tumour reduction and prolonging survival of tumour-bearing mice by augmenting the HDAC inhibitor modulation of the M1 TAM response detailed above [268], PD-1 blockage has also been shown to be effective at aiding the expansion and prolonged potency of CAR T therapy [282]. Unfortunately, in a comprehensive screen of cell surface antigens present on patient-derived DMG cultures, Mount et al. ascertained that both PD-1 and CTLA-4 had relatively low expression [283], indicating that the further targeting of these molecules within this setting, in combination with CAR T therapy, may not be effective. In contrast, Majzner et al. found that cell surface expression of the checkpoint molecule B7-H3 is high on DMGs. The authors went on to show that CAR T cells directed at B7-H3 are capable of crossing the BBB and produce sufficient tumour-killing amounts of IFNγ, IL-2 and TNFα when cocultured with DMG cells [278]. It remains to be seen whether these successful preliminary studies can be recapitulated within an in vivo model of DMGs. In their screen for potential targets for CAR T cell immunotherapy in DMGs, Mount et al. identified disialoganglioside GD2 as being very highly expressed within this disease setting [283]. The upregulation of the GD2 antigen in brain tumours compared to a normal brain makes it an attractive target for immunotherapy [284,285]. Similar to the above study [278], the co-culturing of GD2-CAR T cells with DMG cells triggered the production of IFNγ and IL-2. Furthermore, the authors were able to demonstrate within a range of DMG PDX mouse models that GD2-CAR T cell therapy was accompanied by widespread inflammatory infiltrate to within the tumour microenvironment, effectively clearing tumours, evident as early as day 14 of treatment [283]. They did, however note that tumour clearance was not total, with the persistence of tumour cells that were negative for GD2 expression following GD2-CAR T cell treatment. Worryingly, the authors also noted substantial toxicity occurred in GD2-CAR-T-cell-treated mice during the period of maximal therapeutic effect, occurring from days 10-14. This outcome was attributed to a heightened inflammatory response in brain regions that were susceptible to increased intracranial pressure and lethal transtentorial herniation, such as the thalamus. These occurrences are unfortunately not isolated and are recognised as potential neurotoxic complications of CAR T cell therapy, particularly in combination with checkpoint inhibitors [283]. Although demonstrating potential, the risks of toxicity along with the current scarcity of information of any other potential DMG targets, including immune checkpoint expression, need to be addressed in order to accomplish the sustained level of potency required for effective CAR T therapy in DMGs.

7. Targeting of Neuronal Cell–DMG Interactions

DMGs are highly infiltrative tumours in the brain. At the histological level glioma cells have been observed to display a specific morphology that surrounds neurons, a hallmark now described as Scherer's structures or perineuronal satellitosis [286,287] (Figure 4A). This feature is not unique to neoplastic cells but is also observed in healthy tissues between glial cells and neurons [288,289]. The interaction between oligodendrocyte precursor cells (OPCs) and neurons is essential for the production of myelin, which protects and supports axons during the propagation of action potentials [290]. Increased neuronal activity was found to have mitogenic effects on neural precursor cells (NPCs) and OPCs in juvenile and adult brains [291]. Although the exact cell of origin of DMGs is not understood, NPCs and OPCs have been reported to give rise to gliomagenesis [97,292]. Recent studies through a series of optogenetic experiments demonstrated that neuronal activity could stimulate the growth of HGG and DMG cells through the secretion of synaptic factors such as neuroligin-3 (NLG3). Although the exact receptor at which NLG3 acts upon tumour cells has not been identified, it has been shown that the subsequent activation of focal adhesion kinase (FAK) and downstream signalling through the PI3K/AKT pathway leads to glioma cell proliferation [49]. Subsequently, the same authors demonstrated that HGG/DIPG growth was decreased in *Nlg3* knockout animals. NLG3 release from neurons could be inhibited upon treatment with tetrodotoxin, a voltage-gated sodium channel blocker, indicating that NLG3 release is mediated upon neuronal activity. Furthermore, it was found that NLG3 could be cleaved by a disintegrin and metalloproteinase domain-containing protein 10 (ADAM10) (Figure 4B). Therapeutic inhibition of ADAM10 and ADAM10/17 with GI254023X and INCB7839, respectively, significantly reduced HGG and DMG growth in vivo, as observed by Xenogen imaging. Although treating animals with both inhibitors did not exhibit toxicity, long-term effects on neurofunction need to be investigated carefully [27]. INCB7839 is BBB-permeable and currently under investigation in HGGs, including DIPGs (NCT04295759). Although FAK inhibition could abrogate the effects of NLG3, its therapeutic capacity is limited due to low permeability in infiltrative tumours such as DMGs [293]; as yet, PI3K/AKT/mTOR pathway inhibitors have not been explored for their potential to attenuate synaptic communication within this setting.

Based on these earlier findings, Monje's team hypothesised that DMGs might engage directly in neuron communication through synapse formation [294]. Single-cell transcriptomic analysis of DMG tumours indicated distinct subpopulations with features resembling astrocytes, oligodendrocytes and OPC-like cells, later demonstrating enrichment of synapse-related genes [97,294]. Electron microscopy and electrophysiology experiments indicated the presence of functional synapses between DMG cells and neurons. More specifically, whole-cell patch-clamp experiments measured two distinct electrophysiological responses in DMG cells upon neuronal stimulation: a rapid excitatory postsynaptic current (EPSC, <5 ms) and a rather prolonged (>1 s) current. EPSC was found to be mediated by calcium-permeable (GluA20 α-amino-3-hydroxy-5-methyl-4-isoxazolepropionic acid receptors (AMPARs) and subsequently confirmed to be inhibited by AMPAR antagonists [294] (Figure 4C). Furthermore, treating animals with the AMPAR inhibitor perampanel, an antiepileptic agent, resulted in a significant decrease in proliferative Ki67-positive cells in orthotopic animal models of DMGs. Perampanel has so far been investigated as an antiepileptic agent in brain tumour patients, with promising responses being observed; however, further research is needed to understand which patients may benefit and whether it has anti-glioma properties [295]. HGGs were recently reported to form neurite-like, microtube-connected multicellular structures as a mechanism to communicate and resist treatment [296]. These microtubes were connected through hexameric structures consisting of connexin 43 protein, forming gap channels [296]. Consistent with this notion, the inhibition of gap junctions with meclofenamate repressed the propagation of prolonged currents upon neuronal stimulation and reduced the proliferative index in treated orthotopic DMG animals [294] (Figure 4D). Although these studies collectively demonstrate that neuronal hyperactivity contributes to glioma growth, Yu and colleagues showed that specific PI3K mutations might also influence the neuronal microenvironment [297]. They found that animals with GBM tumours containing specific phosphatidylinositol-4,5-bisphosphate 3-kinase catalytic subunit alpha (*PIK3CA*) mutations (C420R and H1047R) exhibited more seizures, while transcriptomic analysis revealed higher expression levels of genes involved in the formation of synapses [297]. Specifically, in the presence of the C420R variant, further experiments implicated the expression of glypican 3 (GPC3) as the key factor for the increased neuronal hyperactivity. *Gpc3*-knockout glioma cells with *PIK3CA* C420R exhibited prolonged survival compared to wild-type *Gpc3*. Currently, GPC3 inhibition is limited to immunotherapy approaches with antibody-based and CAR T therapies under clinical investigation in adult hepatocellular carcinoma [298]. Given the presence of *PIK3CA* mutations in DMGs, it is still to be confirmed if these variants can initiate neuronal activity as observed for GBMs and whether it is mediated through glypicans. Astrocyte-derived glypicans have been shown to initiate functional synapse formation and increase the recruitment of AMPARs to the synapses [299]; however, this must be yet confirmed in the context of DMGs (Figure 4E). Another intriguing matter is that endogenous polyamines can modulate calcium-permeable AMPARs. Polyamines can enter the water-filled regions of the AMPARs and, with their positive charge, block the flow of small ions such as Na^+ and Ca^{2+} [300]. NASPM, a synthetic polyamine, was found to play a partial neuroprotective role during ischemia in rats [301]. In addition, Venkatesh et al. showed that NASPM treatment inhibited the rapid EPSC but not the prolonged current in glioma cells [294]. As discussed previously, the metabolism of polyamine was found to be upregulated in DMG tumours, and dual inhibition of synthesis and uptake demonstrated significant extension of survival in orthotopic models of DMGs [24]. Although polyamines are known to play an important role in the proliferation of tumour cells, their potential role in modulating neuronal hyperactivity has not been investigated in DMGs. It is possible that at high levels polyamines may play a protective role at the local level where calcium-permeable AMPARs mediate the propagation of action potentials (Figure 4C).

It is currently unknown if other neurotransmitter receptors and molecules promote DMG proliferation through synapse formation. In other aggressive brain tumours, such as GBMs, glutamatergic and dopamine receptors have been implicated in their growth and migration [302] as well as having been recently reviewed in [303,304] (Figure 4C). Downstream mediators of neurotransmitter pathways are starting to be realised as potential pharmacological targets. Based on phosphoproteomic analysis performed across a range of paediatric tumours, calmodulin-dependent protein kinase II alpha (CAMKIIα) was reported to be elevated in the specific "neuronal class" of HGGs, which also exhibited higher expression of genes involved in glutamate neurotransmission and synaptogenesis [297]. CAMKIIα has been shown to play a significant role in synaptic transmission; thus, in the context of brainstem gliomas, it could potentially be implicated in propagating neuronal activity [305,306] (Figure 4C). Currently, highly selective and potent CAMKII inhibitors are not available; however, the development of new inhibitors remains an active area of research for neurological and cardiovascular diseases [307]. Other targets along the CAMKII pathway, such as calmodulin, have not been extensively explored. A few studies suggest antiproliferative, anticancer effects when targeted with antipsychotic agents in subcutaneous GBM models [308,309].

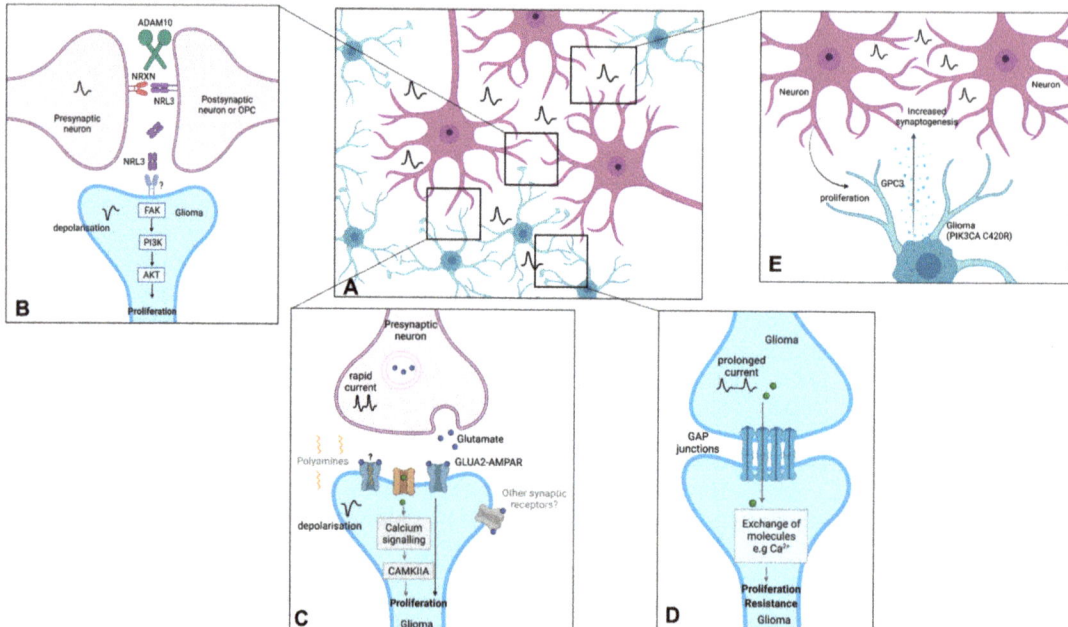

Figure 4. Schematic representation of established and potential interactions between the DMG and neuronal microenvironments. (**A**) DMGs form a complex network involving direct communication with neurons and glioma cells. (**B**) Typically, synaptic neuron interaction occurs through the NLG3/NRXN axis. Metalloproteinase ADAM10 cleaves NLG3 and is subsequently directed towards an unidentified receptor, leading to glioma cell proliferation through the activation of FAK and subsequently the PI3K/AKT pathway. (**C**) A rapid action potential is propagated from presynaptic neurons to DMG cells through calcium-permeable (GluA2) AMPA receptors, leading to glioma proliferation. Other synaptic receptors might be also involved in the propagation of neuron activity as well as downstream calcium signalling pathways mediated by CAMKIIA. Polyamines, short, positively charged molecules recently found to be upregulated in DMGs may also modulate the activity of GLUA2-AMPARs. (**D**) DMGs and HGGs can communicate with each other through gap junctions, promoting proliferation and resistance to radiotherapy. Long potentials were found to be mediated in DMGs through gap junctions. (**E**) Gliomas exhibiting specific PI3K mutations such as a C240R variant may increase synaptogenesis in neurons through the release of GPC3. Abbreviations: neuroligin 3 (NRLG3), neurexin (NRXN), a disintegrin and metalloproteinase domain-containing protein 10 (ADAM10), focal adhesion kinase (FAK), phosphoinositide 3-kinase (PI3K), protein kinase B (AKT), α-amino-3-hydroxy-5-methyl-4-isoxazolepropionic acid receptor (AMPAR), Ca^{2+}/calmodulin-dependent protein kinase II A (CAMKIIα), phosphatidylinositol-4,5-bisphosphate 3-kinase catalytic subunit alpha (PIK3CA) and glypican 3 (GPC3).

Although most recent research efforts have focused on understanding the interactions between neurons and HGGs/DMGs, it is anticipated that the relationship of gliomas with their microenvironment might be more complex. Classically, excessive neuronal activity has been thought to be controlled by specific inhibitory postsynaptic neurons (e.g., GABA-mediated); however, it was recently demonstrated that microglia play a key role in dampening the hyperexcitability of neurons [310]. It was found that microglia suppressed neuronal activity through the conversion of ATP–ADP–AMP through a cascade of purinergic receptor signalling. The subsequent conversion of AMP into adenosine by microglia (and potentially astrocytes) led to the inhibition of the A1 receptor in neurons and consequently a halt in neuronal activity [310]. Microglial dysfunction and specifically microglial activation have been observed in neurological disease settings such as neuroinflammation and epilepsy [311]. Interestingly, microglial activation has been observed in DIPG tumours; however, it is not known if they influence this novel microglial function to enhance their interaction with neurons [26]. Pharmacological targeting of A1 receptors potentially represents a new therapeutic avenue that is worth exploring further.

Apart from the local microenvironment, a rather more distant relationship has also been observed between the neuronal microenvironment and DMGs by influencing their metastasis beyond the brainstem [312]. Qin et al., through a series of biochemical and proteomic experiments, reported that neural precursor cells (NPCs) present in the lateral ventricle subventricular zone (SVZ) released a chemoattractant complex which stimulated the migration and invasion of DMG cells to the SVZ. This chemoattractant complex consisted of neurite-promoting protein pleiotrophin (PTN), heat shock protein 90B (HSP90B), secreted protein acidic and rich in cysteine (SPARC) and SPARC-like protein 1 (SPARCL1). The deletion of either factor of combination could delay the invasion of DMG cells to the SVZ of animals. Although pharmacological inhibition was not possible due to the lack of BBB-permeable HSP90 inhibitors, intracranial injection of a lentivirus expressing sh-RNA targeting the silencing of *hsp90b1* demonstrated a delay in DMG invasion in vivo. As BBB-permeable inhibitors of HSP90 have started emerging, future studies are needed to evaluate if they can inhibit DIPG invasion [313]. Pleiotrophin and midkine (MDK) belong to a family of heparin-binding cytokines influencing many physiological functions, including CNS development and immunity. Both bind to various receptors, including receptor protein tyrosine phosphatase ζ (RPTPζ), which was recently demonstrated in DMG invasion, low-density lipoprotein 1 (LRP1) and anaplastic lymphoma kinase (ALK). Currently, PTN and RPTPζ-targeted therapies are not available as anti-invasion therapeutic options. On the other hand, MDK, particularly the inhibition of its receptor, ALK, has demonstrated potential as a therapeutic option in GBMs [314]. However, it is not currently known if PTN exerts its effects through other receptors in DMGs.

8. Targeting of the Extracellular Matrix

Given the diffuse growth of DMGs in the brain, it is anticipated that it may influence the extracellular matrix (ECM) to promote its invasion of the brain parenchyma. The ECM is a highly organised network consisting of glycoproteins (e.g., fibronectin, laminin and tenascins), fibrous glycoproteins (collagen and laminin) and large amounts of glycosaminoglycans that interact either with proteins or hyaluronan [315]. Although the role of the ECM was mainly thought to be structural, it is now understood that it may influence cancer cell response to environmental changes, thus leading to migration and invasion. Key ECM targets such as tenascin-C (TN-C) have been recently found to be overexpressed in DMG tumours compared to normal brain tissue. In addition, knockdown experiments in primary DMG cultures have been suggestive of an essential role in DMG cell proliferation and migration [316]. Currently, TN-C has been targeted with antibodies; however, although this approach has shown some promise in subcutaneous glioma models, its efficacy has not been demonstrated in orthotopic DMG models, especially when the BBB remains intact [317]. Another potential target for DMG tumours that has recently been explored is the transmembrane receptor CD44. CD44 has been associated with the maintenance of cancer stem cell phenotype, adhesion to hyaluronan and invasion. Particularly in DMG cells, it was explicitly overexpressed in migrating and invading cells [318]. However, its effects on DMG growth and migration through therapeutic targeting has not been investigated in DMGs. Similarly to that mentioned above, TN-C blocking of CD44 with antibodies has demonstrated a reduction in subcutaneous glioma tumour growth while knocking down indicated enhanced sensitivity to cytotoxic agents [319,320]. Overall, targeting ECM components has been a relatively unexplored area of research for DMGs. In contrast, more knowledge has been accumulated for glioblastoma and recently reviewed comprehensively by Mohiuddin and Wakimoto [321]. Of particular interest would be to develop 3D bioengineered models that recapitulate the ECM to elucidate critical components involved in DIPG tumour invasion, migration and ultimately therapeutic targeting.

9. Conclusions

Over the past decade we have gained valuable insights into DMG biology and now recognise the role that histone and other genetic modifications play in the pathogenesis of the disease. Pre-clinically, there has been much success shown in targeting epigenetic dysregulation, cell cycle and proliferation mechanisms in DMGs. Whilst promising, these research endeavours have thus far demonstrated limited translation to effective patient treatment options. This in part may relate to the complex genomic dysregulation of DMGs and development of resistance mechanisms that will ultimately require the investigation of tailored combination therapies. Our understanding of DMG tumorigenicity has recently developed to include a role for the tumour microenvironment, highlighting further potential therapeutic targets involving regulation of the immune system and cross-talk between DMG tumour and neuronal cells. Combined, these facets underscore the potential for a more holistic approach when considering the development of innovative DMG treatment options.

Author Contributions: Conceptualization, D.S.Z., B.S.R.; writing—original draft preparation, E.H., H.H., R.L., A.K., M.T., B.S.R., D.S.Z.; writing—review and editing, E.H., H.H., R.L., M.T., B.S.R., D.S.Z. All authors have read and agreed to the published version of the manuscript.

Funding: This research was funded by Cancer Institute NSW, The DIPG Collaborative, The Cure Starts Now, The Kids' Cancer Project, Isaac McInnes fund, Levi's Project, and Cancer Australia.

Acknowledgments: All figures in this review manuscript were created with BioRender.com (accessed on 10 September 2021).

Conflicts of Interest: The authors declare no conflict of interest.

References

1. Louis, D.N.; Perry, A.; Reifenberger, G.; von Deimling, A.; Figarella-Branger, D.; Cavenee, W.K.; Ohgaki, H.; Wiestler, O.D.; Kleihues, P.; Ellison, D.W. The 2016 World Health Organization Classification of Tumors of the Central Nervous System: A summary. *Acta Neuropathol.* **2016**, *131*, 803–820. [CrossRef] [PubMed]
2. Louis, D.N.; Perry, A.; Wesseling, P.; Brat, D.J.; Cree, I.A.; Figarella-Branger, D.; Hawkins, C.; Ng, H.K.; Pfister, S.M.; Reifenberger, G.; et al. The 2021 WHO Classification of Tumors of the Central Nervous System: A summary. *Neuro-Oncology* **2021**, *23*, 1231–1251. [CrossRef]
3. Espirito Santo, V.; Passos, J.; Nzwalo, H.; Nunes, S.; Salgado, D. Remission of Pediatric Diffuse Intrinsic Pontine Glioma: Case Report and Review of the Literature. *J. Pediatric Neurosci.* **2021**, *16*, 1–4.
4. Warren, K.E. Beyond the Blood:Brain Barrier: The Importance of Central Nervous System (CNS) Pharmacokinetics for the Treatment of CNS Tumors, Including Diffuse Intrinsic Pontine Glioma. *Front. Oncol.* **2018**, *8*, 239. [CrossRef] [PubMed]
5. Wu, G.; Broniscer, A.; McEachron, T.A.; Lu, C.; Paugh, B.S.; Becksfort, J.; Qu, C.; Ding, L.; Huether, R.; Parker, M.; et al. Somatic histone H3 alterations in pediatric diffuse intrinsic pontine gliomas and non-brainstem glioblastomas. *Nat. Genet.* **2012**, *44*, 251–253. [PubMed]
6. Schwartzentruber, J.; Korshunov, A.; Liu, X.-Y.; Jones, D.T.W.; Pfaff, E.; Jacob, K.; Sturm, D.; Fontebasso, A.M.; Quang, D.-A.K.; Tönjes, M.; et al. Driver mutations in histone H3.3 and chromatin remodelling genes in paediatric glioblastoma. *Nature* **2012**, *482*, 226–231. [CrossRef]
7. Khuong-Quang, D.A.; Buczkowicz, P.; Rakopoulos, P.; Liu, X.Y.; Fontebasso, A.M.; Bouffet, E.; Bartels, U.; Albrecht, S.; Schwartzentruber, J.; Letourneau, L.; et al. K27M mutation in histone H3.3 defines clinically and biologically distinct subgroups of pediatric diffuse intrinsic pontine gliomas. *Acta Neuropathol.* **2012**, *124*, 439–447. [CrossRef]
8. Larson, J.D.; Kasper, L.H.; Paugh, B.S.; Jin, H.; Wu, G.; Kwon, C.H.; Fan, Y.; Shaw, T.I.; Silveira, A.B.; Qu, C.; et al. Histone H3.3 K27M Accelerates Spontaneous Brainstem Glioma and Drives Restricted Changes in Bivalent Gene Expression. *Cancer Cell* **2019**, *35*, 140–155.e7. [CrossRef] [PubMed]
9. Cooney, T.M.; Lubanszky, E.; Prasad, R.; Hawkins, C.; Mueller, S. Diffuse midline glioma: Review of epigenetics. *J. Neurooncol.* **2020**, *150*, 27–34. [CrossRef]
10. Fontebasso, A.M.; Liu, X.Y.; Sturm, D.; Jabado, N. Chromatin remodeling defects in pediatric and young adult glioblastoma: A tale of a variant histone 3 tail. *Brain Pathol.* **2013**, *23*, 210–216. [CrossRef]
11. Sievers, P.; Sill, M.; Schrimpf, D.; Stichel, D.; Reuss, D.E.; Sturm, D.; Hench, J.; Frank, S.; Krskova, L.; Vicha, A.; et al. A subset of pediatric-type thalamic gliomas share a distinct DNA methylation profile, H3K27me3 loss and frequent alteration of EGFR. *Neuro-Oncol.* **2021**, *23*, 34–43. [CrossRef]

12. Chan, K.M.; Fang, D.; Gan, H.; Hashizume, R.; Yu, C.; Schroeder, M.; Gupta, N.; Mueller, S.; James, C.D.; Jenkins, R.; et al. The histone H3.3K27M mutation in pediatric glioma reprograms H3K27 methylation and gene expression. *Genes Dev.* **2013**, *27*, 985–990. [CrossRef]
13. Mohammad, F.; Weissmann, S.; Leblanc, B.; Pandey, D.P.; Højfeldt, J.W.; Comet, I.; Zheng, C.; Johansen, J.V.; Rapin, N.; Porse, B.T.; et al. EZH2 is a potential therapeutic target for H3K27M-mutant pediatric gliomas. *Nat. Med.* **2017**, *23*, 483–492. [CrossRef] [PubMed]
14. Knudsen, E.S.; Witkiewicz, A.K. The Strange Case of CDK4/6 Inhibitors: Mechanisms, Resistance, and Combination Strategies. *Trends. Cancer* **2017**, *3*, 39–55. [CrossRef] [PubMed]
15. Hashizume, R. Epigenetic Targeted Therapy for Diffuse Intrinsic Pontine Glioma. *Neurol. Med.-Chir.* **2017**, *57*, 331–342. [CrossRef] [PubMed]
16. Grasso, C.S.; Tang, Y.; Truffaux, N.; Berlow, N.E.; Liu, L.; Debily, M.-A.; Quist, M.J.; Davis, L.E.; Huang, E.C.; Woo, P.J.; et al. Functionally defined therapeutic targets in diffuse intrinsic pontine glioma. *Nat. Med.* **2015**, *21*, 555–559. [CrossRef] [PubMed]
17. Piunti, A.; Hashizume, R.; Morgan, M.A.; Bartom, E.T.; Horbinski, C.M.; Marshall, S.A.; Rendleman, E.J.; Ma, Q.; Takahashi, Y.-H.; Woodfin, A.R.; et al. Therapeutic targeting of polycomb and BET bromodomain proteins in diffuse intrinsic pontine gliomas. *Nat. Med.* **2017**, *23*, 493–500. [CrossRef]
18. Lovén, J.; Hoke, H.A.; Lin, C.Y.; Lau, A.; Orlando, D.A.; Vakoc, C.R.; Bradner, J.E.; Lee, T.I.; Young, R.A. Selective inhibition of tumor oncogenes by disruption of super-enhancers. *Cell* **2013**, *153*, 320–334. [CrossRef] [PubMed]
19. Taylor, I.C.; Hutt-Cabezas, M.; Brandt, W.D.; Kambhampati, M.; Nazarian, J.; Chang, H.T.; Warren, K.E.; Eberhart, C.G.; Raabe, E.H. Disrupting NOTCH Slows Diffuse Intrinsic Pontine Glioma Growth, Enhances Radiation Sensitivity, and Shows Combinatorial Efficacy With Bromodomain Inhibition. *J. Neuropathol. Exp. Neurol.* **2015**, *74*, 778–790. [CrossRef] [PubMed]
20. Gasparian, A.V.; Burkhart, C.A.; Purmal, A.A.; Brodsky, L.; Pal, M.; Saranadasa, M.; Bosykh, D.A.; Commane, M.; Guryanova, O.A.; Pal, S.; et al. Curaxins: Anticancer compounds that simultaneously suppress NF-κB and activate p53 by targeting FACT. *Sci. Transl. Med.* **2011**, *3*, 95ra74–95ra95. [CrossRef] [PubMed]
21. Ehteda, A.; Simon, S.; Franshaw, L.; Giorgi, F.M.; Liu, J.; Joshi, S.; Rouaen, J.R.C.; Pang, C.N.I.; Pandher, R.; Mayoh, C.; et al. Dual targeting of the epigenome via FACT complex and histone deacetylase is a potent treatment strategy for DIPG. *Cell Rep.* **2021**, *35*, 108994. [CrossRef]
22. Chung, C.; Sweha, S.R.; Pratt, D.; Tamrazi, B.; Panwalkar, P.; Banda, A.; Bayliss, J.; Hawes, D.; Yang, F.; Lee, H.J.; et al. Integrated Metabolic and Epigenomic Reprograming by H3K27M Mutations in Diffuse Intrinsic Pontine Gliomas. *Cancer Cell* **2020**, *38*, 334–349.e9. [CrossRef]
23. Tsoli, M.; Liu, J.; Franshaw, L.; Shen, H.; Cheng, C.; Jung, M.; Joshi, S.; Ehteda, A.; Khan, A.; Montero-Carcabosso, A.; et al. Dual targeting of mitochondrial function and mTOR pathway as a therapeutic strategy for diffuse intrinsic pontine glioma. *Oncotarget* **2018**, *9*, 7541–7556. [CrossRef]
24. Khan, A.; Gamble, L.D.; Upton, D.H.; Ung, C.; Yu, D.M.T.; Ehteda, A.; Pandher, R.; Mayoh, C.; Hebert, S.; Jabado, N.; et al. Dual targeting of polyamine synthesis and uptake in diffuse intrinsic pontine gliomas. *Nat. Commun.* **2021**, *12*, 971. [CrossRef]
25. Ross, J.L.; Chen, Z.; Herting, C.J.; Grabovska, Y.; Szulzewsky, F.; Puigdelloses, M.; Monterroza, L.; Switchenko, J.; Wadhwani, N.R.; Cimino, P.J.; et al. Platelet-derived growth factor beta is a potent inflammatory driver in paediatric high-grade glioma. *Brain* **2021**, *144*, 53–69. [CrossRef] [PubMed]
26. Lin, G.L.; Nagaraja, S.; Filbin, M.G.; Suva, M.L.; Vogel, H.; Monje, M. Non-inflammatory tumor microenvironment of diffuse intrinsic pontine glioma. *Acta Neuropathol. Commun.* **2018**, *6*, 51. [CrossRef] [PubMed]
27. Venkatesh, H.S.; Tam, L.T.; Woo, P.J.; Lennon, J.; Nagaraja, S.; Gillespie, S.M.; Ni, J.; Duveau, D.Y.; Morris, P.J.; Zhao, J.J.; et al. Targeting neuronal activity-regulated neuroligin-3 dependency in high-grade glioma. *Nature* **2017**, *549*, 533–537. [CrossRef] [PubMed]
28. Lewis, P.W.; Müller, M.M.; Koletsky, M.S.; Cordero, F.; Lin, S.; Banaszynski, L.A.; Garcia, B.A.; Muir, T.W.; Becher, O.J.; Allis, C.D. Inhibition of PRC2 activity by a gain-of-function H3 mutation found in pediatric glioblastoma. *Science* **2013**, *340*, 857–861. [CrossRef] [PubMed]
29. Bender, S.; Tang, Y.; Lindroth, A.M.; Hovestadt, V.; Jones, D.T.; Kool, M.; Zapatka, M.; Northcott, P.A.; Sturm, D.; Wang, W.; et al. Reduced H3K27me3 and DNA hypomethylation are major drivers of gene expression in K27M mutant pediatric high-grade gliomas. *Cancer Cell* **2013**, *24*, 660–672. [CrossRef]
30. Agger, K.; Cloos, P.A.C.; Christensen, J.; Pasini, D.; Rose, S.; Rappsilber, J.; Issaeva, I.; Canaani, E.; Salcini, A.E.; Helin, K. UTX and JMJD3 are histone H3K27 demethylases involved in HOX gene regulation and development. *Nature* **2007**, *449*, 731–734. [CrossRef]
31. Kruidenier, L.; Chung, C.-w.; Cheng, Z.; Liddle, J.; Che, K.; Joberty, G.; Bantscheff, M.; Bountra, C.; Bridges, A.; Diallo, H.; et al. A selective jumonji H3K27 demethylase inhibitor modulates the proinflammatory macrophage response. *Nature* **2012**, *488*, 404–408. [CrossRef]
32. Hashizume, R.; Andor, N.; Ihara, Y.; Lerner, R.; Gan, H.; Chen, X.; Fang, D.; Huang, X.; Tom, M.W.; Ngo, V.; et al. Pharmacologic inhibition of histone demethylation as a therapy for pediatric brainstem glioma. *Nat. Med.* **2014**, *20*, 1394–1396. [CrossRef] [PubMed]

33. Katagi, H.; Louis, N.; Unruh, D.; Sasaki, T.; He, X.; Zhang, A.; Ma, Q.; Piunti, A.; Shimazu, Y.; Lamano, J.B.; et al. Radiosensitization by Histone H3 Demethylase Inhibition in Diffuse Intrinsic Pontine Glioma. *Clin. Cancer Res.* **2019**, *25*, 5572–5583. [CrossRef] [PubMed]
34. Nikolaev, A.; Fiveash, J.B.; Yang, E.S. Combined Targeting of Mutant p53 and Jumonji Family Histone Demethylase Augments Therapeutic Efficacy of Radiation in H3K27M DIPG. *Int. J. Mol. Sci.* **2020**, *21*, 490. [CrossRef] [PubMed]
35. Wiese, M.; Schill, F.; Sturm, D.; Pfister, S.; Hulleman, E.; Johnsen, S.A.; Kramm, C.M. No Significant Cytotoxic Effect of the EZH2 Inhibitor Tazemetostat (EPZ-6438) on Pediatric Glioma Cells with Wildtype Histone 3 or Mutated Histone 3.3. *Klin. Pädiatrie* **2016**, *228*, 113–117. [CrossRef]
36. Kumar, S.S.; Sengupta, S.; Lee, K.; Hura, N.; Fuller, C.; DeWire, M.; Stevenson, C.B.; Fouladi, M.; Drissi, R. BMI-1 is a potential therapeutic target in diffuse intrinsic pontine glioma. *Oncotarget* **2017**, *8*, 62962–62975. [CrossRef]
37. Balakrishnan, I.; Danis, E.; Pierce, A.; Madhavan, K.; Wang, D.; Dahl, N.; Sanford, B.; Birks, D.K.; Davidson, N.; Metselaar, D.S.; et al. Senescence Induced by BMI1 Inhibition Is a Therapeutic Vulnerability in H3K27M-Mutant DIPG. *Cell Rep.* **2020**, *33*, 108286. [CrossRef] [PubMed]
38. Senthil Kumar, S.; Sengupta, S.; Zhu, X.; Mishra, D.K.; Phoenix, T.; Dyer, L.; Fuller, C.; Stevenson, C.B.; DeWire, M.; Fouladi, M.; et al. Diffuse Intrinsic Pontine Glioma Cells Are Vulnerable to Mitotic Abnormalities Associated with BMI-1 Modulation. *Mol. Cancer Res.* **2020**, *18*, 1711–1723. [CrossRef]
39. Hennika, T.; Hu, G.; Olaciregui, N.G.; Barton, K.L.; Ehteda, A.; Chitranjan, A.; Chang, C.; Gifford, A.J.; Tsoli, M.; Ziegler, D.S.; et al. Pre-Clinical Study of Panobinostat in Xenograft and Genetically Engineered Murine Diffuse Intrinsic Pontine Glioma Models. *PLoS ONE* **2017**, *12*, e0169485. [CrossRef]
40. Nagaraja, S.; Vitanza, N.A.; Woo, P.J.; Taylor, K.R.; Liu, F.; Zhang, L.; Li, M.; Meng, W.; Ponnuswami, A.; Sun, W.; et al. Transcriptional Dependencies in Diffuse Intrinsic Pontine Glioma. *Cancer Cell* **2017**, *31*, 635–652.e6. [CrossRef]
41. Wang, J.; Huang, T.Y.-T.; Hou, Y.; Bartom, E.; Lu, X.; Shilatifard, A.; Yue, F.; Saratsis, A. Epigenomic landscape and 3D genome structure in pediatric high-grade glioma. *Sci. Adv.* **2021**, *7*, eabg4126. [CrossRef]
42. Krug, B.; De Jay, N.; Harutyunyan, A.S.; Deshmukh, S.; Marchione, D.M.; Guilhamon, P.; Bertrand, K.C.; Mikael, L.G.; McConechy, M.K.; Chen, C.C.L.; et al. Pervasive H3K27 Acetylation Leads to ERV Expression and a Therapeutic Vulnerability in H3K27M Gliomas. *Cancer Cell* **2019**, *35*, 782–797.e8. [CrossRef]
43. Zhang, Y.; Dong, W.; Zhu, J.; Wang, L.; Wu, X.; Shan, H. Combination of EZH2 inhibitor and BET inhibitor for treatment of diffuse intrinsic pontine glioma. *Cell Biosci.* **2017**, *7*, 56. [CrossRef] [PubMed]
44. Wiese, M.; Hamdan, F.H.; Kubiak, K.; Diederichs, C.; Gielen, G.H.; Nussbaumer, G.; Carcaboso, A.M.; Hulleman, E.; Johnsen, S.A.; Kramm, C.M. Combined treatment with CBP and BET inhibitors reverses inadvertent activation of detrimental super enhancer programs in DIPG cells. *Cell Death Dis.* **2020**, *11*, 673. [CrossRef] [PubMed]
45. Anastas, J.N.; Zee, B.M.; Kalin, J.H.; Kim, M.; Guo, R.; Alexandrescu, S.; Blanco, M.A.; Giera, S.; Gillespie, S.M.; Das, J.; et al. Re-programing Chromatin with a Bifunctional LSD1/HDAC Inhibitor Induces Therapeutic Differentiation in DIPG. *Cancer Cell* **2019**, *36*, 528–544.e10. [CrossRef] [PubMed]
46. Zhang, P.; de Gooijer, M.C.; Buil, L.C.; Beijnen, J.H.; Li, G.; van Tellingen, O. ABCB1 and ABCG2 restrict the brain penetration of a panel of novel EZH2-Inhibitors. *Int. J. Cancer* **2015**, *137*, 2007–2018. [CrossRef] [PubMed]
47. Piunti, A.; Shilatifard, A. The roles of Polycomb repressive complexes in mammalian development and cancer. *Nat. Rev. Mol. Cell Biol.* **2021**, *22*, 326–345. [CrossRef]
48. Brown, Z.Z.; Müller, M.M.; Jain, S.U.; Allis, C.D.; Lewis, P.W.; Muir, T.W. Strategy for "detoxification" of a cancer-derived histone mutant based on mapping its interaction with the methyltransferase PRC2. *J. Am. Chem. Soc.* **2014**, *136*, 13498–13501. [CrossRef]
49. Venkatesh, H.S.; Johung, T.B.; Caretti, V.; Noll, A.; Tang, Y.; Nagaraja, S.; Gibson, E.M.; Mount, C.W.; Polepalli, J.; Mitra, S.S.; et al. Neuronal Activity Promotes Glioma Growth through Neuroligin-3 Secretion. *Cell* **2015**, *161*, 803–816. [CrossRef]
50. Bailey, C.P.; Figueroa, M.; Gangadharan, A.; Yang, Y.; Romero, M.M.; Kennis, B.A.; Yadavilli, S.; Henry, V.; Collier, T.; Monje, M.; et al. Pharmacologic inhibition of lysine-specific demethylase 1 as a therapeutic and immune-sensitization strategy in pediatric high-grade glioma. *Neuro-Oncology* **2020**, *22*, 1302–1314. [CrossRef] [PubMed]
51. Shi, J.; Vakoc, C.R. The mechanisms behind the therapeutic activity of BET bromodomain inhibition. *Mol. Cell* **2014**, *54*, 728–736. [CrossRef] [PubMed]
52. Xu, Y.; Vakoc, C.R. Targeting Cancer Cells with BET Bromodomain Inhibitors. *Cold Spring Harb. Perspect. Med.* **2017**, *7*, a026674. [CrossRef] [PubMed]
53. Filippakopoulos, P.; Qi, J.; Picaud, S.; Shen, Y.; Smith, W.B.; Fedorov, O.; Morse, E.M.; Keates, T.; Hickman, T.T.; Felletar, I.; et al. Selective inhibition of BET bromodomains. *Nature* **2010**, *468*, 1067–1073. [CrossRef]
54. Vezina, A.; Jackson, S. Scidot-21. Improving drug delivery to glioblastoma by targeting canonical wnt/β-catenin signaling in the blood-brain barrieR. *Neuro-Oncology* **2019**, *21*, vi275–vi276. [CrossRef]
55. Shorstova, T.; Foulkes, W.D.; Witcher, M. Achieving clinical success with BET inhibitors as anti-cancer agents. *Br. J. Cancer* **2021**, *124*, 1478–1490. [CrossRef]
56. Orphanides, G.; LeRoy, G.; Chang, C.H.; Luse, D.S.; Reinberg, D. FACT, a factor that facilitates transcript elongation through nucleosomes. *Cell* **1998**, *92*, 105–116. [CrossRef]
57. Gurova, K.; Chang, H.-W.; Valieva, M.E.; Sandlesh, P.; Studitsky, V.M. Structure and function of the histone chaperone FACT—Resolving FACTual issues. *Biochim. Biophys. Acta Gene Regul. Mech.* **2018**, *1861*, 892–904. [CrossRef]

58. Hsieh, F.-K.; Kulaeva, O.I.; Orlovsky, I.V.; Studitsky, V.M. FACT in Cell Differentiation and Carcinogenesis. *Oncotarget* **2011**, *2*, 830–832. [CrossRef] [PubMed]
59. Garcia, H.; Miecznikowski, J.C.; Safina, A.; Commane, M.; Ruusulehto, A.; Kilpinen, S.; Leach, R.W.; Attwood, K.; Li, Y.; Degan, S.; et al. Facilitates Chromatin Transcription Complex Is an "Accelerator" of Tumor Transformation and Potential Marker and Target of Aggressive Cancers. *Cell Rep.* **2013**, *4*, 159–173. [CrossRef] [PubMed]
60. Chang, H.-W.; Valieva, M.E.; Safina, A.; Chereji, R.V.; Wang, J.; Kulaeva, O.I.; Morozov, A.V.; Kirpichnikov, M.P.; Feofanov, A.V.; Gurova, K.V.; et al. Mechanism of FACT removal from transcribed genes by anticancer drugs curaxins. *Sci. Adv.* **2018**, *4*, eaav2131. [CrossRef]
61. Jeronimo, C.; Watanabe, S.; Kaplan, C.D.; Peterson, C.L.; Robert, F. The Histone Chaperones FACT and Spt6 Restrict H2A.Z from Intragenic Locations. *Mol. Cell* **2015**, *58*, 1113–1123. [CrossRef] [PubMed]
62. Jeronimo, C.; Poitras, C.; Robert, F. Histone Recycling by FACT and Spt6 during Transcription Prevents the Scrambling of Histone Modifications. *Cell Rep.* **2019**, *28*, 1206–1218.e8. [CrossRef]
63. Sarantopoulos, J.; Mahalingam, D.; Sharma, N.; Iyer, R.V.; Ma, W.W.; Ahluwalia, M.S.; Johnson, S.; Purmal, A.; Shpigotskaya, P.; Hards, A.; et al. Results of a completed phase I trial of CBL0137 administered intravenously (IV) to patients (Pts) with advanced solid tumors. *J. Clin. Oncol.* **2020**, *38*, 3583. [CrossRef]
64. Sturm, D.; Witt, H.; Hovestadt, V.; Khuong-Quang, D.A.; Jones, D.T.; Konermann, C.; Pfaff, E.; Tönjes, M.; Sill, M.; Bender, S.; et al. Hotspot mutations in H3F3A and IDH1 define distinct epigenetic and biological subgroups of glioblastoma. *Cancer Cell* **2012**, *22*, 425–437. [CrossRef]
65. Jha, P.; Pia Patric, I.R.; Shukla, S.; Pathak, P.; Pal, J.; Sharma, V.; Thinagararanjan, S.; Santosh, V.; Suri, V.; Sharma, M.C.; et al. Genome-wide methylation profiling identifies an essential role of reactive oxygen species in pediatric glioblastoma multiforme and validates a methylome specific for H3 histone family 3A with absence of G-CIMP/isocitrate dehydrogenase 1 mutation. *Neuro-Oncology* **2014**, *16*, 1607–1617. [CrossRef]
66. Statham, A.L.; Robinson, M.D.; Song, J.Z.; Coolen, M.W.; Stirzaker, C.; Clark, S.J. Bisulfite sequencing of chromatin immunoprecipitated DNA (BisChIP-seq) directly informs methylation status of histone-modified DNA. *Genome Res.* **2012**, *22*, 1120–1127. [CrossRef]
67. Holliday, R.; Pugh, J.E. DNA modification mechanisms and gene activity during development. *Science* **1975**, *187*, 226–232. [CrossRef] [PubMed]
68. Jones, P.A. Functions of DNA methylation: Islands, start sites, gene bodies and beyond. *Nat. Rev. Genet.* **2012**, *13*, 484–492. [CrossRef]
69. Tahiliani, M.; Koh, K.P.; Shen, Y.; Pastor, W.A.; Bandukwala, H.; Brudno, Y.; Agarwal, S.; Iyer, L.M.; Liu, D.R.; Aravind, L.; et al. Conversion of 5-methylcytosine to 5-hydroxymethylcytosine in mammalian DNA by MLL partner TET1. *Science* **2009**, *324*, 930–935. [CrossRef]
70. Ross, S.E.; Bogdanovic, O. TET enzymes, DNA demethylation and pluripotency. *Biochem. Soc. Trans.* **2019**, *47*, 875–885. [CrossRef] [PubMed]
71. Ahsan, S.; Raabe, E.H.; Haffner, M.C.; Vaghasia, A.; Warren, K.E.; Quezado, M.; Ballester, L.Y.; Nazarian, J.; Eberhart, C.G.; Rodriguez, F.J. Increased 5-hydroxymethylcytosine and decreased 5-methylcytosine are indicators of global epigenetic dysregulation in diffuse intrinsic pontine glioma. *Acta Neuropathol. Commun.* **2014**, *2*, 59. [CrossRef]
72. Chua, G.N.L.; Wassarman, K.L.; Sun, H.; Alp, J.A.; Jarczyk, E.I.; Kuzio, N.J.; Bennett, M.J.; Malachowsky, B.G.; Kruse, M.; Kennedy, A.J. Cytosine-Based TET Enzyme Inhibitors. *ACS Med. Chem. Lett.* **2019**, *10*, 180–185. [CrossRef]
73. Hagenbuchner, J.; Ausserlechner, M.J. Targeting transcription factors by small compounds—Current strategies and future implications. *Biochem. Pharmacol.* **2016**, *107*, 1–13. [CrossRef]
74. He, C.; Xu, K.; Zhu, X.; Dunphy, P.S.; Gudenas, B.; Lin, W.; Twarog, N.; Hover, L.D.; Kwon, C.H.; Kasper, L.H.; et al. Patient-derived models recapitulate heterogeneity of molecular signatures and drug response in pediatric high-grade glioma. *Nat. Commun.* **2021**, *12*, 4089. [CrossRef] [PubMed]
75. Dahl, N.A.; Danis, E.; Balakrishnan, I.; Wang, D.; Pierce, A.; Walker, F.M.; Gilani, A.; Serkova, N.J.; Madhavan, K.; Fosmire, S.; et al. Super Elongation Complex as a Targetable Dependency in Diffuse Midline Glioma. *Cell Rep.* **2020**, *31*, 107485. [CrossRef] [PubMed]
76. Lin, C.; Garrett, A.S.; De Kumar, B.; Smith, E.R.; Gogol, M.; Seidel, C.; Krumlauf, R.; Shilatifard, A. Dynamic transcriptional events in embryonic stem cells mediated by the super elongation complex (SEC). *Genes Dev.* **2011**, *25*, 1486–1498. [CrossRef] [PubMed]
77. Chipumuro, E.; Marco, E.; Christensen, C.L.; Kwiatkowski, N.; Zhang, T.; Hatheway, C.M.; Abraham, B.J.; Sharma, B.; Yeung, C.; Altabef, A.; et al. CDK7 inhibition suppresses super-enhancer-linked oncogenic transcription in MYCN-driven cancer. *Cell* **2014**, *159*, 1126–1139. [CrossRef] [PubMed]
78. Kwiatkowski, N.; Zhang, T.; Rahl, P.B.; Abraham, B.J.; Reddy, J.; Ficarro, S.B.; Dastur, A.; Amzallag, A.; Ramaswamy, S.; Tesar, B.; et al. Targeting transcription regulation in cancer with a covalent CDK7 inhibitor. *Nature* **2014**, *511*, 616–620. [CrossRef]
79. Katagi, H.; Takata, N.; Aoi, Y.; Zhang, Y.; Rendleman, E.J.; Blyth, G.T.; Eckerdt, F.D.; Tomita, Y.; Sasaki, T.; Saratsis, A.M.; et al. Therapeutic targeting of transcriptional elongation in diffuse intrinsic pontine glioma. *Neuro-Oncology* **2021**, *23*, 1348–1359. [CrossRef]
80. Garcia-Cuellar, M.P.; Fuller, E.; Mathner, E.; Breitinger, C.; Hetzner, K.; Zeitlmann, L.; Borkhardt, A.; Slany, R.K. Efficacy of cyclin-dependent-kinase 9 inhibitors in a murine model of mixed-lineage leukemia. *Leukemia* **2014**, *28*, 1427–1435. [CrossRef]

81. Yang, W.; Xia, Y.; Hawke, D.; Li, X.; Liang, J.; Xing, D.; Aldape, K.; Hunter, T.; Alfred Yung, W.K.; Lu, Z. PKM2 phosphorylates histone H3 and promotes gene transcription and tumorigenesis. *Cell* **2012**, *150*, 685–696. [CrossRef] [PubMed]
82. Liu, X.; Zhu, Q.; Guo, Y.; Xiao, Z.; Hu, L.; Xu, Q. LncRNA LINC00689 promotes the growth, metastasis and glycolysis of glioma cells by targeting miR-338-3p/PKM2 axis. *Biomed. Pharmacother.* **2019**, *117*, 109069. [CrossRef] [PubMed]
83. Prakasam, G.; Singh, R.K.; Iqbal, M.A.; Saini, S.K.; Tiku, A.B.; Bamezai, R.N.K. Pyruvate kinase M knockdown-induced signaling via AMP-activated protein kinase promotes mitochondrial biogenesis, autophagy, and cancer cell survival. *J. Biol. Chem.* **2017**, *292*, 15561–15576. [CrossRef]
84. Wan, Y.C.E.; Liu, J.; Chan, K.M. Histone H3 Mutations in Cancer. *Curr. Pharmacol. Rep.* **2018**, *4*, 292–300. [CrossRef]
85. Shen, H.; Yu, M.; Tsoli, M.; Chang, C.; Joshi, S.; Liu, J.; Ryall, S.; Chornenkyy, Y.; Siddaway, R.; Hawkins, C.; et al. Targeting reduced mitochondrial DNA quantity as a therapeutic approach in pediatric high-grade gliomas. *Neuro-Oncology* **2020**, *22*, 139–151. [CrossRef]
86. Pegg, A.E. Mammalian polyamine metabolism and function. *IUBMB Life* **2009**, *61*, 880–894. [CrossRef] [PubMed]
87. Truffaux, N.; Philippe, C.; Paulsson, J.; Andreiuolo, F.; Guerrini-Rousseau, L.; Cornilleau, G.; Le Dret, L.; Richon, C.; Lacroix, L.; Puget, S.; et al. Preclinical evaluation of dasatinib alone and in combination with cabozantinib for the treatment of diffuse intrinsic pontine glioma. *Neuro-Oncology* **2015**, *17*, 953–964. [CrossRef] [PubMed]
88. Pollack, I.F.; Jakacki, R.I.; Blaney, S.M.; Hancock, M.L.; Kieran, M.W.; Phillips, P.; Kun, L.E.; Friedman, H.; Packer, R.; Banerjee, A.; et al. Phase I trial of imatinib in children with newly diagnosed brainstem and recurrent malignant gliomas: A Pediatric Brain Tumor Consortium report. *Neuro-Oncology* **2007**, *9*, 145–160. [CrossRef]
89. Broniscer, A.; Baker, S.D.; Wetmore, C.; Pai Panandiker, A.S.; Huang, J.; Davidoff, A.M.; Onar-Thomas, A.; Panetta, J.C.; Chin, T.K.; Merchant, T.E.; et al. Phase I trial, pharmacokinetics, and pharmacodynamics of vandetanib and dasatinib in children with newly diagnosed diffuse intrinsic pontine glioma. *Clin. Cancer Res.* **2013**, *19*, 3050–3058. [CrossRef]
90. Broniscer, A.; Baker, J.N.; Tagen, M.; Onar-Thomas, A.; Gilbertson, R.J.; Davidoff, A.M.; Pai Panandiker, A.S.; Leung, W.; Chin, T.K.; Stewart, C.F.; et al. Phase I study of vandetanib during and after radiotherapy in children with diffuse intrinsic pontine glioma. *J. Clin. Oncol.* **2010**, *28*, 4762–4768. [CrossRef] [PubMed]
91. Geyer, J.R.; Stewart, C.F.; Kocak, M.; Broniscer, A.; Phillips, P.; Douglas, J.G.; Blaney, S.M.; Packer, R.J.; Gururangan, S.; Banerjee, A.; et al. A phase I and biology study of gefitinib and radiation in children with newly diagnosed brain stem gliomas or supratentorial malignant gliomas. *Eur. J. Cancer* **2010**, *46*, 3287–3293. [CrossRef] [PubMed]
92. Geoerger, B.; Hargrave, D.; Thomas, F.; Ndiaye, A.; Frappaz, D.; Andreiuolo, F.; Varlet, P.; Aerts, I.; Riccardi, R.; Jaspan, T.; et al. Innovative Therapies for Children with Cancer pediatric phase I study of erlotinib in brainstem glioma and relapsing/refractory brain tumors. *Neuro-Oncology* **2011**, *13*, 109–118. [CrossRef]
93. Razis, E.; Selviaridis, P.; Labropoulos, S.; Norris, J.L.; Zhu, M.J.; Song, D.D.; Kalebic, T.; Torrens, M.; Kalogera-Fountzila, A.; Karkavelas, G.; et al. Phase II study of neoadjuvant imatinib in glioblastoma: Evaluation of clinical and molecular effects of the treatment. *Clin. Cancer Res.* **2009**, *15*, 6258–6266. [CrossRef] [PubMed]
94. Lassman, A.B.; Pugh, S.L.; Gilbert, M.R.; Aldape, K.D.; Geinoz, S.; Beumer, J.H.; Christner, S.M.; Komaki, R.; DeAngelis, L.M.; Gaur, R.; et al. Phase 2 trial of dasatinib in target-selected patients with recurrent glioblastoma (RTOG 0627). *Neuro-Oncology* **2015**, *17*, 992–998. [CrossRef] [PubMed]
95. Grill, J.; Le Teuff, G.; Nysom, K.; Blomgren, K.; Hargrave, D.; McCowage, G.; Bautista, F.; van Vuurden, D.; Dangouloff-Ros, V.; Puget, S. Pdct-01. Biological medicine for diffuse intrinsic pontine gliomas eradication (biomede): Results of the three-arm biomarker-driven randomized trial in the first 230 patients from europe and australia. *Neuro-Oncology* **2019**, *21*, vi183. [CrossRef]
96. Buczkowicz, P.; Hoeman, C.; Rakopoulos, P.; Pajovic, S.; Letourneau, L.; Dzamba, M.; Morrison, A.; Lewis, P.; Bouffet, E.; Bartels, U.; et al. Genomic analysis of diffuse intrinsic pontine gliomas identifies three molecular subgroups and recurrent activating ACVR1 mutations. *Nat. Genet.* **2014**, *46*, 451–456. [CrossRef] [PubMed]
97. Filbin, M.G.; Tirosh, I.; Hovestadt, V.; Shaw, M.L.; Escalante, L.E.; Mathewson, N.D.; Neftel, C.; Frank, N.; Pelton, K.; Hebert, C.M.; et al. Developmental and oncogenic programs in H3K27M gliomas dissected by single-cell RNA-seq. *Science* **2018**, *360*, 331–335. [CrossRef]
98. Fontebasso, A.M.; Gayden, T.; Nikbakht, H.; Neirinck, M.; Papillon-Cavanagh, S.; Majewski, J.; Jabado, N. Epigenetic dysregulation: A novel pathway of oncogenesis in pediatric brain tumors. *Acta Neuropathol.* **2014**, *128*, 615–627. [CrossRef] [PubMed]
99. Meel, M.H.; Sewing, A.C.P.; Waranecki, P.; Metselaar, D.S.; Wedekind, L.E.; Koster, J.; van Vuurden, D.G.; Kaspers, G.J.L.; Hulleman, E. Culture methods of diffuse intrinsic pontine glioma cells determine response to targeted therapies. *Exp. Cell Res.* **2017**, *360*, 397–403. [CrossRef]
100. Fleischhack, G.; Massimino, M.; Warmuth-Metz, M.; Khuhlaeva, E.; Janssen, G.; Graf, N.; Rutkowski, S.; Beilken, A.; Schmid, I.; Biassoni, V.; et al. Nimotuzumab and radiotherapy for treatment of newly diagnosed diffuse intrinsic pontine glioma (DIPG): A phase III clinical study. *J. Neurooncol.* **2019**, *143*, 107–113. [CrossRef] [PubMed]
101. Halvorson, K.G.; Barton, K.L.; Schroeder, K.; Misuraca, K.L.; Hoeman, C.; Chung, A.; Crabtree, D.M.; Cordero, F.J.; Singh, R.; Spasojevic, I.; et al. A high-throughput in vitro drug screen in a genetically engineered mouse model of diffuse intrinsic pontine glioma identifies BMS-754807 as a promising therapeutic agent. *PLoS ONE* **2015**, *10*, e0118926. [CrossRef] [PubMed]
102. Takei, N.; Nawa, H. mTOR signaling and its roles in normal and abnormal brain development. *Front. Mol. Neurosci.* **2014**, *7*, 28. [CrossRef]

103. Zheng, Y.; Jiang, Y. mTOR Inhibitors at a Glance. *Mol. Cell Pharmacol.* **2015**, *7*, 15–20.
104. Roskoski, R., Jr. Properties of FDA-approved small molecule protein kinase inhibitors. *Pharmacol. Res.* **2019**, *144*, 19–50. [CrossRef] [PubMed]
105. Ebrahimi-Fakhari, D.; Franz, D.N. Pharmacological treatment strategies for subependymal giant cell astrocytoma (SEGA). *Expert Opin. Pharmacother.* **2020**, *21*, 1329–1336. [CrossRef] [PubMed]
106. Paugh, B.S.; Broniscer, A.; Qu, C.; Miller, C.P.; Zhang, J.; Tatevossian, R.G.; Olson, J.M.; Geyer, J.R.; Chi, S.N.; da Silva, N.S.; et al. Genome-wide analyses identify recurrent amplifications of receptor tyrosine kinases and cell-cycle regulatory genes in diffuse intrinsic pontine glioma. *J. Clin. Oncol.* **2011**, *29*, 3999–4006. [CrossRef]
107. Taylor, K.R.; Mackay, A.; Truffaux, N.; Butterfield, Y.; Morozova, O.; Philippe, C.; Castel, D.; Grasso, C.S.; Vinci, M.; Carvalho, D.; et al. Recurrent activating ACVR1 mutations in diffuse intrinsic pontine glioma. *Nat. Genet.* **2014**, *46*, 457–461. [CrossRef]
108. Yang, J.; Nie, J.; Ma, X.; Wei, Y.; Peng, Y.; Wei, X. Targeting PI3K in cancer: Mechanisms and advances in clinical trials. *Mol. Cancer* **2019**, *18*, 26. [CrossRef]
109. Zou, Z.; Tao, T.; Li, H.; Zhu, X. mTOR signaling pathway and mTOR inhibitors in cancer: Progress and challenges. *Cell Biosci.* **2020**, *10*, 31. [CrossRef]
110. Wang, X.; Proud, C.G. mTORC2 is a tyrosine kinase. *Cell Res.* **2016**, *26*, 266. [CrossRef]
111. Saxton, R.A.; Sabatini, D.M. mTOR Signaling in Growth, Metabolism, and Disease. *Cell* **2017**, *168*, 960–976. [CrossRef] [PubMed]
112. Porstmann, T.; Santos, C.R.; Griffiths, B.; Cully, M.; Wu, M.; Leevers, S.; Griffiths, J.R.; Chung, Y.L.; Schulze, A. SREBP activity is regulated by mTORC1 and contributes to Akt-dependent cell growth. *Cell Metab.* **2008**, *8*, 224–236. [CrossRef] [PubMed]
113. Ben-Sahra, I.; Howell, J.J.; Asara, J.M.; Manning, B.D. Stimulation of de novo pyrimidine synthesis by growth signaling through mTOR and S6K1. *Science* **2013**, *339*, 1323–1328. [CrossRef]
114. Robitaille, A.M.; Christen, S.; Shimobayashi, M.; Cornu, M.; Fava, L.L.; Moes, S.; Prescianotto-Baschong, C.; Sauer, U.; Jenoe, P.; Hall, M.N. Quantitative phosphoproteomics reveal mTORC1 activates de novo pyrimidine synthesis. *Science* **2013**, *339*, 1320–1323. [CrossRef] [PubMed]
115. Duvel, K.; Yecies, J.L.; Menon, S.; Raman, P.; Lipovsky, A.I.; Souza, A.L.; Triantafellow, E.; Ma, Q.; Gorski, R.; Cleaver, S.; et al. Activation of a metabolic gene regulatory network downstream of mTOR complex 1. *Mol. Cell.* **2010**, *39*, 171–183. [CrossRef]
116. Martina, J.A.; Chen, Y.; Gucek, M.; Puertollano, R. MTORC1 functions as a transcriptional regulator of autophagy by preventing nuclear transport of TFEB. *Autophagy* **2012**, *8*, 903–914. [CrossRef]
117. Zhao, J.; Zhai, B.; Gygi, S.P.; Goldberg, A.L. mTOR inhibition activates overall protein degradation by the ubiquitin proteasome system as well as by autophagy. *Proc. Natl. Acad. Sci. USA* **2015**, *112*, 15790–15797. [CrossRef]
118. Sarbassov, D.D.; Guertin, D.A.; Ali, S.M.; Sabatini, D.M. Phosphorylation and regulation of Akt/PKB by the rictor-mTOR complex. *Science* **2005**, *307*, 1098–1101. [CrossRef]
119. Garcia-Martinez, J.M.; Alessi, D.R. mTOR complex 2 (mTORC2) controls hydrophobic motif phosphorylation and activation of serum- and glucocorticoid-induced protein kinase 1 (SGK1). *Biochem. J.* **2008**, *416*, 375–385. [CrossRef]
120. Wu, Y.L.; Maachani, U.B.; Schweitzer, M.; Singh, R.; Wang, M.; Chang, R.; Souweidane, M.M. Dual Inhibition of PI3K/AKT and MEK/ERK Pathways Induces Synergistic Antitumor Effects in Diffuse Intrinsic Pontine Glioma Cells. *Transl. Oncol.* **2017**, *10*, 221–228. [CrossRef]
121. Chang, R.; Tosi, U.; Voronina, J.; Adeuyan, O.; Wu, L.Y.; Schweitzer, M.E.; Pisapia, D.J.; Becher, O.J.; Souweidane, M.M.; Maachani, U.B. Combined targeting of PI3K and MEK effector pathways via CED for DIPG therapy. *Neurooncol. Adv.* **2019**, *1*, vdz004. [CrossRef] [PubMed]
122. Pal, S.; Kozono, D.; Yang, X.; Fendler, W.; Fitts, W.; Ni, J.; Alberta, J.A.; Zhao, J.; Liu, K.X.; Bian, J.; et al. Dual HDAC and PI3K Inhibition Abrogates NFkappaB- and FOXM1-Mediated DNA Damage Response to Radiosensitize Pediatric High-Grade Gliomas. *Cancer Res.* **2018**, *78*, 4007–4021. [CrossRef]
123. Asby, D.J.; Killick-Cole, C.L.; Boulter, L.J.; Singleton, W.G.; Asby, C.A.; Wyatt, M.J.; Barua, N.U.; Bienemann, A.S.; Gill, S.S. Combined use of CDK4/6 and mTOR inhibitors induce synergistic growth arrest of diffuse intrinsic pontine glioma cells via mutual downregulation of mTORC1 activity. *Cancer Manag. Res.* **2018**, *10*, 3483–3500. [CrossRef]
124. Flannery, P.C.; DeSisto, J.A.; Amani, V.; Venkataraman, S.; Lemma, R.T.; Prince, E.W.; Donson, A.; Moroze, E.E.; Hoffman, L.; Levy, J.M.M.; et al. Preclinical analysis of MTOR complex 1/2 inhibition in diffuse intrinsic pontine glioma. *Oncol. Rep.* **2018**, *39*, 455–464. [CrossRef] [PubMed]
125. Miyahara, H.; Yadavilli, S.; Natsumeda, M.; Rubens, J.A.; Rodgers, L.; Kambhampati, M.; Taylor, I.C.; Kaur, H.; Asnaghi, L.; Eberhart, C.G.; et al. The dual mTOR kinase inhibitor TAK228 inhibits tumorigenicity and enhances radiosensitization in diffuse intrinsic pontine glioma. *Cancer Lett.* **2017**, *400*, 110–116. [CrossRef]
126. Surowiec, R.K.; Ferris, S.F.; Apfelbaum, A.; Espinoza, C.; Mehta, R.K.; Monchamp, K.; Sirihorachai, V.R.; Bedi, K.; Ljungman, M.; Galban, S. Transcriptomic Analysis of Diffuse Intrinsic Pontine Glioma (DIPG) Identifies a Targetable ALDH-Positive Subset of Highly Tumorigenic Cancer Stem-like Cells. *Mol. Cancer Res.* **2021**, *19*, 223–239. [CrossRef]
127. Becher, O.J.; Millard, N.E.; Modak, S.; Kushner, B.H.; Haque, S.; Spasojevic, I.; Trippett, T.M.; Gilheeney, S.W.; Khakoo, Y.; Lyden, D.C.; et al. A phase I study of single-agent perifosine for recurrent or refractory pediatric CNS and solid tumors. *PLoS ONE* **2017**, *12*, e0178593. [CrossRef] [PubMed]

128. Becher, O.J.; Gilheeney, S.W.; Khakoo, Y.; Lyden, D.C.; Haque, S.; De Braganca, K.C.; Kolesar, J.M.; Huse, J.T.; Modak, S.; Wexler, L.H.; et al. A phase I study of perifosine with temsirolimus for recurrent pediatric solid tumors. *Pediatric Blood Cancer* **2017**, *64*, e26409. [CrossRef]
129. Du, L.; Chen, X.; Cao, Y.; Lu, L.; Zhang, F.; Bornstein, S.; Li, Y.; Owens, P.; Malkoski, S.; Said, S.; et al. Overexpression of PIK3CA in murine head and neck epithelium drives tumor invasion and metastasis through PDK1 and enhanced TGFbeta signaling. *Oncogene* **2016**, *35*, 4641–4652. [CrossRef] [PubMed]
130. Xu, Y.; Pasche, B. TGF-beta signaling alterations and susceptibility to colorectal cancer. *Hum. Mol. Genet.* **2007**, *16*, R14–R20. [CrossRef] [PubMed]
131. Biswas, S.; Trobridge, P.; Romero-Gallo, J.; Billheimer, D.; Myeroff, L.L.; Willson, J.K.; Markowitz, S.D.; Grady, W.M. Mutational inactivation of TGFBR2 in microsatellite unstable colon cancer arises from the cooperation of genomic instability and the clonal outgrowth of transforming growth factor beta resistant cells. *Genes Chromosomes Cancer* **2008**, *47*, 95–106. [CrossRef] [PubMed]
132. Fleming, N.I.; Jorissen, R.N.; Mouradov, D.; Christie, M.; Sakthianandeswaren, A.; Palmieri, M.; Day, F.; Li, S.; Tsui, C.; Lipton, L.; et al. SMAD2, SMAD3 and SMAD4 mutations in colorectal cancer. *Cancer Res.* **2013**, *73*, 725–735. [CrossRef] [PubMed]
133. Mallet, C.; Lamribet, K.; Giraud, S.; Dupuis-Girod, S.; Feige, J.J.; Bailly, S.; Tillet, E. Functional analysis of endoglin mutations from hereditary hemorrhagic telangiectasia type 1 patients reveals different mechanisms for endoglin loss of function. *Hum. Mol. Genet.* **2015**, *24*, 1142–1154. [CrossRef] [PubMed]
134. Weiss, A.; Attisano, L. The TGFbeta superfamily signaling pathway. *Wiley Interdiscip. Rev. Dev. Biol.* **2013**, *2*, 47–63. [CrossRef]
135. Meel, M.H.; Schaper, S.A.; Kaspers, G.J.L.; Hulleman, E. Signaling pathways and mesenchymal transition in pediatric high-grade glioma. *Cell. Mol. Life Sci.* **2018**, *75*, 871–887. [CrossRef]
136. Lamouille, S.; Xu, J.; Derynck, R. Molecular mechanisms of epithelial-mesenchymal transition. *Nat. Rev. Mol. Cell Biol.* **2014**, *15*, 178–196. [CrossRef]
137. Guo, D.; Huang, J.; Gong, J. Bone morphogenetic protein 4 (BMP4) is required for migration and invasion of breast cancer. *Mol. Cell. Biochem.* **2012**, *363*, 179–190. [CrossRef]
138. Paez-Pereda, M.; Giacomini, D.; Refojo, D.; Nagashima, A.C.; Hopfner, U.; Grubler, Y.; Chervin, A.; Goldberg, V.; Goya, R.; Hentges, S.T.; et al. Involvement of bone morphogenetic protein 4 (BMP-4) in pituitary prolactinoma pathogenesis through a Smad/estrogen receptor crosstalk. *Proc. Natl. Acad. Sci. USA* **2003**, *100*, 1034–1039. [CrossRef]
139. Raida, M.; Clement, J.H.; Leek, R.D.; Ameri, K.; Bicknell, R.; Niederwieser, D.; Harris, A.L. Bone morphogenetic protein (BMP-2) and induction of tumor angiogenesis. *J. Cancer Res. Clin. Oncol.* **2005**, *131*, 741–750. [CrossRef]
140. Peng, J.; Yoshioka, Y.; Mandai, M.; Matsumura, N.; Baba, T.; Yamaguchi, K.; Hamanishi, J.; Kharma, B.; Murakami, R.; Abiko, K.; et al. The BMP signaling pathway leads to enhanced proliferation in serous ovarian cancer—A potential therapeutic target. *Mol. Carcinog.* **2016**, *55*, 335–345. [CrossRef]
141. Ghosh-Choudhury, N.; Ghosh-Choudhury, G.; Celeste, A.; Ghosh, P.M.; Moyer, M.; Abboud, S.L.; Kreisberg, J. Bone morphogenetic protein-2 induces cyclin kinase inhibitor p21 and hypophosphorylation of retinoblastoma protein in estradiol-treated MCF-7 human breast cancer cells. *Biochim. Biophys. Acta* **2000**, *1497*, 186–196. [CrossRef]
142. Cao, Y.; Slaney, C.Y.; Bidwell, B.N.; Parker, B.S.; Johnstone, C.N.; Rautela, J.; Eckhardt, B.L.; Anderson, R.L. BMP4 inhibits breast cancer metastasis by blocking myeloid-derived suppressor cell activity. *Cancer Res.* **2014**, *74*, 5091–5102. [CrossRef]
143. Ye, L.; Kynaston, H.; Jiang, W.G. Bone morphogenetic protein-10 suppresses the growth and aggressiveness of prostate cancer cells through a Smad independent pathway. *J. Urol.* **2009**, *181*, 2749–2759. [CrossRef] [PubMed]
144. Chen, A.; Wang, D.; Liu, X.; He, S.; Yu, Z.; Wang, J. Inhibitory effect of BMP-2 on the proliferation of breast cancer cells. *Mol. Med. Rep.* **2012**, *6*, 615–620. [CrossRef] [PubMed]
145. Wrana, J.L. Signaling by the TGFbeta superfamily. *Cold Spring Harb. Perspect. Biol.* **2013**, *5*, a011197. [CrossRef]
146. Wu, G.; Diaz, A.K.; Paugh, B.S.; Rankin, S.L.; Ju, B.; Li, Y.; Zhu, X.; Qu, C.; Chen, X.; Zhang, J.; et al. The genomic landscape of diffuse intrinsic pontine glioma and pediatric non-brainstem high-grade glioma. *Nat. Genet.* **2014**, *46*, 444–450. [PubMed]
147. Fontebasso, A.M.; Papillon-Cavanagh, S.; Schwartzentruber, J.; Nikbakht, H.; Gerges, N.; Fiset, P.O.; Bechet, D.; Faury, D.; De Jay, N.; Ramkissoon, L.A.; et al. Recurrent somatic mutations in ACVR1 in pediatric midline high-grade astrocytoma. *Nat. Genet.* **2014**, *46*, 462–466. [CrossRef]
148. Fukuda, T.; Kohda, M.; Kanomata, K.; Nojima, J.; Nakamura, A.; Kamizono, J.; Noguchi, Y.; Iwakiri, K.; Kondo, T.; Kurose, J.; et al. Constitutively activated ALK2 and increased SMAD1/5 cooperatively induce bone morphogenetic protein signaling in fibrodysplasia ossificans progressiva. *J. Biol. Chem.* **2009**, *284*, 7149–7156. [CrossRef]
149. Shen, Q.; Little, S.C.; Xu, M.; Haupt, J.; Ast, C.; Katagiri, T.; Mundlos, S.; Seemann, P.; Kaplan, F.S.; Mullins, M.C.; et al. The fibrodysplasia ossificans progressiva R206H ACVR1 mutation activates BMP-independent chondrogenesis and zebrafish embryo ventralization. *J. Clin. Investig.* **2009**, *119*, 3462–3472. [CrossRef]
150. Van Dinther, M.; Visser, N.; de Gorter, D.J.; Doorn, J.; Goumans, M.J.; de Boer, J.; ten Dijke, P. ALK2 R206H mutation linked to fibrodysplasia ossificans progressiva confers constitutive activity to the BMP type I receptor and sensitizes mesenchymal cells to BMP-induced osteoblast differentiation and bone formation. *J. Bone Miner. Res.* **2010**, *25*, 1208–1215. [CrossRef]
151. Carvalho, D.; Taylor, K.R.; Olaciregui, N.G.; Molinari, V.; Clarke, M.; Mackay, A.; Ruddle, R.; Henley, A.; Valenti, M.; Hayes, A.; et al. ALK2 inhibitors display beneficial effects in preclinical models of ACVR1 mutant diffuse intrinsic pontine glioma. *Commun. Biol.* **2019**, *2*, 156. [CrossRef]

152. Hino, K.; Ikeya, M.; Horigome, K.; Matsumoto, Y.; Ebise, H.; Nishio, M.; Sekiguchi, K.; Shibata, M.; Nagata, S.; Matsuda, S.; et al. Neofunction of ACVR1 in fibrodysplasia ossificans progressiva. *Proc. Natl. Acad. Sci. USA* **2015**, *112*, 15438–15443. [CrossRef]
153. Ramachandran, A.; Mehic, M.; Wasim, L.; Malinova, D.; Gori, I.; Blaszczyk, B.K.; Carvalho, D.M.; Shore, E.M.; Jones, C.; Hyvonen, M.; et al. Pathogenic ACVR1(R206H) activation by Activin A-induced receptor clustering and autophosphorylation. *EMBO J.* **2021**, *40*, e106317. [CrossRef] [PubMed]
154. Xie, C.; Jiang, W.; Lacroix, J.J.; Luo, Y.; Hao, J. Insight into Molecular Mechanism for Activin A-Induced Bone Morphogenetic Protein Signaling. *Int. J. Mol. Sci.* **2020**, *21*, 6498. [CrossRef]
155. Hoeman, C.M.; Cordero, F.J.; Hu, G.; Misuraca, K.; Romero, M.M.; Cardona, H.J.; Nazarian, J.; Hashizume, R.; McLendon, R.; Yu, P.; et al. ACVR1 R206H cooperates with H3.1K27M in promoting diffuse intrinsic pontine glioma pathogenesis. *Nat. Commun.* **2019**, *10*, 1023. [CrossRef] [PubMed]
156. Hatsell, S.J.; Idone, V.; Wolken, D.M.; Huang, L.; Kim, H.J.; Wang, L.; Wen, X.; Nannuru, K.C.; Jimenez, J.; Xie, L.; et al. ACVR1R206H receptor mutation causes fibrodysplasia ossificans progressiva by imparting responsiveness to activin A. *Sci. Transl. Med.* **2015**, *7*, 303ra137. [CrossRef] [PubMed]
157. Kaplan, F.S.; Le Merrer, M.; Glaser, D.L.; Pignolo, R.J.; Goldsby, R.E.; Kitterman, J.A.; Groppe, J.; Shore, E.M. Fibrodysplasia ossificans progressiva. *Best Pract. Res. Clin. Rheumatol.* **2008**, *22*, 191–205. [CrossRef] [PubMed]
158. Shore, E.M.; Xu, M.; Feldman, G.J.; Fenstermacher, D.A.; Cho, T.J.; Choi, I.H.; Connor, J.M.; Delai, P.; Glaser, D.L.; LeMerrer, M.; et al. A recurrent mutation in the BMP type I receptor ACVR1 causes inherited and sporadic fibrodysplasia ossificans progressiva. *Nat. Genet.* **2006**, *38*, 525–527. [CrossRef]
159. Bocciardi, R.; Bordo, D.; Di Duca, M.; Di Rocco, M.; Ravazzolo, R. Mutational analysis of the ACVR1 gene in Italian patients affected with fibrodysplasia ossificans progressiva: Confirmations and advancements. *Eur. J. Hum. Genet.* **2009**, *17*, 311–318. [CrossRef] [PubMed]
160. Petrie, K.A.; Lee, W.H.; Bullock, A.N.; Pointon, J.J.; Smith, R.; Russell, R.G.; Brown, M.A.; Wordsworth, B.P.; Triffitt, J.T. Novel mutations in ACVR1 result in atypical features in two fibrodysplasia ossificans progressiva patients. *PLoS ONE* **2009**, *4*, e5005. [CrossRef]
161. Fukuda, T.; Kanomata, K.; Nojima, J.; Kokabu, S.; Akita, M.; Ikebuchi, K.; Jimi, E.; Komori, T.; Maruki, Y.; Matsuoka, M.; et al. A unique mutation of ALK2, G356D, found in a patient with fibrodysplasia ossificans progressiva is a moderately activated BMP type I receptor. *Biochem. Biophys. Res. Commun.* **2008**, *377*, 905–909. [CrossRef]
162. Yu, P.B.; Hong, C.C.; Sachidanandan, C.; Babitt, J.L.; Deng, D.Y.; Hoyng, S.A.; Lin, H.Y.; Bloch, K.D.; Peterson, R.T. Dorsomorphin inhibits BMP signals required for embryogenesis and iron metabolism. *Nat. Chem. Biol.* **2008**, *4*, 33–41. [CrossRef]
163. Smil, D.; Wong, J.F.; Williams, E.P.; Adamson, R.J.; Howarth, A.; McLeod, D.A.; Mamai, A.; Kim, S.; Wilson, B.J.; Kiyota, T.; et al. Leveraging an Open Science Drug Discovery Model to Develop CNS-Penetrant ALK2 Inhibitors for the Treatment of Diffuse Intrinsic Pontine Glioma. *J. Med. Chem.* **2020**, *63*, 10061–10085. [CrossRef]
164. Murrell, E.; Tong, J.; Smil, D.; Kiyota, T.; Aman, A.M.; Isaac, M.B.; Watson, I.D.G.; Vasdev, N. Leveraging Open Science Drug Development for PET: Preliminary Neuroimaging of (11)C-Labeled ALK2 Inhibitors. *ACS Med. Chem. Lett.* **2021**, *12*, 846–850. [CrossRef]
165. Ensan, D.; Smil, D.; Zepeda-Velazquez, C.A.; Panagopoulos, D.; Wong, J.F.; Williams, E.P.; Adamson, R.; Bullock, A.N.; Kiyota, T.; Aman, A.; et al. Targeting ALK2: An Open Science Approach to Developing Therapeutics for the Treatment of Diffuse Intrinsic Pontine Glioma. *J. Med. Chem.* **2020**, *63*, 4978–4996. [CrossRef] [PubMed]
166. Mohedas, A.H.; Wang, Y.; Sanvitale, C.E.; Canning, P.; Choi, S.; Xing, X.; Bullock, A.N.; Cuny, G.D.; Yu, P.B. Structure-activity relationship of 3,5-diaryl-2-aminopyridine ALK2 inhibitors reveals unaltered binding affinity for fibrodysplasia ossificans progressiva causing mutants. *J. Med. Chem.* **2014**, *57*, 7900–7915. [CrossRef]
167. Engers, D.W.; Bollinger, S.R.; Felts, A.S.; Vadukoot, A.K.; Williams, C.H.; Blobaum, A.L.; Lindsley, C.W.; Hong, C.C.; Hopkins, C.R. Discovery, synthesis and characterization of a series of 7-aryl-imidazo[1,2-a]pyridine-3-ylquinolines as activin-like kinase (ALK) inhibitors. *Bioorg. Med. Chem. Lett.* **2020**, *30*, 127418. [CrossRef] [PubMed]
168. Fortin, J.; Tian, R.; Zarrabi, I.; Hill, G.; Williams, E.; Sanchez-Duffhues, G.; Thorikay, M.; Ramachandran, P.; Siddaway, R.; Wong, J.F.; et al. Mutant ACVR1 Arrests Glial Cell Differentiation to Drive Tumorigenesis in Pediatric Gliomas. *Cancer Cell* **2020**, *37*, 308–323. [CrossRef] [PubMed]
169. Towner, R.A.; Gillespie, D.L.; Schwager, A.; Saunders, D.G.; Smith, N.; Njoku, C.E.; Krysiak, R.S., III; Larabee, C.; Iqbal, H.; Floyd, R.A.; et al. Regression of glioma tumor growth in F98 and U87 rat glioma models by the Nitrone OKN-007. *Neuro-Oncology* **2013**, *15*, 330–340.e12. [CrossRef]
170. Zheng, X.; Gai, X.; Han, S.; Moser, C.D.; Hu, C.; Shire, A.M.; Floyd, R.A.; Roberts, L.R. The human sulfatase 2 inhibitor 2,4-disulfonylphenyl-tert-butylnitrone (OKN-007) has an antitumor effect in hepatocellular carcinoma mediated via suppression of TGFB1/SMAD2 and Hedgehog/GLI1 signaling. *Genes Chromosomes Cancer* **2013**, *52*, 225–236. [CrossRef]
171. Thomas, L.; Smith, N.; Saunders, D.; Zalles, M.; Gulej, R.; Lerner, M.; Fung, K.M.; Carcaboso, A.M.; Towner, R.A. OKlahoma Nitrone-007: Novel treatment for diffuse intrinsic pontine glioma. *J. Transl. Med.* **2020**, *18*, 424. [CrossRef] [PubMed]
172. Cao, H.; Jin, M.; Gao, M.; Zhou, H.; Tao, Y.J.; Skolnick, J. Differential kinase activity of ACVR1 G328V and R206H mutations with implications to possible TbetaRI cross-talk in diffuse intrinsic pontine glioma. *Sci. Rep.* **2020**, *10*, 6140. [CrossRef]
173. Imamura, T.; Oshima, Y.; Hikita, A. Regulation of TGF-beta family signalling by ubiquitination and deubiquitination. *J. Biochem.* **2013**, *154*, 481–489. [CrossRef]

174. Gibson, P.; Tong, Y.; Robinson, G.; Thompson, M.C.; Currle, D.S.; Eden, C.; Kranenburg, T.A.; Hogg, T.; Poppleton, H.; Martin, J.; et al. Subtypes of medulloblastoma have distinct developmental origins. *Nature* **2010**, *468*, 1095–1099. [CrossRef] [PubMed]
175. Wodarz, A.; Nusse, R. Mechanisms of Wnt signaling in development. *Annu. Rev. Cell Dev. Biol.* **1998**, *14*, 59–88. [CrossRef] [PubMed]
176. Di, K.; Lloyd, G.K.; Abraham, V.; MacLaren, A.; Burrows, F.J.; Desjardins, A.; Trikha, M.; Bota, D.A. Marizomib activity as a single agent in malignant gliomas: Ability to cross the blood-brain barrier. *Neuro-Oncology* **2016**, *18*, 840–848. [CrossRef]
177. Kijima, N.; Kanemura, Y. Molecular Classification of Medulloblastoma. *Neurol. Med. Chir.* **2016**, *56*, 687–697. [CrossRef]
178. Glickman, M.H.; Ciechanover, A. The ubiquitin-proteasome proteolytic pathway: Destruction for the sake of construction. *Physiol. Rev.* **2002**, *82*, 373–428. [CrossRef] [PubMed]
179. Lehman, N.L. The ubiquitin proteasome system in neuropathology. *Acta Neuropathol.* **2009**, *118*, 329–347. [CrossRef]
180. Cavalli, F.M.G.; Remke, M.; Rampasek, L.; Peacock, J.; Shih, D.J.H.; Luu, B.; Garzia, L.; Torchia, J.; Nor, C.; Morrissy, A.S.; et al. Intertumoral Heterogeneity within Medulloblastoma Subgroups. *Cancer Cell* **2017**, *31*, 737–754.e6. [CrossRef] [PubMed]
181. Yang, F.; Jove, V.; Xin, H.; Hedvat, M.; Van Meter, T.E.; Yu, H. Sunitinib induces apoptosis and growth arrest of medulloblastoma tumor cells by inhibiting STAT3 and AKT signaling pathways. *Mol. Cancer Res.* **2010**, *8*, 35–45. [CrossRef]
182. Lin, G.L.; Wilson, K.M.; Ceribelli, M.; Stanton, B.Z.; Woo, P.J.; Kreimer, S.; Qin, E.Y.; Zhang, X.; Lennon, J.; Nagaraja, S.; et al. Therapeutic strategies for diffuse midline glioma from high-throughput combination drug screening. *Sci. Transl. Med.* **2019**, *11*, eaaw0064. [CrossRef] [PubMed]
183. Chen, F.; Zhang, C.; Wu, H.; Ma, Y.; Luo, X.; Gong, X.; Jiang, F.; Gui, Y.; Zhang, H.; Lu, F. The E3 ubiquitin ligase SCF(FBXL14) complex stimulates neuronal differentiation by targeting the Notch signaling factor HES1 for proteolysis. *J. Biol. Chem.* **2017**, *292*, 20100–20112. [CrossRef]
184. Yuan, X.; Wu, H.; Xu, H.; Xiong, H.; Chu, Q.; Yu, S.; Wu, G.S.; Wu, K. Notch signaling: An emerging therapeutic target for cancer treatment. *Cancer Lett.* **2015**, *369*, 20–27. [CrossRef]
185. Bao, S.; Wu, Q.; McLendon, R.E.; Hao, Y.; Shi, Q.; Hjelmeland, A.B.; Dewhirst, M.W.; Bigner, D.D.; Rich, J.N. Glioma stem cells promote radioresistance by preferential activation of the DNA damage response. *Nature* **2006**, *444*, 756–760. [CrossRef]
186. Goffart, N.; Lombard, A.; Lallemand, F.; Kroonen, J.; Nassen, J.; Di Valentin, E.; Berendsen, S.; Dedobbeleer, M.; Willems, E.; Robe, P.; et al. CXCL12 mediates glioblastoma resistance to radiotherapy in the subventricular zone. *Neuro-Oncology* **2017**, *19*, 66–77. [CrossRef] [PubMed]
187. Hussein, D.; Punjaruk, W.; Storer, L.C.; Shaw, L.; Othman, R.; Peet, A.; Miller, S.; Bandopadhyay, G.; Heath, R.; Kumari, R.; et al. Pediatric brain tumor cancer stem cells: Cell cycle dynamics, DNA repair, and etoposide extrusion. *Neuro-Oncology* **2011**, *13*, 70–83. [CrossRef]
188. Chen, K.Y.; Bush, K.; Klein, R.H.; Cervantes, V.; Lewis, N.; Naqvi, A.; Carcaboso, A.M.; Lechpammer, M.; Knoepfler, P.S. Reciprocal H3.3 gene editing identifies K27M and G34R mechanisms in pediatric glioma including NOTCH signaling. *Commun. Biol.* **2020**, *3*, 363. [CrossRef]
189. Galve-Roperh, I.; Sánchez, C.; Cortés, M.L.; del Pulgar, T.G.; Izquierdo, M.; Guzmán, M. Anti-tumoral action of cannabinoids: Involvement of sustained ceramide accumulation and extracellular signal-regulated kinase activation. *Nat. Med.* **2000**, *6*, 313–319. [CrossRef]
190. Carracedo, A.; Lorente, M.; Egia, A.; Blázquez, C.; García, S.; Giroux, V.; Malicet, C.; Villuendas, R.; Gironella, M.; González-Feria, L.; et al. The stress-regulated protein p8 mediates cannabinoid-induced apoptosis of tumor cells. *Cancer Cell* **2006**, *9*, 301–312. [CrossRef] [PubMed]
191. Salazar, M.; Carracedo, A.; Salanueva, Í.J.; Hernández-Tiedra, S.; Egia, A.; Lorente, M.; Vázquez, P.; Torres, S.; Iovanna, J.L.; Guzmán, M.; et al. TRB3 links ER stress to autophagy in cannabinoid antitumoral action. *Autophagy* **2009**, *5*, 1048–1049. [CrossRef]
192. Kyriakou, I.; Yarandi, N.; Polycarpou, E. Efficacy of cannabinoids against glioblastoma multiforme: A systematic review. *Phytomedicine* **2021**, *88*, 153533. [CrossRef] [PubMed]
193. Andradas, C.; Byrne, J.; Kuchibhotla, M.; Ancliffe, M.; Jones, A.C.; Carline, B.; Hii, H.; Truong, A.; Storer, L.C.D.; Ritzmann, T.A.; et al. Assessment of Cannabidiol and Delta9-Tetrahydrocannabiol in Mouse Models of Medulloblastoma and Ependymoma. *Cancers* **2021**, *13*, 330. [CrossRef]
194. Ellert-Miklaszewska, A.; Grajkowska, W.; Gabrusiewicz, K.; Kaminska, B.; Konarska, L. Distinctive pattern of cannabinoid receptor type II (CB2) expression in adult and pediatric brain tumors. *Brain Res.* **2007**, *1137*, 161–169. [CrossRef]
195. Sánchez, C.; de Ceballos, M.L.; del Pulgar, T.G.; Rueda, D.; Corbacho, C.; Velasco, G.; Galve-Roperh, I.; Huffman, J.W.; y Cajal, S.R.; Guzmán, M. Inhibition of glioma growth in vivo by selective activation of the CB2 cannabinoid receptor. *Cancer Res.* **2001**, *61*, 5784–5789. [PubMed]
196. Schley, M.; Ständer, S.; Kerner, J.; Vajkoczy, P.; Schüpfer, G.; Dusch, M.; Schmelz, M.; Konrad, C. Predominant CB2 receptor expression in endothelial cells of glioblastoma in humans. *Brain Res. Bull.* **2009**, *79*, 333–337. [CrossRef] [PubMed]
197. Duchatel, R.J.; Jackson, E.R.; Alvaro, F.; Nixon, B.; Hondermarck, H.; Dun, M.D. Signal Transduction in Diffuse Intrinsic Pontine Glioma. *Proteomics* **2019**, *19*, 1800479. [CrossRef] [PubMed]
198. Andradas, C.; Truong, A.; Byrne, J.; Endersby, R. The Role of Cannabinoids as Anticancer Agents in Pediatric Oncology. *Cancers* **2021**, *13*, 157. [CrossRef]

199. Ananth, P.; Reed-Weston, A.; Wolfe, J. Medical marijuana in pediatric oncology: A review of the evidence and implications for practice. *Pediatric Blood Cancer* **2018**, *65*, e26826. [CrossRef]
200. Matthews, H.K.; Bertoli, C.; de Bruin, R.A.M. Cell cycle control in cancer. *Nat. Rev. Mol. Cell Biol.* **2021**. [CrossRef]
201. Hamilton, E.; Infante, J.R. Targeting CDK4/6 in patients with cancer. *Cancer Treat. Rev.* **2016**, *45*, 129–138. [CrossRef] [PubMed]
202. Chen, P.; Lee, N.V.; Hu, W.; Xu, M.; Ferre, R.A.; Lam, J.; Bergqvist, S.; Solowiej, J.; Diehl, W.; He, Y.A.; et al. Spectrum and Degree of CDK Drug Interactions Predicts Clinical Performance. *Mol. Cancer Ther.* **2016**, *15*, 2273–2281. [CrossRef] [PubMed]
203. Mackay, A.; Burford, A.; Carvalho, D.; Izquierdo, E.; Fazal-Salom, J.; Taylor, K.R.; Bjerke, L.; Clarke, M.; Vinci, M.; Nandhabalan, M.; et al. Integrated Molecular Meta-Analysis of 1000 Pediatric High-Grade and Diffuse Intrinsic Pontine Glioma. *Cancer Cell* **2017**, *32*, 520–537.e5. [CrossRef]
204. Cordero, F.J.; Huang, Z.; Grenier, C.; He, X.; Hu, G.; McLendon, R.E.; Murphy, S.K.; Hashizume, R.; Becher, O.J. Histone H3.3K27M Represses p16 to Accelerate Gliomagenesis in a Murine Model of DIPG. *Mol. Cancer Res.* **2017**, *15*, 1243–1254. [CrossRef] [PubMed]
205. Barton, K.L.; Misuraca, K.; Cordero, F.; Dobrikova, E.; Min, H.D.; Gromeier, M.; Kirsch, D.G.; Becher, O.J. PD-0332991, a CDK4/6 inhibitor, significantly prolongs survival in a genetically engineered mouse model of brainstem glioma. *PLoS ONE* **2013**, *8*, e77639. [CrossRef]
206. Sun, Y.; Sun, Y.; Yan, K.; Li, Z.; Xu, C.; Geng, Y.; Pan, C.; Chen, X.; Zhang, L.; Xi, Q. Potent anti-tumor efficacy of palbociclib in treatment-naive H3.3K27M-mutant diffuse intrinsic pontine glioma. *EBioMedicine* **2019**, *43*, 171–179. [CrossRef]
207. Aoki, Y.; Hashizume, R.; Ozawa, T.; Banerjee, A.; Prados, M.; James, C.D.; Gupta, N. An experimental xenograft mouse model of diffuse pontine glioma designed for therapeutic testing. *J. Neurooncol.* **2012**, *108*, 29–35. [CrossRef]
208. DeWire, M.; Fuller, C.; Hummel, T.R.; Chow, L.M.L.; Salloum, R.; de Blank, P.; Pater, L.; Lawson, S.; Zhu, X.; Dexheimer, P.; et al. A phase I/II study of ribociclib following radiation therapy in children with newly diagnosed diffuse intrinsic pontine glioma (DIPG). *J. Neurooncol.* **2020**, *149*, 511–522. [CrossRef] [PubMed]
209. Van Mater, D.; Gururangan, S.; Becher, O.; Campagne, O.; Leary, S.; Phillips, J.J.; Huang, J.; Lin, T.; Poussaint, T.Y.; Goldman, S.; et al. A phase I trial of the CDK 4/6 inhibitor palbociclib in pediatric patients with progressive brain tumors: A Pediatric Brain Tumor Consortium study (PBTC-042). *Pediatric Blood Cancer* **2021**, *68*, e28879. [CrossRef]
210. Franshaw, L.; Tsoli, M.; Lau, L.M.S.; Ziegler, D.S. Translating palbociclib to the clinic for DIPG—What is truly achievable? *EBioMedicine* **2019**, *45*, 22. [CrossRef]
211. Olmez, I.; Brenneman, B.; Xiao, A.; Serbulea, V.; Benamar, M.; Zhang, Y.; Manigat, L.; Abbas, T.; Lee, J.; Nakano, I.; et al. Combined CDK4/6 and mTOR Inhibition Is Synergistic against Glioblastoma via Multiple Mechanisms. *Clin. Cancer Res.* **2017**, *23*, 6958–6968. [CrossRef] [PubMed]
212. Pedersen, H.; Schmiegelow, K.; Hamerlik, P. Radio-Resistance and DNA Repair in Pediatric Diffuse Midline Gliomas. *Cancers* **2020**, *12*, 2813. [CrossRef]
213. Bryant, H.E.; Schultz, N.; Thomas, H.D.; Parker, K.M.; Flower, D.; Lopez, E.; Kyle, S.; Meuth, M.; Curtin, N.J.; Helleday, T. Specific killing of BRCA2-deficient tumours with inhibitors of poly(ADP-ribose) polymerase. *Nature* **2005**, *434*, 913–917. [CrossRef] [PubMed]
214. Jackson, S.P.; Bartek, J. The DNA-damage response in human biology and disease. *Nature* **2009**, *461*, 1071–1078. [CrossRef] [PubMed]
215. Zarghooni, M.; Bartels, U.; Lee, E.; Buczkowicz, P.; Morrison, A.; Huang, A.; Bouffet, E.; Hawkins, C. Whole-genome profiling of pediatric diffuse intrinsic pontine gliomas highlights platelet-derived growth factor receptor alpha and poly (ADP-ribose) polymerase as potential therapeutic targets. *J. Clin. Oncol.* **2010**, *28*, 1337–1344. [CrossRef] [PubMed]
216. Chornenkyy, Y.; Agnihotri, S.; Yu, M.; Buczkowicz, P.; Rakopoulos, P.; Golbourn, B.; Garzia, L.; Siddaway, R.; Leung, S.; Rutka, J.T.; et al. Poly-ADP-Ribose Polymerase as a Therapeutic Target in Pediatric Diffuse Intrinsic Pontine Glioma and Pediatric High-Grade Astrocytoma. *Mol. Cancer Ther.* **2015**, *14*, 2560–2568. [CrossRef]
217. Zhang, L.; Chen, L.H.; Wan, H.; Yang, R.; Wang, Z.; Feng, J.; Yang, S.; Jones, S.; Wang, S.; Zhou, W.; et al. Exome sequencing identifies somatic gain-of-function PPM1D mutations in brainstem gliomas. *Nat. Genet.* **2014**, *46*, 726–730. [CrossRef]
218. Wang, Z.; Xu, C.; Diplas, B.H.; Moure, C.J.; Chen, C.J.; Chen, L.H.; Du, C.; Zhu, H.; Greer, P.K.; Zhang, L.; et al. Targeting Mutant PPM1D Sensitizes Diffuse Intrinsic Pontine Glioma Cells to the PARP Inhibitor Olaparib. *Mol. Cancer Res.* **2020**, *18*, 968–980. [CrossRef] [PubMed]
219. Chapman, J.R.; Taylor, M.R.; Boulton, S.J. Playing the end game: DNA double-strand break repair pathway choice. *Mol. Cell.* **2012**, *47*, 497–510. [CrossRef]
220. Werbrouck, C.; Evangelista, C.C.S.; Lobon-Iglesias, M.J.; Barret, E.; Le Teuff, G.; Merlevede, J.; Brusini, R.; Kergrohen, T.; Mondini, M.; Bolle, S.; et al. TP53 Pathway Alterations Drive Radioresistance in Diffuse Intrinsic Pontine Gliomas (DIPG). *Clin. Cancer Res.* **2019**, *25*, 6788–6800. [CrossRef] [PubMed]
221. Raso, A.; Vecchio, D.; Cappelli, E.; Ropolo, M.; Poggi, A.; Nozza, P.; Biassoni, R.; Mascelli, S.; Capra, V.; Kalfas, F.; et al. Characterization of glioma stem cells through multiple stem cell markers and their specific sensitization to double-strand break-inducing agents by pharmacological inhibition of ataxia telangiectasia mutated protein. *Brain Pathol.* **2012**, *22*, 677–688. [CrossRef]
222. Vecchio, D.; Daga, A.; Carra, E.; Marubbi, D.; Baio, G.; Neumaier, C.E.; Vagge, S.; Corvo, R.; Pia Brisigotti, M.; Louis Ravetti, J.; et al. Predictability, efficacy and safety of radiosensitization of glioblastoma-initiating cells by the ATM inhibitor KU-60019. *Int. J. Cancer* **2014**, *135*, 479–491. [CrossRef] [PubMed]

223. Cash, T.; Fox, E.; Liu, X.; Minard, C.G.; Reid, J.M.; Scheck, A.C.; Weigel, B.J.; Wetmore, C. A phase 1 study of prexasertib (LY2606368), a CHK1/2 inhibitor, in pediatric patients with recurrent or refractory solid tumors, including CNS tumors: A report from the Children's Oncology Group Pediatric Early Phase Clinical Trials Network (ADVL1515). *Pediatric Blood Cancer* **2021**, *68*, e29065. [CrossRef] [PubMed]
224. Schmidt, M.; Rohe, A.; Platzer, C.; Najjar, A.; Erdmann, F.; Sippl, W. Regulation of G2/M Transition by Inhibition of WEE1 and PKMYT1 Kinases. *Molecules* **2017**, *22*, 2045. [CrossRef] [PubMed]
225. Caretti, V.; Hiddingh, L.; Lagerweij, T.; Schellen, P.; Koken, P.W.; Hulleman, E.; van Vuurden, D.G.; Vandertop, W.P.; Kaspers, G.J.; Noske, D.P.; et al. WEE1 kinase inhibition enhances the radiation response of diffuse intrinsic pontine gliomas. *Mol. Cancer Ther.* **2013**, *12*, 141–150. [CrossRef] [PubMed]
226. Mueller, S.; Hashizume, R.; Yang, X.; Kolkowitz, I.; Olow, A.K.; Phillips, J.; Smirnov, I.; Tom, M.W.; Prados, M.D.; James, C.D.; et al. Targeting Wee1 for the treatment of pediatric high-grade gliomas. *Neuro-Oncology* **2014**, *16*, 352–360. [CrossRef] [PubMed]
227. Perry, J.A.; Kornbluth, S. Cdc25 and Wee1: Analogous opposites? *Cell Div.* **2007**, *2*, 12. [CrossRef]
228. Van Vugt, M.A.; Bras, A.; Medema, R.H. Polo-like kinase-1 controls recovery from a G2 DNA damage-induced arrest in mammalian cells. *Mol. Cell.* **2004**, *15*, 799–811. [CrossRef]
229. Archambault, V.; Glover, D.M. Polo-like kinases: Conservation and divergence in their functions and regulation. *Nat. Rev. Mol. Cell. Biol.* **2009**, *10*, 265–275. [CrossRef]
230. Medema, R.H.; Lin, C.C.; Yang, J.C. Polo-like kinase 1 inhibitors and their potential role in anticancer therapy, with a focus on NSCLC. *Clin. Cancer Res.* **2011**, *17*, 6459–6466. [CrossRef]
231. Toyoshima-Morimoto, F.; Taniguchi, E.; Nishida, E. Plk1 promotes nuclear translocation of human Cdc25C during prophase. *EMBO Rep.* **2002**, *3*, 341–348. [CrossRef] [PubMed]
232. Watanabe, N.; Arai, H.; Nishihara, Y.; Taniguchi, M.; Watanabe, N.; Hunter, T.; Osada, H. M-phase kinases induce phospho-dependent ubiquitination of somatic Wee1 by SCFbeta-TrCP. *Proc. Natl. Acad. Sci. USA* **2004**, *101*, 4419–4424. [CrossRef]
233. Smith, L.; Farzan, R.; Ali, S.; Buluwela, L.; Saurin, A.T.; Meek, D.W. The responses of cancer cells to PLK1 inhibitors reveal a novel protective role for p53 in maintaining centrosome separation. *Sci. Rep.* **2017**, *7*, 16115. [CrossRef] [PubMed]
234. Amani, V.; Prince, E.W.; Alimova, I.; Balakrishnan, I.; Birks, D.; Donson, A.M.; Harris, P.; Levy, J.M.; Handler, M.; Foreman, N.K.; et al. Polo-like Kinase 1 as a potential therapeutic target in Diffuse Intrinsic Pontine Glioma. *BMC Cancer* **2016**, *16*, 647. [CrossRef]
235. Price, G.; Bouras, A.; Hambardzumyan, D.; Hadjipanayis, C.G. Current knowledge on the immune microenvironment and emerging immunotherapies in diffuse midline glioma. *EBioMedicine* **2021**, *69*, 103453. [CrossRef]
236. Caretti, V.; Sewing, A.C.; Lagerweij, T.; Schellen, P.; Bugiani, M.; Jansen, M.H.; van Vuurden, D.G.; Navis, A.C.; Horsman, I.; Vandertop, W.P.; et al. Human pontine glioma cells can induce murine tumors. *Acta Neuropathol.* **2014**, *127*, 897–909. [CrossRef] [PubMed]
237. Wang, Y.; Wang, K.; Fu, J. HDAC6 Mediates Macrophage iNOS Expression and Excessive Nitric Oxide Production in the Blood During Endotoxemia. *Front. Immunol.* **2020**, *11*, 1893. [CrossRef]
238. Xu, H.; Lai, W.; Zhang, Y.; Liu, L.; Luo, X.; Zeng, Y.; Wu, H.; Lan, Q.; Chu, Z. Tumor-associated macrophage-derived IL-6 and IL-8 enhance invasive activity of LoVo cells induced by PRL-3 in a KCNN4 channel-dependent manner. *BMC Cancer* **2014**, *14*, 330. [CrossRef]
239. Fujimoto, H.; Sangai, T.; Ishii, G.; Ikehara, A.; Nagashima, T.; Miyazaki, M.; Ochiai, A. Stromal MCP-1 in mammary tumors induces tumor-associated macrophage infiltration and contributes to tumor progression. *Int. J. Cancer* **2009**, *125*, 1276–1284. [CrossRef] [PubMed]
240. Martinez, F.O.; Sica, A.; Mantovani, A.; Locati, M. Macrophage activation and polarization. *Front. Biosci.* **2008**, *13*, 453–461. [CrossRef] [PubMed]
241. Orecchioni, M.; Ghosheh, Y.; Pramod, A.B.; Ley, K. Macrophage Polarization: Different Gene Signatures in M1(LPS+) vs. Classically and M2(LPS-) vs. Alternatively Activated Macrophages. *Front. Immunol.* **2019**, *10*, 1084. [CrossRef]
242. Andersen, M.N.; Andersen, N.F.; Lauridsen, K.L.; Etzerodt, A.; Sorensen, B.S.; Abildgaard, N.; Plesner, T.; Hokland, M.; Moller, H.J. STAT3 is over-activated within CD163(pos) bone marrow macrophages in both Multiple Myeloma and the benign pre-condition MGUS. *Cancer Immunol. Immunother.* **2021**. [CrossRef] [PubMed]
243. Vasquez-Dunddel, D.; Pan, F.; Zeng, Q.; Gorbounov, M.; Albesiano, E.; Fu, J.; Blosser, R.L.; Tam, A.J.; Bruno, T.; Zhang, H.; et al. STAT3 regulates arginase-I in myeloid-derived suppressor cells from cancer patients. *J. Clin. Investig.* **2013**, *123*, 1580–1589. [CrossRef]
244. Zhang, F.; Wang, H.; Wang, X.; Jiang, G.; Liu, H.; Zhang, G.; Wang, H.; Fang, R.; Bu, X.; Cai, S.; et al. TGF-beta induces M2-like macrophage polarization via SNAIL-mediated suppression of a pro-inflammatory phenotype. *Oncotarget* **2016**, *7*, 52294–52306. [CrossRef]
245. Nakamura, R.; Sene, A.; Santeford, A.; Gdoura, A.; Kubota, S.; Zapata, N.; Apte, R.S. IL10-driven STAT3 signalling in senescent macrophages promotes pathological eye angiogenesis. *Nat. Commun.* **2015**, *6*, 7847. [CrossRef] [PubMed]
246. Huang, L.; Wang, Z.; Chang, Y.; Wang, K.; Kang, X.; Huang, R.; Zhang, Y.; Chen, J.; Zeng, F.; Wu, F.; et al. EFEMP2 indicates assembly of M0 macrophage and more malignant phenotypes of glioma. *Aging* **2020**, *12*, 8397–8412. [CrossRef]

247. Gabrusiewicz, K.; Rodriguez, B.; Wei, J.; Hashimoto, Y.; Healy, L.M.; Maiti, S.N.; Thomas, G.; Zhou, S.; Wang, Q.; Elakkad, A.; et al. Glioblastoma-infiltrated innate immune cells resemble M0 macrophage phenotype. *JCI Insightig.* **2016**, *1*, e85841. [CrossRef] [PubMed]
248. Hattermann, K.; Sebens, S.; Helm, O.; Schmitt, A.D.; Mentlein, R.; Mehdorn, H.M.; Held-Feindt, J. Chemokine expression profile of freshly isolated human glioblastoma-associated macrophages/microglia. *Oncol. Rep.* **2014**, *32*, 270–276. [CrossRef]
249. De Vleeschouwer, S.; Spencer Lopes, I.; Ceuppens, J.L.; Van Gool, S.W. Persistent IL-10 production is required for glioma growth suppressive activity by Th1-directed effector cells after stimulation with tumor lysate-loaded dendritic cells. *J. Neurooncol.* **2007**, *84*, 131–140. [CrossRef] [PubMed]
250. Ngambenjawong, C.; Gustafson, H.H.; Pun, S.H. Progress in tumor-associated macrophage (TAM)-targeted therapeutics. *Adv. Drug. Deliv. Rev.* **2017**, *114*, 206–221. [CrossRef]
251. Chen, W.; Ma, T.; Shen, X.N.; Xia, X.F.; Xu, G.D.; Bai, X.L.; Liang, T.B. Macrophage-induced tumor angiogenesis is regulated by the TSC2-mTOR pathway. *Cancer Res.* **2012**, *72*, 1363–1372. [CrossRef]
252. Hsu, S.P.C.; Chen, Y.C.; Chiang, H.C.; Huang, Y.C.; Huang, C.C.; Wang, H.E.; Wang, Y.S.; Chi, K.H. Rapamycin and hydroxychloroquine combination alters macrophage polarization and sensitizes glioblastoma to immune checkpoint inhibitors. *J. Neurooncol.* **2020**, *146*, 417–426. [CrossRef]
253. Park, J.; Lee, W.; Yun, S.; Kim, S.P.; Kim, K.H.; Kim, J.I.; Kim, S.K.; Wang, K.C.; Lee, J.Y. STAT3 is a key molecule in the oncogenic behavior of diffuse intrinsic pontine glioma. *Oncol. Lett.* **2020**, *20*, 1989–1998. [CrossRef]
254. Gao, Y.; Fang, P.; Li, W.J.; Zhang, J.; Wang, G.P.; Jiang, D.F.; Chen, F.P. LncRNA NEAT1 sponges miR-214 to regulate M2 macrophage polarization by regulation of B7-H3 in multiple myeloma. *Mol. Immunol.* **2020**, *117*, 20–28. [CrossRef]
255. Shin, S.B.; Jang, H.R.; Xu, R.; Won, J.Y.; Yim, H. Active PLK1-driven metastasis is amplified by TGF-beta signaling that forms a positive feedback loop in non-small cell lung cancer. *Oncogene* **2020**, *39*, 767–785. [CrossRef]
256. Mittal, M.; Tiruppathi, C.; Nepal, S.; Zhao, Y.Y.; Grzych, D.; Soni, D.; Prockop, D.J.; Malik, A.B. TNFalpha-stimulated gene-6 (TSG6) activates macrophage phenotype transition to prevent inflammatory lung injury. *Proc. Natl. Acad. Sci. USA* **2016**, *113*, E8151–E8158. [CrossRef]
257. Hu, J.; Wang, G.; Liu, X.; Zhou, L.; Jiang, M.; Yang, L. Polo-like kinase 1 (PLK1) is involved in toll-like receptor (TLR)-mediated TNF-alpha production in monocytic THP-1 cells. *PLoS ONE* **2013**, *8*, e78832.
258. Bode, J.G.; Ehlting, C.; Haussinger, D. The macrophage response towards LPS and its control through the p38(MAPK)-STAT3 axis. *Cell Signal* **2012**, *24*, 1185–1194. [CrossRef]
259. Wanderley, C.W.; Colon, D.F.; Luiz, J.P.M.; Oliveira, F.F.; Viacava, P.R.; Leite, C.A.; Pereira, J.A.; Silva, C.M.; Silva, C.R.; Silva, R.L.; et al. Paclitaxel Reduces Tumor Growth by Reprogramming Tumor-Associated Macrophages to an M1 Profile in a TLR4-Dependent Manner. *Cancer Res.* **2018**, *78*, 5891–5900. [CrossRef]
260. Minturn, J.; Shu, H.-K.; Fisher, M.; Patti, R.; Janss, A.; Allen, J.; Phillips, P.; Belasco, J. Phase i trial of concurrent weekly paclitaxel and radiation therapy for children with newly diagnosed diffuse intrinsic pontine glioma. *Neuro-Oncology* **2012**, *14*, i26–i32.
261. Alexander, E.T.; Minton, A.; Peters, M.C.; Phanstiel, O.t.; Gilmour, S.K. A novel polyamine blockade therapy activates an anti-tumor immune response. *Oncotarget* **2017**, *8*, 84140–84152. [CrossRef]
262. Cavalcante, R.S.; Ishikawa, U.; Silva, E.S.; Silva-Junior, A.A.; Araujo, A.A.; Cruz, L.J.; Chan, A.B.; de Araujo Junior, R.F. STAT3/NF-kappaB signalling disruption in M2 tumour-associated macrophages is a major target of PLGA nanocarriers/PD-L1 antibody immunomodulatory therapy in breast cancer. *Br. J. Pharmacol.* **2021**, *178*, 2284–2304. [CrossRef]
263. Meel, M.H.; de Gooijer, M.C.; Metselaar, D.S.; Sewing, A.C.P.; Zwaan, K.; Waranecki, P.; Breur, M.; Buil, L.C.M.; Lagerweij, T.; Wedekind, L.E.; et al. Combined Therapy of AXL and HDAC Inhibition Reverses Mesenchymal Transition in Diffuse Intrinsic Pontine Glioma. *Clin. Cancer Res.* **2020**, *26*, 3319–3332. [CrossRef] [PubMed]
264. Brenot, A.; Knolhoff, B.L.; DeNardo, D.G.; Longmore, G.D. SNAIL1 action in tumor cells influences macrophage polarization and metastasis in breast cancer through altered GM-CSF secretion. *Oncogenesis* **2018**, *7*, 32. [CrossRef]
265. Leopold Wager, C.M.; Hole, C.R.; Campuzano, A.; Castro-Lopez, N.; Cai, H.; Caballero Van Dyke, M.C.; Wozniak, K.L.; Wang, Y.; Wormley, F.L., Jr. IFN-gamma immune priming of macrophages in vivo induces prolonged STAT1 binding and protection against Cryptococcus neoformans. *PLoS Pathog.* **2018**, *14*, e1007358. [CrossRef]
266. Salmaninejad, A.; Valilou, S.F.; Soltani, A.; Ahmadi, S.; Abarghan, Y.J.; Rosengren, R.J.; Sahebkar, A. Tumor-associated macrophages: Role in cancer development and therapeutic implications. *Cell Oncol.* **2019**, *42*, 591–608. [CrossRef]
267. Tough, D.F. Modulation of T-cell function by type I interferon. *Immunol. Cell Biol.* **2012**, *90*, 492–497. [CrossRef]
268. Li, X.; Su, X.; Liu, R.; Pan, Y.; Fang, J.; Cao, L.; Feng, C.; Shang, Q.; Chen, Y.; Shao, C.; et al. HDAC inhibition potentiates anti-tumor activity of macrophages and enhances anti-PD-L1-mediated tumor suppression. *Oncogene* **2021**, *40*, 1836–1850. [CrossRef]
269. Kythreotou, A.; Siddique, A.; Mauri, F.A.; Bower, M.; Pinato, D.J. Pd-L1. *J. Clin. Pathol.* **2018**, *71*, 189–194. [CrossRef]
270. Jha, P.; Manjunath, N.; Singh, J.; Mani, K.; Garg, A.; Kaur, K.; Sharma, M.C.; Raheja, A.; Suri, A.; Sarkar, C.; et al. Analysis of PD-L1 expression and T cell infiltration in different molecular subgroups of diffuse midline gliomas. *Neuropathology* **2019**, *39*, 413–424. [CrossRef]
271. Liu, S.; Wang, Z.; Wang, Y.; Fan, X.; Zhang, C.; Ma, W.; Qiu, X.; Jiang, T. PD-1 related transcriptome profile and clinical outcome in diffuse gliomas. *Oncoimmunology* **2018**, *7*, e1382792. [CrossRef] [PubMed]

272. Keane, L.; Cheray, M.; Saidi, D.; Kirby, C.; Friess, L.; Gonzalez-Rodriguez, P.; Gerdes, M.E.; Grabert, K.; McColl, B.W.; Joseph, B. Inhibition of microglial EZH2 leads to anti-tumoral effects in pediatric diffuse midline gliomas. *Neurooncol. Adv.* **2021**, *3*, vdab096. [CrossRef] [PubMed]
273. Kitchen, G.B.; Hopwood, T.; Gali Ramamoorthy, T.; Downton, P.; Begley, N.; Hussell, T.; Dockrell, D.H.; Gibbs, J.E.; Ray, D.W.; Loudon, A.S.I. The histone methyltransferase Ezh2 restrains macrophage inflammatory responses. *FASEB J.* **2021**, *35*, e21843. [CrossRef] [PubMed]
274. Wu, A.; Wei, J.; Kong, L.Y.; Wang, Y.; Priebe, W.; Qiao, W.; Sawaya, R.; Heimberger, A.B. Glioma cancer stem cells induce immunosuppressive macrophages/microglia. *Neuro-Oncology* **2010**, *12*, 1113–1125. [CrossRef] [PubMed]
275. Takenaka, M.C.; Gabriely, G.; Rothhammer, V.; Mascanfroni, I.D.; Wheeler, M.A.; Chao, C.C.; Gutierrez-Vazquez, C.; Kenison, J.; Tjon, E.C.; Barroso, A.; et al. Control of tumor-associated macrophages and T cells in glioblastoma via AHR and CD39. *Nat. Neurosci.* **2019**, *22*, 729–740. [CrossRef] [PubMed]
276. Karachi, A.; Dastmalchi, F.; Nazarian, S.; Huang, J.; Sayour, E.J.; Jin, L.; Yang, C.; Mitchell, D.A.; Rahman, M. Optimizing T Cell-Based Therapy for Glioblastoma. *Front. Immunol.* **2021**, *12*, 705580. [CrossRef]
277. Munder, M.; Schneider, H.; Luckner, C.; Giese, T.; Langhans, C.D.; Fuentes, J.M.; Kropf, P.; Mueller, I.; Kolb, A.; Modolell, M.; et al. Suppression of T-cell functions by human granulocyte arginase. *Blood* **2006**, *108*, 1627–1634. [CrossRef]
278. Majzner, R.G.; Theruvath, J.L.; Nellan, A.; Heitzeneder, S.; Cui, Y.; Mount, C.W.; Rietberg, S.P.; Linde, M.H.; Xu, P.; Rota, C.; et al. CAR T Cells Targeting B7-H3, a Pan-Cancer Antigen, Demonstrate Potent Preclinical Activity Against Pediatric Solid Tumors and Brain Tumors. *Clin. Cancer Res.* **2019**, *25*, 2560–2574. [CrossRef] [PubMed]
279. Zhang, H.; Dai, Z.; Wu, W.; Wang, Z.; Zhang, N.; Zhang, L.; Zeng, W.J.; Liu, Z.; Cheng, Q. Regulatory mechanisms of immune checkpoints PD-L1 and CTLA-4 in cancer. *J. Exp. Clin. Cancer Res.* **2021**, *40*, 184. [CrossRef] [PubMed]
280. Ruffo, E.; Wu, R.C.; Bruno, T.C.; Workman, C.J.; Vignali, D.A.A. Lymphocyte-activation gene 3 (LAG3): The next immune checkpoint receptor. *Semin. Immunol.* **2019**, *42*, 101305. [CrossRef] [PubMed]
281. Ninomiya, S.; Narala, N.; Huye, L.; Yagyu, S.; Savoldo, B.; Dotti, G.; Heslop, H.E.; Brenner, M.K.; Rooney, C.M.; Ramos, C.A. Tumor indoleamine 2,3-dioxygenase (IDO) inhibits CD19-CAR T cells and is downregulated by lymphodepleting drugs. *Blood* **2015**, *125*, 3905–3916. [CrossRef]
282. Chong, E.A.; Melenhorst, J.J.; Lacey, S.F.; Ambrose, D.E.; Gonzalez, V.; Levine, B.L.; June, C.H.; Schuster, S.J. PD-1 blockade modulates chimeric antigen receptor (CAR)-modified T cells: Refueling the CAR. *Blood* **2017**, *129*, 1039–1041. [CrossRef]
283. Mount, C.W.; Majzner, R.G.; Sundaresh, S.; Arnold, E.P.; Kadapakkam, M.; Haile, S.; Labanieh, L.; Hulleman, E.; Woo, P.J.; Rietberg, S.P.; et al. Potent antitumor efficacy of anti-GD2 CAR T cells in H3-K27M(+) diffuse midline gliomas. *Nat. Med.* **2018**, *24*, 572–579. [CrossRef]
284. Golinelli, G.; Grisendi, G.; Prapa, M.; Bestagno, M.; Spano, C.; Rossignoli, F.; Bambi, F.; Sardi, I.; Cellini, M.; Horwitz, E.M.; et al. Targeting GD2-positive glioblastoma by chimeric antigen receptor empowered mesenchymal progenitors. *Cancer Gene Ther.* **2020**, *27*, 558–570. [CrossRef]
285. Prapa, M.; Caldrer, S.; Spano, C.; Bestagno, M.; Golinelli, G.; Grisendi, G.; Petrachi, T.; Conte, P.; Horwitz, E.M.; Campana, D.; et al. A novel anti-GD2/4-1BB chimeric antigen receptor triggers neuroblastoma cell killing. *Oncotarget* **2015**, *6*, 24884–24894. [CrossRef]
286. Scherer, H.J. Structureal development in gliomas. *Am. J. Cancer* **1938**, *34*, 333–351.
287. Gillespie, S.; Monje, M. An active role for neurons in glioma progression: Making sense of Scherer's structures. *Neuro-Oncology* **2018**, *20*, 1292–1299. [CrossRef] [PubMed]
288. Brownson, R.H. Perineuronal satellite cells in the motor cortex of aging brains. *J. Neuropathol. Exp. Neurol.* **1956**, *15*, 190–195. [CrossRef]
289. Vijayan, V.K.; Zhou, S.S.; Russell, M.J.; Geddes, J.; Ellis, W.; Cotman, C.W. Perineuronal satellitosis in the human hippocampal formation. *Hippocampus* **1993**, *3*, 239–250. [CrossRef]
290. Baumann, N.; Pham-Dinh, D. Biology of oligodendrocyte and myelin in the mammalian central nervous system. *Physiol. Rev.* **2001**, *81*, 871–927. [CrossRef]
291. Gibson, E.M.; Purger, D.; Mount, C.W.; Goldstein, A.K.; Lin, G.L.; Wood, L.S.; Inema, I.; Miller, S.E.; Bieri, G.; Zuchero, J.B.; et al. Neuronal activity promotes oligodendrogenesis and adaptive myelination in the mammalian brain. *Science* **2014**, *344*, 1252304. [CrossRef]
292. Monje, M.; Mitra, S.S.; Freret, M.E.; Raveh, T.B.; Kim, J.; Masek, M.; Attema, J.L.; Li, G.; Haddix, T.; Edwards, M.S.; et al. Hedgehog-responsive candidate cell of origin for diffuse intrinsic pontine glioma. *Proc. Natl. Acad. Sci. USA* **2011**, *108*, 4453–4458. [CrossRef]
293. Brown, N.F.; Williams, M.; Arkenau, H.T.; Fleming, R.A.; Tolson, J.; Yan, L.; Zhang, J.; Singh, R.; Auger, K.R.; Lenox, L.; et al. A study of the focal adhesion kinase inhibitor GSK2256098 in patients with recurrent glioblastoma with evaluation of tumor penetration of [11C]GSK2256098. *Neuro-Oncology* **2018**, *20*, 1634–1642. [CrossRef]
294. Venkatesh, H.S.; Morishita, W.; Geraghty, A.C.; Silverbush, D.; Gillespie, S.M.; Arzt, M.; Tam, L.T.; Espenel, C.; Ponnuswami, A.; Ni, L.; et al. Electrical and synaptic integration of glioma into neural circuits. *Nature* **2019**, *573*, 539–545. [CrossRef]
295. Coppola, A.; Zarabla, A.; Maialetti, A.; Villani, V.; Koudriavtseva, T.; Russo, E.; Nozzolillo, A.; Sueri, C.; Belcastro, V.; Balestrini, S.; et al. Perampanel Confirms to Be Effective and Well-Tolerated as an Add-On Treatment in Patients with Brain Tumor-Related Epilepsy (PERADET Study). *Front. Neurol.* **2020**, *11*, 592. [CrossRef] [PubMed]

296. Osswald, M.; Jung, E.; Sahm, F.; Solecki, G.; Venkataramani, V.; Blaes, J.; Weil, S.; Horstmann, H.; Wiestler, B.; Syed, M.; et al. Brain tumour cells interconnect to a functional and resistant network. *Nature* **2015**, *528*, 93–98. [CrossRef]
297. Yu, K.; Lin, C.J.; Hatcher, A.; Lozzi, B.; Kong, K.; Huang-Hobbs, E.; Cheng, Y.T.; Beechar, V.B.; Zhu, W.; Zhang, Y.; et al. PIK3CA variants selectively initiate brain hyperactivity during gliomagenesis. *Nature* **2020**, *578*, 166–171. [CrossRef] [PubMed]
298. Huang, S.L.; Wang, Y.M.; Wang, Q.Y.; Feng, G.G.; Wu, F.Q.; Yang, L.M.; Zhang, X.H.; Xin, H.W. Mechanisms and Clinical Trials of Hepatocellular Carcinoma Immunotherapy. *Front. Genet.* **2021**, *12*, 691391. [CrossRef] [PubMed]
299. Allen, N.J.; Bennett, M.L.; Foo, L.C.; Wang, G.X.; Chakraborty, C.; Smith, S.J.; Barres, B.A. Astrocyte glypicans 4 and 6 promote formation of excitatory synapses via GluA1 AMPA receptors. *Nature* **2012**, *486*, 410–414. [CrossRef]
300. Rozov, A.; Zakharova, Y.; Vazetdinova, A.; Valiullina-Rakhmatullina, F. The Role of Polyamine-Dependent Facilitation of Calcium Permeable AMPARs in Short-Term Synaptic Enhancement. *Front. Cell Neurosci.* **2018**, *12*, 345. [CrossRef] [PubMed]
301. Noh, K.M.; Yokota, H.; Mashiko, T.; Castillo, P.E.; Zukin, R.S.; Bennett, M.V. Blockade of calcium-permeable AMPA receptors protects hippocampal neurons against global ischemia-induced death. *Proc. Natl. Acad. Sci. USA* **2005**, *102*, 12230–12235. [CrossRef] [PubMed]
302. Dolma, S.; Selvadurai, H.J.; Lan, X.; Lee, L.; Kushida, M.; Voisin, V.; Whetstone, H.; So, M.; Aviv, T.; Park, N.; et al. Inhibition of Dopamine Receptor D4 Impedes Autophagic Flux, Proliferation, and Survival of Glioblastoma Stem Cells. *Cancer Cell* **2016**, *29*, 859–873. [CrossRef] [PubMed]
303. Venkataramani, V.; Tanev, D.I.; Kuner, T.; Wick, W.; Winkler, F. Synaptic input to brain tumors: Clinical implications. *Neuro-Oncology* **2021**, *23*, 23–33. [CrossRef]
304. Corsi, L.; Mescola, A.; Alessandrini, A. Glutamate Receptors and Glioblastoma Multiforme: An Old "Route" for New Perspectives. *Int. J. Mol. Sci.* **2019**, *20*, 1796. [CrossRef] [PubMed]
305. Zoidl, G.R.; Spray, D.C. The Roles of Calmodulin and CaMKII in Cx36 Plasticity. *Int. J. Mol. Sci.* **2021**, *22*, 4473. [CrossRef]
306. Giese, K.P. The role of CaMKII autophosphorylation for NMDA receptor-dependent synaptic potentiation. *Neuropharmacology* **2021**, *193*, 108616. [CrossRef]
307. Pellicena, P.; Schulman, H. CaMKII inhibitors: From research tools to therapeutic agents. *Front. Pharmacol.* **2014**, *5*, 21. [CrossRef]
308. Azab, M.A.; Alomari, A.; Azzam, A.Y. Featuring how calcium channels and calmodulin affect glioblastoma behavior. A review article. *Cancer Treat. Res. Commun.* **2020**, *25*, 100255. [CrossRef]
309. Kang, S.; Hong, J.; Lee, J.M.; Moon, H.E.; Jeon, B.; Choi, J.; Yoon, N.A.; Paek, S.H.; Roh, E.J.; Lee, C.J.; et al. Trifluoperazine, a Well-Known Antipsychotic, Inhibits Glioblastoma Invasion by Binding to Calmodulin and Disinhibiting Calcium Release Channel IP3R. *Mol. Cancer Ther.* **2017**, *16*, 217–227. [CrossRef]
310. Badimon, A.; Strasburger, H.J.; Ayata, P.; Chen, X.; Nair, A.; Ikegami, A.; Hwang, P.; Chan, A.T.; Graves, S.M.; Uweru, J.O.; et al. Negative feedback control of neuronal activity by microglia. *Nature* **2020**, *586*, 417–423. [CrossRef]
311. Altmann, A.; Ryten, M.; Di Nunzio, M.; Ravizza, T.; Tolomeo, D.; Reynolds, R.H.; Somani, A.; Bacigaluppi, M.; Iori, V.; Micotti, E.; et al. A systems-level analysis highlights microglial activation as a modifying factor in common epilepsies. *Neuropathol. Appl. Neurobiol.* **2021**. [CrossRef]
312. Qin, E.Y.; Cooper, D.D.; Abbott, K.L.; Lennon, J.; Nagaraja, S.; Mackay, A.; Jones, C.; Vogel, H.; Jackson, P.K.; Monje, M. Neural Precursor-Derived Pleiotrophin Mediates Subventricular Zone Invasion by Glioma. *Cell* **2017**, *170*, 845–859.e19. [CrossRef]
313. Chen, H.; Gong, Y.; Ma, Y.; Thompson, R.C.; Wang, J.; Cheng, Z.; Xue, L. A Brain-Penetrating Hsp90 Inhibitor NXD30001 Inhibits Glioblastoma as a Monotherapy or in Combination with Radiation. *Front. Pharmacol.* **2020**, *11*, 974. [CrossRef]
314. Lopez-Valero, I.; Davila, D.; Gonzalez-Martinez, J.; Salvador-Tormo, N.; Lorente, M.; Saiz-Ladera, C.; Torres, S.; Gabicagogeascoa, E.; Hernandez-Tiedra, S.; Garcia-Taboada, E.; et al. Midkine signaling maintains the self-renewal and tumorigenic capacity of glioma initiating cells. *Theranostics* **2020**, *10*, 5120–5136. [CrossRef]
315. Novak, U.; Kaye, A.H. Extracellular matrix and the brain: Components and function. *J. Clin. Neurosci.* **2000**, *7*, 280–290. [CrossRef]
316. Qi, J.; Esfahani, D.R.; Huang, T.; Ozark, P.; Bartom, E.; Hashizume, R.; Bonner, E.R.; An, S.; Horbinski, C.M.; James, C.D.; et al. Tenascin-C expression contributes to pediatric brainstem glioma tumor phenotype and represents a novel biomarker of disease. *Acta Neuropathol. Commun.* **2019**, *7*, 75. [CrossRef] [PubMed]
317. Brack, S.S.; Silacci, M.; Birchler, M.; Neri, D. Tumor-targeting properties of novel antibodies specific to the large isoform of tenascin-C. *Clin. Cancer Res.* **2006**, *12*, 3200–3208. [CrossRef]
318. Pericoli, G.; Ferretti, R.; Moore, A.S.; Vinci, M. Live-3D-Cell Immunocytochemistry Assays of Pediatric Diffuse Midline Glioma. *J. Vis. Exp.* **2021**, *177*, e63091. [CrossRef] [PubMed]
319. Wolf, K.J.; Shukla, P.; Springer, K.; Lee, S.; Coombes, J.D.; Choy, C.J.; Kenny, S.J.; Xu, K.; Kumar, S. A mode of cell adhesion and migration facilitated by CD44-dependent microtentacles. *Proc. Natl. Acad. Sci. USA* **2020**, *117*, 11432–11443. [CrossRef] [PubMed]
320. Xu, Y.; Stamenkovic, I.; Yu, Q. CD44 attenuates activation of the hippo signaling pathway and is a prime therapeutic target for glioblastoma. *Cancer Res.* **2010**, *70*, 2455–2464. [CrossRef] [PubMed]
321. Mohiuddin, E.; Wakimoto, H. Extracellular matrix in glioblastoma: Opportunities for emerging therapeutic approaches. *Am. J. Cancer Res.* **2021**, *11*, 3742–3754. [PubMed]

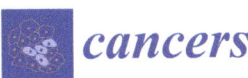

Review

Update on Novel Therapeutics for Primary CNS Lymphoma

Lauren R. Schaff * and Christian Grommes

Memorial Sloan Kettering Cancer Center, Department of Neurology, Weill Cornell Medicine, New York, NY 10065, USA; GrommesC@mskcc.org
* Correspondence: SchaffL@mskcc.org; Tel.: +1-212-610-0485

Simple Summary: Primary central nervous system lymphoma is a rare and aggressive form of non-Hodgkin lymphoma. While it is highly responsive to first-line chemo and radiation treatments, rates of relapse are high, demonstrating the need for improved therapeutic strategies. Recent advancements in the understanding of the pathophysiology of this disease have led to the identification of new potential treatment targets and the development of novel agents. This review aims to discuss different targeted strategies and review some of the data supporting these approaches, and discusses recently completed and ongoing clinical trials using these novel agents.

Abstract: Primary central nervous system lymphoma (PCNSL) is a rare lymphoma isolated to the central nervous system or vitreoretinal space. Standard treatment consists of cytotoxic methotrexate-based chemotherapy, with or without radiation. Despite high rates of response, relapse is common, highlighting the need for novel therapeutic approaches. Recent advances in the understanding of PCNSL have elucidated mechanisms of pathogenesis and resistance including activation of the B-cell receptor and mammalian target of rapamycin pathways. Novel treatment strategies such as the Bruton's tyrosine kinase (BTK) inhibitor ibrutinib, phosphatidylinositol-3 kinase (PI3K) inhibitors, and immunomodulatory drugs are promising. Increasingly, evidence suggests immune evasion plays a role in PCNSL pathogenesis and several immunotherapeutic strategies including checkpoint inhibition and targeted chimeric antigen receptor T (CAR-T) cells are under investigation. This review provides a discussion on the challenges in development of targeted therapeutic strategies, an update on recent treatment advances, and offers a look toward ongoing clinical studies.

Keywords: PCNSL; CNS lymphoma; methotrexate; novel therapies; novel therapeutics

1. Introduction

Primary central nervous system lymphoma (PCNSL) is a rare variant of extra-nodal non-Hodgkin lymphoma that affects only the central nervous system (CNS) and/or vitreoretinal space in the absence of systemic involvement. This differs from secondary CNS lymphoma (SCNSL) in which CNS disease may represent progression or a relapse of a systemic lymphoma that may harbor different genetic features. CNS lymphoma affects approximately 1600 people per year in the United States and is more common in the elderly, with a median age of 67 at diagnosis [1]. Immunodeficiency is a risk factor for PCNSL, but the disease may also occur sporadically in immunocompetent patients. This review will focus on advances in the treatment of immunocompetent patients with PCNSL.

The presentation of PCNSL may be varied and diagnosis requires a high degree of clinical suspicion. Symptoms may be focal, related to direct tumor involvement of the eye, brain, or spinal cord, or may be non-specific. Up to 50% of the time, patients present with cognitive decline and behavioral changes that may not prompt immediate neuro-imaging [2]. When imaging is obtained, magnetic resonance imaging (MRI) with and without contrast is the modality of choice. PCNSL often presents with characteristic homogeneously enhancing, diffusion restricting, deep brain lesions. Full disease staging requires an MRI of the spine, a lumbar puncture, and a slit lamp examination. To differentiate a

Citation: Schaff, L.R.; Grommes, C. Update on Novel Therapeutics for Primary CNS Lymphoma. *Cancers* **2021**, *13*, 5372. https://doi.org/10.3390/cancers13215372

Academic Editor: Elisabetta Abruzzese

Received: 6 October 2021
Accepted: 20 October 2021
Published: 26 October 2021

Publisher's Note: MDPI stays neutral with regard to jurisdictional claims in published maps and institutional affiliations.

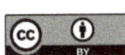

Copyright: © 2021 by the authors. Licensee MDPI, Basel, Switzerland. This article is an open access article distributed under the terms and conditions of the Creative Commons Attribution (CC BY) license (https://creativecommons.org/licenses/by/4.0/).

PCNSL from SCNSL, systemic work up is required. A positron emission tomography (PET) scan of the body should be performed. If a PET cannot be obtained, patients should undergo computed tomography (CT) of the chest/abdomen/pelvis to look for lymphadenopathy, paired with a bone marrow biopsy and a testicular ultrasound in men.

PCNSL is highly chemo- and radio-responsive. While surgical sampling is often required for diagnosis, tissue studies suggest involvement of the whole brain [3]. Multiple retrospective studies have failed to demonstrate a survival benefit with extensive surgery [2,4,5] and as a result, resection is typically not pursued.

Chemotherapy alone, particularly methotrexate (MTX)-based treatment, results in dramatic clinical and radiographic responses, often inducing remission. While MTX is broadly considered an important component of first-line treatment, there is a lack of consensus regarding the optimal chemotherapy regimen. Polychemotherapy regimens that include MTX are associated with improved response rates and progression-free survival (PFS) as compared to MTX monotherapy [6]. However, there is a paucity of prospective randomized data comparing MTX-based regimens and as a result, different practice approaches have developed. Common regimens include rituximab/MTX/procarbazine/vincristine (R-MPV) [7], MTX/temozolomide/rituximab) (MT-R) [8], MTX/cytarabine/thiotepa/rituximab (MA-TRix) [9], rituximab/MTX/carmustine/teniposide/prednisolone (R-MBVP) [10], and rituximab/MTX (R-M) [11]. The optimal dose of MTX is not known, though most practitioners agree that a dose of at least 3 g/m^2 is required for adequate penetration of the CNS [12]. Some regimens utilize dosages up to 8 g/m^2 [8] though toxicity often necessitates dose reductions and there is no clear benefit to these higher doses. Ultimately, choice of regimen often comes down to institutional and practitioner preference.

Without a consolidation strategy to follow MTX-based chemotherapy, the likelihood of PCNSL relapse is high, with a median PFS of 21.5 months after a complete response (CR) [13]. Historically, consolidation consisted of whole brain radiation therapy (WBRT) though it is unclear whether WBRT results in an overall survival (OS) benefit and it is associated with long-term neurotoxicity [13]. Whether a lower than standard dose of WBRT adequately addresses the issue of neurotoxicity remains to be seen [14]. Increasingly, myeloablative high-dose chemotherapy followed by autologous stem cell transplant (HDC-ASCT) is the preferred consolidation strategy for eligible patients. Such an approach after MTX-based therapy yields response rates of more than 90% [15] with median PFS of 74 months in one study [15] and not-reached in others [16,17]. For patients who are elderly or frail, non-myeloablative chemotherapy with high-dose cytarabine with or without etoposide may be considered [8,10,18]. Maintenance chemotherapy in lieu of consolidation is also a reasonable treatment approach [19,20]. In clinical trials, targeted or immunotherapies are also being explored for this purpose.

Despite aggressive treatment for PCNSL, approximately 15% of patients have refractory disease [21] and relapse rates are high, particularly in patents who are not candidates for HDC-ASCT. Traditional strategies for salvage therapy include MTX-rechallenge [22,23], alternate cytotoxic chemotherapy regimens [24–26], and WBRT [27,28]. Prognosis for relapsed disease is poor with a PFS of only about a year with aggressive salvage therapy [29]. As a result, there is a desperate need for novel therapeutic strategies. Recent developments in the understanding of the pathogenesis of PCNSL have led to the investigation and use of new, targeted approaches.

2. Pathophysiology

A vast majority of PCNSL cases are comprised of a diffuse large B cell lymphoma (DLBCL) and express pan-B cell markers CD20, CD19, CD22, and CD79a. Other lymphomatous malignancies such as T-cell lymphoma, Burkitt lymphoma, and lower grade lymphoproliferative neoplasms have been described but are less common and may warrant special considerations with regard to treatment strategy.

Histologically, DLBCL in the brain is highly proliferative with an angiocentric growth pattern. Based on the Hans criteria [30] and immunohistochemistry, a majority (>75%)

of PCNSL cases are classified as activated B-cell-like (ABC)/nongerminal center subtype [31–33]. However further evidence with immunoglobulin heavy chain gene mutational signatures and immunophenotyping suggest PCNSL has germinal center origin or exposure [31,34–37] and increasingly, there is evidence PCNSL may demonstrate an overlapping state of differentiation with concurrent expression of germinal center markers such as BCL6 and activation markers such as cyclin D2 or MUM1/Interferon Regulatory Factor 4 (IRF4) [31,38]. Ultimately the relevance of differentiating between ABC or germinal center subtype in PCNSL is unclear and unlike in systemic lymphoma where the ABC subtype confers a poorer prognosis, there is no clear survival advantage associated with any particular subtype of PCNSL [39].

Single nucleotide variants and copy number alterations are frequent genetic events in PCNSL. *MYD88*, *CD79B*, *CARD11*, and *TNFAIP3* are amongst the most frequently mutated genes. Systemically, *MYD88* mutations are associated with the ABC subtype; but in PCNSL, *MYD88*, and *CD79B* have been described in both ABC and GCB subtypes of disease. *MYD88* missense mutations (most common L265P [40]) lead to constitutive activation of the TLR pathway [41], while alterations in *CD79B* activate the BCR pathway [42]. Mutations in the coiled-coil domain of *CARD11* result in downstream activation of both pathways [43] while alterations to *TNFAIP3* can result in a loss of pathway inhibition. Ultimately, the BCR/TLR pathways result in upregulation of nuclear factor kappaB (NFκB), a protein transcription factor that promotes neoplastic proliferation and prevents apoptosis [44]. Copy number alterations may also contribute to pathogenesis. Losses are common at 6p21.33 (*HLA-B*, *HLA-C*), 6q21-23 (*TNFAIP3*), and 9p21.3 (*CDKN2A*). Copy number gains may be seen at 12q (*MDM2*, *CDK4*) and 9p24.1 (*PD-L1*, *PD-L2*). Somatic hypermutation (SHM) is also thought to play a role in PCNSL pathogenesis and may offer further rationale for use of immunotherapy. Genetic features of vitreoretinal lymphoma (VRL) have significant overlap with PCNSL, and result in probable activation of the TLR pathway. Mutations in *MYD88* may be more common in VRL (and not limited to L265P) while *CD79B* mutations appear less common [45]. SHM genes may be similarly mutated.

Increasingly, evidence suggests the tumor microenvironment also plays an important role in PCNSL. IL-10 is a cytokine that may serve as a prognostic biomarker and also appears to lead to activation of signal transducer and activator of transcription 3 (STAT3) [46]. The Janus kinase 2 (JAK2)/STAT3 pathway results in transcription of target genes involved in cellular proliferation, survival, and angiogenesis. STAT3 is expressed in a variety of malignancies including PCNSL [46]. Tumor-associated macrophages (TAMs) interact with PCNSL cells and promote tumor invasion, proliferation, and an immunosuppressed environment. Quantification of TAMs may be important in prognosis [47]. TAMs also overexpress *PD-L1*, suggesting a potential target for immunotherapy.

Overall, PCNSL appears to be biologically distinct from systemic lymphoma and is increasingly considered a separate entity [48–50]. Genetic alterations seen in PCNSL including activation of the B-cell receptor (BCR) and Toll-like receptor (TLR) signaling pathways most closely resemble those observed in testicular lymphoma [51–53], suggesting similar pathogenesis between these two immunoprivileged sites. Improved understanding of the unique molecular profile of PCNSL has allowed for the recent investigation of multiple targeted strategies (Table 1).

Table 1. Recent prospective trials of novel agents.

Author	Year	Agent(s)	Phase	Evaluable Patients	Disease Status	Median Age, y	ORR (PR + CR)	mPFS, mo	mOS, mo
Korfel [54]	2016	Temsirolimus	2	37	R/R	70	20/37 (54%)	2.1	3.7
Grommes [55]	2017	Ibrutinib	1	20 (13 PCNSL)	R/R	69	10/13 (77%)	4.6	15

Table 1. Cont.

Author	Year	Agent(s)	Phase	Evaluable Patients	Disease Status	Median Age, y	ORR (PR + CR)	mPFS, mo	mOS, mo
Lionakis [40]	2017	TMZ, etoposide, liposomal doxorubicin, dexamethasone, rituximab, ibrutinib	1b	18	R/R, new	66	15/18 (83%)	15.3 in R/R	NR
Rubenstein [56]	2018	Lenalidomide + rituximab; lenalidomide maintenance	1	14 (7 PCNSL)	R/R	66	6/7 (86%)	6	NS
Tun [57]	2018	Pomalidomide + dexamethasone	1	25 (23 PCNSL)	R/R	NS, >60	11/23 (48%)	5.3	NS
Ghesquieres [58]	2019	Lenalidomide + rituximab	2	45 (34 PCNSL)	R/R	69	22/34 (65%)	3.9	NS
Grommes [59]	2019	Ibrutinib + M(3.5) + rituximab	1b	15 (9 PCNSL)	R/R	62	8/9 (89%)	NR	NR
Soussain [60]	2019	Ibrutinib	2	44	R/R	70	26/44 (59%)	4.8	19.2
Narita [61]	2021	Tirabrutinib	1/2	44	R/R	60	28/44 (64%)	2.9	NR

CR: complete response; M: methotrexate; mOS: median overall survival; mo: months mPFS: median progression-free survival; NR: not reached; NS: not specified; ORR: overall response rate; PCNSL: primary central nervous system lymphoma; PR: partial response; R/R: relapsed/refractory; TMZ: temozolomide; y: years.

3. Molecular Targets

3.1. BCR/TLR Pathway

Discovery of alterations involving the BCR and TLR pathways has led to the most significant recent breakthroughs in the treatment of PCNSL. The BCR signaling pathway can be targeted at different signaling nodes. Upstream, the pathway may be downregulated through targeting phosphatidylinositol-3 kinase (PI3K). Downstream, immunomodulatory drugs like lenalidomide may be used to inhibit IRF4, which affects NFκB function. Proteosome inhibitors may prevent release of NFκB to the nucleus, where it results in alteration of gene expression. Unfortunately, proteasome inhibitors are often too bulky to cross the blood–brain barrier (BBB).

Bruton's tyrosine kinase (BTK), the central signaling node of the pathway, can be targeted with ibrutinib. A prospective study of ibrutinib 560 mg daily in 52 patients with relapsed/refractory PCNSL demonstrated a response rate of 52% [60]. A higher dose of 840 mg daily may result in increased cerebrospinal fluid (CSF) concentration and remains well tolerated [55,59] though the clinical benefit of this higher dosing schedule is unknown and additional data suggests the enzymatic IC_{50} is not proportional to dose [40]. Response to ibrutinib occurs quickly with one 'window study' demonstrating a response rate of 83% to only two weeks of single-agent ibrutinib, prior to the addition of further chemotherapy [40]. Notably, these high response rates are in contrast the experience in systemic lymphoma where single agent ibrutinib may result in a response rate of only 25% [62]. While this may be in part due a higher incidence of BCR/TLR alterations in PCNSL such as *MYD88*, it is important to note that even PCNSL patients without obvious genomic alterations in the BCR pathway demonstrate ibrutinib response [60]. It is also worth noting that while concurrent *CD79B* and *MYD88* mutations appear to sensitize systemic lymphoma to ibrutinib [62], this same combination was associated with a poorer response in CNS disease, perhaps due to decreased dependence on the BCR pathway [55]. These mutations appear to coincide in approximately 37% of cases of PCNSL [40]. *CARD11* and *TNFAIP3* mutations are potential sources of ibrutinib resistance given their activity downstream BTK. While this has been described in systemic lymphoma [62,63] and PCNSL with ibrutinib monotherapy [55], adequate responses were seen in patients with these potential resistance mechanisms when ibrutinib was used in combination with cytotoxic chemotherapy [59].

Despite high rates of radiographic response, the progression-free survival provided by ibrutinib monotherapy is less than 5 months, suggesting early development of resistance [55,60]. With ibrutinib combination treatment, that PFS is extended to approximately 9 months in pre-treated patients [59]. Multiple studies are now incorporating ibrutinib into combination therapy, paired with agents such as lenalidomide (NCT03703167), copanlisib (NCT03581942), checkpoint inhibition (NCT04421560, NCT03770416), and traditional chemotherapy (NCT04066920, NCT02315326).

Ibrutinib has been incorporated to the National Comprehensive Cancer Network (NCCN) guidelines for treatment of relapsed/refractory PCNSL. Studies investigating ibrutinib for use in newly diagnosed patients are currently underway (Table 2). Some newly diagnosed patients were included in a study of ibrutinib in combination with temozolomide, etoposide, liposomal doxorubicin, rituximab, and intrathecal cytarabine (DA-TEDDI-R) but the regimen was associated with high rates of toxicity, specifically aspergillosis in 39% of treated patients [40]. The same combination is now being used with prophylactic anti-fungal agents (NCT02203526). In the upfront setting, ibrutinib is also being studied in combination with MTX, vincristine, procarbazine, rituximab (NCT02315326, NCT04446962), and is being studied as maintenance therapy following response to induction therapy (NCT02623010).

Table 2. Ongoing trials of novel agents.

Agents	Clinicaltrails.Gov ID	Trial Start	Phase	Target Accrual	Eligible Age	Country
Upfront Induction						
Rituximab, MTX, lenalidomide, nivolumab	NCT04609046	2020	1	27	18+	USA
Rituximab, MTX, procarbazine, vincristine; and lenalidomide or ibrutinib	NCT04446962	2020	1b/2	128	18 to 60	France
Rituximab, MTX ± lenalidomide	NCT04481815	2020	2	240	18 to 75	China
Rituximab, lenalidomide, MTX, and TMZ	NCT04737889	2021	2	30	18 to 70	China
Rituximab, MTX, procarbazine, vincristine, and ibrutinib	NCT02315326	2021	2	30	18+	USA
Upfront Maintenance						
Nivolumab maintenance	NCT04022980	2019	1b	20	65+	USA
MTX, rituximab, lenalidomide, with lenalidomide maintenance	NCT04120350	2019	1b/2	47	18 to 75	China
Rituximab, MTX, with ibrutinib maintenance	NCT02623010	2016	2	30	60 to 85	Israel
MTX or TMZ-based therapy with procarbazine or lenalidomide maintenance	NCT03495960	2019	2	208	70+	Italy
Lenalidomide/rituximab maintenance	NCT04627753	2020	2	30	19+	Korea
Nivolumab maintenance	NCT04401774	2020	2	25	18+	USA
Relapsed/Refractory Disease						
TMZ, etoposide, liposomal doxorubicin, dexamethasone, ibrutinib, rituximab, IT-cytarabine	NCT02203526	2014	1	93	18+	USA

Table 2. Cont.

Agents	Clinicaltrails.Gov ID	Trial Start	Phase	Target Accrual	Eligible Age	Country
Tisagenlecleucel	NCT04134117	2019	1	6	18+	USA
Acalabrutinib and durvalumab	NCT04462328	2020	1	21	18+	USA
Fludarabine, cyclophosphamide, axicabtagene ciloleucel	NCT04608487	2020	1	18	18+	USA
Ibrutinib with rituximab and lenalidomide	NCT03703167	2019	1b	40	18+	USA
Copanlisib with ibrutinib	NCT03581942	2018	1b/2	45	18+	USA
Pembrolizumab, ibrutinib, and rituximab	NCT04421560	2020	1b/2	37	18+	USA
PQR309	NCT02669511	2015	2	21	18+	Germany
Nivolumab	NCT02857426	2016	2	47	18+	USA
Abemaciclib	NCT03220646	2017	2	10	18+	USA
Ibrutinib, rituximab, ifosfamide and etoposide, with ibrutinib maintenance	NCT04066920	2019	2	30	20 to 79	Korea
Nivolumab and ibrutinib	NCT03770416	2019	2	40	18+	USA
Nivolumab and pomalidomide	NCT03798314	2019	1	3	18+	USA
Acalabrutinib	NCT04548648	2020	2	32	18+	USA
Ibrutinib versus lenalidomide, with MTX, rituximab, etoposide	NCT04129710	2020	2	120	18 to 75	China
Orelabrutinib	NCT04438044	2020	2	39	18 to 75	China
Paxalisib	NCT04906096	2021	2	25	18+	USA
Tirabrutinib	NCT04947319	2021	2	44	18+	USA

IT: intrathecal; MTX: methotrexate; TMZ: temozolomide.

It is unclear whether the next generation of BTK inhibitors such as tirabrutinib and acalabrutinib will offer any advantage over ibrutinib. Tirabrutinib was recently studied in a phase I/II dose escalation trial in Japan for treatment of relapsed/refractory PCNSL. Overall response rate (ORR) was 64% though PFS was only 2.9 months. Tirabrutinib is highly selective for BTK, theoretically reducing toxicity. Nevertheless, nearly half the patients (47.7%) experienced a grade 3 or greater adverse event including three cases of grade 3 skin reaction (2, erythema multiforme) and one case of a grade 5 interstitial lung disease and concurrent *Pneumocystis jirovecii* (PJP) in a patient not treated with PJP prophylaxis [61]. A phase II study in the United States is anticipated (NCT04947319). Acalabrutinib, another second generation BTK inhibitor, is currently being studied in patients with relapsed/refractory primary and secondary CNS lymphoma (NCT04548648, NCT04462328).

3.2. PI3K/mTOR Pathway

PI3K is a family of kinases that function as second messengers in multiple signal transduction pathways. Mammalian target of rapamycin (mTOR) is a ubiquitously expressed member of the PI3K family of proteins and a potential therapeutic target. The PI3K/AKT/mTOR pathway is highly conserved regulating cell growth and proliferation [64]. It functions via influence on BTK resulting in activation of NFκB via the BCR pathway but also leads to the activation of independent signaling pathways [41,42]. Inhibition of mTOR has demonstrated modest activity in the treatment of mantle cell lymphoma and systemic DLBCL [65,66].

Temsirolimus, an mTOR inhibitor, was the first targeted agent studied in the treatment of PCNSL. A phase 2 study of relapsed/refractory PCNSL patients yielded a response rate of 54%, notably higher than that observed with systemic lymphoma, but with a PFS of only 2.1 months. Importantly, CSF pharmacokinetics in fourteen samples failed to confirm presence of temsirolimus in all but one specimen which contained a marginal concentration of drug [54]. This was in contrast to a glioma study which demonstrated presence of intratumoral temsirolimus with tissue/blood concentration ratios ranging from 0.69–3.37 [67]. The mismatch between observed response and duration of control may speak to the importance of selecting a therapeutic agent that will treat both the intraparenchymal and leptomeningeal compartments or be a function of early development of resistance mechanisms.

A study of buparlisib, a pan-PI3K inhibitor resulted in even lower response rates (25%) [68]. Again, while pharmacokinetic data from a surgical glioma study demonstrate intratumoral concentrations on par with those in plasma [69], CSF concentrations were subtherapeutic in the CNS lymphoma population [68]. Further complicating the picture is evidence indicating incomplete blockade of the PI3K/AKT/mTOR pathway, even when intratumoral concentrations are achieved [69].

Current studies are underway with additional agents targeting this pathway. PQR309, a dual PI3K/mTOR inhibitor, has shown promise in the preclinical setting. Paxalisib is a PI3K/mTOR inhibitor with CNS penetrance. Each are being studied as monotherapy for patients with relapsed/refractory PCNSL (NCT02669511, NCT04906096). Copanlisib, another PI3K inhibitor, is being used in combination with ibrutinib (NCT03581942) in order to address increased activation of the PI3K/AKT/mTOR pathway observed in CD79B mutant lymphomas. Preclinical data suggest synergistic cell death with dual PI3K pathway inhibition and ibrutinib [55].

3.3. Immunomedulatory Drugs

Lenalidomide and pomalidomide are second and third generation immunomodulatory drugs (IMiDs) with the potential for direct and indirect antineoplastic effects. IMiDs suppress IRF4 which interfaces with NFκB, as well as MYC, frequently upregulated in PCNSL [8]. They also block the PI3K/AKT pathway, resulting in anti-angiogenic effects [70], and appear to impact the immune microenvironment by modulating tumor-associated macrophages [71].

Lenalidomide has been studied as monotherapy for treatment of recurrent/relapsed PCNSL and SCNSL. Response was seen in 9 of 14 patients (64%) including within the leptomeningeal and ocular compartments. CSF analysis suggested dose-dependent increases in lenalidomide concentration with a CSF/plasma partition coefficient of >20% following the 15 and 20 mg dose levels [56]. A phase 2 study of lenalidomide in combination with systemic rituximab for relapsed/refractory PCNSL yielded an ORR 35.6% with median PFS and OS 7.8 and 17.7 months with a follow up of 19.2 months [58]. The combination was well tolerated and is now being studied in conjunction with ibrutinib (NCT03703167) for treatment of relapsed/refractory PCNSL. A retrospective study of rituximab/lenalidomide/ibrutinib demonstrated response in 8 of 14 heavily pre-treated patients [72]. Multiple combinations using lenalidomide are being studied for both newly diagnosed and relapsed disease (Table 2).

Another potential role for lenalidomide is use as a maintenance agent. In a retrospective study, low doses of 5–10 mg daily appeared to potentiate response to salvage therapy, resulting in longer PFS following salvage therapy than with initial treatment [56]. A small prospective cohort of lenalidomide maintenance following induction therapy with lenalidomide and rituximab induction did not yield as positive results [58]. The role of lenalidomide maintenance following induction treatment for newly diagnosed disease is currently under investigation (NCT04120350, NCT03495960, NCT04627753).

Pomalidomide is a third-generation agent that was studied in combination with dexamethasone in a phase I study of relapsed/refractory PCNSL and primary VRL patients [57]. ORR was 48% with a PFS of 5.3 months in all-comers and 9 months in responders. Notably, one patient had pseudoprogression after 4 cycles of treatment. CSF analysis was performed in one patient; pomalidomide was detected with a CSF-to-plasma ration of 19 and 17% [57], consistent with pre-clinical data [71]. Pomalidomide is now being studied in combination with immunotherapy (NCT03798314).

IMiDs seem to be fairly well tolerated with toxicities most commonly consisting of marrow suppression, infection, and fatigue.

4. Targeting the Immune System

Increasingly, evidence suggests immune evasion and immune response modulation play a role in PCNSL pathogenesis and *PD-L1* upregulation has been well-described [52]. Two small retrospective studies have reported encouraging outcomes. Nayak et al., treated five patients (four PCNSL, one isolated SCNSL from testicular primary) with the anti-PD-1 agent nivolumab. All five had objective radiographic responses with four patients achieving a CR. PFS appeared promising at >13 months in all patients, and all were alive at a median follow up of 17 months [73]. The study was of course limited by its retrospective nature and several patients received either concurrent therapy (rituximab) or had initiated nivolumab immediately following brain radiation. Still, it lent support for further investigation into use of immunotherapy. A second, more recent retrospective study reported six patients with PCNSL (3) and isolated SCNSL (3) treated with anti-PD-1 therapy, pembrolizumab (5) or nivolumab (1). Ambady et al., achieved CR in three of six patients and reported progressive disease in the remaining. Interestingly, one patient who achieved an initial CR progressed after therapy was discontinued but was able to re-attain a CR upon re-initiation of immunotherapy [74]. PD-1 blockade tends to be well-tolerated and has the potential to offer a viable alternative treatment strategy to patients who are elderly or frail. Prospective studies are ongoing exploring its use as monotherapy (NCT02857426) and in conjunction with other agents such as ibrutinib (NCT03770416, NCT04421560), lenalidomide (NCT04609046), or pomalidomide (NCT03798314). PD-1 blockade is also being explored as a potential maintenance or consolidation strategy (NCT04401774, NCT04022980).

Targeting tumors with chimeric antigen receptor T (CAR-T) cells is a novel strategy that utilizes a patients' own genetically engineered T cells to identify and bind a tumor-specific target antigen. CD19-targeted CAR-T cells have been studied in systemic DLBCL with encouraging results [75]. Initially patients with CNS disease were excluded from studies out of concern for neurotoxicity and the potential for limited efficacy at immunoprivileged sites. However, CAR-T cells have been identified in the CSF [75] and an index patient with SCNSL and concurrent systemic disease demonstrated a CR in the brain following treatment with CD-19 directed CAR-T cell therapy [76]. More recently, a retrospective report of patients with SCNSL treated with off-label tisagenlecleucel, another CD19-directed CAR-T, yielded responses in four of eight patients (two CR, two partial response at 28 days) [77]. Notably T-cell expansion was evident even in patients with isolated CNS disease. The treatment was tolerated well with no reports of greater than grade 1 neurotoxicity [77]. Preliminary data from an ongoing clinical trial enrolling patients with PCNSL reported high rates of toxicity with all patients developing at least grade 1 cytokine release syndrome and neurotoxicity, though all toxicities were reversible [78]. At initial disease response, three of five patients had achieved CR while the remaining 2 appeared to have stable disease. Additional prospective studies of CD19 CAR-T agents tisagenlecleucel (NCT04134117) and axicabtagene ciloleucel (NCT04608487) are underway in patients with CNS lymphoma, with results eagerly awaited. Newer generations of CAR-T cells are in development and may allow for modulation of the tumor microenvironment simultaneous with direct tumor killing. This newer generation of agents known as T-cells redirected for antigen-unrestricted cytokine-initiated killing (TRUCKs) express an additional transgenic inducible-cytokine to be released upon tumor-antigen binding, inducing a pro-inflammatory response and potentially mitigating the immunosuppressive lymphoma microenvironment [79].

Bi-specific T-cell engagers (BiTEs) are engineered bi-specific monoclonal antibodies with two single-chain variable domains of different antibodies. One domain targets the

CD3 receptor on T cells while the other targets a tumor-specific antigen. BiTEs form a link between T cells and tumor, triggering cellular death via target cell lysis in the absence of regular major histocompatibility complex (MHC) class I/peptide antigen recognition [80]. Blinatumomab, a CD19/CD3-BiTE has been approved for use in the treatment of B-cell precursor acute lymphoblastic leukemia with minimal residual disease. It and a variety of CD20/CD3-BiTEs are undergoing investigation for treatment of systemic DLBCL [81]. At this time, studies are not enrolling patients with CNS disease due to concerns for neurotoxicity; however, this may be a treatment strategy in the future.

5. Other Targets

Other potential therapeutic targets are being explored in PCSNL. Loss of CDKN2A is frequently observed [52] and may be targeted by cyclin dependent kinase inhibitors. A small prospective study of abemaciclib in CNS lymphoma is ongoing (NCT03220646). Venetoclax, a targeted agent against BCL-2, appears to penetrate the BBB—though at lower concentrations—and may have some efficacy in CNS lymphoproliferative disease [82,83]. A prospective study of venetoclax with obinutuzumab, an anti-CD20 monoclonal antibody, was halted due to low enrollment (NCT04073147).

Selinexor, an inhibitor of exportin 1, blocks nuclear export, leading to accumulation of tumor suppressor proteins in the nucleus and resultant cell death. It is currently approved for the treatment of refractory multiple myeloma, relapsed systemic diffuse large B-cell lymphoma, and is planned to be studied for treatment of PCNSL. Pre-clinical data suggest selinexor may have synergy with ibrutinib, potentially paving the way for future studies [84].

6. Challenges to Drug Development and Delivery

Development of new targeted treatments has been difficult. One challenge is that PCNSL is a rare disease, limiting the ability to perform statistically significant head-to-head comparisons of treatment strategies. Prior to large-scale clinical studies however, it is important to achieve adequate understanding of drug pharmacokinetics in the CNS. Many targeted drugs such as proteasome inhibitors are too large to penetrate the BBB. Increasingly, it is being recognized that drug concentrations need to be explored in both the leptomeningeal compartment and intraparenchymal tumor tissue as one appears to be a poor surrogate for the other. Differences in concentration may be a result of frequent breakdown of the BBB in intraparenchymal disease.

Penetration of the BBB remains a challenge in the treatment of CNS malignancies, including PCNSL. One potential strategy to enhance drug delivery is disruption of the BBB, which can potentially be achieved with drugs, ultrasound, or osmotic disruption. One multi-center study of BBB disruption (BBBD) using mannitol followed by intra-arterial (IA) MTX yielded an ORR of 81.9% (CRR 57.8%) with an OS of 3.1 years [85]. This compared favorably to historical controls, particularly considering that approximately half the patients enrolled did not undergo consolidation treatment. Another strategy for BBBD include delivery of low doses of tumor necrosis factor-alpha (TNF) to the vasculature. This has been followed by delivery of systemic lymphoma regimens with otherwise poor CNS penetration (rituximab/cyclophosphamide/doxorubicin/vincristine/prednisone or R-CHOP) with good response rates [86].

Development of drug resistance is also a complicating factor, particularly for molecular strategies targeting only a single pathway. Combination studies are one potential strategy to reduce resistance. For example, while ibrutinib is associated with a short PFS when used as monotherapy, response appears more durable when it is used in combination. As a result, ibrutinib is now under investigation as part of a number of potential treatment regimens (Table 2). These studies are ongoing, and it remains to be seen whether this strategy will improve efficacy and long-term control in PCNSL.

7. Future Directions

The efficacy of MTX has meant that the investigation of most of these novel treatment strategies has been in the relapsed/refractory setting. Only recently are studies starting to incorporate the use of some of these newer agents into upfront treatment, and largely in combination with MTX. It remains to be seen whether any of these agents will obviate the need for MTX and for the most part, this is not being studied except in patients who are considered ineligible for MTX-based therapy. While MTX is effective, it necessitates frequent hospitalizations, leading to time away from work and family. Additionally, it confers risk of MTX-related toxicity, as well as complications associated with inpatient admission such as delirium, urinary tract infections, and thromboembolic events. Many of the novel therapies are oral and most can be administered in the outpatient setting. If they prove to be as effective as MTX, this may lead to a new treatment paradigm for PCNSL.

As we continue to develop novel strategies for this disease, it will become increasingly important to develop minimally invasive biomarkers. Traditionally, patients are monitored for recurrence with routine MRIs and possibly CSF sampling and ocular exams, depending on their presentation. Monitoring of biomarkers such as interleukin-10 (IL-10) may help monitor treatment response and allow for early detection of relapse [56,87]. Detection of circulating tumor DNA (ctDNA) may serve a similar role while allowing for detection and confirmation of genetic arrangements. While this technology has been unsuccessful in the serum of patients with PCNSL [88] in CSF, ctDNA has been used to detect molecular alterations [59,89]. Studies are ongoing to determine whether detection of ctDNA in the CSF is of prognostic import and can be used to monitor treatment response (NCT04401774). Monitoring of ctDNA in the CSF may also allow for monitoring of the presence of targetable mutations.

8. Conclusions

Advances in our understanding of the molecular drivers of PCNSL have led to the development of novel drug strategies. We must ensure these drugs penetrate the CNS, create responses, and that these responses are durable. Combination therapy may be one way to avoid early resistance. Harnessing of the immune system is another strategy. Further genetic characterization and monitoring will be crucial in furthering our understanding and predicting response.

Author Contributions: Conceptualization, L.R.S. and C.G.; Investigation, L.R.S. and C.G.; Resources, L.R.S. and C.G.; Writing—original draft preparation, L.R.S.; Writing—review and editing, L.R.S. and C.G. All authors have read and agreed to the published version of the manuscript.

Funding: This article was supported, in part, by the MSK Cancer Center Support Grant (P30 CA008748), National Institute of Health. CG was supported by grants from Cycle for Survival Equinox and the Leukemia & Lymphoma Society.

Conflicts of Interest: L.R.S. served as a consultant for Debiopharm and receives research funding from BTG, plc. C.G. is a consultant for BTG, KITE, and ONO.

References

1. Ostrom, Q.T.; Patil, N.; Cioffi, G.; Waite, K.; Kruchko, C.; Barnholtz-Sloan, J.S. Corrigendum to: CBTRUS Statistical Report: Primary Brain and Other Central Nervous System Tumors Diagnosed in the United States in 2013–2017. *Neuro-Oncology* **2020**, *22*, iv1–iv96. [CrossRef] [PubMed]
2. Bataille, B.; Delwail, V.; Menet, E.; Vandermarcq, P.; Ingrand, P.; Wager, M.; Guy, G.; Lapierre, F. Primary intracerebral malignant lymphoma: Report of 248 cases. *J. Neurosurg.* **2000**, *92*, 261–266. [CrossRef]
3. Lai, R.; Rosenblum, M.K.; DeAngelis, L.M. Primary CNS lymphoma: A whole-brain disease? *Neurology* **2002**, *59*, 1557–1562. [CrossRef] [PubMed]
4. Bellinzona, M.; Roser, F.; Ostertag, H.; Gaab, R.; Saini, M. Surgical removal of primary central nervous system lymphomas (PCNSL) presenting as space occupying lesions: A series of 33 cases. *Eur. J. Surg. Oncol.* **2005**, *31*, 100–105. [CrossRef] [PubMed]
5. Reni, M.; Ferreri, A.J.M.; Garancini, M.P.; Villa, E. Therapeutic management of primary central nervous system lymphoma in immunocompetent patients: Results of a critical review of the literature. *Ann. Oncol.* **1997**, *8*, 227–234. [CrossRef] [PubMed]

6. Ferreri, A.J.; Reni, M.; Foppoli, M.; Martelli, M.; Pangalis, G.; Frezzato, M.; Cabras, M.G.; Fabbri, A.; Corazzelli, G.; Ilariucci, F.; et al. High-dose cytarabine plus high-dose methotrexate versus high-dose methotrexate alone in patients with primary CNS lymphoma: A randomised phase 2 trial. *Lancet* **2009**, *374*, 1512–1520. [CrossRef]
7. Morris, P.G.; Correa, D.D.; Yahalom, J.; Raizer, J.J.; Schiff, D.; Grant, B.; Grimm, S.; Lai, R.K.; Reiner, A.; Panageas, K.; et al. Rituximab, Methotrexate, Procarbazine, and Vincristine Followed by Consolidation Reduced-Dose Whole-Brain Radiotherapy and Cytarabine in Newly Diagnosed Primary CNS Lymphoma: Final Results and Long-Term Outcome. *J. Clin. Oncol.* **2013**, *31*, 3971–3979. [CrossRef] [PubMed]
8. Rubenstein, J.L.; Hsi, E.D.; Johnson, J.L.; Jung, S.-H.; Nakashima, M.O.; Grant, B.; Cheson, B.D.; Kaplan, L.D. Intensive Chemotherapy and Immunotherapy in Patients with Newly Diagnosed Primary CNS Lymphoma: CALGB 50202 (Alliance 50202). *J. Clin. Oncol.* **2013**, *31*, 3061–3068. [CrossRef] [PubMed]
9. Ferreri, A.J.M.; Cwynarski, K.; Pulczynski, E.; Ponzoni, M.; Deckert, M.; Politi, L.S.; Torri, V.; Fox, C.P.; La Rosée, P.; Schorb, E.; et al. Chemoimmunotherapy with methotrexate, cytarabine, thiotepa, and rituximab (MATRix regimen) in patients with primary CNS lymphoma: Results of the first randomisation of the International Extranodal Lymphoma Study Group-32 (IELSG32) phase 2 trial. *Lancet Haematol.* **2016**, *3*, e217–e227. [CrossRef]
10. Bromberg, J.E.C.; Issa, S.; Bakunina, K.; Minnema, M.C.; Seute, T.; Durian, M.; Cull, G.; Schouten, H.C.; Stevens, W.B.C.; Zijlstra, J.M.; et al. Rituximab in patients with primary CNS lymphoma (HOVON 105/ALLG NHL 24): A randomised, open-label, phase 3 intergroup study. *Lancet Oncol.* **2019**, *20*, 216–228. [CrossRef]
11. Chamberlain, M.C.; Johnston, S.K. High-dose methotrexate and rituximab with deferred radiotherapy for newly diagnosed primary B-cell CNS lymphoma. *Neuro-Oncology* **2010**, *12*, 736–744. [CrossRef] [PubMed]
12. Reni, M.; Ferreri, A.J.; Guha-Thakurta, N.; Blay, J.-Y.; Dell'Oro, S.; Biron, P.; Hochberg, F.H. Clinical relevance of consolidation radiotherapy and other main therapeutic issues in primary central nervous system lymphomas treated with upfront high-dose methotrexate. *Int. J. Radiat. Oncol.* **2001**, *51*, 419–425. [CrossRef]
13. Thiel, E.; Korfel, A.; Martus, P.; Kanz, L.; Griesinger, F.; Rauch, M.; Röth, A.; Hertenstein, B.; von Toll, T.; Hundsberger, T.; et al. High-dose methotrexate with or without whole brain radiotherapy for primary CNS lymphoma (G-PCNSL-SG-1): A phase 3, randomised, non-inferiority trial. *Lancet Oncol.* **2010**, *11*, 1036–1047.
14. Omuro, A.M.P.; DeAngelis, L.M.; Karrison, T.; Bovi, J.; Rosenblum, M.; Corn, B.W.; Correa, D.; Wefel, J.S.; Aneja, S.; Grommes, C.; et al. Randomized phase II study of rituximab, methotrexate (MTX), procarbazine, vincristine, and cytarabine (R-MPV-A) with and without low-dose whole-brain radiotherapy (LD-WBRT) for newly diagnosed primary CNS lymphoma (PCNSL). *J. Clin. Oncol.* **2020**, *38*, 2501. [CrossRef]
15. Illerhaus, G.; Kasenda, B.; Ihorst, G.; Egerer, G.; Lamprecht, M.; Keller, U.; Wolf, H.-H.; Hirt, C.; Stilgenbauer, S.; Binder, M.; et al. High-dose chemotherapy with autologous haemopoietic stem cell transplantation for newly diagnosed primary CNS lymphoma: A prospective, single-arm, phase 2 trial. *Lancet Haematol.* **2016**, *3*, e388–e397. [CrossRef] [PubMed]
16. Omuro, A.; Correa, D.D.; DeAngelis, L.M.; Moskowitz, C.H.; Matasar, M.J.; Kaley, T.J.; Gavrilovic, I.T.; Nolan, C.; Pentsova, E.; Grommes, C.C.; et al. R-MPV followed by high-dose chemotherapy with TBC and autologous stem-cell transplant for newly diagnosed primary CNS lymphoma. *Blood* **2015**, *125*, 1403–1410. [CrossRef] [PubMed]
17. Houillier, C.; Taillandier, L.; Dureau, S.; Lamy, T.; Laadhari, M.; Chinot, O.; Moluçon-Chabrot, C.; Soubeyran, P.; Gressin, R.; Choquet, S.; et al. Radiotherapy or Autologous Stem-Cell Transplantation for Primary CNS Lymphoma in Patients 60 Years of Age and Younger: Results of the Intergroup ANOCEF-GOELAMS Randomized Phase II PRECIS Study. *J. Clin. Oncol.* **2019**, *37*, 823–833. [CrossRef] [PubMed]
18. Omuro, A.; Chinot, O.; Taillandier, L.; Ghesquieres, H.; Soussain, C.; Delwail, V.; Lamy, T.; Gressin, R.; Choquet, S.; Soubeyran, P.-L.; et al. Methotrexate and temozolomide versus methotrexate, procarbazine, vincristine, and cytarabine for primary CNS lymphoma in an elderly population: An intergroup ANOCEF-GOELAMS randomised phase 2 trial. *Lancet Haematol.* **2015**, *2*, e251–e259. [CrossRef]
19. Ambady, P.; Fu, R.; Szidonya, L.; Peereboom, D.M.; Doolittle, N.D.; Neuwelt, E.A. Impact of maintenance rituximab on duration of response in primary central nervous system lymphoma. *J. Neuro-Oncol.* **2020**, *147*, 171–176. [CrossRef] [PubMed]
20. Pulczynski, E.J.; Kuittinen, O.; Erlanson, M.; Hagberg, H.; Fosså, A.; Eriksson, M.; Nordstrøm, M.; Østenstad, B.; Fluge, Ø.; Leppä, S.; et al. Successful change of treatment strategy in elderly patients with primary central nervous system lymphoma by de-escalating induction and introducing temozolomide maintenance: Results from a phase II study by The Nordic Lymphoma Group. *Haematologica* **2014**, *100*, 534–540. [CrossRef] [PubMed]
21. Jahnke, K.; Thiel, E.; Martus, P.; Herrlinger, U.; Weller, M.; Fischer, L.; Korfel, A.; on behalf of the German Primary Central Nervous System Lymphoma Study Group (G-PCNSL-SG). Relapse of primary central nervous system lymphoma: Clinical features, outcome and prognostic factors. *J. Neuro-Oncol.* **2006**, *80*, 159–165. [CrossRef] [PubMed]
22. Plotkin, S.R.; Betensky, R.A.; Hochberg, F.H.; Grossman, S.A.; Lesser, G.J.; Nabors, L.; Chon, B.; Batchelor, T.T. Treatment of Relapsed Central Nervous System Lymphoma with High-Dose Methotrexate. *Clin. Cancer Res.* **2004**, *10*, 5643–5646. [CrossRef]
23. Pentsova, E.; DeAngelis, L.; Omuro, A. Methotrexate re-challenge for recurrent primary central nervous system lymphoma. *J. Neuro-Oncol.* **2014**, *117*, 161–165. [CrossRef]

24. Mappa, S.; Marturano, E.; Licata, G.; Frezzato, M.; Frungillo, N.; Ilariucci, F.; Stelitano, C.; Ferrari, A.; Sorarù, M.; Vianello, F.; et al. Salvage chemoimmunotherapy with rituximab, ifosfamide and etoposide (R-IE regimen) in patients with primary CNS lymphoma relapsed or refractory to high-dose methotrexate-based chemotherapy. *Hematol. Oncol.* **2012**, *31*, 143–150. [CrossRef] [PubMed]
25. Choi, M.K.; Kang, E.S.; Kim, D.W.; Ko, Y.H.; Seok, H.; Park, J.H.; Pyo, D.H.; Lim, D.H.; Kim, S.J.; Kim, W.S. Treatment outcome of relapsed/refractory primary central nervous system diffuse large B-cell lymphoma: A single-center experience of autologous stem cell transplantation. *Int. J. Hematol.* **2013**, *98*, 346–354. [CrossRef] [PubMed]
26. Soussain, C.; Hoang-Xuan, K.; Taillandier, L.; Fourme, E.; Choquet, S.; Witz, F.; Casasnovas, O.; Dupriez, B.; Souleau, B.; Taksin, A.-L.; et al. Intensive Chemotherapy Followed by Hematopoietic Stem-Cell Rescue for Refractory and Recurrent Primary CNS and Intraocular Lymphoma: Société Française de Greffe de Moëlle Osseuse-Thérapie Cellulaire. *J. Clin. Oncol.* **2008**, *26*, 2512–2518. [CrossRef] [PubMed]
27. Hottinger, A.F.; DeAngelis, L.M.; Yahalom, J.; Abrey, L.E. Salvage whole brain radiotherapy for recurrent or refractory primary CNS lymphoma. *Neurology* **2007**, *69*, 1178–1182. [CrossRef]
28. Nguyen, P.L.; Chakravarti, A.; Finkelstein, D.M.; Hochberg, F.H.; Batchelor, T.T.; Loeffler, J.S. Results of Whole-Brain Radiation as Salvage of Methotrexate Failure for Immunocompetent Patients with Primary CNS Lymphoma. *J. Clin. Oncol.* **2005**, *23*, 1507–1513. [CrossRef] [PubMed]
29. Langner-Lemercier, S.; Houillier, C.; Soussain, C.; Ghesquières, H.; Chinot, O.; Taillandier, L.; Soubeyran, P.-L.; Lamy, T.; Morschhauser, F.; Benouaich-Amiel, A.; et al. Primary CNS lymphoma at first relapse/progression: Characteristics, management, and outcome of 256 patients from the French LOC network. *Neuro-Oncology* **2016**, *18*, 1297–1303. [CrossRef] [PubMed]
30. Hans, C.P.; Weisenburger, D.D.; Greiner, T.C.; Gascoyne, R.D.; Delabie, J.; Ott, G.; Müller-Hermelink, H.K.; Campo, E.; Braziel, R.M.; Jaffe, E.S.; et al. Confirmation of the molecular classification of diffuse large B-cell lymphoma by immunohistochemistry using a tissue microarray. *Blood* **2004**, *103*, 275–282. [CrossRef]
31. Camilleri-Broët, S.; Crinière, E.; Broet, P.; Delwail, V.; Mokhtari, K.; Moreau, A.; Kujas, M.; Raphaël, M.; Iraqi, W.; Sautes-Fridman, C.; et al. A uniform activated B-cell–like immunophenotype might explain the poor prognosis of primary central nervous system lymphomas: Analysis of 83 cases. *Blood* **2005**, *107*, 190–196. [CrossRef] [PubMed]
32. Liu, J.; Wang, Y.; Liu, Y.; Liu, Z.; Cui, Q.; Ji, N.; Sun, S.; Wang, B.; Wang, Y.; Sun, X.; et al. Immunohistochemical profile and prognostic significance in primary central nervous system lymphoma: Analysis of 89 cases. *Oncol. Lett.* **2017**, *14*, 5505–5512. [CrossRef] [PubMed]
33. Raoux, D.; Duband, S.; Forest, F.; Trombert, B.; Chambonnière, M.-L.; Dumollard, J.-M.; Khaddage, A.; Gentil-Perret, A.; Péoc'H, M. Primary central nervous system lymphoma: Immunohistochemical profile and prognostic significance. *Neuropathology* **2009**, *30*, 232–240. [CrossRef]
34. Thompsett, A.R.; Ellison, D.W.; Stevenson, F.; Zhu, D. V(H) gene sequences from primary central nervous system lymphomas indicate derivation from highly mutated germinal center B cells with ongoing mutational activity. *Blood* **1999**, *94*, 1738–1746. [CrossRef] [PubMed]
35. Montesinos-Rongen, M.; Küppers, R.; Schlüter, D.; Spieker, T.; Van Roost, D.; Schaller, C.; Reifenberger, G.; Wiestler, O.D.; Deckert-Schlüter, M. Primary Central Nervous System Lymphomas Are Derived from Germinal-Center B Cells and Show a Preferential Usage of the V4–34 Gene Segment. *Am. J. Pathol.* **1999**, *155*, 2077–2086. [CrossRef]
36. LaRocca, L.M.; Capello, D.; Rinelli, A.; Nori, S.; Antinori, A.; Gloghini, A.; Cingolani, A.; Migliazza, A.; Saglio, G.; Cammilleri-Broet, S.; et al. The molecular and phenotypic profile of primary central nervous system lymphoma identifies distinct categories of the disease and is consistent with histogenetic derivation from germinal center-related B cells. *Blood* **1998**, *92*, 1011–1019. [PubMed]
37. Sugita, Y.; Tokunaga, O.; Nakashima, A.; Shigemori, M. SHP-1 expression in primary central nervous system B-cell lymphomas in immunocompetent patients reflects maturation stage of normal B cell counterparts. *Pathol. Int.* **2004**, *54*, 659–666. [CrossRef] [PubMed]
38. Rubenstein, J.L.; Fridlyand, J.; Shen, A.; Aldape, K.; Ginzinger, D.; Batchelor, T.; Treseler, P.; Berger, M.; McDermott, M.; Prados, M.; et al. Gene expression and angiotropism in primary CNS lymphoma. *Blood* **2006**, *107*, 3716–3723. [CrossRef]
39. Bödör, C.; Alpar, D.; Marosvári, D.; Galik, B.; Rajnai, H.; Bátai, B.; Nagy, Á.; Kajtár, B.; Burján, A.; Deák, B.; et al. Molecular Subtypes and Genomic Profile of Primary Central Nervous System Lymphoma. *J. Neuropathol. Exp. Neurol.* **2019**, *79*, 176–183. [CrossRef] [PubMed]
40. Lionakis, M.S.; Dunleavy, K.; Roschewski, M.; Widemann, B.C.; Butman, J.A.; Schmitz, R.; Yang, Y.; Cole, D.E.; Melani, C.; Higham, C.S.; et al. Inhibition of B Cell Receptor Signaling by Ibrutinib in Primary CNS Lymphoma. *Cancer Cell* **2017**, *31*, 833–843.e5. [CrossRef] [PubMed]
41. Ngo, V.; Young, R.M.; Schmitz, R.; Jhavar, S.; Xiao, W.; Lim, K.-H.; Kohlhammer, H.; Xu, W.; Yang, Y.; Zhao, H.; et al. Oncogenically active MYD88 mutations in human lymphoma. *Nature* **2010**, *470*, 115–119. [CrossRef]
42. Davis, R.E.; Ngo, V.; Lenz, G.; Tolar, P.; Young, R.M.; Romesser, P.; Kohlhammer, H.; Lamy, L.; Zhao, H.; Yang, Y.; et al. Chronic active B-cell-receptor signalling in diffuse large B-cell lymphoma. *Nature* **2010**, *463*, 88–92. [CrossRef]
43. Lenz, G.; Davis, R.E.; Ngo, V.N.; Lam, L.; George, T.C.; Wright, G.W.; Dave, S.S.; Zhao, H.; Xu, W.; Rosenwald, A.; et al. Oncogenic CARD11 Mutations in Human Diffuse Large B Cell Lymphoma. *Science* **2008**, *319*, 1676–1679. [CrossRef]

44. Nagel, D.; Vincendeau, M.; Eitelhuber, A.C.; Krappmann, D. Mechanisms and consequences of constitutive NF-kappaB activation in B-cell lymphoid malignancies. *Oncogene* **2014**, *33*, 5655–5665. [CrossRef]
45. Lee, J.; Kim, B.; Lee, H.; Park, H.; Byeon, S.H.; Choi, J.R.; Lee, S.C.; Lee, S.-T.; Lee, C.S. Whole exome sequencing identifies mutational signatures of vitreoretinal lymphoma. *Haematologica* **2020**, *105*, e458–e460. [CrossRef] [PubMed]
46. Mizowaki, T.; Sasayama, T.; Tanaka, K.; Mizukawa, K.; Takata, K.; Nakamizo, S.; Tanaka, H.; Nagashima, H.; Nishihara, M.; Hirose, T.; et al. STAT3 activation is associated with cerebrospinal fluid interleukin-10 (IL-10) in primary central nervous system diffuse large B cell lymphoma. *J. Neuro-Oncol.* **2015**, *124*, 165–174. [CrossRef] [PubMed]
47. You, H.; Wei, L.; Kaminska, B. Emerging insights into origin and pathobiology of primary central nervous system lymphoma. *Cancer Lett.* **2021**, *509*, 121–129. [CrossRef] [PubMed]
48. Fukumura, K.; Kawazu, M.; Kojima, S.; Ueno, T.; Sai, E.; Soda, M.; Ueda, H.; Yasuda, T.; Yamaguchi, H.; Lee, J.; et al. Genomic characterization of primary central nervous system lymphoma. *Acta Neuropathol.* **2016**, *131*, 865–875. [CrossRef]
49. Braggio, E.; Van Wier, S.; Ojha, J.; McPhail, E.; Asmann, Y.W.; Egan, J.; Ayres-Silva, J.; Schiff, D.; Lopes, M.B.; Decker, P.A.; et al. Genome-Wide Analysis Uncovers Novel Recurrent Alterations in Primary Central Nervous System Lymphomas. *Clin. Cancer Res.* **2015**, *21*, 3986–3994. [CrossRef] [PubMed]
50. Vater, I.; Montesinosrongen, M.; Schlesner, M.; Haake, A.R.; Purschke, F.G.; Sprute, R.; Mettenmeyer, N.; Nazzal, I.; Nagel, I.; Gutwein, J.; et al. The mutational pattern of primary lymphoma of the central nervous system determined by whole-exome sequencing. *Leukemia* **2014**, *29*, 677–685. [CrossRef] [PubMed]
51. Kraan, W.; Horlings, H.M.; Van Keimpema, M.; Schildertol, E.J.M.; Oud, M.E.C.M.; Scheepstra, C.; Kluin, P.M.; Kersten, M.J.; Spaargaren, M.; Pals, S.T. High prevalence of oncogenic MYD88 and CD79B mutations in diffuse large B-cell lymphomas presenting at immune-privileged sites. *Blood Cancer J.* **2013**, *3*, e139. [CrossRef] [PubMed]
52. Chapuy, B.; Roemer, M.G.M.; Stewart, C.; Tan, Y.; Abo, R.P.; Zhang, L.; Dunford, A.J.; Meredith, D.M.; Thorner, A.R.; Jordanova, E.S.; et al. Targetable genetic features of primary testicular and primary central nervous system lymphomas. *Blood* **2016**, *127*, 869–881. [CrossRef]
53. Booman, M.; Szuhai, K.; Rosenwald, A.; Hartmann, E.; Kluin-Nelemans, J.C.; De Jong, D.; Schuuring, E.; Kluin, P.M. Genomic alterations and gene expression in primary diffuse large B-cell lymphomas of immune-privileged sites: The importance of apoptosis and immunomodulatory pathways. *J. Pathol.* **2008**, *216*, 209–217. [CrossRef] [PubMed]
54. Korfel, A.; Schlegel, U.; Herrlinger, U.; Dreyling, M.; Schmidt, C.; von Baumgarten, L.; Pezzutto, A.; Grobosch, T.; Kebir, S.; Thiel, E.; et al. Phase II Trial of Temsirolimus for Relapsed/Refractory Primary CNS Lymphoma. *J. Clin. Oncol.* **2016**, *34*, 1757–1763. [CrossRef] [PubMed]
55. Grommes, C.; Pastore, A.; Palaskas, N.; Tang, S.S.; Campos, C.; Schartz, D.; Codega, P.; Nichol, D.; Clark, O.; Hsieh, W.-Y.; et al. Ibrutinib Unmasks Critical Role of Bruton Tyrosine Kinase in Primary CNS Lymphoma. *Cancer Discov.* **2017**, *7*, 1018–1029. [CrossRef] [PubMed]
56. Rubenstein, J.L.; Geng, H.; Fraser, E.J.; Formaker, P.; Chen, L.; Sharma, J.; Killea, P.; Choi, K.; Ventura, J.; Kurhanewicz, J.; et al. Phase 1 investigation of lenalidomide/rituximab plus outcomes of lenalidomide maintenance in relapsed CNS lymphoma. *Blood Adv.* **2018**, *2*, 1595–1607. [CrossRef]
57. Tun, H.W.; Johnston, P.B.; DeAngelis, L.M.; Atherton, P.J.; Pederson, L.D.; Koenig, P.A.; Reeder, C.B.; Omuro, A.M.P.; Schiff, D.; O'Neill, B.; et al. Phase 1 study of pomalidomide and dexamethasone for relapsed/refractory primary CNS or vitreoretinal lymphoma. *Blood* **2018**, *132*, 2240–2248. [CrossRef] [PubMed]
58. Ghesquieres, H.; Chevrier, M.; Laadhari, M.; Chinot, O.; Choquet, S.; Molurçon-Chabrot, C.; Beauchesne, P.; Gressin, R.; Morschhauser, F.; Schmitt, A.; et al. Lenalidomide in combination with intravenous rituximab (REVRI) in relapsed/refractory primary CNS lymphoma or primary intraocular lymphoma: A multicenter prospective 'proof of concept' phase II study of the French Oculo-Cerebral lymphoma (LOC) Network and the Lymphoma Study Association (LYSA). *Ann. Oncol.* **2019**, *30*, 621–628. [CrossRef] [PubMed]
59. Grommes, C.; Tang, S.S.; Wolfe, J.; Kaley, T.J.; Daras, M.; Pentsova, E.I.; Piotrowski, A.F.; Stone, J.; Lin, A.; Nolan, C.P.; et al. Phase 1b trial of an ibrutinib-based combination therapy in recurrent/refractory CNS lymphoma. *Blood* **2019**, *133*, 436–445. [CrossRef] [PubMed]
60. Soussain, C.; Choquet, S.; Blonski, M.; Leclercq, D.; Houillier, C.; Rezai, K.; Bijou, F.; Houot, R.; Boyle, E.; Gressin, R.; et al. Ibrutinib monotherapy for relapse or refractory primary CNS lymphoma and primary vitreoretinal lymphoma: Final analysis of the phase II 'proof-of-concept' iLOC study by the Lymphoma study association (LYSA) and the French oculo-cerebral lymphoma (LOC) network. *Eur. J. Cancer* **2019**, *117*, 121–130. [CrossRef]
61. Narita, Y.; Nagane, M.; Mishima, K.; Terui, Y.; Arakawa, Y.; Yonezawa, H.; Asai, K.; Fukuhara, N.; Sugiyama, K.; Shinojima, N.; et al. Phase I/II study of tirabrutinib, a second-generation Bruton's tyrosine kinase inhibitor, in relapsed/refractory primary central nervous system lymphoma. *Neuro-Oncology* **2020**, *23*, 122–133. [CrossRef]
62. Wilson, W.H.; Young, R.M.; Schmitz, R.; Yang, Y.; Pittaluga, S.; Wright, G.; Lih, C.-J.; Williams, P.M.; Shaffer, A.L.; Gerecitano, J.; et al. Targeting B cell receptor signaling with ibrutinib in diffuse large B cell lymphoma. *Nat. Med.* **2015**, *21*, 922–926. [CrossRef] [PubMed]
63. Wu, C.; de Miranda, N.; Chen, L.; Wasik, A.M.; Mansouri, L.; Jurczak, W.; Galazka, K.; Dlugosz-Danecka, M.; Machaczka, M.; Zhang, H.; et al. Genetic heterogeneity in primary and relapsed mantle cell lymphomas: Impact of recurrent CARD11 mutations. *Oncotarget* **2016**, *7*, 38180–38190. [CrossRef]

64. Fingar, D.C.; Blenis, J. Target of rapamycin (TOR): An integrator of nutrient and growth factor signals and coordinator of cell growth and cell cycle progression. *Oncogene* **2004**, *23*, 3151–3171. [CrossRef] [PubMed]
65. Hess, G.; Herbrecht, R.; Romaguera, J.; Verhoef, G.; Crump, M.; Gisselbrecht, C.; Laurell, A.; Offner, F.; Strahs, A.; Berkenblit, A.; et al. Phase III study to evaluate temsirolimus compared with investigator's choice therapy for the treatment of relapsed or refractory mantle cell lymphoma. *J. Clin. Oncol.* **2009**, *27*, 3822–3829. [CrossRef] [PubMed]
66. Smith, S.M.; van Besien, K.; Karrison, T.; Dancey, J.; McLaughlin, P.; Younes, A.; Smith, S.; Stiff, P.; Lester, E.; Modi, S.; et al. Temsirolimus has activity in non-mantle cell non-Hodgkin's lymphoma subtypes: The University of Chicago phase II consortium. *J. Clin. Oncol.* **2010**, *28*, 4740–4746. [PubMed]
67. Kuhn, J.G.; Chang, S.M.; Wen, P.Y.; Cloughesy, T.F.; Greenberg, H.; Schiff, D.; Conrad, C.; Fink, K.L.; Robins, H.I.; Mehta, M.; et al. Pharmacokinetic and tumor distribution characteristics of temsirolimus in patients with recurrent malignant glioma. *Clin. Cancer Res.* **2007**, *13*, 7401–7406. [CrossRef] [PubMed]
68. Grommes, C.; Pentsova, E. ACTR-11. Phase II study of single agent buparlisib in recurrent/refractory primary (PCNSL) and secondary CNS lymphoma (SCNSL). *Neuro-Oncology* **2016**, *18*, vi3. [CrossRef]
69. Wen, P.Y.; Touat, M.; Alexander, B.M.; Mellinghoff, I.K.; Ramkissoon, S.; McCluskey, C.S.; Pelton, K.; Haidar, S.; Basu, S.S.; Gaffey, S.C.; et al. Buparlisib in Patients with Recurrent Glioblastoma Harboring Phosphatidylinositol 3-Kinase Pathway Activation: An Open-Label, Multicenter, Multi-Arm, Phase II Trial. *J. Clin. Oncol.* **2019**, *37*, 741–750. [CrossRef] [PubMed]
70. Dredge, K.; Horsfall, R.; Robinson, S.P.; Zhang, L.-H.; Lu, L.; Tang, Y.; Shirley, M.A.; Muller, G.; Schafer, P.; Stirling, D.; et al. Orally administered lenalidomide (CC-5013) is anti-angiogenic in vivo and inhibits endothelial cell migration and Akt phosphorylation in vitro. *Microvasc. Res.* **2005**, *69*, 56–63. [CrossRef] [PubMed]
71. Li, Z.; Qiu, Y.; Personett, D.; Huang, P.; Edenfield, B.; Katz, J.; Babusis, D.; Tang, Y.; Shirely, M.A.; Moghaddam, M.F.; et al. Pomalidomide Shows Significant Therapeutic Activity against CNS Lymphoma with a Major Impact on the Tumor Microenvironment in Murine Models. *PLoS ONE* **2013**, *8*, e71754. [CrossRef] [PubMed]
72. Houillier, C.; Chabrot, C.M.; Moles-Moreau, M.; Willems, L.; Ahle, G.; Waultier-Rascalou, A.; Fornecker, L.M.; Hoang-Xuan, K.; Soussain, C. Rituximab-Lenalidomide-Ibrutinib Combination for Relapsed/Refractory Primary CNS Lymphoma: A case Series of the LOC Network. *Neurology* **2021**, *97*, 628–631. [CrossRef] [PubMed]
73. Nayak, L.; Iwamoto, F.M.; LaCasce, A.; Mukundan, S.; Roemer, M.G.M.; Chapuy, B.; Armand, P.; Rodig, S.J.; Shipp, M.A. PD-1 blockade with nivolumab in relapsed/refractory primary central nervous system and testicular lymphoma. *Blood* **2017**, *129*, 3071–3073. [CrossRef] [PubMed]
74. Ambady, P.; Szidonya, L.; Firkins, J.; James, J.; Johansson, K.; White, T.; Jezierski, C.; Doolittle, N.D.; Neuwelt, E.A. Combination immunotherapy as a non-chemotherapy alternative for refractory or recurrent CNS lymphoma. *Leuk. Lymphoma* **2018**, *60*, 515–518. [CrossRef] [PubMed]
75. Kochenderfer, J.N.; Dudley, M.E.; Kassim, S.H.; Somerville, R.P.; Carpenter, R.O.; Stetler-Stevenson, M.; Yang, J.C.; Phan, G.Q.; Hughes, M.S.; Sherry, R.M.; et al. Chemotherapy-Refractory Diffuse Large B-Cell Lymphoma and Indolent B-Cell Malignancies Can Be Effectively Treated with Autologous T Cells Expressing an Anti-CD19 Chimeric Antigen Receptor. *J. Clin. Oncol.* **2015**, *33*, 540–549. [CrossRef]
76. Abramson, J.S.; McGree, B.; Noyes, S.; Plummer, S.; Wong, C.; Chen, Y.-B.; Palmer, E.; Albertson, T.; Ferry, J.A.; Arrillaga-Romany, I.C. Anti-CD19 CAR T Cells in CNS Diffuse Large-B-Cell Lymphoma. *N. Engl. J. Med.* **2017**, *377*, 783–784. [CrossRef] [PubMed]
77. Frigault, M.J.; Dietrich, J.; Martinez-Lage, M.; Leick, M.; Choi, B.D.; DeFilipp, Z.; Chen, Y.-B.; Abramson, J.; Crombie, J.; Armand, P.; et al. Tisagenlecleucel CAR T-cell therapy in secondary CNS lymphoma. *Blood* **2019**, *134*, 860–866. [CrossRef]
78. Siddiqi, T.; Wang, X.; Blanchard, M.S.; Wagner, J.; Popplewell, L.; Budde, L.; Stiller, T.; Clark, M.C.; Lim, L.; Vyas, V.; et al. CD19 directed CAR T cell therapy for treatment of primary CNS lymphoma. *Blood Adv.* **2021**, *5*, 4059–4063. [CrossRef] [PubMed]
79. Chmielewski, M.; Abken, H. TRUCKs: The fourth generation of CARs. *Expert Opin. Biol. Ther.* **2015**, *15*, 1145–1154. [CrossRef] [PubMed]
80. Baeuerle, P.A.; Reinhardt, C. Bispecific T-Cell Engaging Antibodies for Cancer Therapy. *Cancer Res.* **2009**, *69*, 4941–4944. [CrossRef]
81. Schuster, S.J. Bispecific antibodies for the treatment of lymphomas: Promises and challenges. *Hematol. Oncol.* **2021**, *39*, 113–116. [CrossRef]
82. Reda, G.; Cassin, R.; Dovrtelova, G.; Matteo, C.; Giannotta, J.; D'Incalci, M.; Cortelezzi, A.; Zucchetti, M. Venetoclax penetrates in cerebrospinal fluid and may be effective in chronic lymphocytic leukemia with central nervous system involvement. *Haematologica* **2019**, *104*, e222–e223. [CrossRef] [PubMed]
83. Zhang, X.; Chen, J.; Wang, W.; Li, X.; Tan, Y.; Zhang, X.; Qian, W. Treatment of Central Nervous System Relapse in Acute Promyelocytic Leukemia by Venetoclax: A Case Report. *Front. Oncol.* **2021**, *11*, 693670. [CrossRef] [PubMed]
84. Kapoor, I.; Li, Y.; Sharma, A.; Zhu, H.; Bodo, J.; Xu, W.; Hsi, E.D.; Hill, B.T.; Almasan, A. Resistance to BTK inhibition by ibrutinib can be overcome by preventing FOXO3a nuclear export and PI3K/AKT activation in B-cell lymphoid malignancies. *Cell Death Dis.* **2019**, *10*, 1–12. [CrossRef] [PubMed]
85. Angelov, L.; Doolittle, N.D.; Kraemer, D.F.; Siegal, T.; Barnett, G.H.; Peereboom, D.M.; Stevens, G.; McGregor, J.; Jahnke, K.; Lacy, C.A.; et al. Blood-Brain Barrier Disruption and Intra-Arterial Methotrexate-Based Therapy for Newly Diagnosed Primary CNS Lymphoma: A Multi-Institutional Experience. *J. Clin. Oncol.* **2009**, *27*, 3503–3509. [CrossRef] [PubMed]

86. Ferreri, A.J.M.; Calimeri, T.; Ponzoni, M.; Curnis, F.; Conte, G.M.; Scarano, E.; Rrapaj, E.; De Lorenzo, D.; Cattaneo, D.; Fallanca, F.; et al. Improving the antitumor activity of R-CHOP with NGR-hTNF in primary CNS lymphoma: Final results of a phase 2 trial. *Blood Adv.* **2020**, *4*, 3648–3658. [CrossRef]
87. Sasayama, T.; Nakamizo, S.; Nishihara, M.; Kawamura, A.; Tanaka, H.; Mizukawa, K.; Miyake, S.; Taniguchi, M.; Hosoda, K.; Kohmura, E. Cerebrospinal fluid interleukin-10 is a potentially useful biomarker in immunocompetent primary central nervous system lymphoma (PCNSL). *Neuro-Oncology* **2011**, *14*, 368–380. [CrossRef] [PubMed]
88. Montesinos-Rongen, M.; Brunn, A.; Tuchscherer, A.; Borchmann, P.; Schorb, E.; Kasenda, B.; Altmüller, J.; Illerhaus, G.; Ruge, M.I.; Maarouf, M.; et al. Analysis of Driver Mutational Hot Spots in Blood-Derived Cell-Free DNA of Patients with Primary Central Nervous System Lymphoma Obtained before Intracerebral Biopsy. *J. Mol. Diagn.* **2020**, *22*, 1300–1307. [CrossRef] [PubMed]
89. Hiemcke-Jiwa, L.S.; Leguit, R.J.; Snijders, T.; Jiwa, N.M.; Kuiper, J.J.; de Weger, R.A.; Minnema, M.C.; Huibers, M.M. Molecular analysis in liquid biopsies for diagnostics of primary central nervous system lymphoma: Review of literature and future opportunities. *Crit. Rev. Oncol.* **2018**, *127*, 56–65. [CrossRef]

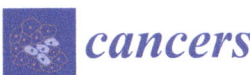

Review

Enhancing T Cell Chemotaxis and Infiltration in Glioblastoma

Kirit Singh *, Kelly M. Hotchkiss, Kisha K. Patel, Daniel S. Wilkinson, Aditya A. Mohan, Sarah L. Cook and John H. Sampson *

Duke Brain Tumor Immunotherapy Program, Department of Neurosurgery, Duke University Medical Center, Durham, NC 27710, USA; kelly.hotchkiss@duke.edu (K.M.H.); kisha.patel@duke.edu (K.K.P.); daniel.wilkinson@duke.edu (D.S.W.); aditya.mohan@duke.edu (A.A.M.); sarah.quackenbush@duke.edu (S.L.C.)
* Correspondence: kirit.singh@duke.edu (K.S.); john.sampson@duke.edu (J.H.S.)

Simple Summary: Immunotherapy in glioblastoma has so far failed to yield a survival benefit. This failure can be attributed to a paucity of immune cells at the tumor site which can be reinvigorated to kill tumor cells. Therefore, driving effector immune cells such as cytotoxic T lymphocytes to the tumor is a necessary pre-requisite of any effective immunotherapy approach. In this review, we will discuss therapeutic approaches possible for trafficking T cells from the periphery to travel through the blood–brain barrier and tissue of the brain to reach the tumor.

Abstract: Glioblastoma is an immunologically 'cold' tumor, which are characterized by absent or minimal numbers of tumor-infiltrating lymphocytes (TILs). For those tumors that have been invaded by lymphocytes, they are profoundly exhausted and ineffective. While many immunotherapy approaches seek to reinvigorate immune cells at the tumor, this requires TILs to be present. Therefore, to unleash the full potential of immunotherapy in glioblastoma, the trafficking of lymphocytes to the tumor is highly desirable. However, the process of T cell recruitment into the central nervous system (CNS) is tightly regulated. Naïve T cells may undergo an initial licensing process to enter the migratory phenotype necessary to enter the CNS. T cells then must express appropriate integrins and selectin ligands to interact with transmembrane proteins at the blood–brain barrier (BBB). Finally, they must interact with antigen-presenting cells and undergo further licensing to enter the parenchyma. These T cells must then navigate the tumor microenvironment, which is rich in immunosuppressive factors. Altered tumoral metabolism also interferes with T cell motility. In this review, we will describe these processes and their mediators, along with potential therapeutic approaches to enhance trafficking. We also discuss safety considerations for such approaches as well as potential counteragents.

Keywords: immunotherapy; glioblastoma; blood–brain barrier; central nervous system; T cells; T lymphocytes

Citation: Singh, K.; Hotchkiss, K.M.; Patel, K.K.; Wilkinson, D.S.; Mohan, A.A.; Cook, S.L.; Sampson, J.H. Enhancing T Cell Chemotaxis and Infiltration in Glioblastoma. *Cancers* **2021**, *13*, 5367. https://doi.org/10.3390/cancers13215367

Academic Editor: Edward Pan

Received: 27 September 2021
Accepted: 25 October 2021
Published: 26 October 2021

Publisher's Note: MDPI stays neutral with regard to jurisdictional claims in published maps and institutional affiliations.

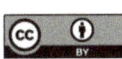

Copyright: © 2021 by the authors. Licensee MDPI, Basel, Switzerland. This article is an open access article distributed under the terms and conditions of the Creative Commons Attribution (CC BY) license (https://creativecommons.org/licenses/by/4.0/).

1. Introduction

Immune surveillance of the central nervous system (CNS) is essential for environmental homeostasis and pathogen clearance. Without immune surveillance, opportunistic infections in the CNS commonly develop [1]. However, the entry of immune cells into the CNS is tightly controlled by the blood–brain barrier (BBB) and the blood–cerebrospinal fluid (BCSF) barrier. These formidable barriers lack fenestrations, exhibit a low degree of pinocytosis, and are sealed together by a network of intracellular junctions [2,3]. While this close control is desirable in health to avoid runaway immune responses in the CNS, restricted immune cell entry severely hampers the effectiveness of immunotherapy in glioblastoma [4]. This is further complicated by the immunosuppressive tumor microenvironment (TME), which consists of endothelial cells, pericytes, fibroblasts, and regulatory immune cells [5]. The TME drives effector immune cell exhaustion, thereby shielding solid malignancies from immune attack [6]. While immune checkpoint inhibition (ICI) seeks to reverse this exhausted state and 'release the brakes' on regional T cells, it is notable that the evaluation of resected stage IV gliomas are either devoid or demonstrate limited numbers of tumor-infiltrating lymphocytes (TILs) [7,8]. This would suggest that ICI will struggle owing to the lack of targets to reinvigorate. Indeed, initial trials of ICI in glioblastoma have failed [9]. However, when ICI is combined with increased numbers of functional TILs in pre-clinical models, long-term survival can be achieved [10,11]. Therefore, we require therapeutic strategies that can both recruit effector cells to the tumor site and ensure they remain functional.

While the CNS does host several immune cell classes, including T cells, these immune cells are clustered away from the tumor-bearing parenchyma in regions such as the choroid plexus, the meninges (containing the subarachnoid and perivascular spaces), and the CSF [12–17]. The clinical implications of this clustering were recognized as long ago as 1923, where Murphy and Sturm confirmed Shirai's initial finding that foreign tumors in the parenchyma could grow, but tumors implanted close to the ventricles (and thus the immune interfaces) were rejected [18]. Fortunately, immune responses in the CNS can be bolstered by an adaptive response originating from the periphery. Medawar demonstrated in 1948 that tumors implanted into brain tissue can be rejected following exposure to tumor antigens outside of the CNS [19]. Recruitment of peripheral T cells into the parenchyma also occurs in multiple sclerosis (MS) and its animal analogue experimental autoimmune encephalitis (EAE) [20].

Even though adaptive immune clearance of tumors is possible, glioblastoma possesses several mechanisms that suppress the recruitment and functioning of T cells. Glioblastoma expresses decreased levels of lymphangiogenesis-promoting factors such as VEGF-C, reducing potential routes for T cell ingress, while the highly immunosuppressive tumor microenvironment (TME) blunts the response of any lymphocytes that reach the tumor [21–23]. Therefore, in this review we will discuss the physiological processes that drive T cell trafficking from the periphery, tumoral infiltration, and potential therapeutic options for their enhancement. We will also discuss safety considerations, given the potential for T cell infiltration to drive inflammation and neurodegeneration in the CNS [24,25].

2. T Cell Trafficking from the Periphery to the Blood–Brain Barrier

The mechanism by which T cells leave the circulation and enter inflamed tissues is well characterized and has been reviewed in detail elsewhere [26–28]. In brief, the expression of selectins on endothelial cells results in the slowing and rolling of leukocytes. The leukocyte crawls along the endothelial layer, where stimulating chemokines trigger the activation of integrins, which ultimately result in the leukocyte being firmly captured [29–31]. Engagement of endothelial adhesion molecules by integrins results in immune cells being drawn to endothelial junctions, permitting their diapedesis (crossing) into the tissue [32]. T cell trafficking across the BBB involves a similar process of rolling, capture, and diapedesis [33]. However, certain aspects of this process differ from the periphery. In the resting state, the constitutive expression of selectin is largely absent in the CNS, with the exception of blood vessels in the sub arachnoid space [34,35]. T cell rolling on the BBB is instead driven by the cell surface integrin LFA-1, which binds to intercellular adhesion molecule-1 (ICAM-1) on the endothelium. These T cells are captured and cross via G protein-coupled receptor (GPCR) signaling [36].

In the pathological state, the release of inflammatory cytokines induces the expression of chemokines and adhesion molecules that recruit effector T cells to the CNS [37,38]. Transcription and expression of E- or P-selectins on the BBB adheres to P-selectin glycoprotein ligand-1 on $CD8^+$ T cells, inducing their slowing on the endothelial surface [39]. Binding is again mediated by GPCR signaling, which activates the integrins LFA-1 and VLA-4 on the T cells that bind to ICAM-1 and VCAM-1, respectively [40]. Other factors at the BBB also interact with VLA-4, including transmembrane proteins described as junctional adhesional molecules (JAM). So far, JAM-B and JAML have been implicated in CD8 chemotaxis—blockade of JAM-B results in the reduced CNS infiltration of $CD8^+$ T cells [41,42]. Atypical chemokine receptor-1 (ACKR1) also mediates trafficking in the inflammatory state, transporting pro-infiltrative chemokines to the luminal aspect of the BBB [43]. Interleukin (IL)-1 signaling in BBB endothelial cells is associated with upregulated expression of VCAM-1, ICAM-1, and ACKR1 and therefore may offer a potential strategy for enhancing T cell capture if delivered intra-tumorally [44]. Frewert et al. reported that intra-tumoral infusion of IL-1β or interferon-γ via convection enhanced delivery enhanced the number of CD4$^+$ and CD8$^+$ TILs in a rat glioma model [45]. This may therefore be a rational combinatorial approach alongside ICI.

It should be noted that the expression of these adhesion molecules is also influenced by perivascular stromal cells such as regional pericytes [46,47]. In health, these cells coordinate with endothelial cells to control both the development and permeability of the vasculature [48]. Pericytes also inhibit endocytosis by endothelial cells, limiting transcellular routes of migration [49,50]. Indeed, mice deficient in pericytes display significantly increased expression of VCAM-1 and ICAM-1 on the BBB endothelium, resulting in a mass influx of leukocytes [51]. In the tumor setting, overgrowth of pericytes derived from glioma stem cells (GSCs) results in the blockage of the entrance of therapeutic drugs such as temozolomide (TMZ) [52]. Pericyte coverage is inversely correlated with survival in patients with glioblastoma following chemotherapy [53]. Interestingly, selective targeting of these cells using ibrutinib was shown to enhance delivery of TMZ in orthotopic models of glioma by disrupting the blood–tumor barrier [53]. This may also have a double effect of interrupting the pericyte secretion of CCL5, which acts on CCR5 on glioblastoma cells, inducing resistance to TMZ by promoting DNA damage repair mechanisms [54]. However, pericytes can re-organize themselves to cover areas of deficient coverage and their function may be compensated for by other local cells such as astrocytes [55].

The CCL5–CCR5 axis is also associated with enhanced regulatory T cell recruitment [56]. CCR5 antagonists such as maraviroc (licensed for HIV-1) have been found to deplete regulatory T cells, which express CCR5/CXCR4 ratios differently to T effector cells [57,58]. Blockade of CCR5 has also been demonstrated to reduce the growth of orthotopically injected colon cancer cells by limiting cancer-associated fibroblast accumulation. Maraviroc has also been shown to reverse CCL5 resistance to TMZ and is also BBB penetrable with a favorable safety profile, making this an agent of significant interest as part of future combinatorial approaches [54,59,60]. CCR5 also binds CCL3 and CCL4 and the interaction between CCR5 and its ligands appears to have location-specific pro or anti-tumor effects [61]. For example, CCL4 can help to recruit cytolytic CCR5$^+$ T cells in esophageal squamous cell carcinoma, but the CCL4–CCR5 interaction can enhance the invasion ability of glioblastoma in vitro [62,63].

To determine how best to drive T cells into the CNS, we need to identify the optimal pro-infiltrative phenotype of lymphocytes. A high expression of integrins and chemokine receptors as seen in autoimmune disease is likely beneficial for enhancing T cell chemotaxis in glioblastoma. When reviewing T cell phenotypes that predominate in autoimmune diseases, CNS-infiltrative lymphocytes are predictably dominated by effector memory T cells (CD62L$_{Lo}$ and CCR7$_{Lo}$) [64–69]. While sensitizing T cells in the periphery would be ideal, the high degree of heterogeneity in glioblastoma makes it impossible to identify a universal target [70]. A more optimal approach would be trafficking antigen-naïve T cells that can interact with antigen-presenting cells (APCs) that endogenously present tumor antigen. This strategy benefits from the fact that T cells do not require target antigen recognition before they are able to cross the BBB [71]. In glioblastoma, T cells primed in tumor-draining cervical lymph nodes strongly upregulated VLA-4, leading to preferential infiltration of the CNS [72]. Therefore, activating tumor-antigen naïve T cells to express VLA-4 will help to achieve this objective. Administration of IL-12 to mice bearing multiple tumor types appeared to enhance the induction of LFA-1 and VLA-4 and subsequently T cell migration, resulting in tumor regression [73]. However, this response differed across tumor types, with IL-12 resulting in largely CD4 migration in fibrosarcoma but pre-dominantly

CD8 migration in ovarian cancer, and further work is required to determine its impact in glioblastoma [73].

While antigen specificity is not a pre-requisite of migration into the CNS, it is interesting to note that adoptively transferred tumor-naïve T cells appear to undergo a period of residence in the lungs, where their gene expression profile switches to a migratory phenotype [74]. Determining mediators of this 'licensing' process may therefore yield useful therapeutic targets of interest. Before entering the lungs, adoptively transferred T cells predominantly migrate towards homeostatic chemokines CCL19 and CCL21 (expressed in bronchus-associated lymphoid tissues). After transiting through the lungs, T cell homing shifts towards chemokine gradients associated with inflammation such as CXCL11 and CCL5 [74]. CXCL11 binds the chemokine receptor CXCR3 (expressed on effector T cells), and this binding can promote T cell infiltration into tumors [75]. Conversely, inhibition of CXCR3 binding results in reduced invasion of effector T cells [76].

CXCR3 binds three ligands: CXCL9, CXCL10, and CXCL11. While CXCL11 binds CXCR3 with higher affinity, it also can induce receptor internalization and promote a regulatory T cell lineage [75]. Instead, CXCL10 may be a more suitable therapeutic approach, as CXCL10 induces moderate receptor internalization and still enhances T cell infiltration [77]. This was demonstrated in intracranial melanoma models, where the absence of CXCL10 was associated with decreased numbers of CD8$^+$ TILs [78]. Although glioma does express CXCL10, this is accompanied by the expression of dipeptidylpeptidase (DPP)-4, which cleaves CXCL10 [79]. DPP-4 blockade has been shown to increase the numbers of TILs, but when considering therapeutic blockade, it must be noted that DPP-4 also inhibits glioma proliferation independently of its enzymatic activity [80,81]. An alternative approach to inducing expression of CXCL10 is the use of poly-ICLC, which has been found to significantly increase the frequency of TILs when combined with peptide vaccination against glioma [82]. An overview of peripheral T cell chemotaxis and BBB penetrance is shown in Figure 1.

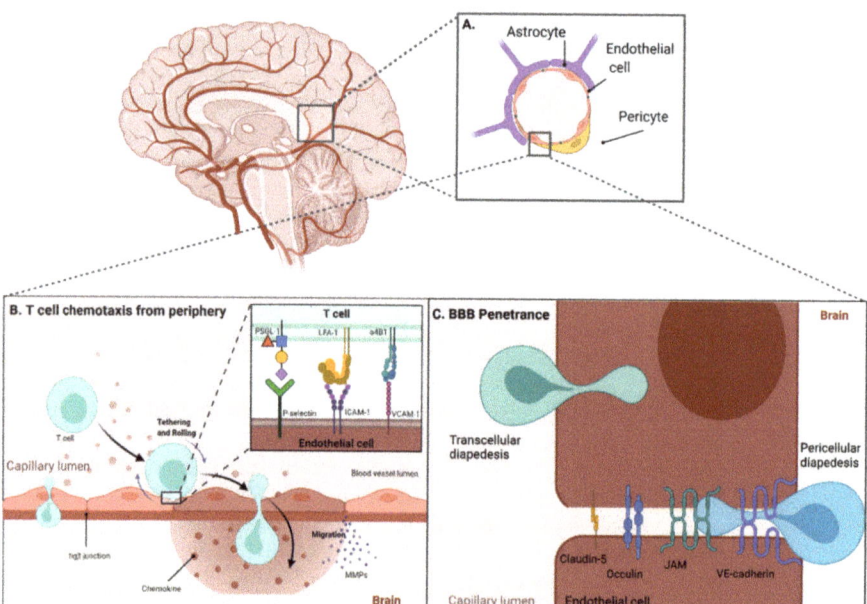

Figure 1. (**A**) The BBB consists of endothelial cells held together by tight junctions surrounded by pericytes and astrocytes. (**B**) T cell chemotaxis across the BBB is facilitated by expression of tethering molecules (P-selectin, ICAM-1, VCAM-1, etc.) on endothelial cell surfaces that bind to integrins on circulating T cells (LFA-1, $\alpha 4\beta 1$, etc.) to slow and allow cells to roll across the membrane surface. (**C**) T cells can cross the endothelial cells either between cells (paracellular) through tight junctions or through individual cells (transcellular) to migrate into the brain. Produced using Biorender.

3. Blood–Brain Barrier Specific Targets

Following the shift towards a pro-infiltrative phenotype, T cells must cross the BBB. Although glioblastoma is a disease state in which the BBB is disrupted, regions of the tumor are likely surrounded by intact portions of barrier [83]. These privileged regions may act as the site of regrowth, shielded from immunotherapeutic attack [8,83]. Such privileged regions correspond with the non-contrast enhancing infiltrating edge, which can form the site of recurrence following core resection [84]. Infiltrating glioma cells at the leading edge demonstrate upregulated fibroblast growth factor-mediated signaling that promotes tumorigenesis [85]. The changes in cellular phenotype at the leading edge are driven by histone deacetylase signaling from the tumor core [86]. This results in a permanent alteration at the border to a pro-infiltrative milieu of glioma-initiating cells, which does not reverse following resection of the core [86]. Immune cell populations differ at this interface zone also. Spatial single-cell RNA-Seq analysis performed by Darmanis et al. revealed that tumor associated macrophages (TAMs) dominated the core while brain-derived microglia dominated the peritumoral zone [87]. These both have key roles in T cell activity at the tumor site. Macrophages can express the cytokine TGF-β, which enhances glioblastoma cell growth, migration, and invasion and downregulates antitumor immunity [88,89]. Microglia in the peritumoral zone show an increased expression of ligands for T cell exhaustion-associated receptors such as PD1 and CTLA4 [87]. Microglia also express CCL2 and CCL5 which, as mentioned previously, enhances regulatory T cell recruitment and myeloid-derived suppressor cells [56,90]. Notably, CCL5 also acts as an auto-stimulatory signal for GBM cells by binding to the non-conventional receptor CD44, resulting in increased cell survival, invasion, and proliferation [91]. Therefore, targeting this zone of recurrence and immune exhaustion protected by intact barrier is key to enhancing the efficacy of immunotherapy. However, achieving this requires CTLs to traffic through the BBB.

The BBB is a highly regulated physical and metabolic barrier which extends from the CNS microvasculature to the endothelial cells of postcapillary venules [92]. During neuro-inflammation the permeability of the endothelial cells changes to allow for the entrance of lymphocytes into the CNS. This is achieved by changes in BBB junctional morphology that allow lymphocytes access either by squeezing between endothelial cells (paracellular diapedesis) or crossing through pores in the endothelial cell membrane (transcellular diapedesis) [93]. Recent single-cell RNA sequencing of the neuro-vasculature also shows enhanced endothelial cell expression of MHC class II genes in the disease state. The endothelial cell signature also changes from CNS specific to mirroring the periphery, thereby promoting immune trafficking from the blood (preprint [94]). The endothelial cells of the BBB are sealed by adherens junctions, a continuous series of complex tight junctions, and recently discovered tricellular junctions [95]. In the inflammatory state, these tricellular junctions have been suggested to be the primary site of cellular migration, through the downregulation of proteins (tricellulin and angulins) which normally maintain their morphology [95,96]. Interestingly, recombinant CCL2 and CCL5 administration was demonstrated in vitro to enhance T cell diapedesis through tricellular junctions. This may therefore offer a therapeutic strategy specifically to enhance paracellular crossing at the BBB, although their effect on recruiting regulatory T cells must also be considered [95,96].

Tight junctions can also be targeted to allow for entry of therapeutic agents [97,98]. These junctions are maintained on the basolateral side by the transmembrane adhesion proteins VE-cadherin and platelet endothelial cell adhesion molecule (PECAM)-1 [99,100]. The apical side of endothelial tight junctions is secured by occludin and claudin-1/3/5/12 [101]. Together, these proteins seal the tight junctions together by binding with each other on opposite endothelial cells, reducing the intercellular distance [101]. Claudin-5 is the most commonly expressed protein in tight junctions [101], and can be targeted with recombinant protein inhibitors such as the non-toxic C-terminal domain of the *Clostridium Perfringens* enterotoxin [102]. This can reversibly open endothelial tight junctions and allow ingress of therapeutic agents. Targeting of claudin-5 in vitro results in reduced paracellular diapedesis of lymphocytes while increasing transcellular diapedesis [103]. Other studies have also shown that knockout of adhesion molecules such as PECAM-1 does not result in enhanced paracellular movement, but instead increases migration via cell membrane channels [104]. Taken together, it becomes apparent that functional tight junction regulating proteins are required for paracellular diapedesis, and that disruption of these proteins may shift trafficking towards endocytic lymphocyte migration patterns similar to those found in neuroinflammatory CNS states [93].

The process of transcellular diapedesis is mediated by endocytosis at the endothelial cell membrane. This endocytosis occurs through vesicles containing caveolin (Cav)-1, which are increased in number during disease states such as EAE [105,106]. Regions of the BBB rich in Cav1 upregulate expression of adhesion receptors such as ICAM-1, capturing T cells at regions of the BBB where endocytic vesicles are present [107]. Interestingly, in inflammatory conditions such as EAE, ICAM-1 is highly expressed on the endothelium, and this over-expression promotes transcellular diapedesis. This contrasts with the resting state where low/intermediate expression of ICAM-1 favors paracellular diapedesis [108]. Therefore, promoting the expression of LFA-1 on T cells which can bind to over-expressed ICAM-1 may enhance T cell trafficking (therapeutic approaches described in the previous section). However, whether this effect also extends to $CD8^+$ T cells in the context of glioblastoma is unclear.

Differential trafficking of T cell subsets was also demonstrated by experiments using $Cav1^{-/-}$ mice which induced almost total loss of Th1 transcellular migration but did not impair migration of Th17 cells [109]. In EAE, Th17 T cells have been demonstrated to use CCR6 to bind CCL20 produced by the choroid plexus epithelial cells to gain access to the ventricular CSF [110,111]. When considering the CCR6–CCL20 axis for therapeutic targeting in glioblastoma, $CD8^+CCR6^+$ T cells also migrate towards CCL20 and blockade of CCL20 or CCR6 has also been demonstrated to reduce neuroinflammation in murine models of subarachnoid hemorrhage [112,113]. However, over-expression of CCL20 by tumors also correlates with tumor progression in multiple cancer types, as well as decreased survival [114]. Importantly though, the tumor-promoting effects of CCR6 signaling appear to rely on $CCR6^+$ stromal cells but not $CCR6^+$ immune cells [114]. Upregulation of CCR6 on immune cells may therefore be the more prudent therapeutic approach for enhancing T cell infiltration while maintaining tumor control. Transforming growth factor (TGF)-β has been shown to promote CCR6 expression on human CD4 T cells but is also implicated in the promotion of regulatory FOXP3 expression [115]. However, TGF-β priming also generates a fractional population of $CCR6^+FOXP3^-$ cells [116]. Further selection of this population would therefore be desirable to achieve a pro-infiltrative, effector T cell phenotype. Models of EAE have also found that increased expression of CCL19 and CCL21 from mononuclear inflammatory cells binds $CCR7^+$ T cells in the CSF [117]. CCL19 has been shown to enhance the frequency of antigen responsive IFN-γ$^+$ $CD8^+$ T cells in viral infection and CCR7 chemotaxis may be stimulated in vitro using by-products of coagulation factor XIIa (high-molecular-weight kininogen domain 5) [118,119]. However, CCL19 may also promote the migration of regulatory T cells ($CD4^+CD25^+FoxP3^+$) and therefore its usefulness in glioblastoma is unclear [120].

While these mechanisms are of interest therapeutically to allow T cells to cross the BBB from the periphery, this is only the initial step in accessing the parenchyma. Interaction with professional antigen-presenting cells in the perivascular spaces is a key step before penetration of the glia limitans, which lines the blood vessels and the surface of the brain [121].

4. The Glia Limitans—Accessing the Parenchyma

Between the outer BBB and the parenchyma lies the glia limitans. The glia limitans is formed by astrocyte foot processes associating with the basal lamina of the parenchyma [110]. It is divided into two membranes: the glia limitans perivascularis (surrounding blood vessels) and the glia limitans superficialis (covering the surface of the brain) [122]. In much of the brain, these two membranes lie so closely together that they are indistinguishable, but beyond the capillaries at the venules, inflammation can cause these two membranes to separate, forming a perivascular space. This space communicates with the CSF and allows for APCs to present antigens to entering T cells [123]. This interaction is critical in allowing T cells to access the parenchyma—indeed, the effects of T cells in EAE only begin once immune cells have crossed the glia limitans [124]. The APC–T cell interaction drives the production of further pro-inflammatory cytokines which triggers the recruitment of more immune cells [111,125]. Interestingly, while the initial T cells that enter these perivascular spaces tend to have increased expression of CCR6, further recruitment occurs in a CCR6-independent manner [110,111]. This would suggest that CCR6$^+$ T cells form part of an initial 'licensing' step and that their interaction with APCs in the perivascular spaces facilitates further entry of T cells in a non-CCR6-specific manner.

In normal physiology, T cell crossing at the glia limitans is mediated by the expression of laminins [126]. For example, the parenchymal membrane of the glia limitans contains $\alpha 1$ and $\alpha 2$ laminins [127], which CD4$^+$ T cells are unable to bind in the non-inflammatory state. However, in EAE, CD4$^+$ T cells can bypass this control mechanism by using matrix metalloproteinases (MMPs) which disrupt the astrocytic foot processes, breaking down barrier integrity and allowing for T cell ingress [124]. While this might suggest that MMP agonism may be an attractive prospect for opening the glia limitans, MMPs are involved in the angiogenesis and invasion of glioma [128]. Inhibition of MMP was even trialed using a broad-spectrum MMP inhibitor, but this resulted in widespread reports of musculoskeletal toxicity due to on-target, off-tumor effects [129,130]. Given these experiences, it is unlikely that MMP agonism in glioblastoma will be a desirable therapeutic target.

Another mediator of T cell entry into the parenchyma is CXCL12. In murine models, T cells have been noted to be held in perivascular spaces due to expression of CXCL12 [131]. This 'hold' is released in inflammatory conditions, as increased levels of IL-17 drive the expression of CXCR7 on endothelial cells, resulting in the internalization of CXCL12 [132]. This leads to increased CXCR4 expression on T cells and subsequent T cell entry into the parenchyma [131,132]. However, when considering the downregulation of CXCL12 as a therapeutic strategy, it is worth noting that recent studies evaluating T cell responses to viral infection in vitro have found that CXCL12 at the BBB endothelium can promote CD8$^+$ migration across the BCSF interface, suggestive of a location-dependent role [133]. A summary of these selected targets and therapeutic considerations is shown in Table 1.

Table 1. A summary of selected factors that may enhance trafficking and infiltration of T cells across the BBB.

Interactor	Behavior	Therapeutic Considerations	References
		T cell processes	
LFA-1	T cell integrin which binds ICAM-1. Promotes T cell capture and rolling in inflammatory and non-inflammatory state.	IL-12 induces LFA-1 expression and can enhance T cell migration in several murine malignancies.	[36,73]
VLA-4 ($\alpha 4\beta 1$)	Integrin on T cell which binds VCAM-1 in the inflammatory state and interacts with other transmembrane proteins (JAM-B, JAML, etc.).	IL-12 induces LFA-1 and VLA-4 expression and enhances T cell migration in several murine malignancies. Effect may be malignancy dependent.	[41,42,73]
CXCR3 (3 ligands)	CXCL9: Polarizes T cells to a Th1/Th17 phenotype.	Mediated lymphocyte infiltration and suppresses tumor growth in cutaneous fibrosarcoma.	[134]
	CXCL10: Only moderately induces CXCR3 internalization and enhances T cell infiltration.	DPP-4 blockade increases TILs but is also tumorigenic (independent of enzymatic function). Combinatorial poly-ICLC enhances CXCL10 expression.	[81–83]
	CXCL11: Binds CXCR3 strongly and induces receptor internalization.	Promotes lineage of regulatory T cells.	[75]

Table 1. Cont.

Interactor	Behavior	Therapeutic Considerations	References
CCR4	CCL2, CCL22 (and others): Overexpressed on glioma cells, recruits regulatory T cells.	CCR4-CCL22 signaling recruits regulatory T cells. Blockade of CCR4 in vitro can reduce regulatory T cell migration. TMZ can also mitigate production of CCL2.	[135,136]
CCR5	Binds CCL3, CCL4, and CCL5. May help to recruit cytolytic T cells but also regulatory T cells.	CCL4 can help recruit cytolytic CCR5$^+$ T cells in esophageal squamous cell carcinoma but CCL4–CCR5 interaction can enhance the invasion ability of glioblastoma in vitro. CCL5 is also associated with enhanced T cell diapedesis at tricellular junctions. However, CCL5 also binds CD44 on GBM cells to drive proliferation and survival and is produced by perivascular stromal cells such as pericytes. Blockade of CCR5 (maraviroc) may limit cancer-associated fibroblast accumulation.	[54,62,63,91,95]
CCR6	Binds CCL20 expressed at the choroid plexus. CD8$^+$ T cells migrate to CCL20 in murine SAH.	TGF-β promotes CCR6 expression but also is implicated in the promotion of FOXP3$^+$ cells. However, a fraction of the population is CCR6$^+$FOXP3$^-$. CCR6 T cells may also be involved with licensing further recruitment to perivascular spaces.	[115,116]
CCR7	Present on activated CD8 T cells (and central memory T cells).	Interacts with CCL19 and may mediate integrin activation on immune cells or diapedesis. Chemotaxis may be enhanced by a peptide derived from the byproduct of coagulation factor XIIa cleavage. May also promote regulatory T cells.	[117,119,120]
Blood–brain barrier processes			
E/P-Selectin	Expressed in inflammatory state only. Binds PSGL-1$^+$ CD8 T cells, slowing them on BBB endothelium.	Expression enhanced in response to inflammatory cytokines (e.g., IL-1 or TNF α). IL-1 has been delivered via CED in rat models of glioma.	[45,137]
Claudin-5, PECAM-1	Commonly expressed proteins involved in sealing tight junctions at BBB.	Modified Clostridium perfringens enterotoxin can reversibly open tight junctions. May drive T cells to transcellular migration.	[93,103,104]
ACKR1	Trafficking of pro-infiltrative chemokines from abluminal to luminal surface of BBB.	IL-1 signaling associated with upregulated expression ACKR1 (along with VCAM-1, ICAM-1). Trialed using CED in rat glioma.	[45]
Caveolin-1	Expressed in endocytic vesicles at BBB and acts as a mediator of transcellular diapedesis.	Regions of BBB rich in CAV-1 are also rich in ICAM-1. Enhancing ICAM-1 on BBB (e.g., via IL-1) may capture more T cells that can undergo para and transcellular diapedesis.	[108]
CXCL12	Acts as a T cell, holding factor cells in perivascular spaces. Expression of CXCR7 on endothelial cells internalizes CXCL12.	IL-17 drives expression of CXCR7 on endothelial cells and CXCR4 on T cells which licenses their entry into the parenchyma. However, CXCL12 may promote CD8$^+$ migration across BCSF barrier—may be a location-specific role.	[131–133]

This table only provides selected examples and is not exhaustive.

5. T Cell Trafficking through the Parenchyma

Once past the glia limitans, effector T cells must reach and infiltrate the tumor to exert their cytotoxic effect. As discussed in the introduction, glioblastoma can restrict T cell trafficking due to the downregulated expression of VEGF-C, resulting in restricted lymphangiogenesis [22]. Notably, in patients treated with neoadjuvant anti-PD-1, VEGF-C expression was highly correlated with increased infiltration of T cells [138]. Thus, restoring levels of lymphangiogenesis-promoting factors such as VEGF-C could also enhance T cell homing and infiltration to the tumor. This is supported by the findings of Song et al., who demonstrated that intra-cisterna magna injections of an adeno-associated viral vector coding for VEGF-C could remodel meningeal lymphatic vessels in murine models of glioma [22]. Further enhanced expression of VEGF-C in lymphatic endothelial cells could potentiate the effect of checkpoint blockade due to enhanced T cell infiltration [22].

T cell motility is also dependent on metabolic pathways that are often usurped by rapidly proliferating tumors. Tumor cells demonstrate increased glucose uptake and lactose production, even in the presence of oxygen and functioning mitochondria (known as the Warburg effect) [139,140]. This affords the tumor and other rapidly proliferating cells essential anabolic precursors for cell proliferation [140]. The increased glucose demand by tumor cells therefore decreases the amount available for circulating T cells to maintain effector and migratory function [141]. Aerobic glycolysis is the main source of ATP production in leukocytes, which is required for the energetic demands of migration [142,143]. Inhibition of the T cell glycolytic pathway through administration of 2-DG and rapamycin causes a decrease in naïve T cell motility, demonstrating the importance of glucose in T cell homing [144,145]. The associated build-up of lactate caused by the Warburg effect also results in decreased migration of $CD4^+$ T cells and a loss of cytolytic function of $CD8^+$ T cells by interfering with T cell glycolysis [145–148]. However, this effect can be reversed, as demonstrated in an animal model of peritonitis where antibody-mediated blockade of lactate transporters on T cells allowed them to maintain their migratory potential [149]. Expression of CTLA-4 decreases the expression of the glucose transporter GLUT-1 on T cells, and further decreases effector function, implying that combinatorial approaches using checkpoint blockade may aid with T cell trafficking as well as reinvigoration of function [142,150]. However, recent work suggests that exhausted human $CD8^+$ T cells may actually become more mobile [151]. CTLA-4 signaling can lead to a RAP1-mediated increase in LFA-1 binding, which can induce migration [152]. This has potential implications for considering which form of ICI would best work with a tumor where T cell trafficking poses a significant challenge. An overview of the metabolic pathways limiting T cell efficacy in glioblastoma is shown in Figure 2.

Another mediator of T cell glycolysis is the PI3K/AKT/mTOR pathway, whose activation can also downregulate the expression of adhesion and migration molecules CD62L, CCR7, and S1P1 in $CD8^+$ T cells [142,153]. Loss of S1P1 has been shown to mediate T cell sequestration in bone marrow in glioblastoma, while $S1P1^+$ cells are resistant to sequestration and can return into the circulation [142,154–156]. Therefore, reversing sequestration will be critical for future immunotherapy efficacy and is currently the subject of ongoing therapeutic investigation [157]. While one approach may be to inhibit the PI3K/AKT/mTOR pathway, this inhibition must be selective, as AKT possesses three isoforms which have varying pro- and anti-tumor effects. AKT signaling also plays an important role for the development of effector-like memory $CD8^+$ T cells necessary for tumor immune surveillance [158]. Interestingly, recent work has described small-molecule inhibitors that may be capable of targeting pathogenic AKT isoforms only (AKT1 and AKT2) while leaving the tumor-suppressive functionality of AKT3 intact [159,160]. Indeed, specific AKT1 and 2 inhibition has been associated with enhanced central memory $CD8^+$ T cell proliferation with prolonged cytokine and Granzyme B production, making this a potential future therapeutic strategy [158–161].

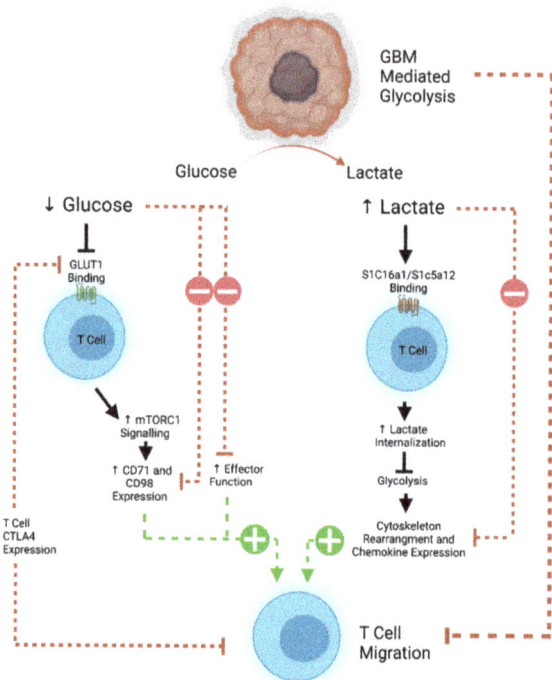

Figure 2. Glioblastoma effects on T cell metabolism and motility. As a rapidly dividing tumor, glioblastoma rapidly takes up glucose and produces lactate (the Warburg effect). Lack of glucose results in decreased GLUT1 binding (also downregulated by CTLA4) and downregulates effector function and motility. Increased lactate is internalized in T cells, where it also inhibits glycolysis and interferes with cytoskeleton rearrangement, resulting in decreased T cell migration. Produced using Biorender.

6. The Tumor Microenvironment

Once T cells traffic past the BBB and through the parenchyma, they will encounter the highly immunosuppressive tumor microenvironment. This is made up of regulatory T cells (CD4$^+$CD25$^+$FOXP3$^+$), tumor-associated macrophages (TAMs) and myeloid-derived suppressor cells (MDSCs), as well as other stromal cells such as GSC-derived pericytes [23,162]. These can all work to suppress effector T cell function. Regulatory T cells induce T cell exhaustion and apoptosis, signaling via programmed death-ligand 1 (PD-L1), cytotoxic T-lymphocyte-associated protein 4 (CTLA-4), lymphocyte activation gene 3 (LAG-3), T cell immunoglobulin and mucin domain-containing protein 3 (TIM-3), and others [163,164]. They also can dampen the production of inflammatory cytokines and CTL proliferation by downregulating interleukin-2 and interferon-γ [165]. Gliomas are adept at recruiting regulatory T cells to the microenvironment by over-production of factors such as indoleamine 2,3 -dioxygenase-1 (IDO-1) [166]. As mentioned previously, GSC-derived pericytes also secrete CCL5, which can promote the recruitment of regulatory T cells to the TME [54]. Stromal cells in the microenvironment also produce highly immunosuppressive cytokines, such as transforming growth factor β (TGFβ) and interleukin-10 (IL-10) [167,168].

Despite the numerous targets for blockade, it is notable that ICI and the interruption of pro-tumor metabolic pathways have failed as a monotherapy [9,169]. Increasingly, attention is turning towards combinatorial therapies, where multiple drivers of T cell exhaustion can be blocked simultaneously [170]. This includes using bispecific antibodies against TGF-β and PD-L1 or against PD-L1 and the anti-agonist CD27 [171–173]. These approaches are currently being evaluated in Phase I trials in advanced solid tumors (NCT04429542, NCT04440943). Cytokine modulation approaches are also a potential avenue for enhancing T cell activity in the TME, as seen in 'armored' CAR-T constructs. The addition of IL-12, IL-15, or IL-18 along with antigen specificity to T cells appears to result in greater CTL activity and anti-tumor efficacy [174–176]. A high percentage of regulatory T cells in the peripheral blood of GBM patients express CCR4 compared to controls (74 vs. 43%) [135]. CCL4 binds CCL22 (and others), which has been shown to be overexpressed in freshly resected human glioma cells, and blockade of CCR4 in vitro can significantly reduce regulatory T cell migration [135]. Targeting fibroblast activation proteins or introducing heparinase-expressing agents may also help to disrupt immunosuppressive stromal elements [146,177,178]. Intratumoral APCs are also necessary to stimulate and retain infiltrating lymphocytes at the tumor site, as well as carrying antigens to draining lymph nodes and cross priming peripheral CD8 T cells [179–181]. The administration of intratumoral FMS-like tyrosine kinase 3 ligand (Flt3L) and poly I:C has been shown to expand and mature dendritic cell precursors, resulting in greater antitumor efficacy when combined with immunotherapies such as PD-L1 blockade or oncolytic herpes simplex viruses [179,182].

Standard-of-care therapies also can help drive a more potent immune response. Temozolomide (TMZ) is an alkylating chemotherapy whose main function is to induce DNA double-stranded breaks, resulting in tumor cell death [183]. Interestingly, TMZ can also help to reduce the numbers of peripheral regulatory T cells, as well as interrupting their migration [136,184]. In disease states such as glioblastoma, tumor cells and platelet-derived growth factor receptor beta (PDGFRβ)-expressing cells of the neurovascular sub-units (such as pericytes and perivascular fibroblast-like cells) produce CCL2 to recruit regulatory T cells and dampen the effector response [185]. TMZ interrupts the CCL2–CCR4 axis, thereby reducing this effect [136,184]. Combining immunotherapy with radiotherapy also can help to polarize the T cell response to a cytotoxic phenotype by inducing greater T cell receptor diversity and expanding the numbers of tumor-infiltrating lymphocytes and effector memory T cells [186]. In pre-clinical murine models of glioma, radiotherapy combined with antibodies against markers of exhaustion such as TIM-3 and PD-1 was able to produce long-term survival [11].

7. Modeling the BBB

Animal and in vitro models have contributed greatly to our knowledge regarding the cell and protein interactions required to cross the BBB. Rudimentary animal models from the 1980s first established how BBB permeability could change in response to systemic compounds by tracking the CNS uptake of Evan's Blue dye following intravenous infusion [187–190]. These models established protocols to visualize membrane cellular components and tissue hierarchy through fluorescent microscopy and histology, allowing for the elucidation of fundamental mechanisms behind membrane permeability. Such models included mice with proteins essential for T cell chemotaxis across the BBB knocked out, including tight junction proteins claudin 5 [100] and occludin [191]. Unfortunately, full knockout of these proteins results in non-viable pups or other dysfunctional phenotypes, suggesting the importance of tight junction proteins in development. Additional knockout mice focusing on proteins involved in T cell rolling, p-selectin, and its ligand PSGL-1 [192] were developed and confirmed less BBB breakdown and leukocyte trafficking into the CNS. Similarly, the use of antibody natalizumab to block the α4 subunit on T cells has been successful in preventing BBB chemotaxis in MS [193]. Genetic models targeting pericyte and astrocyte function have also been generated to establish how these cell types support BBB formation in development and regulate tight junctions in injury and disease. The use of two-photon microscopy has allowed for imaging at depths up to 1mm, but real-time high-resolution imaging and cell tracking capabilities are limited. Animal models closely mimic BBB features by including all cell types within the vascular interface, fluid flow and biochemical concentrations. However, there are still challenges translating in vivo finding to clinical significance. Genetic, molecular, and immunological differences between humans and rodents, as well as high cost and ethical concerns with animal testing, have generated a need for robust in vitro models.

In vitro models of the BBB range from simple endothelial cell monolayers to complex three-dimensional systems with fluid flow and ionic gradients [194,195]. These models have the advantage of using human cells as well as being cost effective and allowing for high-throughput screening of a variety of different conditions or molecules. Transwell, hydrogels, and microfluidic devices with three or four different cell types have been created in attempts to best mimic native BBB function. Simplified in vitro models allow for researchers to specifically modify or track elements of the BBB. Cell types used in these models have traditionally been primary brain endothelial cells or immortalized cell lines. Immune factors affecting BBB permeability have been most studied with BECs due to their accurate expression of chemokine and cytokine receptors. Interestingly, these models found CCL2 to cause redistribution of tight junction proteins, such as claudin-5 and occluding, under physiological and pathological conditions [196,197], which gives insight into the mechanism of increased T cell chemotaxis during inflammation and elevated CCL2. Brain-cancer-specific models have focused on integrating vasculature and tumor cells to test the toxicity of therapeutics prior to animal studies [198,199]. These models recapitulated the three-dimensional structure of a brain tumor but used lung fibroblasts, HUVECs, and gelatin, which may not accurately represent the blood–brain barrier and brain microenvironment. The development of induced pluripotent stem cells (iPSCs) has allowed for genetically identical personalized in vitro models to test drug and cell interactions with BBB of specific individuals and disease conditions [200]. Overall, both in vivo and in vitro models of the BBB have limitations but can provide valuable insight to improve T cell chemotaxis in GBM.

8. Safety

While this review has largely focused on strategies by which T cells can be recruited and restored to a cytotoxic effector status, it must be noted that rapid increases in activated T cells in the circulation can potentially lead to cytokine release syndrome (CRS), mediated by the release of pro-inflammatory cytokines such as IL-6 [201]. Therefore, when considering therapies that will increase circulating activated T cells and subsequent CNS T cell infiltration, careful consideration must be given to the safety of any such approach. Such therapies may lead to systemic and neurological complications, even when not used specifically to treat CNS malignancies.

This is demonstrated by the example of clinically used therapeutics such as ipilimumab, which re-invigorates T cells by blockade of CTLA-4 [202]. Ipilimumab has been associated with pituitary inflammation (hypophysitis), occurring in up to 17% of patients receiving ipilimumab treatment [203,204]. Similar syndromes are also observed when using anti-PD-1 and anti-PD-L1 therapies, albeit at a lower frequency compared to anti-CTLA-4 [205]. The mechanism of how ipilimumab causes hypophysitis remains unclear, but it is speculated that ipilimumab can release the brakes on T cells that target and destroy pituitary cells, or that expression of CTLA-4 on pituitary cells leads to complement fixation mediated by ipilimumab, resulting in the destruction of pituitary cells [206,207]. In rarer circumstances (less than 0.2% of patients), ICI, especially ipilimumab or combination ipilimumab/nivolumab (anti-PD-1), has caused aseptic meningitis and encephalitis [208–212]. Like with hypophysitis, the exact mechanism is unclear. However, in the case of encephalitis, there is evidence that the effect is autoimmune in origin, as some patients treated with ICI exhibit autoantibodies to the NMDA receptor, a characteristic of other autoimmune encephalopathies [213,214]. ICI has also reportedly induced new CNS demyelination and exacerbated existing CNS demyelination in MS patients [215,216]. These rare, but serious neurological deficits resulting from systemic ICI emphasize the need for careful monitoring of patients receiving therapies that enhance T cell trafficking and function.

The experience of treatments using adoptively transferred chimeric antigen receptor (CAR) T cells in extracranial and intracranial malignancies can also be illustrative for potential systemic and neurological toxicities. The most common CAR-related toxicity is cytokine release syndrome (CRS), occurring in up to 37–93% of patients with lymphoma or leukemia receiving CD19 CARs [217]. As described previously, CRS is caused by rapid activation of CAR T cells upon administration and subsequent release of pro-inflammatory cytokines, such as IL-6 [201]. High levels of serum IL-6 were found to correlate with severe CRS, which led to the FDA approval of tocilizumab, an anti-IL-6 receptor antagonist [218]. Strategies to reduce CRS include administering lower doses of CAR T cells over multiple infusions as opposed to one single bolus [219,220].

Neurological-specific toxicities after CAR administration are also possible. Immune effector cell-associated neurotoxicity syndrome (ICANS) can develop in around 50% of patients following systemic CAR infusion [221]. ICANS manifests with minor symptoms such as lethargy and confusion but can also cause seizures and coma. The pathophysiology of ICANS remains unclear, but evidence suggests that release of pro-inflammatory cytokines, such as IL-6 and IL-1β, by CAR T cells can disrupt the BBB, resulting in the accumulation of CAR T cells and pro-inflammatory cytokines in the CNS [222]. Klinger et al. recently described a mechanism whereby CD19 bi-specific T cell engagers (blinatumomab) can induce T cell adhesion to endothelial cells of the BBB followed by T cell migration into the perivascular space in a CD19-independent manner. Once past the BBB, they may encounter rare target CD19 cells in the CNS and release pro-inflammatory cytokines, triggering ICANS-like symptoms [223]. However, unlike CRS, ICANS does not respond to tocilizumab treatment, and symptoms are typically managed with corticosteroids or cessation of therapy [224]. Klinger et al. also reported that the non-specific entry of CD19 T cells into the CNS could be abrogated by the administration of anti-adhesion agents (anti-VLA4, natalizumab), offering another potential therapeutic if toxicity occurs [223]. In summary, while enhanced T cell chemotaxis and infiltration of glioblastoma are necessary for effective immune-mediated treatment of tumors, this must be carefully balanced with the risks described above.

9. Conclusions

For immunotherapy in glioblastoma to be successful, sustained recruitment of effector lymphocytes from the periphery to the tumor is necessary. However, achieving this in a unique immune environment such as the CNS must overcome both physical and chemical barriers. In this review, we have described the process by which effector T cells can be recruited from the periphery and what modifications may result in a pro-infiltrative phenotype. We have described both T cell and BBB factors that would be desirable therapeutic targets and set out strategies by which this may be achieved. Adhesional factors on the BBB endothelium such as ICAM-1, VCAM-1, or ACKR1 may be upregulated by IL-1β or IFN-γ, which can be delivered via convection-enhanced delivery (CED) directly to the tumor site. Delivery of these cytokines and other inflammatory factors can have profound effects on increasing BBB penetration and the migration potential of T cells. Induced expression of CXCL10 by using poly-ICLC can also interact with CXCR3 on effector T cells, prompting their infiltration into tumor. Co-culture with IL-12 may help drive the expression of key integrins such as LFA-1 on the surface of T cells in preparation for adoptive transfer to further enhance their adhesive capabilities. CCL2 and CCL5 may promote paracellular diapedesis through tricellular junctions in the BBB endothelium, while TGF-β priming of T cells can increase their CCR6 expression, which can promote transcellular crossing. However, CCL2 and CCL5 may also mediate regulatory T cell recruitment, perhaps necessitating co-administration with checkpoint blockade. Subsequent navigation through the glia limitans may be aided by IL-17-mediated downregulation of CXCL12, although this may be a location-specific effect. Once inside the parenchyma, lymphangiogenesis-promoting factors such as VEGF-C may further enhance trafficking of T cells to the tumor. Metabolic mediators such as the PI3K/AKT/mTOR pathway may also be therapeutically targeted using small-molecule inhibitors of the AKT1 and AKT2 isoforms. Combinatorial approaches to stimulate T cells and block checkpoint inhibition will likely be necessary to overcome the microenvironment. This may be achieved using novel bispecific constructs or co-administration with immune stimulatory cytokines such as IL-12, IL-15, or IL-18. Standard-of-care therapies such as TMZ and radiotherapy may also help to blockade regulatory T cell recruitment and drive a more diverse and potent T cell response. Importantly, however, any approach that enhances T cell infiltration into the CNS must consider safety, and although there are therapeutic options for adverse events, future trial designs using pro-infiltrative therapies should err on the side of caution. Nevertheless, enhanced T cell trafficking and infiltration of glioblastoma is essential for immunotherapeutic efficacy. While ICI seeks to 'release the brakes' on T cell activity, in the case of glioblastoma, we must first drive T cells to the tumor.

Author Contributions: K.S., writing—original draft preparation, review and editing, visualization, project administration, revision. K.M.H., writing—original draft preparation, review and editing, visualization, revision. K.K.P., writing—original draft preparation, D.S.W., writing—original draft preparation. A.A.M., visualization. S.L.C., writing—review and editing. J.H.S., supervision. All authors have read and agreed to the published version of the manuscript.

Funding: This work was supported by grants from the National Institutes of Health (NIH) (U01NS090284 (JHS) and P50CA190991(JHS)).

Conflicts of Interest: K.S., K.M.H., K.K.P., D.S.W., A.A.M. and S.L.C. report no conflict of interest. J.H.S. has an equity interest in Istari Oncology, which has licensed intellectual property from Duke related to the use of poliovirus and D2C7 in the treatment of glioblastoma. J.H.S. is an inventor on patents related to the PEP-CMV DC vaccine with tetanus, as well as the poliovirus vaccine and D2C7 in the treatment of glioblastoma. J.H.S. has an equity interest in Annias Immunotherapeutics, which has licensed intellectual property from Duke related to the use of the pepCMV vaccine in the treatment of glioblastoma.

References

1. Klein, R.S.; Hunter, C.A. Protective and Pathological Immunity during Central Nervous System Infections. *Immunity* **2017**, *46*, 891–909. [CrossRef]
2. Daneman, R.; Prat, A. The blood-brain barrier. *Cold Spring Harb. Perspect. Biol.* **2015**, *7*, a020412. [CrossRef] [PubMed]
3. Engelhardt, B.; Sorokin, L. The blood-brain and the blood-cerebrospinal fluid barriers: Function and dysfunction. *Semin. Immunopathol.* **2009**, *31*, 497–511. [CrossRef] [PubMed]
4. Khasraw, M.; Reardon, D.A.; Weller, M.; Sampson, J.H. PD-1 Inhibitors: Do they have a Future in the Treatment of Glioblastoma? *Clin. Cancer Res. Off. J. Am. Assoc. Cancer Res.* **2020**, *26*, 5287–5296. [CrossRef]
5. Quail, D.F.; Joyce, J.A. Microenvironmental regulation of tumor progression and metastasis. *Nat. Med.* **2013**, *19*, 1423–1437. [CrossRef]
6. Quail, D.F.; Joyce, J.A. The Microenvironmental Landscape of Brain Tumors. *Cancer Cell* **2017**, *31*, 326–341. [CrossRef] [PubMed]
7. Yeung, J.T.; Hamilton, R.L.; Ohnishi, K.; Ikeura, M.; Potter, D.M.; Nikiforova, M.N.; Ferrone, S.; Jakacki, R.I.; Pollack, I.F.; Okada, H. LOH in the HLA Class I Region at 6p21 Is Associated with Shorter Survival in Newly Diagnosed Adult Glioblastoma. *Clin. Cancer Res.* **2013**, *19*, 1816–1826. [CrossRef] [PubMed]
8. Johanns, T.M.; Bowman-Kirigin, J.A.; Liu, C.; Dunn, G.P. Targeting Neoantigens in Glioblastoma: An Overview of Cancer Immunogenomics and Translational Implications. *Neurosurgery* **2017**, *64*, 165–176. [CrossRef]
9. Reardon, D.A.; Brandes, A.A.; Omuro, A.; Mulholland, P.; Lim, M.; Wick, A.; Baehring, J.; Ahluwalia, M.S.; Roth, P.; Bähr, O.; et al. Effect of Nivolumab vs Bevacizumab in Patients With Recurrent Glioblastoma: The CheckMate 143 Phase 3 Randomized Clinical Trial. *JAMA Oncol.* **2020**, *6*, 1003–1010. [CrossRef] [PubMed]
10. Garzon-Muvdi, T.; Theodros, D.; Luksik, A.S.; Maxwell, R.; Kim, E.; Jackson, C.M.; Belcaid, Z.; Ganguly, S.; Tyler, B.; Brem, H.; et al. Dendritic cell activation enhances anti-PD-1 mediated immunotherapy against glioblastoma. *Oncotarget* **2018**, *9*, 20681–20697. [CrossRef] [PubMed]
11. Kim, J.E.; Patel, M.A.; Mangraviti, A.; Kim, E.S.; Theodros, D.; Velarde, E.; Liu, A.; Sankey, E.W.; Tam, A.; Xu, H.; et al. Combination Therapy with Anti-PD-1, Anti-TIM-3, and Focal Radiation Results in Regression of Murine Gliomas. *Clin. Cancer Res.* **2017**, *23*, 124–136. [CrossRef] [PubMed]
12. Ellwardt, E.; Walsh, J.T.; Kipnis, J.; Zipp, F. Understanding the Role of T Cells in CNS Homeostasis. *Trends Immunol.* **2016**, *37*, 154–165. [CrossRef] [PubMed]
13. Ziv, Y.; Ron, N.; Butovsky, O.; Landa, G.; Sudai, E.; Greenberg, N.; Cohen, H.; Kipnis, J.; Schwartz, M. Immune cells contribute to the maintenance of neurogenesis and spatial learning abilities in adulthood. *Nat. Neurosci.* **2006**, *9*, 268–275. [CrossRef]

14. Kipnis, J.; Cohen, H.; Cardon, M.; Ziv, Y.; Schwartz, M. T cell deficiency leads to cognitive dysfunction: Implications for therapeutic vaccination for schizophrenia and other psychiatric conditions. *Proc. Natl. Acad. Sci. USA* **2004**, *101*, 8180–8185. [CrossRef] [PubMed]
15. Engelhardt, B.; Vajkoczy, P.; Weller, R.O. The movers and shapers in immune privilege of the CNS. *Nat. Immunol.* **2017**, *18*, 123–131. [CrossRef] [PubMed]
16. Baruch, K.; Schwartz, M. CNS-specific T cells shape brain function via the choroid plexus. *Brain Behav. Immun.* **2013**, *34*, 11–16. [CrossRef] [PubMed]
17. Korin, B.; Ben-Shaanan, T.L.; Schiller, M.; Dubovik, T.; Azulay-Debby, H.; Boshnak, N.T.; Koren, T.; Rolls, A. High-dimensional, single-cell characterization of the brain's immune compartment. *Nat. Neurosci.* **2017**, *20*, 1300–1309. [CrossRef] [PubMed]
18. Murphy, J.B.; Sturm, E. Conditions determining the transplantability of tissues in the brain. *J. Exp. Med.* **1923**, *38*, 183–197. [CrossRef] [PubMed]
19. Medawar, P.B. Immunity to homologous grafted skin; the fate of skin homografts transplanted to the brain, to subcutaneous tissue, and to the anterior chamber of the eye. *Br. J. Exp. Pathol.* **1948**, *29*, 58–69. [PubMed]
20. Schläger, C.; Körner, H.; Krueger, M.; Vidoli, S.; Haberl, M.; Mielke, D.; Brylla, E.; Issekutz, T.; Cabañas, C.; Nelson, P.J.; et al. Effector T-cell trafficking between the leptomeninges and the cerebrospinal fluid. *Nature* **2016**, *530*, 349–353. [CrossRef] [PubMed]
21. Hu, X.; Deng, Q.; Ma, L.; Li, Q.; Chen, Y.; Liao, Y.; Zhou, F.; Zhang, C.; Shao, L.; Feng, J.; et al. Meningeal lymphatic vessels regulate brain tumor drainage and immunity. *Cell Res.* **2020**, *30*, 229–243. [CrossRef] [PubMed]
22. Song, E.; Mao, T.; Dong, H.; Boisserand, L.S.B.; Antila, S.; Bosenberg, M.; Alitalo, K.; Thomas, J.-L.; Iwasaki, A. VEGF-C-driven lymphatic drainage enables immunosurveillance of brain tumours. *Nature* **2020**, *577*, 689–694. [CrossRef] [PubMed]
23. Tomaszewski, W.; Sanchez-Perez, L.; Gajewski, T.F.; Sampson, J.H. Brain Tumor Microenvironment and Host State: Implications for Immunotherapy. *Clin. Cancer Res.* **2019**, *25*, 4202–4210. [CrossRef] [PubMed]
24. González, H.; Pacheco, R. T-cell-mediated regulation of neuroinflammation involved in neurodegenerative diseases. *J. Neuroinflamm.* **2014**, *11*, 201. [CrossRef] [PubMed]
25. Sommer, A.; Winner, B.; Prots, I. The Trojan horse—Neuroinflammatory impact of T cells in neurodegenerative diseases. *Mol. Neurodegener.* **2017**, *12*, 78. [CrossRef] [PubMed]
26. Muller, W.A. Getting leukocytes to the site of inflammation. *Vet. Pathol.* **2013**, *50*, 7–22. [CrossRef] [PubMed]
27. Lawrence, M.B.; Springer, T.A. Leukocytes roll on a selectin at physiologic flow rates: Distinction from and prerequisite for adhesion through integrins. *Cell* **1991**, *65*, 859–873. [CrossRef]
28. Von Andrian, U.H.; Chambers, J.D.; McEvoy, L.M.; Bargatze, R.F.; Arfors, K.E.; Butcher, E.C. Two-step model of leukocyte-endothelial cell interaction in inflammation: Distinct roles for LECAM-1 and the leukocyte beta 2 integrins in vivo. *Proc. Natl. Acad. Sci. USA* **1991**, *88*, 7538–7542. [CrossRef] [PubMed]
29. Ley, K.; Laudanna, C.; Cybulsky, M.I.; Nourshargh, S. Getting to the site of inflammation: The leukocyte adhesion cascade updated. *Nat. Rev. Immunol.* **2007**, *7*, 678–689. [CrossRef] [PubMed]
30. Nourshargh, S.; Alon, R. Leukocyte Migration into Inflamed Tissues. *Immunity* **2014**, *41*, 694–707. [CrossRef]
31. Montresor, A.; Toffali, L.; Constantin, G.; Laudanna, C. Chemokines and the signaling modules regulating integrin affinity. *Front. Immunol.* **2012**, *3*, 127. [CrossRef] [PubMed]
32. Kim, S.H.J.; Hammer, D.A. Integrin cross-talk modulates stiffness-independent motility of $CD4^+$ T lymphocytes. *Mol. Biol. Cell* **2021**, *32*, 1749–1757. [CrossRef]
33. Marchetti, L.; Engelhardt, B. Immune cell trafficking across the blood-brain barrier in the absence and presence of neuroinflammation. *Vasc. Biol.* **2020**, *2*, H1–H18. [CrossRef]
34. Nourshargh, S.; Hordijk, P.L.; Sixt, M. Breaching multiple barriers: Leukocyte motility through venular walls and the interstitium. *Nat. Rev. Mol. Cell Biol.* **2010**, *11*, 366–378. [CrossRef] [PubMed]
35. Engelhardt, B.; Ransohoff, R.M. Capture, crawl, cross: The T cell code to breach the blood–brain barriers. *Trends Immunol.* **2012**, *33*, 579–589. [CrossRef] [PubMed]
36. Vajkoczy, P.; Laschinger, M.; Engelhardt, B. α4-integrin-VCAM-1 binding mediates G protein–independent capture of encephalitogenic T cell blasts to CNS white matter microvessels. *J. Clin. Investig.* **2001**, *108*, 557–565. [CrossRef] [PubMed]
37. Sporici, R.; Issekutz, T.B. CXCR3 blockade inhibits T-cell migration into the CNS during EAE and prevents development of adoptively transferred, but not actively induced, disease. *Eur. J. Immunol.* **2010**, *40*, 2751–2761. [CrossRef]
38. Murphy, C.A.; Hoek, R.M.; Wiekowski, M.T.; Lira, S.A.; Sedgwick, J.D. Interactions between hemopoietically derived TNF and central nervous system-resident glial chemokines underlie initiation of autoimmune inflammation in the brain. *J. Immunol.* **2002**, *169*, 7054–7062. [CrossRef] [PubMed]
39. Battistini, L.; Piccio, L.; Rossi, B.; Bach, S.; Galgani, S.; Gasperini, C.; Ottoboni, L.; Ciabini, D.; Caramia, M.D.; Bernardi, G.; et al. $CD8^+$ T cells from patients with acute multiple sclerosis display selective increase of adhesiveness in brain venules: A critical role for P-selectin glycoprotein ligand-1. *Blood* **2003**, *101*, 4775–4782. [CrossRef] [PubMed]
40. Steiner, O.; Coisne, C.; Cecchelli, R.; Boscacci, R.; Deutsch, U.; Engelhardt, B.; Lyck, R. Differential roles for endothelial ICAM-1, ICAM-2, and VCAM-1 in shear-resistant T cell arrest, polarization, and directed crawling on blood-brain barrier endothelium. *J. Immunol.* **2010**, *185*, 4846–4855. [CrossRef] [PubMed]

41. Martin-Blondel, G.; Pignolet, B.; Tietz, S.; Yshii, L.; Gebauer, C.; Perinat, T.; Van Weddingen, I.; Blatti, C.; Engelhardt, B.; Liblau, R. Migration of encephalitogenic CD8 T cells into the central nervous system is dependent on the α4β1-integrin. *Eur. J. Immunol.* **2015**, *45*, 3302–3312. [CrossRef]
42. Alvarez, J.I.; Kébir, H.; Cheslow, L.; Charabati, M.; Chabarati, M.; Larochelle, C.; Prat, A. JAML mediates monocyte and CD8 T cell migration across the brain endothelium. *Ann. Clin. Transl. Neurol.* **2015**, *2*, 1032–1037. [CrossRef]
43. Minten, C.; Alt, C.; Gentner, M.; Frei, E.; Deutsch, U.; Lyck, R.; Schaeren-Wiemers, N.; Rot, A.; Engelhardt, B. DARC shuttles inflammatory chemokines across the blood-brain barrier during autoimmune central nervous system inflammation. *Brain* **2014**, *137*, 1454–1469. [CrossRef] [PubMed]
44. Hauptmann, J.; Johann, L.; Marini, F.; Kitic, M.; Colombo, E.; Mufazalov, I.A.; Krueger, M.; Karram, K.; Moos, S.; Wanke, F.; et al. Interleukin-1 promotes autoimmune neuroinflammation by suppressing endothelial heme oxygenase-1 at the blood-brain barrier. *Acta Neuropathol.* **2020**, *140*, 549–567. [CrossRef]
45. Frewert, S.; Stockhammer, F.; Warschewske, G.; Zenclussen, A.C.; Rupprecht, S.; Volk, H.D.; Woiciechowsky, C. Intratumoral infusion of interleukin-1beta and interferon-gamma induces tumor invasion with macrophages and lymphocytes in a rat glioma model. *Neurosci. Lett.* **2004**, *364*, 145–148. [CrossRef] [PubMed]
46. Armulik, A.; Genové, G.; Mäe, M.; Nisancioglu, M.H.; Wallgard, E.; Niaudet, C.; He, L.; Norlin, J.; Lindblom, P.; Strittmatter, K.; et al. Pericytes regulate the blood-brain barrier. *Nature* **2010**, *468*, 557–561. [CrossRef]
47. Daneman, R.; Zhou, L.; Kebede, A.A.; Barres, B.A. Pericytes are required for blood-brain barrier integrity during embryogenesis. *Nature* **2010**, *468*, 562–566. [CrossRef] [PubMed]
48. Nikolakopoulou, A.M.; Montagne, A.; Kisler, K.; Dai, Z.; Wang, Y.; Huuskonen, M.T.; Sagare, A.P.; Lazic, D.; Sweeney, M.D.; Kong, P.; et al. Pericyte loss leads to circulatory failure and pleiotrophin depletion causing neuron loss. *Nat. Neurosci.* **2019**, *22*, 1089–1098. [CrossRef]
49. Ben-Zvi, A.; Lacoste, B.; Kur, E.; Andreone, B.J.; Mayshar, Y.; Yan, H.; Gu, C. Mfsd2a is critical for the formation and function of the blood–brain barrier. *Nature* **2014**, *509*, 507–511. [CrossRef]
50. Shulman, Z.; Cohen, S.J.; Roediger, B.; Kalchenko, V.; Jain, R.; Grabovsky, V.; Klein, E.; Shinder, V.; Stoler-Barak, L.; Feigelson, S.W.; et al. Transendothelial migration of lymphocytes mediated by intraendothelial vesicle stores rather than by extracellular chemokine depots. *Nat. Immunol.* **2012**, *13*, 67–76. [CrossRef]
51. Török, O.; Schreiner, B.; Schaffenrath, J.; Tsai, H.-C.; Maheshwari, U.; Stifter, S.A.; Welsh, C.; Amorim, A.; Sridhar, S.; Utz, S.G.; et al. Pericytes regulate vascular immune homeostasis in the CNS. *Proc. Natl. Acad. Sci. USA* **2021**, *118*, e2016587118. [CrossRef]
52. Park, J.S.; Kim, I.K.; Han, S.; Park, I.; Kim, C.; Bae, J.; Oh, S.J.; Lee, S.; Kim, J.H.; Woo, D.C.; et al. Normalization of Tumor Vessels by Tie2 Activation and Ang2 Inhibition Enhances Drug Delivery and Produces a Favorable Tumor Microenvironment. *Cancer Cell* **2016**, *30*, 953–967. [CrossRef]
53. Zhou, W.; Chen, C.; Shi, Y.; Wu, Q.; Gimple, R.C.; Fang, X.; Huang, Z.; Zhai, K.; Ke, S.Q.; Ping, Y.F.; et al. Targeting Glioma Stem Cell-Derived Pericytes Disrupts the Blood-Tumor Barrier and Improves Chemotherapeutic Efficacy. *Cell Stem Cell* **2017**, *21*, 591–603.e594. [CrossRef]
54. Zhang, X.-N.; Yang, K.-D.; Chen, C.; He, Z.-C.; Wang, Q.-H.; Feng, H.; Lv, S.-Q.; Wang, Y.; Mao, M.; Liu, Q.; et al. Pericytes augment glioblastoma cell resistance to temozolomide through CCL5-CCR5 paracrine signaling. *Cell Res.* **2021**, *31*, 1072–1087. [CrossRef] [PubMed]
55. Berthiaume, A.A.; Grant, R.I.; McDowell, K.P.; Underly, R.G.; Hartmann, D.A.; Levy, M.; Bhat, N.R.; Shih, A.Y. Dynamic Remodeling of Pericytes In Vivo Maintains Capillary Coverage in the Adult Mouse Brain. *Cell Rep.* **2018**, *22*, 8–16. [CrossRef] [PubMed]
56. Schlecker, E.; Stojanovic, A.; Eisen, C.; Quack, C.; Falk, C.S.; Umansky, V.; Cerwenka, A. Tumor-infiltrating monocytic myeloid-derived suppressor cells mediate CCR5-dependent recruitment of regulatory T cells favoring tumor growth. *J. Immunol.* **2012**, *189*, 5602–5611. [CrossRef]
57. Pozo-Balado, M.M.; Martínez-Bonet, M.; Rosado, I.; Ruiz-Mateos, E.; Méndez-Lagares, G.; Rodríguez-Méndez, M.M.; Vidal, F.; Muñoz-Fernández, M.A.; Pacheco, Y.M.; Leal, M. Maraviroc Reduces the Regulatory T-Cell Frequency in Antiretroviral-Naive HIV-Infected Subjects. *J. Infect. Dis.* **2014**, *210*, 890–898. [CrossRef] [PubMed]
58. Moreno-Fernandez, M.E.; Zapata, W.; Blackard, J.T.; Franchini, G.; Chougnet, C.A. Human regulatory T cells are targets for human immunodeficiency Virus (HIV) infection, and their susceptibility differs depending on the HIV type 1 strain. *J. Virol.* **2009**, *83*, 12925–12933. [CrossRef]
59. Halama, N.; Zoernig, I.; Berthel, A.; Kahlert, C.; Klupp, F.; Suarez-Carmona, M.; Suetterlin, T.; Brand, K.; Krauss, J.; Lasitschka, F.; et al. Tumoral Immune Cell Exploitation in Colorectal Cancer Metastases Can Be Targeted Effectively by Anti-CCR5 Therapy in Cancer Patients. *Cancer Cell* **2016**, *29*, 587–601. [CrossRef]
60. Joy, M.T.; Ben Assayag, E.; Shabashov-Stone, D.; Liraz-Zaltsman, S.; Mazzitelli, J.; Arenas, M.; Abduljawad, N.; Kliper, E.; Korczyn, A.D.; Thareja, N.S.; et al. CCR5 Is a Therapeutic Target for Recovery after Stroke and Traumatic Brain Injury. *Cell* **2019**, *176*, 1143–1157.e1113. [CrossRef] [PubMed]
61. Struyf, S.; Menten, P.; Lenaerts, J.P.; Put, W.; D'Haese, A.; De Clercq, E.; Schols, D.; Proost, P.; Van Damme, J. Diverging binding capacities of natural LD78beta isoforms of macrophage inflammatory protein-1alpha to the CC chemokine receptors 1, 3 and 5 affect their anti-HIV-1 activity and chemotactic potencies for neutrophils and eosinophils. *Eur. J. Immunol.* **2001**, *31*, 2170–2178. [CrossRef]

62. Liu, J.Y.; Li, F.; Wang, L.P.; Chen, X.F.; Wang, D.; Cao, L.; Ping, Y.; Zhao, S.; Li, B.; Thorne, S.H.; et al. CTL- vs Treg lymphocyte-attracting chemokines, CCL4 and CCL20, are strong reciprocal predictive markers for survival of patients with oesophageal squamous cell carcinoma. *Br. J. Cancer* **2015**, *113*, 747–755. [CrossRef] [PubMed]
63. Wang, Y.; Liu, T.; Yang, N.; Xu, S.; Li, X.; Wang, D. Hypoxia and macrophages promote glioblastoma invasion by the CCL4-CCR5 axis. *Oncol. Rep.* **2016**, *36*, 3522–3528. [CrossRef] [PubMed]
64. Sallusto, F.; Lenig, D.; Förster, R.; Lipp, M.; Lanzavecchia, A. Two subsets of memory T lymphocytes with distinct homing potentials and effector functions. *Nature* **1999**, *401*, 708–712. [CrossRef]
65. Joshi, N.S.; Cui, W.; Chandele, A.; Lee, H.K.; Urso, D.R.; Hagman, J.; Gapin, L.; Kaech, S.M. Inflammation directs memory precursor and short-lived effector CD8(+) T cell fates via the graded expression of T-bet transcription factor. *Immunity* **2007**, *27*, 281–295. [CrossRef]
66. Intlekofer, A.M.; Takemoto, N.; Wherry, E.J.; Longworth, S.A.; Northrup, J.T.; Palanivel, V.R.; Mullen, A.C.; Gasink, C.R.; Kaech, S.M.; Miller, J.D.; et al. Effector and memory CD8$^+$ T cell fate coupled by T-bet and eomesodermin. *Nat. Immunol.* **2005**, *6*, 1236–1244. [CrossRef]
67. Rutishauser, R.L.; Martins, G.A.; Kalachikov, S.; Chandele, A.; Parish, I.A.; Meffre, E.; Jacob, J.; Calame, K.; Kaech, S.M. Transcriptional repressor Blimp-1 promotes CD8(+) T cell terminal differentiation and represses the acquisition of central memory T cell properties. *Immunity* **2009**, *31*, 296–308. [CrossRef]
68. Cannarile, M.A.; Lind, N.A.; Rivera, R.; Sheridan, A.D.; Camfield, K.A.; Wu, B.B.; Cheung, K.P.; Ding, Z.; Goldrath, A.W. Transcriptional regulator Id2 mediates CD8$^+$ T cell immunity. *Nat. Immunol.* **2006**, *7*, 1317–1325. [CrossRef] [PubMed]
69. Yang, C.Y.; Best, J.A.; Knell, J.; Yang, E.; Sheridan, A.D.; Jesionek, A.K.; Li, H.S.; Rivera, R.R.; Lind, K.C.; D'Cruz, L.M.; et al. The transcriptional regulators Id2 and Id3 control the formation of distinct memory CD8$^+$ T cell subsets. *Nat. Immunol.* **2011**, *12*, 1221–1229. [CrossRef] [PubMed]
70. Soeda, A.; Hara, A.; Kunisada, T.; Yoshimura, S.-i.; Iwama, T.; Park, D.M. The Evidence of Glioblastoma Heterogeneity. *Sci. Rep.* **2015**, *5*, 1–7. [CrossRef]
71. Hickey, W.F.; Hsu, B.L.; Kimura, H. T-lymphocyte entry into the central nervous system. *J. Neurosci. Res.* **1991**, *28*, 254–260. [CrossRef] [PubMed]
72. Calzascia, T.; Masson, F.; Di Berardino-Besson, W.; Contassot, E.; Wilmotte, R.; Aurrand-Lions, M.; Rüegg, C.; Dietrich, P.Y.; Walker, P.R. Homing phenotypes of tumor-specific CD8 T cells are predetermined at the tumor site by crosspresenting APCs. *Immunity* **2005**, *22*, 175–184. [CrossRef]
73. Ogawa, M.; Tsutsui, T.; Zou, J.P.; Mu, J.; Wijesuriya, R.; Yu, W.G.; Herrmann, S.; Kubo, T.; Fujiwara, H.; Hamaoka, T. Enhanced induction of very late antigen 4/lymphocyte function-associated antigen 1-dependent T-cell migration to tumor sites following administration of interleukin 12. *Cancer Res.* **1997**, *57*, 2216–2222. [PubMed]
74. Odoardi, F.; Sie, C.; Streyl, K.; Ulaganathan, V.K.; Schläger, C.; Lodygin, D.; Heckelsmiller, K.; Nietfeld, W.; Ellwart, J.; Klinkert, W.E.; et al. T cells become licensed in the lung to enter the central nervous system. *Nature* **2012**, *488*, 675–679. [CrossRef] [PubMed]
75. Karin, N. CXCR3 Ligands in Cancer and Autoimmunity, Chemoattraction of Effector T Cells, and Beyond. *Front. Immunol.* **2020**, *11*, 976. [CrossRef] [PubMed]
76. Korn, T.; Kallies, A. T cell responses in the central nervous system. *Nat. Rev. Immunol.* **2017**, *17*, 179–194. [CrossRef]
77. Smith, J.S.; Alagesan, P.; Desai, N.K.; Pack, T.F.; Wu, J.-H.; Inoue, A.; Freedman, N.J.; Rajagopal, S. CXC motif chemokine receptor 3 splice variants differentially activate beta-arrestins to regulate downstream signaling pathways. *Mol. Pharmacol.* **2017**, *92*, 136–150. [CrossRef]
78. Nishimura, F.; Dusak, J.E.; Eguchi, J.; Zhu, X.; Gambotto, A.; Storkus, W.J.; Okada, H. Adoptive transfer of type 1 CTL mediates effective anti–central nervous system tumor response: Critical roles of IFN-inducible protein-10. *Cancer Res.* **2006**, *66*, 4478–4487. [CrossRef]
79. Maru, S.V.; Holloway, K.A.; Flynn, G.; Lancashire, C.L.; Loughlin, A.J.; Male, D.K.; Romero, I.A. Chemokine production and chemokine receptor expression by human glioma cells: Role of CXCL10 in tumour cell proliferation. *J. Neuroimmunol.* **2008**, *199*, 35–45. [CrossRef]
80. Barreira da Silva, R.; Laird, M.E.; Yatim, N.; Fiette, L.; Ingersoll, M.A.; Albert, M.L. Dipeptidylpeptidase 4 inhibition enhances lymphocyte trafficking, improving both naturally occurring tumor immunity and immunotherapy. *Nat. Immunol.* **2015**, *16*, 850–858. [CrossRef] [PubMed]
81. Busek, P.; Stremenova, J.; Sromova, L.; Hilser, M.; Balaziova, E.; Kosek, D.; Trylcova, J.; Strnad, H.; Krepela, E.; Sedo, A. Dipeptidyl peptidase-IV inhibits glioma cell growth independent of its enzymatic activity. *Int. J. Biochem. Cell Biol.* **2012**, *44*, 738–747. [CrossRef]
82. Zhu, X.; Fallert-Junecko, B.A.; Fujita, M.; Ueda, R.; Kohanbash, G.; Kastenhuber, E.R.; McDonald, H.A.; Liu, Y.; Kalinski, P.; Reinhart, T.A.; et al. Poly-ICLC promotes the infiltration of effector T cells into intracranial gliomas via induction of CXCL10 in IFN-alpha and IFN-gamma dependent manners. *Cancer Immunol. Immunother.* **2010**, *59*, 1401–1409. [CrossRef]
83. Sarkaria, J.N.; Hu, L.S.; Parney, I.F.; Pafundi, D.H.; Brinkmann, D.H.; Laack, N.N.; Giannini, C.; Burns, T.C.; Kizilbash, S.H.; Laramy, J.K.; et al. Is the blood-brain barrier really disrupted in all glioblastomas? A critical assessment of existing clinical data. *Neuro-Oncology* **2018**, *20*, 184–191. [CrossRef] [PubMed]
84. Kotrotsou, A.; Elakkad, A.; Sun, J.; Thomas, G.A.; Yang, D.; Abrol, S.; Wei, W.; Weinberg, J.S.; Bakhtiari, A.S.; Kircher, M.F.; et al. Multi-center study finds postoperative residual non-enhancing component of glioblastoma as a new determinant of patient outcome. *J. Neuro-Oncol.* **2018**, *139*, 125–133. [CrossRef] [PubMed]
85. Turner, N.; Grose, R. Fibroblast growth factor signalling: From development to cancer. *Nat. Rev. Cancer* **2010**, *10*, 116–129. [CrossRef] [PubMed]

86. Bastola, S.; Pavlyukov, M.S.; Yamashita, D.; Ghosh, S.; Cho, H.; Kagaya, N.; Zhang, Z.; Minata, M.; Lee, Y.; Sadahiro, H.; et al. Glioma-initiating cells at tumor edge gain signals from tumor core cells to promote their malignancy. *Nat. Commun.* **2020**, *11*, 4660. [CrossRef] [PubMed]
87. Darmanis, S.; Sloan, S.A.; Croote, D.; Mignardi, M.; Chernikova, S.; Samghababi, P.; Zhang, Y.; Neff, N.; Kowarsky, M.; Caneda, C.; et al. Single-Cell RNA-Seq Analysis of Infiltrating Neoplastic Cells at the Migrating Front of Human Glioblastoma. *Cell Rep.* **2017**, *21*, 1399–1410. [CrossRef]
88. Platten, M.; Wick, W.; Weller, M. Malignant glioma biology: Role for TGF-β in growth, motility, angiogenesis, and immune escape. *Microsc. Res. Tech.* **2001**, *52*, 401–410. [CrossRef]
89. Li, C.; Jiang, P.; Wei, S.; Xu, X.; Wang, J. Regulatory T cells in tumor microenvironment: New mechanisms, potential therapeutic strategies and future prospects. *Mol. Cancer* **2020**, *19*, 116. [CrossRef] [PubMed]
90. Chang, A.L.; Miska, J.; Wainwright, D.A.; Dey, M.; Rivetta, C.V.; Yu, D.; Kanojia, D.; Pituch, K.C.; Qiao, J.; Pytel, P.; et al. CCL2 Produced by the Glioma Microenvironment Is Essential for the Recruitment of Regulatory T Cells and Myeloid-Derived Suppressor Cells. *Cancer Res.* **2016**, *76*, 5671–5682. [CrossRef] [PubMed]
91. Pan, Y.; Smithson, L.J.; Ma, Y.; Hambardzumyan, D.; Gutmann, D.H. Ccl5 establishes an autocrine high-grade glioma growth regulatory circuit critical for mesenchymal glioblastoma survival. *Oncotarget* **2017**, *8*, 32977–32989. [CrossRef]
92. Vanlandewijck, M.; He, L.; Mäe, M.A.; Andrae, J.; Ando, K.; Del Gaudio, F.; Nahar, K.; Lebouvier, T.; Laviña, B.; Gouveia, L.; et al. A molecular atlas of cell types and zonation in the brain vasculature. *Nature* **2018**, *554*, 475–480. [CrossRef] [PubMed]
93. Wolburg, H.; Wolburg-Buchholz, K.; Engelhardt, B. Diapedesis of mononuclear cells across cerebral venules during experimental autoimmune encephalomyelitis leaves tight junctions intact. *Acta Neuropathol.* **2005**, *109*, 181–190. [CrossRef]
94. Wälchli, T.; Ghobrial, M.; Schwab, M.; Takada, S.; Zhong, H.; Suntharalingham, S.; Vetiska, S.; Rodrigues Rodrigues, D.; Rehrauer, H.; Wu, R.; et al. Molecular atlas of the human brain vasculature at the single-cell level. *bioRxiv* **2021**. [CrossRef]
95. Castro Dias, M.; Odriozola Quesada, A.; Soldati, S.; Bösch, F.; Gruber, I.; Hildbrand, T.; Sönmez, D.; Khire, T.; Witz, G.; McGrath, J.L.; et al. Brain endothelial tricellular junctions as novel sites for T cell diapedesis across the blood-brain barrier. *J. Cell Sci.* **2021**, *134*, jcs253880. [CrossRef] [PubMed]
96. Ikenouchi, J.; Furuse, M.; Furuse, K.; Sasaki, H.; Tsukita, S.; Tsukita, S. Tricellulin constitutes a novel barrier at tricellular contacts of epithelial cells. *J. Cell Biol.* **2005**, *171*, 939–945. [CrossRef]
97. Fujita, K.; Katahira, J.; Horiguchi, Y.; Sonoda, N.; Furuse, M.; Tsukita, S. *Clostridium Perfringens* enterotoxin binds to the second extracellular loop of claudin-3, a tight junction integral membrane protein. *FEBS Lett.* **2000**, *476*, 258–261. [CrossRef]
98. Veshnyakova, A.; Piontek, J.; Protze, J.; Waziri, N.; Heise, I.; Krause, G. Mechanism of *Clostridium Perfringens* enterotoxin interaction with claudin-3/-4 protein suggests structural modifications of the toxin to target specific claudins. *J. Biol. Chem.* **2012**, *287*, 1698–1708. [CrossRef] [PubMed]
99. Taddei, A.; Giampietro, C.; Conti, A.; Orsenigo, F.; Breviario, F.; Pirazzoli, V.; Potente, M.; Daly, C.; Dimmeler, S.; Dejana, E. Endothelial adherens junctions control tight junctions by VE-cadherin-mediated upregulation of claudin-5. *Nat. Cell Biol.* **2008**, *10*, 923–934. [CrossRef]
100. Nitta, T.; Hata, M.; Gotoh, S.; Seo, Y.; Sasaki, H.; Hashimoto, N.; Furuse, M.; Tsukita, S. Size-selective loosening of the blood-brain barrier in claudin-5-deficient mice. *J. Cell Biol.* **2003**, *161*, 653–660. [CrossRef] [PubMed]
101. Greene, C.; Hanley, N.; Campbell, M. Claudin-5: Gatekeeper of neurological function. *Fluids Barriers CNS* **2019**, *16*, 3. [CrossRef]
102. Neuhaus, W.; Piontek, A.; Protze, J.; Eichner, M.; Mahringer, A.; Subileau, E.A.; Lee, I.M.; Schulzke, J.D.; Krause, G.; Piontek, J. Reversible opening of the blood-brain barrier by claudin-5-binding variants of *Clostridium Perfringens* enterotoxin's claudin-binding domain. *Biomaterials* **2018**, *161*, 129–143. [CrossRef]
103. Paul, D.; Baena, V.; Ge, S.; Jiang, X.; Jellison, E.R.; Kiprono, T.; Agalliu, D.; Pachter, J.S. Appearance of claudin-5(+) leukocytes in the central nervous system during neuroinflammation: A novel role for endothelial-derived extracellular vesicles. *J. Neuroinflamm.* **2016**, *13*, 292. [CrossRef] [PubMed]
104. Wimmer, I.; Tietz, S.; Nishihara, H.; Deutsch, U.; Sallusto, F.; Gosselet, F.; Lyck, R.; Muller, W.A.; Lassmann, H.; Engelhardt, B. PECAM-1 Stabilizes Blood-Brain Barrier Integrity and Favors Paracellular T-Cell Diapedesis Across the Blood-Brain Barrier During Neuroinflammation. *Front. Immunol.* **2019**, *10*, 711. [CrossRef]
105. Nag, S. Ultracytochemical studies of the compromised blood-brain barrier. *Methods Mol. Med.* **2003**, *89*, 145–160. [CrossRef] [PubMed]
106. Claudio, L.; Brosnan, C.F. Effects of prazosin on the blood-brain barrier during experimental autoimmune encephalomyelitis. *Brain Res.* **1992**, *594*, 233–243. [CrossRef]
107. Millán, J.; Hewlett, L.; Glyn, M.; Toomre, D.; Clark, P.; Ridley, A.J. Lymphocyte transcellular migration occurs through recruitment of endothelial ICAM-1 to caveola- and F-actin-rich domains. *Nat. Cell Biol.* **2006**, *8*, 113–123. [CrossRef]
108. Abadier, M.; Haghayegh Jahromi, N.; Cardoso Alves, L.; Boscacci, R.; Vestweber, D.; Barnum, S.; Deutsch, U.; Engelhardt, B.; Lyck, R. Cell surface levels of endothelial ICAM-1 influence the transcellular or paracellular T-cell diapedesis across the blood–brain barrier. *Eur. J. Immunol.* **2015**, *45*, 1043–1058. [CrossRef] [PubMed]
109. Lutz, S.E.; Smith, J.R.; Kim, D.H.; Olson, C.V.L.; Ellefsen, K.; Bates, J.M.; Gandhi, S.P.; Agalliu, D. Caveolin1 Is Required for Th1 Cell Infiltration, but Not Tight Junction Remodeling, at the Blood-Brain Barrier in Autoimmune Neuroinflammation. *Cell Rep.* **2017**, *21*, 2104–2117. [CrossRef]
110. Engelhardt, B.; Carare, R.O.; Bechmann, I.; Flügel, A.; Laman, J.D.; Weller, R.O. Vascular, glial, and lymphatic immune gateways of the central nervous system. *Acta Neuropathol.* **2016**, *132*, 317–338. [CrossRef]

111. Reboldi, A.; Coisne, C.; Baumjohann, D.; Benvenuto, F.; Bottinelli, D.; Lira, S.; Uccelli, A.; Lanzavecchia, A.; Engelhardt, B.; Sallusto, F. C-C chemokine receptor 6-regulated entry of TH-17 cells into the CNS through the choroid plexus is required for the initiation of EAE. *Nat. Immunol.* **2009**, *10*, 514–523. [CrossRef] [PubMed]
112. Kondo, T.; Takata, H.; Takiguchi, M. Functional expression of chemokine receptor CCR6 on human effector memory CD8$^+$ T cells. *Eur. J. Immunol.* **2007**, *37*, 54–65. [CrossRef] [PubMed]
113. Liao, L.-S.; Zhang, M.-W.; Gu, Y.-J.; Sun, X.-C. Targeting CCL20 inhibits subarachnoid hemorrhage-related neuroinflammation in mice. *Aging* **2020**, *12*, 14849–14862. [CrossRef] [PubMed]
114. Hippe, A.; Braun, S.A.; Oláh, P.; Gerber, P.A.; Schorr, A.; Seeliger, S.; Holtz, S.; Jannasch, K.; Pivarcsi, A.; Buhren, B.; et al. EGFR/Ras-induced CCL20 production modulates the tumour microenvironment. *Br. J. Cancer* **2020**, *123*, 942–954. [CrossRef]
115. Fantini, M.C.; Becker, C.; Monteleone, G.; Pallone, F.; Galle, P.R.; Neurath, M.F. Cutting edge: TGF-beta induces a regulatory phenotype in CD4$^+$CD25$^-$ T cells through Foxp3 induction and down-regulation of Smad7. *J. Immunol.* **2004**, *172*, 5149–5153. [CrossRef]
116. Rivino, L.; Gruarin, P.; Häringer, B.; Steinfelder, S.; Lozza, L.; Steckel, B.; Weick, A.; Sugliano, E.; Jarrossay, D.; Kühl, A.A.; et al. CCR6 is expressed on an IL-10–producing, autoreactive memory T cell population with context-dependent regulatory function. *J. Exp. Med.* **2010**, *207*, 565–577. [CrossRef]
117. Krumbholz, M.; Theil, D.; Steinmeyer, F.; Cepok, S.; Hemmer, B.; Hofbauer, M.; Farina, C.; Derfuss, T.; Junker, A.; Arzberger, T.; et al. CCL19 is constitutively expressed in the CNS, up-regulated in neuroinflammation, active and also inactive multiple sclerosis lesions. *J. Neuroimmunol.* **2007**, *190*, 72–79. [CrossRef]
118. Yan, Y.; Zhao, W.; Liu, W.; Li, Y.; Wang, X.; Xun, J.; Davgadorj, C. CCL19 enhances CD8(+) T-cell responses and accelerates HBV clearance. *J. Gastroenterol.* **2021**, *56*, 769–785. [CrossRef]
119. Ponda, M.P.; Breslow, J.L. Serum stimulation of CCR7 chemotaxis due to coagulation factor XIIa-dependent production of high-molecular-weight kininogen domain 5. *Proc. Natl. Acad. Sci. USA* **2016**, *113*, E7059–E7068. [CrossRef]
120. Schneider, M.A.; Meingassner, J.G.; Lipp, M.; Moore, H.D.; Rot, A. CCR7 is required for the in vivo function of CD4$^+$ CD25$^+$ regulatory T cells. *J. Exp. Med.* **2007**, *204*, 735–745. [CrossRef]
121. Greter, M.; Heppner, F.L.; Lemos, M.P.; Odermatt, B.M.; Goebels, N.; Laufer, T.; Noelle, R.J.; Becher, B. Dendritic cells permit immune invasion of the CNS in an animal model of multiple sclerosis. *Nat. Med.* **2005**, *11*, 328–334. [CrossRef]
122. Owens, T.; Bechmann, I.; Engelhardt, B. Perivascular Spaces and the Two Steps to Neuroinflammation. *J. Neuropathol. Exp. Neurol.* **2008**, *67*, 1113–1121. [CrossRef]
123. Mundt, S.; Mrdjen, D.; Utz, S.G.; Greter, M.; Schreiner, B.; Becher, B. Conventional DCs sample and present myelin antigens in the healthy CNS and allow parenchymal T cell entry to initiate neuroinflammation. *Sci. Immunol.* **2019**, *4*. [CrossRef]
124. Agrawal, S.; Anderson, P.; Durbeej, M.; van Rooijen, N.; Ivars, F.; Opdenakker, G.; Sorokin, L.M. Dystroglycan is selectively cleaved at the parenchymal basement membrane at sites of leukocyte extravasation in experimental autoimmune encephalomyelitis. *J. Exp. Med.* **2006**, *203*, 1007–1019. [CrossRef]
125. Tzartos, J.S.; Friese, M.A.; Craner, M.J.; Palace, J.; Newcombe, J.; Esiri, M.M.; Fugger, L. Interleukin-17 production in central nervous system-infiltrating T cells and glial cells is associated with active disease in multiple sclerosis. *Am. J. Pathol.* **2008**, *172*, 146–155. [CrossRef]
126. Zhang, X.; Wang, Y.; Song, J.; Gerwien, H.; Chuquisana, O.; Chashchina, A.; Denz, C.; Sorokin, L. The endothelial basement membrane acts as a checkpoint for entry of pathogenic T cells into the brain. *J. Exp. Med.* **2020**, *217*, e20191339. [CrossRef]
127. Sixt, M.; Engelhardt, B.; Pausch, F.; Hallmann, R.; Wendler, O.; Sorokin, L.M. Endothelial cell laminin isoforms, laminins 8 and 10, play decisive roles in T cell recruitment across the blood-brain barrier in experimental autoimmune encephalomyelitis. *J. Cell Biol.* **2001**, *153*, 933–946. [CrossRef] [PubMed]
128. Pullen, N.A.; Anand, M.; Cooper, P.S.; Fillmore, H.L. Matrix metalloproteinase-1 expression enhances tumorigenicity as well as tumor-related angiogenesis and is inversely associated with TIMP-4 expression in a model of glioblastoma. *J. Neuro-Oncol.* **2012**, *106*, 461–471. [CrossRef]
129. Steward, W.P.; Thomas, A.L. Marimastat: The clinical development of a matrix metalloproteinase inhibitor. *Expert Opin. Investig. Drugs* **2000**, *9*, 2913–2922. [CrossRef] [PubMed]
130. Butler, G.S.; Overall, C.M. Updated biological roles for matrix metalloproteinases and new "intracellular" substrates revealed by degradomics. *Biochemistry* **2009**, *48*, 10830–10845. [CrossRef]
131. McCandless, E.E.; Wang, Q.; Woerner, B.M.; Harper, J.M.; Klein, R.S. CXCL12 limits inflammation by localizing mononuclear infiltrates to the perivascular space during experimental autoimmune encephalomyelitis. *J. Immunol.* **2006**, *177*, 8053–8064. [CrossRef]
132. Cruz-Orengo, L.; Holman, D.W.; Dorsey, D.; Zhou, L.; Zhang, P.; Wright, M.; McCandless, E.E.; Patel, J.R.; Luker, G.D.; Littman, D.R.; et al. CXCR7 influences leukocyte entry into the CNS parenchyma by controlling abluminal CXCL12 abundance during autoimmunity. *J. Exp. Med.* **2011**, *208*, 327–339. [CrossRef]
133. Wiatr, M.; Stump-Guthier, C.; Latorre, D.; Uhlig, S.; Weiss, C.; Ilonen, J.; Engelhardt, B.; Ishikawa, H.; Schwerk, C.; Schroten, H.; et al. Distinct migratory pattern of naive and effector T cells through the blood-CSF barrier following Echovirus 30 infection. *J. Neuroinflamm.* **2019**, *16*, 232. [CrossRef] [PubMed]
134. Zohar, Y.; Wildbaum, G.; Novak, R.; Salzman, A.L.; Thelen, M.; Alon, R.; Barshesket, Y.; Karp, C.L.; Karin, N. CXCL11-dependent induction of FOXP3-negative regulatory T cells suppresses autoimmune encephalomyelitis. *J. Clin. Investig.* **2014**, *124*, 2009–2022. [CrossRef]

135. Haynes, A.B.; Weiser, T.G.; Berry, W.R.; Lipsitz, S.R.; Breizat, A.H.; Dellinger, E.P.; Herbosa, T.; Joseph, S.; Kibatala, P.L.; Lapitan, M.C.; et al. A surgical safety checklist to reduce morbidity and mortality in a global population. *New Engl. J. Med.* **2009**, *360*, 491–499. [CrossRef]
136. Jordan, J.T.; Sun, W.; Hussain, S.F.; DeAngulo, G.; Prabhu, S.S.; Heimberger, A.B. Preferential migration of regulatory T cells mediated by glioma-secreted chemokines can be blocked with chemotherapy. *Cancer Immunol. Immunother.* **2008**, *57*, 123–131. [CrossRef] [PubMed]
137. Gotsch, U.; Jäger, U.; Dominis, M.; Vestweber, D. Expression of P-selectin on endothelial cells is upregulated by LPS and TNF-alpha in vivo. *Cell Adhes. Commun.* **1994**, *2*, 7–14. [CrossRef] [PubMed]
138. Cloughesy, T.F.; Mochizuki, A.Y.; Orpilla, J.R.; Hugo, W.; Lee, A.H.; Davidson, T.B.; Wang, A.C.; Ellingson, B.M.; Rytlewski, J.A.; Sanders, C.M.; et al. Neoadjuvant anti-PD-1 immunotherapy promotes a survival benefit with intratumoral and systemic immune responses in recurrent glioblastoma. *Nat. Med.* **2019**, *25*, 477–486. [CrossRef] [PubMed]
139. Strickland, M.; Stoll, E.A. Metabolic Reprogramming in Glioma. *Front. Cell Dev. Biol.* **2017**, *5*, 43. [CrossRef] [PubMed]
140. Poff, A.; Koutnik, A.P.; Egan, K.M.; Sahebjam, S.; D'Agostino, D.; Kumar, N.B. Targeting the Warburg effect for cancer treatment: Ketogenic diets for management of glioma. *Semin. Cancer Biol.* **2019**, *56*, 135–148. [CrossRef]
141. Macintyre, A.N.; Gerriets, V.A.; Nichols, A.G.; Michalek, R.D.; Rudolph, M.C.; Deoliveira, D.; Anderson, S.M.; Abel, E.D.; Chen, B.J.; Hale, L.P.; et al. The glucose transporter Glut1 is selectively essential for CD4 T cell activation and effector function. *Cell Metab.* **2014**, *20*, 61–72. [CrossRef] [PubMed]
142. Mauro, C.; Fu, H.; Marelli-Berg, F.M. T cell trafficking and metabolism: Novel mechanisms and targets for immunomodulation. *Curr. Opin. Pharm.* **2012**, *12*, 452–457. [CrossRef] [PubMed]
143. Marelli-Berg, F.M.; Jangani, M. Metabolic regulation of leukocyte motility and migration. *J. Leukoc. Biol.* **2018**, *104*, 285–293. [CrossRef]
144. Chapman, N.M.; Boothby, M.R.; Chi, H. Metabolic coordination of T cell quiescence and activation. *Nat. Rev. Immunol.* **2020**, *20*, 55–70. [CrossRef] [PubMed]
145. Lim, A.R.; Rathmell, W.K.; Rathmell, J.C. The tumor microenvironment as a metabolic barrier to effector T cells and immunotherapy. *Elife* **2020**, *9*, e55185. [CrossRef] [PubMed]
146. Haas, R.; Smith, J.; Rocher-Ros, V.; Nadkarni, S.; Montero-Melendez, T.; D'Acquisto, F.; Bland, E.J.; Bombardieri, M.; Pitzalis, C.; Perretti, M.; et al. Lactate Regulates Metabolic and Pro-inflammatory Circuits in Control of T Cell Migration and Effector Functions. *PLoS Biol.* **2015**, *13*, e1002202. [CrossRef]
147. Fischer, K.; Hoffmann, P.; Voelkl, S.; Meidenbauer, N.; Ammer, J.; Edinger, M.; Gottfried, E.; Schwarz, S.; Rothe, G.; Hoves, S.; et al. Inhibitory effect of tumor cell-derived lactic acid on human T cells. *Blood* **2007**, *109*, 3812–3819. [CrossRef] [PubMed]
148. Hu, J.; Mao, Y.; Li, M.; Lu, Y. The profile of Th17 subset in glioma. *Int. Immunopharmacol.* **2011**, *11*, 1173–1179. [CrossRef] [PubMed]
149. Kramer, P.A.; Chacko, B.K.; George, D.J.; Zhi, D.; Wei, C.C.; Dell'Italia, L.J.; Melby, S.J.; George, J.F.; Darley-Usmar, V.M. Decreased Bioenergetic Health Index in monocytes isolated from the pericardial fluid and blood of post-operative cardiac surgery patients. *Biosci. Rep.* **2015**, *35*, e00237. [CrossRef]
150. Oelkrug, C.; Ramage, J.M. Enhancement of T cell recruitment and infiltration into tumours. *Clin. Exp. Immunol.* **2014**, *178*, 1–8. [CrossRef]
151. You, R.; Artichoker, J.; Fries, A.; Edwards, A.W.; Combes, A.J.; Reeder, G.C.; Samad, B.; Krummel, M.F. Active surveillance characterizes human intratumoral T cell exhaustion. *J. Clin. Investig.* **2021**, *131*. [CrossRef]
152. Kloog, Y.; Mor, A. Cytotoxic-T-lymphocyte antigen 4 receptor signaling for lymphocyte adhesion is mediated by C3G and Rap1. *Mol. Cell. Biol.* **2014**, *34*, 978–988. [CrossRef]
153. Finlay, D.; Cantrell, D.A. Metabolism, migration and memory in cytotoxic T cells. *Nat. Rev. Immunol.* **2011**, *11*, 109–117. [CrossRef]
154. Garris, C.S.; Blaho, V.A.; Hla, T.; Han, M.H. Sphingosine-1-phosphate receptor 1 signalling in T cells: Trafficking and beyond. *Immunology* **2014**, *142*, 347–353. [CrossRef] [PubMed]
155. Chongsathidkiet, P.; Jackson, C.; Koyama, S.; Loebel, F.; Cui, X.; Farber, S.H.; Woroniecka, K.; Elsamadicy, A.A.; Dechant, C.A.; Kemeny, H.R.; et al. Sequestration of T cells in bone marrow in the setting of glioblastoma and other intracranial tumors. *Nat. Med.* **2018**, *24*, 1459–1468. [CrossRef]
156. Wilkinson, D.S.; Chongsathidkiet, P.; Dechant, C.; Fecci, P. Sphingosine-1-phosphate receptor 1 (S1P1) loss mediates T cell sequestration in bone marrow in the setting of intracranial tumors: A novel mode of cancer-induced immunosuppression. *J. Immunol.* **2019**, *202*, 138.135.
157. Wilkinson, D.S.; Champion, C.; Chongsathidkiet, P.; Wang, H.; Laskowitz, D.; Fecci, P. Bone marrow T cell sequestration as a novel mode of CNS immune privilege. *J. Immunol.* **2020**, *204*, 78.14.
158. Rogel, A.; Willoughby, J.E.; Buchan, S.L.; Leonard, H.J.; Thirdborough, S.M.; Al-Shamkhani, A. Akt signaling is critical for memory CD8(+) T-cell development and tumor immune surveillance. *Proc. Natl. Acad. Sci. USA* **2017**, *114*, E1178–E1187. [CrossRef] [PubMed]
159. Joy, A.; Kapoor, M.; Georges, J.; Butler, L.; Chang, Y.; Li, C.; Crouch, A.; Smirnov, I.; Nakada, M.; Hepler, J.; et al. The role of AKT isoforms in glioblastoma: AKT3 delays tumor progression. *J. Neuro-Oncol.* **2016**, *130*, 43–52. [CrossRef]
160. Quambusch, L.; Depta, L.; Landel, I.; Lubeck, M.; Kirschner, T.; Nabert, J.; Uhlenbrock, N.; Weisner, J.; Kostka, M.; Levy, L.M.; et al. Cellular model system to dissect the isoform-selectivity of Akt inhibitors. *Nat. Commun.* **2021**, *12*, 5297. [CrossRef]
161. Abu Eid, R.; Friedman, K.M.; Mkrtichyan, M.; Walens, A.; King, W.; Janik, J.; Khleif, S.N. Akt1 and -2 inhibition diminishes terminal differentiation and enhances central memory CD8(+) T-cell proliferation and survival. *Oncoimmunology* **2015**, *4*, e1005448. [CrossRef]
162. Guedan, S.; Ruella, M.; June, C.H. Emerging Cellular Therapies for Cancer. *Annu. Rev. Immunol.* **2019**, *37*, 145–171. [CrossRef]

163. Kmiecik, J.; Poli, A.; Brons, N.H.; Waha, A.; Eide, G.E.; Enger, P.; Zimmer, J.; Chekenya, M. Elevated CD3+ and CD8+ tumor-infiltrating immune cells correlate with prolonged survival in glioblastoma patients despite integrated immunosuppressive mechanisms in the tumor microenvironment and at the systemic level. *J. Neuroimmunol.* **2013**, *264*, 71–83. [CrossRef]
164. El Andaloussi, A.; Lesniak, M.S. An increase in CD4+CD25+FOXP3+ regulatory T cells in tumor-infiltrating lymphocytes of human glioblastoma multiforme. *Neuro-Oncology* **2006**, *8*, 234–243. [CrossRef]
165. Thornton, A.M.; Shevach, E.M. CD4+CD25+ immunoregulatory T cells suppress polyclonal T cell activation in vitro by inhibiting interleukin 2 production. *J. Exp. Med.* **1998**, *188*, 287–296. [CrossRef] [PubMed]
166. Uyttenhove, C.; Pilotte, L.; Théate, I.; Stroobant, V.; Colau, D.; Parmentier, N.; Boon, T.; Van den Eynde, B.J. Evidence for a tumoral immune resistance mechanism based on tryptophan degradation by indoleamine 2,3-dioxygenase. *Nat. Med.* **2003**, *9*, 1269–1274. [CrossRef]
167. Vitkovic, L.; Maeda, S.; Sternberg, E. Anti-inflammatory cytokines: Expression and action in the brain. *Neuroimmunomodulation* **2001**, *9*, 295–312. [CrossRef]
168. Gong, D.; Shi, W.; Yi, S.J.; Chen, H.; Groffen, J.; Heisterkamp, N. TGFβ signaling plays a critical role in promoting alternative macrophage activation. *BMC Immunol.* **2012**, *13*, 31. [CrossRef] [PubMed]
169. Long, G.V.; Dummer, R.; Hamid, O.; Gajewski, T.F.; Caglevic, C.; Dalle, S.; Arance, A.; Carlino, M.S.; Grob, J.-J.; Kim, T.M.; et al. Epacadostat plus pembrolizumab versus placebo plus pembrolizumab in patients with unresectable or metastatic melanoma (ECHO-301/KEYNOTE-252): A phase 3, randomised, double-blind study. *Lancet Oncol.* **2019**, *20*, 1083–1097. [CrossRef]
170. Singh, K.; Batich, K.A.; Wen, P.Y.; Tan, A.C.; Bagley, S.J.; Lim, I.M.; Platten, M.; Colman, H.; Ashley, D.M.; Chang, S.M.; et al. Designing Clinical Trials for Combination Immunotherapy: A Framework for Glioblastoma. *Clin. Cancer Res.* **2021**. [CrossRef] [PubMed]
171. Study of Safety and Tolerability of BCA101 Alone and in Combination with Pembrolizumab in Patients With EGFR-driven Advanced Solid Tumors—Full Text View—ClinicalTrials.gov. Available online: https://clinicaltrials.gov/ct2/show/NCT04429542 (accessed on 30 December 2020).
172. Tesselaar, K.; Gravestein, L.A.; van Schijndel, G.M.; Borst, J.; van Lier, R.A. Characterization of murine CD70, the ligand of the TNF receptor family member CD27. *J. Immunol.* **1997**, *159*, 4959–4965. [PubMed]
173. Hintzen, R.Q.; Lens, S.M.; Lammers, K.; Kuiper, H.; Beckmann, M.P.; van Lier, R.A. Engagement of CD27 with its ligand CD70 provides a second signal for T cell activation. *J. Immunol.* **1995**, *154*, 2612–2623. [PubMed]
174. Slaney, C.Y.; Wang, P.; Darcy, P.K.; Kershaw, M.H. CARs versus BiTEs: A Comparison between T Cell-Redirection Strategies for Cancer Treatment. *Cancer Discov.* **2018**, *8*, 924–934. [CrossRef]
175. Hurton, L.V.; Singh, H.; Najjar, A.M.; Switzer, K.C.; Mi, T.; Maiti, S.; Olivares, S.; Rabinovich, B.; Huls, H.; Forget, M.A.; et al. Tethered IL-15 augments antitumor activity and promotes a stem-cell memory subset in tumor-specific T cells. *Proc. Natl. Acad. Sci. USA* **2016**, *113*, E7788–E7797. [CrossRef]
176. Avanzi, M.P.; Yeku, O.; Li, X.; Wijewarnasuriya, D.P.; van Leeuwen, D.G.; Cheung, K.; Park, H.; Purdon, T.J.; Daniyan, A.F.; Spitzer, M.H.; et al. Engineered Tumor-Targeted T Cells Mediate Enhanced Anti-Tumor Efficacy Both Directly and through Activation of the Endogenous Immune System. *Cell Rep.* **2018**, *23*, 2130–2141. [CrossRef] [PubMed]
177. Caruana, I.; Savoldo, B.; Hoyos, V.; Weber, G.; Liu, H.; Kim, E.S.; Ittmann, M.M.; Marchetti, D.; Dotti, G. Heparanase promotes tumor infiltration and antitumor activity of CAR-redirected T lymphocytes. *Nat. Med.* **2015**, *21*, 524–529. [CrossRef] [PubMed]
178. Wang, L.C.; Lo, A.; Scholler, J.; Sun, J.; Majumdar, R.S.; Kapoor, V.; Antzis, M.; Cotner, C.E.; Johnson, L.A.; Durham, A.C.; et al. Targeting fibroblast activation protein in tumor stroma with chimeric antigen receptor T cells can inhibit tumor growth and augment host immunity without severe toxicity. *Cancer Immunol. Res.* **2014**, *2*, 154–166. [CrossRef] [PubMed]
179. Salmon, H.; Idoyaga, J.; Rahman, A.; Leboeuf, M.; Remark, R.; Jordan, S.; Casanova-Acebes, M.; Khudoynazarova, M.; Agudo, J.; Tung, N.; et al. Expansion and Activation of CD103(+) Dendritic Cell Progenitors at the Tumor Site Enhances Tumor Responses to Therapeutic PD-L1 and BRAF Inhibition. *Immunity* **2016**, *44*, 924–938. [CrossRef]
180. Pellegatta, S.; Poliani, P.L.; Stucchi, E.; Corno, D.; Colombo, C.A.; Orzan, F.; Ravanini, M.; Finocchiaro, G. Intra-tumoral dendritic cells increase efficacy of peripheral vaccination by modulation of glioma microenvironment. *Neuro-Oncology* **2010**, *12*, 377–388. [CrossRef]
181. Calzascia, T.; Di Berardino-Besson, W.; Wilmotte, R.; Masson, F.; de Tribolet, N.; Dietrich, P.Y.; Walker, P.R. Cutting edge: Cross-presentation as a mechanism for efficient recruitment of tumor-specific CTL to the brain. *J. Immunol.* **2003**, *171*, 2187–2191. [CrossRef]
182. Barnard, Z.; Wakimoto, H.; Zaupa, C.; Patel, A.P.; Klehm, J.; Martuza, R.L.; Rabkin, S.D.; Curry, W.T., Jr. Expression of FMS-like tyrosine kinase 3 ligand by oncolytic herpes simplex virus type I prolongs survival in mice bearing established syngeneic intracranial malignant glioma. *Neurosurgery* **2012**, *71*, 741–748. [CrossRef] [PubMed]
183. Wick, A.; Felsberg, J.; Steinbach, J.P.; Herrlinger, U.; Platten, M.; Blaschke, B.; Meyermann, R.; Reifenberger, G.; Weller, M.; Wick, W. Efficacy and tolerability of temozolomide in an alternating weekly regimen in patients with recurrent glioma. *J. Clin. Oncol.* **2007**, *25*, 3357–3361. [CrossRef]
184. Heimberger, A.B.; Sun, W.; Hussain, S.F.; Dey, M.; Crutcher, L.; Aldape, K.; Gilbert, M.; Hassenbusch, S.J.; Sawaya, R.; Schmittling, B.; et al. Immunological responses in a patient with glioblastoma multiforme treated with sequential courses of temozolomide and immunotherapy: Case study. *Neuro-Oncology* **2008**, *10*, 98–103. [CrossRef] [PubMed]
185. Duan, L.; Zhang, X.D.; Miao, W.Y.; Sun, Y.J.; Xiong, G.; Wu, Q.; Li, G.; Yang, P.; Yu, H.; Li, H.; et al. PDGFRβ Cells Rapidly Relay Inflammatory Signal from the Circulatory System to Neurons via Chemokine CCL2. *Neuron* **2018**, *100*, 183–200.e8. [CrossRef] [PubMed]
186. Twyman-Saint Victor, C.; Rech, A.J.; Maity, A.; Rengan, R.; Pauken, K.E.; Stelekati, E.; Benci, J.L.; Xu, B.; Dada, H.; Odorizzi, P.M.; et al. Radiation and dual checkpoint blockade activate non-redundant immune mechanisms in cancer. *Nature* **2015**, *520*, 373–377. [CrossRef]

187. Wiranowska, M.; Wilson, T.C.; Bencze, K.S.; Prockop, L.D. A mouse model for the study of blood-brain barrier permeability. *J. Neurosci. Methods* **1988**, *26*, 105–109. [CrossRef]
188. Wiranowska, M. Blood-brain barrier and treatment of central nervous system tumors. *J. Fla. Med. Assoc.* **1992**, *79*, 707–710.
189. Cook, P.R.; Myers, D.; Barker, M.; Jones, J.G. Blood-brain barrier to pertechnetate following drug-induced hypotension. *Br. J. Anaesth.* **1989**, *62*, 402–408. [CrossRef]
190. Wiranowska, M.; Gonzalvo, A.A.; Saporta, S.; Gonzalez, O.R.; Prockop, L.D. Evaluation of blood-brain barrier permeability and the effect of interferon in mouse glioma model. *J. Neurooncol.* **1992**, *14*, 225–236. [CrossRef]
191. Saitou, M.; Furuse, M.; Sasaki, H.; Schulzke, J.D.; Fromm, M.; Takano, H.; Noda, T.; Tsukita, S. Complex phenotype of mice lacking occludin, a component of tight junction strands. *Mol. Biol. Cell* **2000**, *11*, 4131–4142. [CrossRef]
192. Jin, A.Y.; Tuor, U.I.; Rushforth, D.; Kaur, J.; Muller, R.N.; Petterson, J.L.; Boutry, S.; Barber, P.A. Reduced blood brain barrier breakdown in P-selectin deficient mice following transient ischemic stroke: A future therapeutic target for treatment of stroke. *BMC Neurosci.* **2010**, *11*, 12. [CrossRef] [PubMed]
193. Hutchinson, M. Natalizumab: A new treatment for relapsing remitting multiple sclerosis. *Clin. Risk Manag.* **2007**, *3*, 259–268. [CrossRef] [PubMed]
194. Cakir, B.; Xiang, Y.; Tanaka, Y.; Kural, M.H.; Parent, M.; Kang, Y.J.; Chapeton, K.; Patterson, B.; Yuan, Y.; He, C.S.; et al. Engineering of human brain organoids with a functional vascular-like system. *Nat. Methods* **2019**, *16*, 1169–1175. [CrossRef] [PubMed]
195. Pham, M.T.; Pollock, K.M.; Rose, M.D.; Cary, W.A.; Stewart, H.R.; Zhou, P.; Nolta, J.A.; Waldau, B. Generation of human vascularized brain organoids. *Neuroreport* **2018**, *29*, 588–593. [CrossRef] [PubMed]
196. Stamatovic, S.M.; Keep, R.F.; Wang, M.M.; Jankovic, I.; Andjelkovic, A.V. Caveolae-mediated internalization of occludin and claudin-5 during CCL2-induced tight junction remodeling in brain endothelial cells. *J. Biol. Chem.* **2009**, *284*, 19053–19066. [CrossRef]
197. Stamatovic, S.M.; Dimitrijevic, O.B.; Keep, R.F.; Andjelkovic, A.V. Protein kinase Calpha-RhoA cross-talk in CCL2-induced alterations in brain endothelial permeability. *J. Biol. Chem.* **2006**, *281*, 8379–8388. [CrossRef]
198. Ngo, M.T.; Harley, B.A.C. Perivascular signals alter global gene expression profile of glioblastoma and response to temozolomide in a gelatin hydrogel. *Biomaterials* **2019**, *198*, 122–134. [CrossRef]
199. Ozturk, M.S.; Lee, V.K.; Zou, H.; Friedel, R.H.; Intes, X.; Dai, G. High-resolution tomographic analysis of in vitro 3D glioblastoma tumor model under long-term drug treatment. *Sci. Adv.* **2020**, *6*, eaay7513. [CrossRef] [PubMed]
200. Plummer, S.; Wallace, S.; Ball, G.; Lloyd, R.; Schiapparelli, P.; Quinones-Hinojosa, A.; Hartung, T.; Pamies, D. A Human iPSC-derived 3D platform using primary brain cancer cells to study drug development and personalized medicine. *Sci. Rep.* **2019**, *9*, 1407. [CrossRef] [PubMed]
201. Lee, D.W.; Gardner, R.; Porter, D.L.; Louis, C.U.; Ahmed, N.; Jensen, M.; Grupp, S.A.; Mackall, C.L. Current concepts in the diagnosis and management of cytokine release syndrome. *Blood* **2014**, *124*, 188–195. [CrossRef] [PubMed]
202. Leach, D.R.; Krummel, M.F.; Allison, J.P. Enhancement of antitumor immunity by CTLA-4 blockade. *Science* **1996**, *271*, 1734–1736. [CrossRef]
203. Dillard, T.; Yedinak, C.G.; Alumkal, J.; Fleseriu, M. Anti-CTLA-4 antibody therapy associated autoimmune hypophysitis: Serious immune related adverse events across a spectrum of cancer subtypes. *Pituitary* **2010**, *13*, 29–38. [CrossRef] [PubMed]
204. Chodakiewitz, Y.; Brown, S.; Boxerman, J.L.; Brody, J.M.; Rogg, J.M. Ipilimumab treatment associated pituitary hypophysitis: Clinical presentation and imaging diagnosis. *Clin. Neurol. Neurosurg.* **2014**, *125*, 125–130. [CrossRef]
205. Lupi, I.; Brancatella, A.; Cosottini, M.; Viola, N.; Lanzolla, G.; Sgro, D.; Dalmazi, G.D.; Latrofa, F.; Caturegli, P.; Marcocci, C. Clinical heterogeneity of hypophysitis secondary to PD-1/PD-L1 blockade: Insights from four cases. *Endocrinol. Diabetes Metab. Case Rep.* **2019**, *2019*. [CrossRef] [PubMed]
206. Mahzari, M.; Liu, D.; Arnaout, A.; Lochnan, H. Immune checkpoint inhibitor therapy associated hypophysitis. *Clin. Med. Insights Endocrinol. Diabetes* **2015**, *8*, 21–28. [CrossRef]
207. Iwama, S.; De Remigis, A.; Callahan, M.K.; Slovin, S.F.; Wolchok, J.D.; Caturegli, P. Pituitary expression of CTLA-4 mediates hypophysitis secondary to administration of CTLA-4 blocking antibody. *Sci. Transl. Med.* **2014**, *6*, 230ra245. [CrossRef] [PubMed]
208. Bossart, S.; Thurneysen, S.; Rushing, E.; Frontzek, K.; Leske, H.; Mihic-Probst, D.; Nagel, H.W.; Mangana, J.; Goldinger, S.M.; Dummer, R. Case Report: Encephalitis, with Brainstem Involvement, Following Checkpoint Inhibitor Therapy in Metastatic Melanoma. *Oncologist* **2017**, *22*, 749–753. [CrossRef]
209. Robert, L.; Langner-Lemercier, S.; Angibaud, A.; Sale, A.; Thepault, F.; Corre, R.; Lena, H.; Ricordel, C. Immune-related Encephalitis in Two Patients Treated With Immune Checkpoint Inhibitor. *Clin. Lung Cancer* **2020**, *21*, e474–e477. [CrossRef] [PubMed]
210. Cabral, G.; Ladeira, F.; Gil, N. Nivolumab-induced seronegative encephalitis. *J. Neuroimmunol.* **2020**, *347*, 577350. [CrossRef]
211. Astaras, C.; de Micheli, R.; Moura, B.; Hundsberger, T.; Hottinger, A.F. Neurological Adverse Events Associated with Immune Checkpoint Inhibitors: Diagnosis and Management. *Curr. Neurol. Neurosci. Rep.* **2018**, *18*, 3. [CrossRef]
212. Dalakas, M.C. Neurological complications of immune checkpoint inhibitors: What happens when you 'take the brakes off' the immune system. *Adv. Neurol. Disord.* **2018**, *11*, 1756286418799864. [CrossRef]
213. Feng, S.; Coward, J.; McCaffrey, E.; Coucher, J.; Kalokerinos, P.; O'Byrne, K. Pembrolizumab-Induced Encephalopathy: A Review of Neurological Toxicities with Immune Checkpoint Inhibitors. *J. Thorac. Oncol.* **2017**, *12*, 1626–1635. [CrossRef]
214. Dalmau, J.; Bataller, L. Limbic encephalitis: The new cell membrane antigens and a proposal of clinical-immunological classification with therapeutic implications. *Neurologia* **2007**, *22*, 526–537. [PubMed]

215. Pillonel, V.; Dunet, V.; Hottinger, A.F.; Berthod, G.; Schiappacasse, L.; Peters, S.; Michielin, O.; Aedo-Lopez, V. Multiple nivolumab-induced CNS demyelination with spontaneous resolution in an asymptomatic metastatic melanoma patient. *J. Immunother. Cancer* **2019**, *7*, 336. [CrossRef] [PubMed]
216. Gettings, E.J.; Hackett, C.T.; Scott, T.F. Severe relapse in a multiple sclerosis patient associated with ipilimumab treatment of melanoma. *Mult. Scler.* **2015**, *21*, 670. [CrossRef]
217. Santomasso, B.; Bachier, C.; Westin, J.; Rezvani, K.; Shpall, E.J. The Other Side of CAR T-Cell Therapy: Cytokine Release Syndrome, Neurologic Toxicity, and Financial Burden. *Am. Soc. Clin. Oncol. Educ. Book* **2019**, *39*, 433–444. [CrossRef] [PubMed]
218. Norelli, M.; Camisa, B.; Barbiera, G.; Falcone, L.; Purevdorj, A.; Genua, M.; Sanvito, F.; Ponzoni, M.; Doglioni, C.; Cristofori, P.; et al. Monocyte-derived IL-1 and IL-6 are differentially required for cytokine-release syndrome and neurotoxicity due to CAR T cells. *Nat. Med.* **2018**, *24*, 739–748. [CrossRef] [PubMed]
219. Brown, C.E.; Alizadeh, D.; Starr, R.; Weng, L.; Wagner, J.R.; Naranjo, A.; Ostberg, J.R.; Blanchard, M.S.; Kilpatrick, J.; Simpson, J.; et al. Regression of Glioblastoma after Chimeric Antigen Receptor T-Cell Therapy. *New Engl. J. Med.* **2016**, *375*, 2561–2569. [CrossRef]
220. Akhavan, D.; Alizadeh, D.; Wang, D.; Weist, M.R.; Shepphird, J.K.; Brown, C.E. CAR T cells for brain tumors: Lessons learned and road ahead. *Immunol. Rev.* **2019**, *290*, 60–84. [CrossRef]
221. Pennisi, M.; Jain, T.; Santomasso, B.D.; Mead, E.; Wudhikarn, K.; Silverberg, M.L.; Batlevi, Y.; Shouval, R.; Devlin, S.M.; Batlevi, C.; et al. Comparing CAR T-cell toxicity grading systems: Application of the ASTCT grading system and implications for management. *Blood Adv.* **2020**, *4*, 676–686. [CrossRef] [PubMed]
222. Gust, J.; Hay, K.A.; Hanafi, L.A.; Li, D.; Myerson, D.; Gonzalez-Cuyar, L.F.; Yeung, C.; Liles, W.C.; Wurfel, M.; Lopez, J.A.; et al. Endothelial Activation and Blood-Brain Barrier Disruption in Neurotoxicity after Adoptive Immunotherapy with CD19 CAR-T Cells. *Cancer Discov.* **2017**, *7*, 1404–1419. [CrossRef] [PubMed]
223. Klinger, M.; Zugmaier, G.; Nagele, V.; Goebeler, M.E.; Brandl, C.; Stelljes, M.; Lassmann, H.; von Stackelberg, A.; Bargou, R.C.; Kufer, P. Adhesion of T Cells to Endothelial Cells Facilitates Blinatumomab-Associated Neurologic Adverse Events. *Cancer Res.* **2020**, *80*, 91–101. [CrossRef] [PubMed]
224. Neelapu, S.S.; Tummala, S.; Kebriaei, P.; Wierda, W.; Gutierrez, C.; Locke, F.L.; Komanduri, K.V.; Lin, Y.; Jain, N.; Daver, N.; et al. Chimeric antigen receptor T-cell therapy—assessment and management of toxicities. *Nat. Rev. Clin. Oncol.* **2018**, *15*, 47–62. [CrossRef] [PubMed]

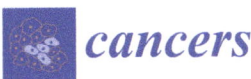

Article

Multi-Platform Classification of IDH-Wild-Type Glioblastoma Based on ERK/MAPK Pathway: Diagnostic, Prognostic and Therapeutic Implications

Maria-Magdalena Georgescu

NeuroMarkers PLLC, Houston, TX 77025, USA; mmgeorgescu@yahoo.com; Tel.: +1-281-433-0492

Simple Summary: This study presents a unified classification of glioblastoma that streams multi-platform data from genomic, transcriptomic, histologic, and demographic analyses into targetable glioblastoma subgroups connected by signaling through canonical growth pathways. This structured and clear analysis addresses the current needs of neuro-oncological practice and offers practical guidelines for the diagnosis, prognosis, and therapeutic targeting of glioblastoma, being thus of great benefit to both patients and brain tumor practitioners alike.

Abstract: Glioblastoma is the most aggressive and frequent glioma in the adult population. Because current therapy regimens confer only minimal survival benefit, molecular subgrouping to stratify patient prognosis and therapy design is warranted. This study presents a multi-platform classification of glioblastoma by analyzing a large, ethnicity-inclusive 101-adult-patient cohort. It defines seven non-redundant IDH-wild-type glioblastoma molecular subgroups, G1–G7, corresponding to the upstream receptor tyrosine kinase (RTK) and RAS-RAF segment of the ERK/MAPK signal transduction pathway. These glioblastoma molecular subgroups are classified as G1/EGFR, G2/FGFR3, G3/NF1, G4/RAF, G5/PDGFRA, G6/Multi-RTK, and G7/Other. The comprehensive genomic analysis was refined by expression landscaping of all RTK genes, as well as of the major associated growth pathway mediators, and used to hierarchically cluster the subgroups. Parallel demographic, clinical, and histologic pattern analyses were merged with the molecular subgrouping to yield the first inclusive multi-platform classification for IDH-wild-type glioblastoma. This straightforward classification with diagnostic and prognostic significance may be readily used in neuro-oncological practice and lays the foundation for personalized targeted therapy approaches.

Keywords: glioblastoma molecular classification; ERK/MAPK pathway; PI3K/PTEN pathway; receptor tyrosine kinase; EGFR; PDGFRA; FGFR3; MET; EPHB2; NF1

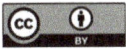

1. Introduction

Glioblastoma is the most frequent malignant primary brain neoplasm in adults, with an incidence of 3–4 cases per 100,000 population, and 41% survival at 1 year [1]. The 2016 World Health Organization (WHO) Classification of Tumors of the Central Nervous System recognizes IDH-wild-type and IDH-mutant glioblastomas as separate molecular entities, with significant survival differences [2]. IDH-wild-type glioblastomas comprise over 90% of glioblastomas and show *TERT* promoter mutations, *CDKN2A/B* homozygous loss, *EGFR* amplification, *TP53* and *PTEN* mutations, as most frequent common and mostly concurrent alterations [2]. These mutations address basic cancer cell maintenance requirements: telomere extension by *TERT* overexpression, cell cycle progression by *CDKN2A/B* cell cycle-dependent kinase (CDK) 4/6 inhibitors loss and *TP53* alterations, the latter being also involved in gatekeeping the DNA-damage response (DDR), and cell survival by inactivation of PTEN, the main inhibitor of the phosphatidyl inositol 3-OH kinase (PI3K) proliferative and anti-apoptotic pathway [3,4]. EGFR is the most frequently altered receptor tyrosine kinase (RTK) in glioblastoma, but amplification and activating mutation or fusions have been also reported in other RTKs, such as PDGFRA, MET, FGFR, and NTRK1 [2].

The RTKs are categorized into 19 well-defined classes based on sequence and structural similarity of their ligand-binding extracellular domains [5]. The intracellular domains contain the highly homologous tyrosine kinase domain and more specific juxtamembrane and carboxyl (C)-terminal regions that contain tyrosine motifs. Upon ligand binding leading to RTK dimerization and activation, the phosphorylation of tyrosine motifs triggers the activation of downstream signaling pathways by docking SH2-domain-containing adaptor and enzymatic proteins. The extracellular signal-regulated kinase/mitogen-activated protein kinase (ERK/MAPK) and PI3K/AKT/mTOR are two parallel signaling pathways controlling proliferation, survival, metabolism, and invasion of cancer cells that are commonly activated by RTKs, whereas Src, STAT, and phospholipase C-γ pathways are additional pathways activated by most RTKs.

There are four conventional MAPK families: ERK1/2, p38, JUNK, and ERK5, all phosphorylated and activated by upstream kinases or MAP2Ks, in turn, phosphorylated and activated by a third layer of upstream MAP3Ks [6]. Within the ERK1/2 MAPK cascade, RTKs activate Ras, which, in its active GTP-bound form, binds and activates Raf kinases (MAP3K), which activate MEK1/2 (MAP2K), which further activate ERK1/2 (MAPK). Phosphorylated ERKs translocate to the nucleus to activate transcription factors or remain cytoplasmic to activate substrates involved in cell growth. The pathway is negatively controlled upstream by direct inhibition through NF1, a Ras GTPase-activating protein (GAP) but also by feedback loops resulting from ERK-dependent transcription of the ERK phosphatases DUSP4/5/6 and the Sprouty family members [7–10]. In contrast, the PI3K/AKT/mTOR pathway is a heterogeneous pathway involving both protein and lipid signal transduction mediators and is directly inhibited by the PTEN tumor suppressor, acting upstream as phosphoinositide phosphatase counteracting the effect of PI3K [3].

By using an integrated approach interrogating a controlled glioblastoma patient cohort, I propose a simplified multi-platform classification of glioblastoma tailored to map the ERK/MAPK pathway activation, with important implications for precision therapy.

2. Materials and Methods

Tumor specimens, histology and, immunohistochemistry (IHC): Surgical resection, biopsy or autopsy specimens were obtained from patients with glioblastoma, as previously described, in accordance with hospital regulations [7,11,12]. With one exception, the IDH-wild-type cases illustrated in this study correspond to first-diagnosis, untreated tumors. Formalin-fixed paraffin-embedded (FFPE) sections were stained with hematoxylin-eosin (H&E). Images were acquired with the Nikon Eclipse Ci microscope equipped with the Nikon Digital Sight DS-Fi2 camera (Nikon Instruments Inc., Melville, NY, USA), as previously described [13]. For histologic pattern analysis, digital images were acquired from all cases at various magnifications. Representative tumor fields were chosen, aiming at the viable tumor core, away from areas of necrosis and normal brain interface. The images were processed in batch for level adjustment and displayed stacked in an extended image library for comparison. For difficult patterns, both digitalized images and slides were cross-examined. IHC was performed on selected sections, as described [11,13]. The following primary antibodies were used: histone H3-K27M (Millipore/Sigma, Burlington, MA, USA), IDH1-R132H (DIA-H09, Dianova, Hamburg, Germany), p53 (DO-7), Ki-67 (30-9) (Roche/Ventana Medical Systems Inc., Tucson, AZ, USA), GFAP (EP672Y) (Ventana/Cell Marque, Rocklin, CA, USA).

Next-generation sequencing (NGS) and copy number (CN) variation: Nucleic acids were extracted from FFPE samples, as previously described [11]. Variant analysis and interpretation following NGS using the xT 596-gene or xE whole-exome panels (Tempus Labs, Chicago, IL, USA) or the customized 295-gene panel were performed as previously described [7,11,12]. CN analysis was performed as previously described [7,14]. Gene amplification was called for CN ≥ 7, and loss of heterozygosity (LOH) for alterations with loss of one allele. The tumor mutation burden is expressed as single-nucleotide protein-altering mutations per megabase DNA. The MGMT promoter methylation assay was performed by quantitative methylation-specific PCR using DNA extracted from FFPE samples (Integrated Oncology, Phoenix, AZ, USA).

Transcriptomics: Whole transcriptome RNA sequencing with RNA fusion detection was performed at Tempus Labs for all glioblastoma samples with more than 30% tumor on FFPE sections as described [7]. The expression was analyzed by a proprietary protocol. Briefly, the threshold for total RNA counts was set at $\geq$500 in at least one tumor sample, and pseudogenes and Y-chromosome genes were excluded. A $\geq$5-fold overexpression threshold was set for the average tumor values from subgroups relative to precursor low-grade control values, as previously described [7].

Statistical analysis: Differences between groups were assessed by using unpaired two-tailed t-test with or without Welch's correction for variances significantly different, as described [15]. Multivariable correlation matrices and hierarchical clustering were generated for the glioblastoma subgroups by using the Pearson correlation coefficient. Kaplan–Meier survival analyses using the Log-rank (Mantel–Cox) test were performed as previously described [16,17]. Statistical significance was considered for $p < 0.05$. Confidence intervals for all tests were 95%. The graphic, statistic, and hierarchical clustering software included Microsoft Excel (Microsoft Corp., Redmond, WA, USA), GraphPad Prism (Version 8.3.0, GraphPad Software, La Jolla, CA, USA), and Instant Clue [18].

3. Results

3.1. Non-Redundant Molecular Classification of Glioblastoma Based on ERK/MAPK Pathway

The tumors from a 101-adult-patient cohort with WHO grade IV diffuse glioma were initially classified based on IHC into IDH wild-type glioblastoma (90 cases), IDH-mutant glioblastoma (eight cases), and diffuse midline glioma (DMG) with histone H3 K27M mutation (three cases) (Figure 1A). NGS genomic results were obtained for 112 tumors from 97 patients and whole transcriptomics results were obtained for 82 tumors from 70 of these patients. The integrated genomic and transcriptomic analysis of the tumors showed *EGFR*, *PDGFRA*, *FGFR3*, *NF1*, and *BRAF/RAF1* mutually exclusive alterations within the glioblastoma IDH-wild-type category (Figure 1 and Table S1). An additional subgroup, Multi-RTK, showed alterations in multiple RTKs, including *MET*. The combined NF1, RAF, and RTK alterations from EGFR, PDGFRA, FGFR3, and Multi-RTK subgroups that activate the ERK/MAPK signaling pathway (Figure 1B) accounted for 85% of the glioblastoma IDH-wild-type cases. In the remaining cases, alterations targeting the ERK/MAPK pathway were not found, and this subset, labeled as Other, represented approximately 15% of IDH-wild-type glioblastoma cases (Figure 1A).

The RTK subgroups accounted for 63.2% of the glioblastoma IDH-wild-type cases, and the EGFR subgroup alone, for 41.4%, being thus the largest of all glioblastoma molecular subgroups (Figure 1A). The vast majority of the EGFR tumors from 91.7% of EGFR subgroup cases harbored *EGFR* amplification (EGFR↑), and only three cases showed *EGFR* gain-of-function mutations without amplification (EGFRm) (Table S1). Two tumors, EGFR#5 and EGFR#33, were multifocal with the main focus showing *EGFR* amplification and a secondary focus showing *EGFR* mutation without amplification. Interestingly, the majority of tumors with *EGFR* amplification also showed another *EGFR* genetic alteration, such as the splice variants vIII, vIVa, pathogenic mutations with or without amplification, C-terminal deletion, or *EGFR-SEPT14*, *EGFR-VOPP1*, *CTDSP2-EGFR*, and *SEC61G-EGFR* fusions. The next largest RTK subgroups are the PDGFRA and Multi-RTK, each accounting for 8% (Figure 1A). *PDGFRA* amplification with or without adjacent *KIT* and *KDR* amplification was the most frequent genetic alteration in the PDGFRA subgroup, and was found in 85.7% of the PDGFRA subgroup cases. As observed for *EGFR*, simultaneous *PDGFRA* amplification and missense mutations were frequently noted (Table S1). A common type of missense mutation targeted the di-sulfide bond cysteines of the extracellular domains of both EGFR and PDGFRα. The Multi-RTK subgroup is an eclectic group harboring various combinations of RTK alterations. It included three cases with *PDGFRA* amplification without overexpression. The smallest RTK subgroup is composed of cases with FGFR3 fusions or mutations (Table S1) and it has been characterized in detail elsewhere [7].

The NF1 and RAF subgroups accounted for almost one-quarter of the glioblastoma IDH-wild-type cases, with the NF1 subgroup being the second largest after the EGFR subgroup (Figure 1A). Two of the 15 NF1 cases were syndromic, and these patients presented other neurofibromatosis type 1 manifestations in addition to brain tumors. Almost all NF1 tumors had two *NF1* hits, either by different mutations or by LOH (Table S1). Twenty distinct *NF1* alterations were detected, most resulting in protein truncation. Among these, two *NF1* frameshift fusions were noted, underscoring the importance of fusion detection for correct classification in the NF1 subgroup. All four tumors in the RAF subgroup also showed distinct gain-of-function mutations, three in *BRAF*, and one in *RAF1*, the latter accompanied by gene amplification (Table S1).

The landscape of RTK expression in the glioblastoma subgroups was compiled by examining the relative expression levels of all the members from the 19 RTK classes (Table S2 and Figure S1). In the EGFR subgroup, *EGFR* high overexpression was associated with gene amplification in all but one case, with an average of 26 ± 3.7 and a range between 4.5- and 72-fold overexpression (Figure 1C,D). Conversely, low or no *EGFR* overexpression characterized the samples displaying activating *EGFR* gain-of-function mutations in the absence of amplification, indicating a strong correlation between *EGFR* amplification and overexpression in the EGFR subgroup. Moderate levels of EGFR overexpression were present in some cases of the Multi-RTK subgroup, and only in isolated cases in other subgroups, in the absence of gene amplification. In contrast to *EGFR*, only two-thirds of the cases with *PDGFRA* amplification showed overexpression, with an average of 16.8 ± 3 and a range between 4.9- and 25.7-fold (Figure 1C,D). The remaining one-third of cases were classified in the Multi-RTK subgroup, as they showed genetic alterations and/or overexpression of other major RTKs, most commonly *MET*, but also *EGFR*, *KIT*, *FGFR2*, *NTRK1*, *EPHA3*, and *EPHB2* (Figure 1C,D and Table S1). The *KIT* and *KDR* gene loci are contiguous with the *PDGFRA* locus, and their amplifications showed generally the same expression trend as *PDGFRA*, except for the Multi-RTK#1 case that showed high *KIT* overexpression in the absence of gene amplification. *MET* amplification was detected in two cases from the Multi-RTK subgroup and correlated with over 40-fold expression levels. Relatively high *MET* overexpression levels were also noted in four additional cases, ranging from 5.4- to 28-fold, without amplification but with low CN gain on chromosome 7. In the PDGFRA#4 case, *MET* overexpression was most likely caused by the presence of a *PTPRZ1-MET* fusion, as *PTPRZ1* is among the highest expressed genes in glioma, and the fusion places *MET* under the control of the *PTPRZ1* promoter (Table S1). *FGFR2* was the only other RTK with amplification and very high overexpression in the cohort, and the IDH#1 case harboring it has been previously described [7].

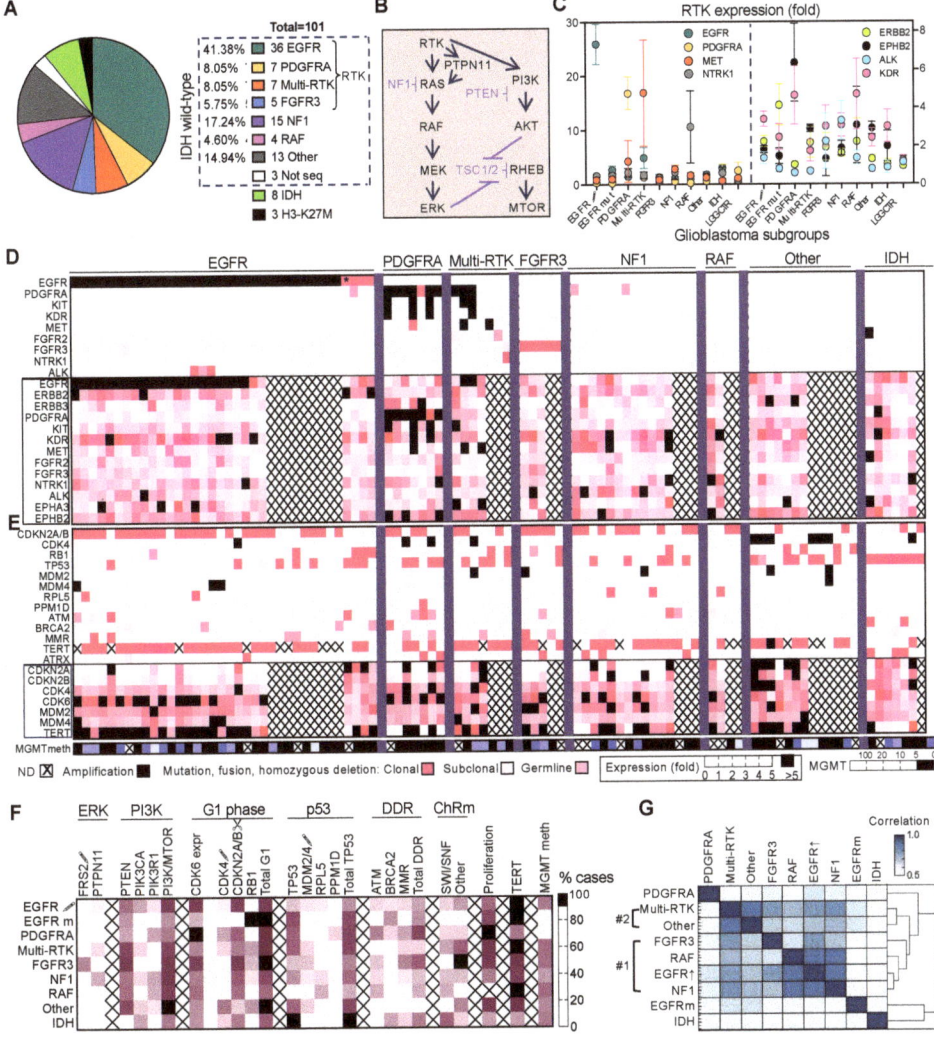

Figure 1. Glioblastoma molecular subgroups—molecular characteristics and pathway-based clustering. (**A**) Subgrouping of the glioblastoma cohort in non-overlapping molecular alterations corresponding to ERK/MAPK signaling pathway. (**B**) Diagram of the canonical ERK/MAPK and PI3K signaling pathways. Inhibitors are indicated in purple; arrows and blunt arrows represent activation or inhibition, respectively. (**C**) RTK fold-expression in glioblastoma subgroups, as mean ± SEM values, showing RTKs with high or intermediate overexpression on the left or right y-axis, respectively. EGFR↑, EGFR with gene amplification; EGFRm, EGFR with mutation only; LGG CTR, low-grade glioma expression control subgroup. (**D**,**E**) Heatmaps of subgrouped individual tumors showing mutation–expression correlations for RTKs (**D**) and cell cycle G1 phase, p53, DDR and telomere elongation pathways (**E**). Colored or black squares mark presence of genomic alterations in the upper part of the heatmaps. Asterisk (*) marks the multifocal EGFR#33 case with EGFR amplification in the main focus and EGFR mutation in the secondary focus, for which the expression profile is shown. Genes boxed in pink show expression data. MGMT promoter methylation (meth) is also shown, with positive values ≥ 5. ND, not determined. (**F**) Heatmap of % cases with indicated alterations grouped in pathways, based on the values from Table 1 for the glioblastoma subgroups. ↑, gene amplification (CN ≥ 7); ↓, homozygous loss; ChRm, chromatin remodeling. The gene composition of the DDR and ChRm pathways is described in Table 1. Mean CDK6 and proliferation markers expression values are also included. (**G**) Hierarchical clustering of glioblastoma subgroups by multivariable Pearson correlation analysis. Note two subgroup clusters #1 and #2, and individual segregation of the PDGFRA, EGFRm and IDH subgroups.

Table 1. Mutation percent (%) frequency in glioblastoma subgroups.

Gene	Total IDH wt $n=87$	EGFR ↑ $n=33$	EGFR m $n=3$	PDGFRA $n=7$	Multi-RTK $n=7$	FGFR3 $n=5$	NF1 $n=15$	RAF $n=4$	Other $n=13$	IDH m $n=7$
TERT [1]	85 (81.2)	96.4	100	42.9	100	80	73.3	100	81.8	28.6
PTEN	53	48.5	33.3	28.6	71.4	80	46.7	50	69.2	0
PIK3CA	18.4	27.3	0	0	14.3	0	13.3	0	15.4	28.6
PIK3R1	12.6	9.1	0	28.6	0	0	26.7	25	7.7	0
PI3K/mTOR [2]	75.9	75.8	33.3	42.9	71.4	80	80	75	100	42.9
CDKN2A ↓	55.2	72.7	0	57.1	42.9	80	60	50	15.4	42.9
CDK4 ↑	11.5	3	0	28.6	14.3	0	0	0	46.2	14.3
RB1	12.6	0	100	0	28.6	20	6.7	0	30.8	0
G1 phase [3]	79.3	75.8	100	85.7	85.7	100	66.7	50	92.3	57.1
TP53	33.3	18.2	66.7	57.1	57.1	20	33.3	0	53.8	100
MDM2 ↑	5.7	0	0	0	14.3	20	6.7	0	15.4	0
MDM4 ↑	4.6	9.1	0	0	0	0	0	0	7.7	0
RPL5	5.7	6.1	0	0	0	0	13.3	25	0	0
PPM1D	1.1	0	0	14.3	0	0	0	0	0	0
TP53 path [4]	49.4	33.3	66.7	71.4	71.4	40	53.3	25	69.2	100
ATM	12.6	12.1	0	42.9	0	20	13.3	0	0	0
BRCA2	5.7	9.1	33.3	14.3	0	0	0	0	0	28.6
MMR [5]	11.5	12.1	0	28.6	14.3	40	6.7	0	0	14.3
DDR path [6]	26.4	27.3	33.3	71.4	14.3	60	20	25	0	42.9
STAG2	12.6	15.2	0	14.3	14.3	20	13.3	0	0	0
SWI/SNF [7]	13.8	15.2	0	14.3	28.6	0	20	25	0	57.1
Other ChRm [8]	32.2	30.3	0	14.3	57.1	100	20	0	38.5	14.3
MGMT methyl	36.1	43.3	0	0	50	50	27.3	50	36.4	42.9

Wt, wild-type; ↑, gene amplification; ↓, homozygous CN loss; m, point mutation; path, pathway; DDR, DNA damage response; MMR, mismatch repair; ChRm, chromatin remodeling; methyl, methylation. The highest % for a certain alteration is indicated in bold. [1] % cases with cumulated TERT promoter mutation and TERT overexpression in the absence of mutation. The value in brackets corresponds to the total % cases with TERT promoter mutations only. [2] % cases with at least one alteration in PTEN, PIK3CA, PIK3R1, TSC2, or MTOR. [3] % cases with CDKN2A homozygous loss, CDK4 amplification, or RB1 mutation. [4] % cases with TP53, MDM2, MDM4, RPL5, and PPM1D alterations. [5] % cases with either MSH6, MSH5, PMS2, or MLH3 pathogenic mutations. [6] % cases with at least one alteration in ATM, BRCA2, or MMR genes. [7] % cases with SWI/SNF complex ARID1A, ARID1B, ARID2, SMARCA1, SMARCA4, or PBRM1 pathogenic mutations. [8] % cases with either YEATS4 amplification or DNM3TA, TET2, EZH2, SUZ12, ASXL1, ASXL2, KDM5C, KDM6A, KMT2C, KMT2D, or CREBBP pathogenic mutations.

A number of RTKs showed >5-fold overexpression in some cases in the absence of gene amplification (Figure 1C,D and Figure S1). The other three members of the EGFR RTK class appeared upregulated differentially in the various glioblastoma subgroups, with ERBB2 mild overexpression in the EGFR subgroup, especially associated with EGFRm cases, ERBB3 mild overexpression in PDGFRA and Other subgroups, and ERBB4, in the IDH subgroup. NTRK1 was upregulated in isolated cases in almost all glioblastoma subgroups but more prominently in the two cases with RNA expression data from the RAF subgroup. NTRK1 genetic alterations were noted in only one case, the Multi-RTK#7 that showed LMNA-NTRK1 fusion. Two of the ephrin class RTKs, EPHA3, and EPHB2, also showed overexpression in scattered cases across the glioblastoma subgroups but more prominently in the Multi-RTK and PDGFRA subgroups, respectively. Similarly, ALK showed overexpression in a few isolated cases and more clustered in the NF1 subgroup. Three EGFR cases also showed ALK variants of unknown significance or likely pathogenic (Table S1). Interestingly, KDR, besides the 10-fold overexpression in the cancer cells from the PDGFRA#4 and #6 cases with gene amplification, showed mild to moderate overexpression without gene amplification, with a 7.7-fold upper range, in the majority of cases from many subgroups. Most likely, this overexpression stems from the endothelial compartment, reflecting the active vascular proliferation program in these tumors. Interestingly, the pseudokinase RTKs PTK7, ROR1, and ROR2 that activate the Wnt pathway rather than the canonical MAPK and PI3K pathways [19] were mildly to moderately overexpressed in all glioblastoma subgroups (Figure S1).

3.2. Glioblastoma Subgroup Clustering Based on Pathway Analysis

The most frequent genetic alterations from glioblastoma were mapped to the different molecular subgroups (Table 1). *TERT* promoter mutations were the most frequent alteration, accounting for 81.2% of cases. *TERT* overexpression usually correlated with promoter mutations but also showed high values in a few cases without *TERT* promoter mutations (Figure 1E). *ATRX* mutations were rare and mostly complementary to *TERT* mutations. In general, *TERT* overexpression was the main mechanism of telomere elongation in IDH wild-type glioblastoma, except for the PDGFRA subgroup. The PI3K/mTOR canonical pathway showed genomic alterations in 76% of IDH-wild-type glioblastoma cases, mainly through *PTEN* mutations in 53% of cases (Table 1). The *PTEN* alterations peaked in the FGFR3, Multi-RTK, and Other subgroups. In contrast, *PIK3CA* mutations were rather clustered in the EGFR subgroup, and *PIK3R1* mutations, in the PDGFRA and NF1 subgroups.

Mutations in the cell cycle G1 phase genes *CDKN2A/2B*, *CDK4*, and *RB1* were mutually exclusive in this series, except for two heterozygous germline *RB1* point mutations, and were present in 79.3% of glioblastoma IDH-wild-type cases (Table 1 and Figure 1E). With one exception in the FGFR3 subgroup previously discussed [7], all *CDKN2A* homozygous losses were extended to the *CDKN2B* adjacent gene. Moreover, there was a perfect correlation between *CDKN2A/2B* homozygous loss and decreased RNA expression levels, although decreased levels were also seen in the absence of gene loss in two IDH-wild-type and one IDH-mutant glioblastoma cases. The type of mutated G1 phase gene was relatively specific in some subgroups. In particular, in the EGFR subgroup, EGFR↑ cases showed preferential *CDKN2A/2B* homozygous loss and EGFRm cases showed *RB1* inactivating mutations with LOH. The cases with *CDK4* amplification clustered in the Other subgroup that contained six of the ten total IDH-wild-type glioblastoma cases with *CDK4* amplification. This subgroup also presented cases with *RB1* mutation and only a minority with *CDKN2A/2B* loss. *CDK4* amplification correlated perfectly with overexpression. The other G1 phase kinase gene, *CDK6*, showed overexpression in the absence of genomic abnormalities especially in the PDGFRA, EGFR↑, and FGFR3 subgroups (Figure 1E,F).

The p53 cell cycle and cell proliferation gatekeeping pathway, defined here by mutations in *TP53* itself, as well as mutually exclusive mutations in *MDM2*, *MDM4*, *RPL5*, and *PPM1D*, was altered in approximately half of the IDH-wild-type and all IDH-mutant glioblastoma cases (Table 1 and Figure 1E). The *CDKN2A* gene locus also encodes p14ARF, a regulator of MDM2 that promotes its degradation and therefore stabilization of p53 [20]. With the exception of the NF1 and IDH subgroups, mutations in *TP53* tended to occur in the cases without *CDKN2A* loss, explaining the inverse relationship in mutation frequency between *TP53* and *CDKN2A* in most subgroups. Interestingly, *MDM4* mutations clustered in the EGFR subgroup and *MDM2* mutations were exclusively noted in the non-EGFR subgroups. Mutations in DDR genes *ATM* and *BRCA2* and in mismatch repair genes were clustered in the PDGFRA, IDH, and FGFR3 subgroups, respectively. In contrast, mutations of *STAG2*, encoding a subunit of the cohesin complex controlling sister chromatid separation during cell division, were scattered among almost all glioblastoma subgroups. Gene mutations in multiple chromatin remodeling mediators were present in all FGFR3 cases, and mutations especially in components of the SWI/SNF complex were noted in over half of IDH subgroup cases.

Overall, the tumor mutation burden of the subgroups was similar, with median values between 2.8 and 5.8 mutations/megabase DNA (Figure S2). Only three tumors representing 3.2% of the cohort had high tumor mutation burden values over 10 mutations/megabase DNA.

The relative specificity of mutation partition prompted the assembly of a correlation matrix for glioblastoma subgroup hierarchical clustering (Figure 1F). Besides gene mutations in the pathways discussed above, and *CDK6* average expression, two additional parameters were included, *MGMT* promoter methylation and proliferation. As compared to roughly half of the tumors in the Multi-RTK, FGFR3, RAF, but also EGFR↑ subgroups, none of the tumors from EGFRm or PDGFRA subgroups showed *MGMT* promoter methylation (Table 1 and Figure 1E). The extent of *MGMT* promoter methylation was also variable, with some tumors displaying only marginally positive values. The proliferation was assessed for the cases with expression data as a compound parameter, including the *MKI67* expression, and showed the highest average value in the PDGFRA subgroup (Figure S3). The distribution of the individual proliferation values in some subgroups was not gaussian, and especially for the EGFR↑ subgroup, two clusters could be separated, in correlation with *EGFR* overexpression values.

Hierarchical clustering showed the IDH subgroup separated from the IDH-wild-type subgroups, as expected (Figures 2G and S4). Surprisingly, the EGFRm subgroup was also isolated from other subgroups. Another subgroup that segregated sharply from the rest was the PDGFRA subgroup. Unexpectedly, the EGFR↑ and NF1 subgroups clustered with the highest correlation coefficient, followed by the RAF subgroup. The FGFR3 subgroup more distantly clustered with the former three subgroups, whereas the Multi-RTK and Other subgroups formed a separate molecular cluster.

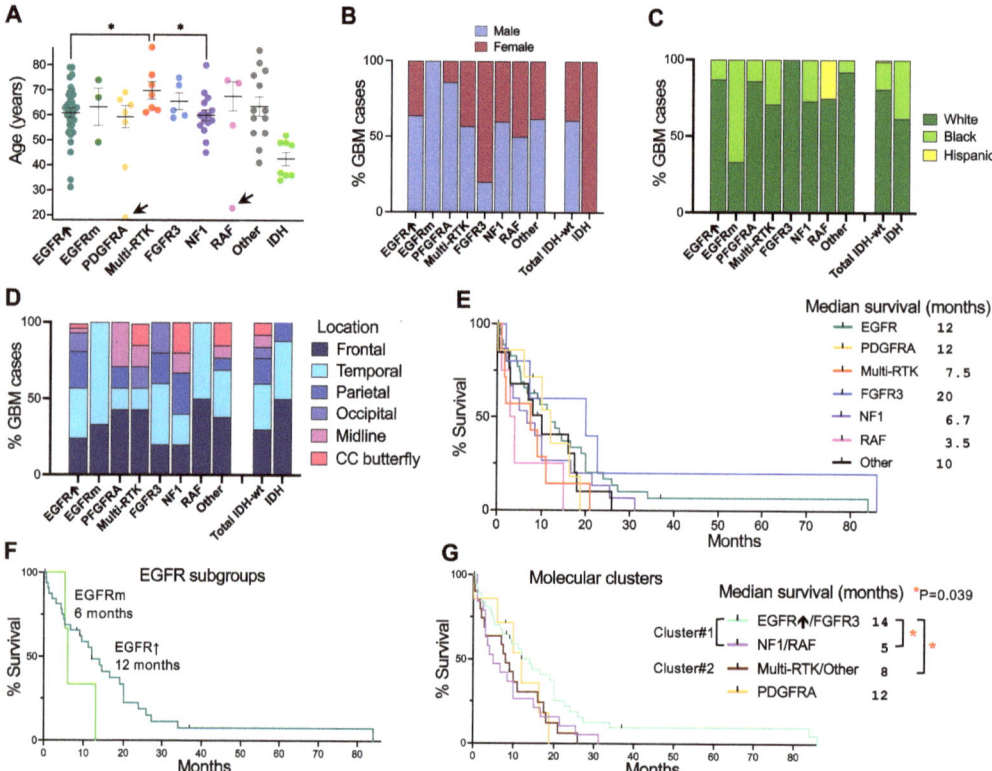

Figure 2. Demographic analysis of glioblastoma subgroups. (**A**) Mean ± SEM of individual age values excluding the outliers indicated by arrows. Statistically significant differences between IDH-wild-type subgroups are indicated by asterisks. (**B**) Sex distribution in glioblastoma subgroups. (**C**) Ethnic/race distribution in glioblastoma subgroups. (**D**) Tumor location distribution showing hemispheric and midline locations, the latter encompassing basal ganglia, pineal gland, and cerebellum. Corpus callosum (CC) symmetric or asymmetric butterfly glioblastoma is shown separately. (**E–G**) Kaplan–Meier survival curves for the 7 IDH-wild-type glioblastoma subgroups (**E**), separated EGFR subgroups (**F**), and molecular clusters (**G**). Median survival and statistical significance (*p*-values and asterisks) are indicated.

3.3. Glioblastoma Subgroup Demographic Characterization

The IDH-wild-type glioblastoma subgroups showed generally similar age central tendency parameters, with median and mean age values ranging from 60 to 62 and 59.3 to 63.7 years, respectively, for the most numerous subgroups, except for the Multi-RTK subgroup that showed significantly higher values, with a median of 68 and mean of 70 years (Figure 2A). The median and mean age for the IDH subgroup coincided, at 42 years, significantly lower than for the IDH-wild-type glioblastoma subgroups, aligning with other reports [2]. The male-to-female sex distribution of IDH-wild-type cases was 1.57:1, comparable with the reported ratio [2], but there was a bias towards 100% females in the IDH-mutant subgroup compared to the 0.96:1 reported ratio, probably at least partly due to the small sample (N = 8) (Figure 2B). The main deviations from the male-to-female ratio were noted in the PDGFRA and FGFR3 subgroups that showed bias towards males or females, respectively. The cohort comprised mainly Caucasian/White and African-American/Black patients, at a white-to-black ratio of 4.67:1 for IDH-wild-type glioblastoma and 1.7:1 for IDH-mutant glioblastoma (Figure 2C). Most IDH-wild-type subgroups had a similar ratio to the main group, except for the EGFRm subgroup which stood out with two African-American/Black out of three patients.

In the adult glioblastoma cohort, all except for one NF1 cerebellar tumor were supratentorial. This contrasted with the three histone H3-K27M-mutant DMG cases, of which two were spinal. The IDH-wild-type cases were evenly distributed between the frontal lobe (30%), temporal lobe (30%), and other locations, of which the parietal lobe was preponderant (17%) (Figure 2D). Midline locations comprised thalamus/internal capsule, pineal gland, and cerebellum, and were relatively rare, except in the PDGFRA subgroup that contained two tumors in the thalamus/internal capsule. Corpus callosum butterfly location was considered a separate location, as patients showing these tumors fare poorly, and isolated cases were seen in the major subgroups, with two cases clustered in the NF1 subgroup. In general, the location distribution varied among subgroups, with a preponderance of frontal cases in the PDGFRA, Multi-RTK, and IDH subgroups (Figure 2D).

The survival, as measured from the first surgery until death, in the IDH-wild-type glioblastoma cohort was 37.9% at 1 year, slightly lower than the reported one of 41% [1], and the median survival was 9.5 months. The best median survival was noted in the FGFR3 subgroup, at 20 months, followed by EGFR and PDGFRA, at 12 months (Figure 2E). The two longest-surviving patients, reaching 7 years, had tumors mapping to the FGFR3 and EGFR subgroups. The poorest median survival was observed in the RAF subgroup, at 3.5 months, followed by the NF1, Multi-RTK, and Other subgroups, at 6.7, 7.5, and 10 months, respectively. Further examination of the EGFRm subgroup showed a median survival of 6 months (Figure 2F). The molecular cluster #1 showed survival heterogeneity, with the EGFR↑ and FGFR3 subgroups showing longer median survival, compounded at 14 months, and the NF1 and RAF subgroups showing significantly shorter median survival ($p = 0.039$), compounded at 5 months (Figure 2G). The molecular cluster #2 composed of the Multi-RTK and Other subgroups showed also significantly lower survival than the EGFR↑/FGFR3 combined subgroups ($p = 0.039$), with a compound value at 8 months.

3.4. Enrichment of Histologic Patterns in Molecular Glioblastoma Subgroups

The three WHO-recognized IDH-wild-type histologic variants, giant cell, gliosarcoma, and epithelioid [2], were scattered in the cohort at relatively low frequencies of 3.6%, 4.8%, and 6%, respectively (Figure 3A). The remaining samples were classified into nine additional patterns and further categorized on glioblastoma subgroups (Figure 3A). Four subgroups—EGFR, Other, NF1, and RAF—showed significant enrichment for a more specific pattern. The most frequent histologic pattern was seen in over half of the EGFR subgroup cases and appeared to also be specific, hence called "EGFR" (Figure 3A,B). It consisted of monomorphic cells with minimally discernible cytoplasm, blending in an eosinophilic extracellular matrix (ECM), with small, round, or slightly elongated nuclei with vesicular chromatin (Figure 3B, Figures S5 and S6). The second most frequent pattern had high-grade neuroendocrine (HGNE)/embryonal features previously described for the IDH#1 case [7], with pseudorosetting in most cases, and constituted about half of the PDGFRA and Other subgroup cases (Figure 3A,C, Figures S5 and S6). A similar pattern, called HGNE precursor (Pre-HGNE), had related cellular features to HGNE, except for a lack of nuclear molding, slightly vesicular chromatin, and lack of myxoid ECM (Figure S5). This pattern was also enriched in the PDGFRA and Other subgroups, but was also seen scattered in other subgroups. The third most common pattern was represented by cells with small, mostly round, hyperchromatic/dark nuclei with regular contours. It corresponded to all older adult RAF cases, where the nuclei were also surrounded by halos (Figure 3A,D, Figures S5 and S6). This pattern was also scattered in other subgroups and especially enriched in the EGFRm subgroup. Another histologic pattern that was almost entirely seen in the NF1 subgroup in approximately half of the cases was the fibroblastic type, with spindle cells embedded in eosinophilic or myxoid ECM (Figure 1A,D, Figures S5 and S6). The histology of the FGFR3 subgroup was described elsewhere [7] and, in the context of the entire cohort, showed overlap with EGFR, in a pattern called EGFR/FGFR, with a similar EGFR cell morphology pattern and prominent, intersecting capillary network (Figures S5 and S6). However, two FGFR3 cases constituting the FGFR small pattern appeared to show more specific nuclear characteristics, featuring small, finely stippled round or ovoid nuclei, and an ECM richer in hematoxylin-reacting components (Figures S5 and S6). As expected, the Multi-RTK subgroup showed a variation of patterns and included two of the three cases of giant cell glioblastoma from the cohort (Figures S5 and S6). These findings showed that the EGFR, PDGFRA, NF1, RAF, and Other subgroups were enriched in a defined histologic pattern, with the EGFR and fibroblastic patterns relatively specific for the EGFR↑ and NF1 subgroups, respectively.

To assess whether there were additional histologic–molecular associations, the 12 patterns were further clustered in five histologic clusters based on morphological similarities: #1/EGFR-like, #2/Small neuronal-like, #3/Anaplastic, #4/Spindle and #5/Epithelioid (Figure 3A,F). Case-by-case histologic cluster correlations with the most common mutations showed best correlations with cell cycle G1-phase mediators and *TP53* mutations. The EGFR-like histologic cluster was almost exclusively seen in the context of *CDKN2A/2B* homozygous loss and usually the absence of *TP53* mutations. *CDK4* mutations were only seen in the anaplastic cluster, usually associated with *TP53* or *MDM2* alterations. However, the anaplastic cluster was a feature of the PDGFRA subgroup, regardless of other alterations. The epithelioid cluster was associated with *TP53* mutations in 70% of cases, and with *RB1* mutations in 40% of the cases (Figure 3F).

GFAP IHC was performed for almost all cases, and showed reactivity in the majority of tumors, as expected (Figure 3F). The Multi-RTK, Other, and RAF subgroups showed lower or absent GFAP staining in 50%, 67%, and 71% of cases, respectively, suggesting lack of astrocytic differentiation in these subgroups.

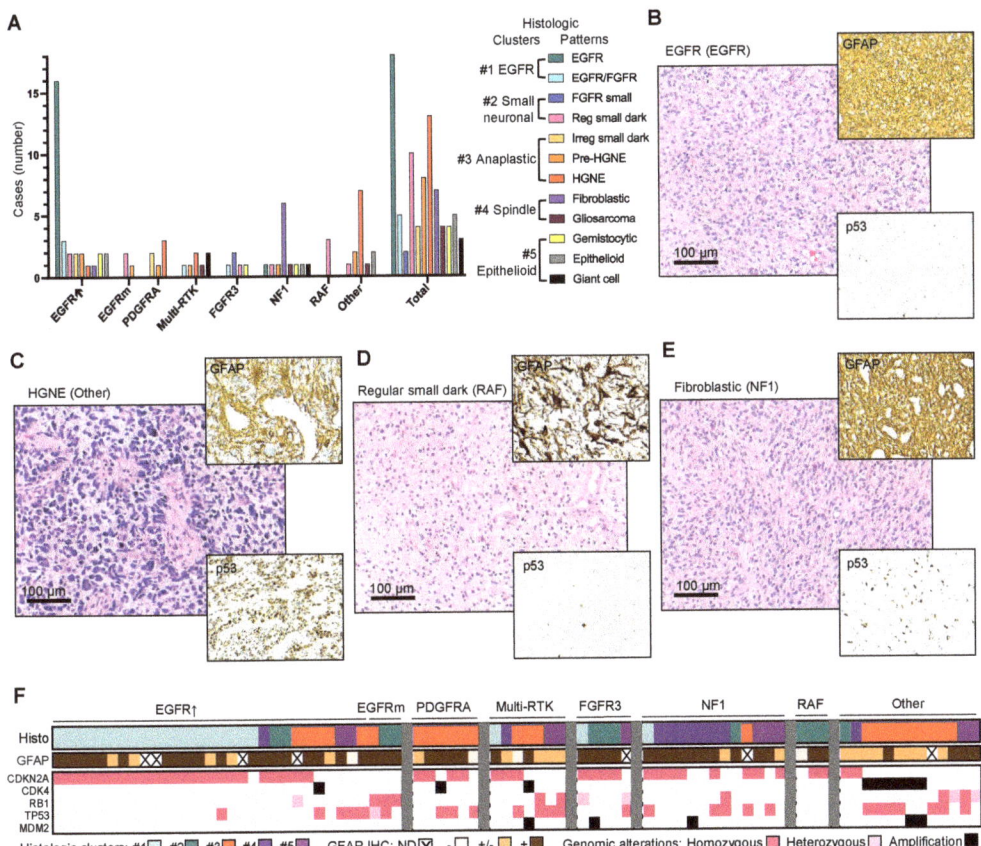

Figure 3. Histologic patterns and clusters in IDH-wild-type glioblastoma subgroups. (**A**) Bar graph showing histologic pattern distribution in the molecular glioblastoma subgroups and the total distribution in the cohort. Reg, regular nuclear contour; irreg, irregular nuclear contour; HGNE, high-grade neuroendocrine. (**B–E**) Representative H&E morphological appearances of the most common histological patterns. The molecular subgroup corresponding to the case is indicated in parenthesis. IHC with GFAP and p53 antibodies is shown in insets. (**F**) Histologic–molecular correlations. Histologic cluster distribution in individual cases from the IDH-wild-type glioblastoma subgroups shown in association with cell cycle G1 phase and p53 pathway mutations. The five histologic clusters (histo) are illustrated in (**A**).

4. Discussion

The WHO 2016 molecular subgrouping into IDH-wild-type and IDH-mutant glioblastoma emphasizes a significantly longer survival for the IDH-mutant subgroup, due to a slower tumor growth rate, and is reflected in a more insidious onset [21]. IDH-mutant cases represent approximately 10% of all glioblastoma cases [2] and 8% in this study. Except for a small number of cases, now classified as DMG with histone H3-K27M mutation, representing 4% in this study, there is no comprehensive histo-molecular classification for the IDH- and H3-wild-type glioblastoma cases approximating 90% of glioblastoma. Attempts have been made to distinguish histologic variants, and there are three variants of very rare incidence recognized in the WHO 2016 classification of brain tumors: gliosarcoma, giant cell, and epithelioid glioblastoma [2]. For the latter, the molecular association with *BRAF* p.V600E mutation in 50% of cases was noted [22]. Recent histologic–molecular correlations have also focused on the phenotype associated with *FGFR3* fusions in glioblastoma [7,23,24]. The efforts for molecularly classifying glioblastoma have been recently reviewed [25] and are based on a bioinformatics study categorizing in three different clusters the tumors with

EGFR, NF1, and PDGFRA/IDH genetic alterations [26]. However, a more refined and inclusive molecular classification is warranted due to the lack of prognosis stratification for glioblastoma patients, and to the lack of efficacious specific therapies. In addition, developments in personalized medicine for other solid tumors and the availability of alternative targeted treatments for these demand a closer look at glioblastoma in order to design similar targeted therapies.

This study represents a novel, stepwise, comprehensive classification of glioblastoma and includes pertinent genomic, transcriptomic, demographic, clinical, and histologic information (Figure 4A). It assigns all the glioblastoma cases to seven molecular subgroups, G1–G7, and shows their prognostic stratification. The classification was performed on a relatively large controlled cohort compared to cohorts from other studies [25]. Importantly, the cohort is representative for a mixed demographic population, including both Caucasian/White and African-American/Black ethnicities, providing thus more inclusive information than previously analyzed cohorts. The classification is based on my observation of the presence of non-redundant genomic alterations that activate RTKs and the upper segment of the MAPK/ERK pathway, whereas genomic alterations activating the PI3K pathway coexist with RTK alterations in a relatively even distribution (Figure 4A). The RTK subgroups G1/EGFR, G2/FGFR3, G5/PDGFRA, and G6/Multi-RTK accounted for roughly two-thirds of the glioblastoma IDH-wild-type cases, indicating a major role of RTKs in the pathogenesis of glioblastoma. An additional approximately 20% of cases were due to alteration in the upper segment of the ERK signaling pathway, namely NF1 tumor suppressor, in the subgroup G3/NF1, or RAF family members, in the subgroup G4/RAF. The remaining cases formed a separate subgroup, G7/Other, in which only genomic alterations of the PI3K pathway were apparent.

Hierarchical clustering analysis based on the main molecular characteristics of the subgroups showed two clusters and three independent subgroups (Figure 4A). The independent subgroups were the IDH, PDGFRA, and EGFRm. Whereas the IDH subgroup has been singled out in many studies because of its distinct better patient survival and lower tumor proliferation rate [21], the lack of clustering of PDGFRA and especially of EGFRm with other RTK subgroups is surprising. The main features of the IDH-wild-type glioblastoma subgroups are illustrated in Figure 4A. The G5/PDGFRA was the only subgroup that showed a majority of cases without *TERT* alterations as a mechanism of telomere elongation, an observation noted first by Higa et al. [27]. It also showed relatively few PI3K pathway alterations, equally divided between *PTEN* and *PIK3R1*. The histology was aggressive but the survival was not shorter than that for the G1/EGFR subgroup. The G1/EGFRm is a novel, very small subgroup, and will need further characterization to confirm the preliminary results presented in this study. It featured a shorter survival, the only predominant inclusion of African American/Black patients, a relatively aggressive histology, and *RB1* and *TP53* mutations, in contrast to the main G1/EGFR↑ subgroup.

The two clusters contained two or more subgroups. The largest subgroup, G1/EGFR↑, clustered closely with the G3/NF1 and G4/RAF subgroups, and more distantly with the G2/FGFR3 subgroup, in the molecular cluster#1. The G1/EGFR↑ subgroup showed the second-longest survival after the G2/FGFR3 subgroup, which was the subgroup with the longest survival, in concordance with a previous report [28]. The longest survivors of the cohort belonged to these two subgroups, with two survivors reaching 7 years, representing 2.2% of the IDH-wild-type cohort. Although the G3/NF1 subgroup alone showed similar survival relative to non-NF1 cases (not shown), as previously reported for the TCGA dataset [29], the combined G3/NF1-G4/RAF subgroups showed significantly shorter survival compared to the combined G1/EGFR↑-G2/FGFR3 subgroups, indicating a worse prognosis overall for patients with mutations in the upper segment of the ERK/MAPK pathway. The G2/FGFR3 subgroup was enriched in female patients, similar to the IDH subgroup, and in contrast to all other glioblastoma subgroups. Surprisingly, the histology of this subgroup was variable, with the small neuronal-like morphology as the most frequent. In contrast, both G1/EGFR and G3/NF1 subgroups showed a quasi-pathognomonic morphology in half of the tumors. All four subgroups from the molecular cluster #1 showed similar activation profiles of the major pathways: high incidence of PI3K pathway mutations, represented mainly by *PTEN* but also by *PIK3CA* and *PIK3R1* mutations, high incidence of *CDKN2A* homozygous loss coupled with *CDK6* overexpression, and conversely, low incidence of *TP53* mutations.

A

	Subgroups	G1/EGFRm	Molecular cluster#1					Molecular cluster#2	
			G1/EGFR↑	G2/FGFR3	G3/NF1	G4/RAF	G5/PDGFRA	G6/Multi-RTK	G7/Other
Demographics	Incidence	Very rare 3%	Frequent 41%	Rare 5.7%	Moderate 17%	Very rare 4.6%	Rare 8%	Rare 8%	Moderate 15%
	Prognosis Median survival	Poor 6	Intermediate 12	Best 20	Poor 6.7	Very poor 3.5	Intermediate 12	Poor 7.5	Poor 10
	Sex	M	M>F	F>>M	M>F	M=F	M>>F	M>F	M>F
	Race	B>W	W>>B	W	W>B	W*	W>>B	W>B	W>>B
Tumors	Midline location	No	Rare	No	Highest	No	Yes	Yes	Yes
	Histology	Neuro>Ana	EGFR>>Ana	Neuro*	Spindle>>Epith	Neuro	Anaplastic	Ana>Epith	Ana>>Epith
	RTK overexpr	ERBB2	**EGFR**, KDR	KDR	ALK, MET, KDR	NTRK1, KDR	PDGFRA, KIT, EPHB2, **KDR**	**MET**, EGFR, EPHB2	EPHB2
Molecular alterations	TERT	All	All*	4/5	3/4	All	<1/2	All	4/5
	PI3K pathway	Low PTEN	High PTEN>PIK3CA	High PTEN	High PTEN>PIK3R1	High PTEN>PIK3R1	Moderate PTEN=PIK3R1	High PTEN*	Highest PTEN*
	G1 phase	Highest RB1	High CDKN2A*	Highest CDKN2A*	High CDKN2A*	Moderate CDKN2A	High CDKN2A>CDK4	High CDKN2A>RB1	Very high CDK4>RB1
	p53 pathway	High TP53	Low TP53>MDM4	Moderate TP53=MDM2	Moderate TP53>RPL5	Low RPL5	High TP53>>PPM1D	High TP53>>MDM2	High TP53>>MDM2
	MGMT methyl	None	1/2	1/2	1/3	1/2	None	1/2	1/3

B

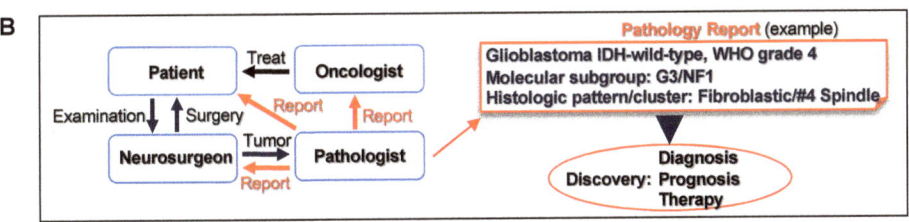

Figure 4. ERK/MAPK-based glioblastoma classification. (**A**) Multi-platform characterization of the IDH-wild-type glioblastoma G1–G7 molecular subgroups showing main demographic, histologic, RTK expression, and growth pathway mutation analysis: light blue and peach shading indicate molecular cluster#1 and #2, respectively; yellow shading highlights some characteristic features of the subgroup. M, male; F, female; B, African-American/Black; W, Caucasian/White. The midline location comprises all midline structures including the corpus callosum. Histologic clusters: Neuro, Small neuronal; Ana, Anaplastic; Epith, Epithelioid. RTK overexpression (overexpr) shows the most commonly upregulated RTKs; in bold are RTKs with gene amplifications. The mutation frequency is considered: highest, 100% cases; very high, >90% cases; high, ≥66.7% cases; moderate, between 33.3% and 66.7% cases; low, ≤33.3% cases. Asterisks (*) mark the presence of other minor components within the subgroup when only one parameter is shown. (**B**) Implementation of the glioblastoma classification in clinical practice and discovery. Schematic flowchart shows the management of the glioblastoma patient by the brain tumor team. An example of pathology report is shown, with incorporation of the glioblastoma molecular subgroup and histologic pattern and cluster.

The molecular cluster#2 comprised cases with similar demographic and histologic characteristics, including relatively poor survival, classified separately into the G6/Multi-

RTK and G7/Other subgroups. The molecular signature was also similar for the PI3K and p53 pathways, with a high incidence of *PTEN* and *TP53* mutations, but showed clustering of *CDK4* amplification in the G7/Other subgroup. Although the G6/Multi-RTK subgroup appeared heterogeneous, with concurrent genomic alterations and overexpression of a wide range of RTKs, it may represent a good target for the multi-RTK therapy that has shown some success in recurrent glioblastoma [30].

This classification required both genomic and transcriptomic information. The transcriptomic analysis uncovered pathogenic fusions with subgrouping relevance, and examined the translation of CN alterations into gene expression levels, as we have previously shown that gene amplification does not always result in mRNA overexpression [7]. The landscaping of RTK expression and correlation with genomic alterations has not been performed previously in glioblastoma. Its major findings are (1) lack of overlap between *EGFR*, *PDGFRA*, and *FGFR3* alterations, including overexpression; (2) good correlation between *EGFR* amplification and high overexpression in the vast majority of cases; a similar correlation for *MET* and *FGFR2*-amplified cases was also found; (3) presence of a small subgroup characterized by *EGFR* activating mutations without gene amplification or high overexpression; (4) lack of correlation between *PDGFRA* locus amplification, including *KIT* and *KDR*, and overexpression, requiring correct assignment of cases with high *PDGF RA* overexpression in the G5/PDGFRA subgroup and of the *PDGFRA*-amplified non-overexpressing cases in the G6/Multi-RTK subgroup; (5) *KDR* overexpression in the majority of cases and at higher levels in the molecular cluster#1, most likely in the vascular compartment; (6) overexpression without amplification of additional RTKs in many cases, such as *NTRK1*, *ERBB2/ERBB3*, *EPHA3/EPHB2* and *ALK*, some showing subgroup specificity (Figure 4A).

The RTK landscaping, pathway associations, and subgrouping efforts presented here also carry a major impact for the clinical management of glioblastoma, including diagnosis, prognosis, and therapy (Figure 4B). Although many clinical trials targeting a plethora of pathways are ongoing in glioblastoma [31] and aim at the major pathways presented here, correct patient inclusion is crucial for regimen success. For example, the G1/EGFRm subgroup may represent a more promising target to EGFR inhibitors than the larger G1/EGFR↑ subgroup, similarly to non-small cell lung carcinomas with *EGFR* mutations. Likewise, PDGFRα inhibitors may not work for tumors with *PDGFRA* amplification without overexpression. Specific RTK inhibitors are available not only for the RTKs with genomic alterations for which drug trials are usually designed, such as EGFR, PDGFRα, FGFR2 and FGFR3, NTRK1, and MET, but also for RTKs with overexpression with or without mutations of unknown significance, such as ALK, ERBB2 (Her2/Neu), and EPHA3 [32]. Together with new targets revealed in this study, such as EPHB2, these RTKs also warrant consideration for glioblastoma therapy. Moreover, efforts should include RTK family or multi-RTK strategies to cover convergent growth signaling from multiple RTKs, and testing for RTK reprogramming leading to drug resistance [14,33]. Open questions remain, such as the use of combination therapy for targeting downstream or parallel growth pathways. Of these, the PI3K pathway may represent a selective target for the tumors composing the G7/Other subgroup that apparently rely predominantly on this canonical growth pathway.

5. Conclusions

In conclusion, I presented here a comprehensive multi-platform glioblastoma classification with large patient inclusion and immediate field applicability for diagnosis and prognosis (Figure 4). The incorporation of this novel classification in the pathology report will foster discovery by immediate molecular subgroup stratification, data sorting, and personalized follow-up of patients. This classification complements and expands the previous efforts for a better understanding of this deadly disease, and lays the foundation for precision therapy design.

Supplementary Materials: The following are available online at https://www.mdpi.com/article/10.3390/cancers13184532/s1, Figure S1: Glioblastoma subgroups—landscape of RTK expression, Figure S2: Glioblastoma subgroups—tumor mutation burden, Figure S3: Glioblastoma subgroups—proliferation, Figure S4: Glioblastoma subgroups—correlation matrix, Figure S5: Glioblastoma IDH-wild-type—characteristic nuclear morphology of the histologic patterns, Figure S6: Glioblastoma IDH-wild-type—correspondence between histologic patterns and molecular subgroups, Table S1: Glioblastoma genomic alterations, Table S2: RTK classes and genes.

Funding: This work was supported by an award from NeuroMarkers PLLC [NM2021-1] to MMG.

Institutional Review Board Statement: The study was conducted according to the guidelines of the Declaration of Helsinki, and approved by the Institutional Review Board of NeuroMarkers PLLC (protocol code 2019/GBM—16 October 2019). The inclusion of patients was performed in accordance to institutional ethical guidelines and regulations.

Informed Consent Statement: The patients or patients' next of kin consented for research and publication.

Data Availability Statement: Supporting data for this manuscript are available in the Supplementary Material and upon request to the corresponding author. Physicians may also contact the author for hands-on help in reporting the glioblastoma subgroups.

Acknowledgments: This work is dedicated to my best childhood friend's mother who died of glioblastoma, and to all the patients in this study. Special acknowledgements go to the patients' families and friends, for their helpful comments and their support for this work. I am grateful to Kathrin H. Kirsch and Adriana Olar for their insightful suggestions and critical reading of the revised manuscript, and to Randy Legerski for scientific English language check and for his kind donation covering publication charges.

Conflicts of Interest: The author declares no conflict of interest.

Abbreviations

C-	carboxyl
CN	copy number
DDR	DNA damage response
ECM	extracellular matrix
EGFR	epidermal growth factor receptor; EGFR↑, EGFR with gene amplification with or without other genetic alterations; EGFRm, EGFR with gene mutation only
ERK/MAPK	extracellular signal-regulated kinase/mitogen-activated protein kinase
FFPE	formalin-fixed paraffin-embedded
FGFR	fibroblast growth factor receptor
GFAP	glial fibrillary acidic protein
H&E	hematoxylin eosin
IDH	isocitrate dehydrogenase
IHC	immunohistochemistry
LOH	loss of heterozygosity
NF1	neurofibromatosis type 1
NGS	next generation sequencing
PDGFR	platelet-derived growth factor receptor
PI3K	phosphatidylinositol 3-OH kinase
RTK	receptor tyrosine kinase
WHO	World Health Organization

References

1. Ostrom, Q.T.; Truitt, G.; Gittleman, H.; Brat, D.J.; Kruchko, C.; Wilson, R.; Barnholtz-Sloan, J.S. Relative survival after diagnosis with a primary brain or other central nervous system tumor in the National Program of Cancer Registries, 2004 to 2014. *Neuro-Oncol. Pr.* **2020**, *7*, 306–312. [CrossRef]
2. Louis, D.N.; Ohgaki, H.; Wiestler, O.D.; Caveneee, W.K. *WHO Classification of Tumors of the Central Nervous System*; IARC: Lyon, France, 2016.
3. Georgescu, M.-M. PTEN Tumor Suppressor Network in PI3K-Akt Pathway Control. *Genes Cancer* **2010**, *1*, 1170–1177. [CrossRef] [PubMed]

4. Hanahan, D.; Weinberg, R.A. Hallmarks of cancer: The next generation. *Cell* **2011**, *144*, 646–674. [CrossRef] [PubMed]
5. Ségaliny, A.I.; Tellez-Gabriel, M.; Heymann, M.-F.; Heymann, D. Receptor tyrosine kinases: Characterisation, mechanism of action and therapeutic interests for bone cancers. *J. Bone Oncol.* **2015**, *4*, 1–12. [CrossRef] [PubMed]
6. Cargnello, M.; Roux, P.P. Activation and function of the MAPKs and their substrates, the MAPK-activated protein kinases. *Microbiol. Mol. Biol. Rev.* **2011**, *75*, 50–83. [CrossRef]
7. Georgescu, M.-M.; Islam, M.Z.; Li, Y.; Traylor, J.; Nanda, A. Novel targetable FGFR2 and FGFR3 alterations in glioblastoma associate with aggressive phenotype and distinct gene expression programs. *Acta Neuropathol. Commun.* **2021**, *9*, 1–17. [CrossRef] [PubMed]
8. Kawazoe, T.; Taniguchi, K. The Sprouty/Spred family as tumor suppressors: Coming of age. *Cancer Sci.* **2019**, *110*, 1525–1535. [CrossRef]
9. Kidger, A.M.; Keyse, S.M. The regulation of oncogenic Ras/ERK signalling by dual-specificity mitogen activated protein kinase phosphatases (MKPs). *Semin. Cell Dev. Biol.* **2016**, *50*, 125–132. [CrossRef] [PubMed]
10. Ratner, N.; Miller, S.J. A RASopathy gene commonly mutated in cancer: The neurofibromatosis type 1 tumour suppressor. *Nat. Rev. Cancer* **2015**, *15*, 290–301. [CrossRef]
11. Georgescu, M.-M.; Li, Y.; Islam, M.; Notarianni, C.; Sun, H.; Olar, A.; Fuller, G.N. Mutations of the MAPK/TSC/mTOR pathway characterize periventricular glioblastoma with epithelioid SEGA-like morphology-morphological and therapeutic implications. *Oncotarget* **2019**, *10*, 4038–4052. [CrossRef]
12. Georgescu, M.M.; Olar, A. Genetic and histologic spatiotemporal evolution of recurrent, multifocal, multicentric and metastatic glioblastoma. *Acta Neuropathol. Commun.* **2020**, *8*, 1–9. [CrossRef]
13. Georgescu, M.-M.; Olar, A.; Mobley, B.C.; Faust, P.L.; Raisanen, J.M. Epithelial differentiation with microlumen formation in meningioma: Diagnostic utility of NHERF1/EBP50 immunohistochemistry. *Oncotarget* **2018**, *9*, 28652–28665. [CrossRef]
14. Georgescu, M.-M.; Islam, M.Z.; Li, Y.; Circu, M.L.; Traylor, J.; Notarianni, C.M.; Kline, C.N.; Burns, D.K. Global activation of oncogenic pathways underlies therapy resistance in diffuse midline glioma. *Acta Neuropathol. Commun.* **2020**, *8*, 1–17. [CrossRef]
15. Agarwal, N.K.; Zhu, X.; Gagea, M.; White, C.L., 3rd; Cote, G.; Georgescu, M.M. PHLPP2 suppresses the NF-kappaB pathway by inactivating IKKbeta kinase. *Oncotarget* **2014**, *5*, 815–823. [CrossRef]
16. Georgescu, M.M.; Gagea, M.; Cote, G. NHERF1/EBP50 Suppresses Wnt-beta-Catenin Pathway-Driven Intestinal Neoplasia. *Neoplasia* **2016**, *18*, 512–523. [CrossRef] [PubMed]
17. Georgescu, M.-M.; Nanda, A.; Li, Y.; Mobley, B.C.; Faust, P.L.; Raisanen, J.M.; Olar, A. Mutation Status and Epithelial Differentiation Stratify Recurrence Risk in Chordoid Meningioma—A Multicenter Study with High Prognostic Relevance. *Cancers* **2020**, *12*, 225. [CrossRef] [PubMed]
18. Nolte, H.; MacVicar, T.D.; Tellkamp, F.; Krüger, M. Instant Clue: A Software Suite for Interactive Data Visualization and Analysis. *Sci. Rep.* **2018**, *8*, 12648. [CrossRef]
19. Katoh, M. Canonical and non-canonical WNT signaling in cancer stem cells and their niches: Cellular heterogeneity, omics reprogramming, targeted therapy and tumor plasticity (Review). *Int. J. Oncol.* **2017**, *51*, 1357–1369. [CrossRef]
20. Dobbelstein, M.; Levine, A.J. Mdm2: Open questions. *Cancer Sci.* **2020**, *111*, 2203–2211. [CrossRef]
21. Ohgaki, H.; Kleihues, P. The definition of primary and secondary glioblastoma. *Clin. Cancer Res.* **2013**, *19*, 764–772. [CrossRef] [PubMed]
22. Kleinschmidt-DeMasters, B.K.; Aisner, D.L.; Birks, D.K.; Foreman, N. Epithelioid GBMs Show a High Percentage of BRAF V600E Mutation. *Am. J. Surg. Pathol.* **2013**, *37*, 685–698. [CrossRef]
23. Bielle, F.; Di Stefano, A.L.; Meyronet, D.; Picca, A.; Villa, C.; Bernier, M.; Schmitt, Y.; Giry, M.; Rousseau, A.; Figarella-Branger, D.; et al. Diffuse gliomas with FGFR3-TACC3 fusion have characteristic histopathological and molecular features. *Brain Pathol.* **2018**, *28*, 674–683. [CrossRef] [PubMed]
24. Gilani, A.; Davies, K.D.; Kleinschmidt-DeMasters, B.K. Can adult IDH-wildtype glioblastomas with FGFR3:TACC3 fusions be reliably predicted by histological features? *Clin. Neuropathol.* **2021**, *40*, 165–167. [CrossRef] [PubMed]
25. Tilak, M.; Holborn, J.; New, L.; Lalonde, J.; Jones, N. Receptor Tyrosine Kinase Signaling and Targeting in Glioblastoma Multiforme. *Int. J. Mol. Sci.* **2021**, *22*, 1831. [CrossRef]
26. Verhaak, R.G.W.; Hoadley, K.A.; Purdom, E.; Wang, V.; Qi, Y.; Wilkerson, M.D.; Miller, C.R.; Ding, L.; Golub, T.; Mesirov, J.P.; et al. Integrated Genomic Analysis Identifies Clinically Relevant Subtypes of Glioblastoma Characterized by Abnormalities in PDGFRA, IDH1, EGFR, and NF1. *Cancer Cell* **2010**, *17*, 98–110. [CrossRef]
27. Higa, N.; Akahane, T.; Yokoyama, S.; Yonezawa, H.; Uchida, H.; Takajo, T.; Kirishima, M.; Hamada, T.; Matsuo, K.; Fujio, S.; et al. A tailored next-generation sequencing panel identified distinct subtypes of wildtype IDH and TERT promoter glioblastomas. *Cancer Sci.* **2020**, *111*, 3902–3911. [CrossRef] [PubMed]
28. Di Stefano, A.L.; Picca, A.; Saragoussi, E.; Bielle, F.; Ducray, F.; Villa, C.; Eoli, M.; Paterra, R.; Bellu, L.; Mathon, B.; et al. Clinical, molecular, and radiomic profile of gliomas with FGFR3-TACC3 fusions. *Neuro. Oncol.* **2020**, *22*, 1614–1624. [CrossRef]
29. Vizcaíno, M.A.; Shah, S.; Eberhart, C.G.; Rodriguez, F.J. Clinicopathologic implications of NF1 gene alterations in diffuse gliomas. *Hum. Pathol.* **2015**, *46*, 1323–1330. [CrossRef] [PubMed]
30. Lombardi, G.; De Salvo, G.L.; Brandes, A.A.; Eoli, M.; Rudà, R.; Faedi, M.; Lolli, I.; Pace, A.; Daniele, B.; Pasqualetti, F.; et al. Regorafenib compared with lomustine in patients with relapsed glioblastoma (REGOMA): A multicentre, open-label, randomised, controlled, phase 2 trial. *Lancet Oncol.* **2019**, *20*, 110–119. [CrossRef]

31. Cruz Da Silva, E.; Mercier, M.C.; Etienne-Selloum, N.; Dontenwill, M.; Choulier, L. A Systematic Review of Glioblastoma-Targeted Therapies in Phases II, III, IV Clinical Trials. *Cancers* **2021**, *13*, 1795. [CrossRef]
32. Taylor, O.G.; Brzozowski, J.S.; Skelding, K.A. Glioblastoma Multiforme: An Overview of Emerging Therapeutic Targets. *Front. Oncol.* **2019**, *9*, 963. [CrossRef] [PubMed]
33. Kleczko, E.K.; Heasley, L.E. Mechanisms of rapid cancer cell reprogramming initiated by targeted receptor tyrosine kinase inhibitors and inherent therapeutic vulnerabilities. *Mol. Cancer* **2018**, *17*. [CrossRef] [PubMed]

MDPI
St. Alban-Anlage 66
4052 Basel
Switzerland
www.mdpi.com

Cancers Editorial Office
E-mail: cancers@mdpi.com
www.mdpi.com/journal/cancers

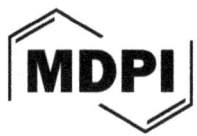

Disclaimer/Publisher's Note: The statements, opinions and data contained in all publications are solely those of the individual author(s) and contributor(s) and not of MDPI and/or the editor(s). MDPI and/or the editor(s) disclaim responsibility for any injury to people or property resulting from any ideas, methods, instructions or products referred to in the content.

www.ingramcontent.com/pod-product-compliance
Lightning Source LLC
LaVergne TN
LVHW070237100526
838202LV00015B/2144